Nguyen Duc Anh
Chicago Sept 97

Atlas of
CUTANEOUS
SURGERY

Atlas of
CUTANEOUS
SURGERY

JUNE K. ROBINSON, M.D.
Professor of Dermatology and Surgery
Departments of Dermatology and Surgery
Northwestern University Medical School
Chicago, Illinois

KENNETH A. ARNDT, M.D.
Dermatologist-in-Chief
Beth Israel Hospital
Professor of Dermatology
Harvard Medical School
Boston, Massachusetts

PHILIP E. LeBOIT, M.D.
Associate Professor of Pathology and Dermatology
University of California, San Francisco
San Francisco, California

BRUCE U. WINTROUB, M.D.
Professor and Chairman
Department of Dermatology
Associate Dean
School of Medicine
University of California, San Francisco
San Francisco, California

ILLUSTRATOR   Lauren E. Shavell

W.B. SAUNDERS COMPANY
A Division of Harcourt Brace & Company
Philadelphia • London • Toronto • Montreal • Sydney • Tokyo

W.B. SAUNDERS COMPANY
A Division of Harcourt Brace & Company

The Curtis Center
Independence Square West
Philadelphia, Pennsylvania 19106

Library of Congress Cataloging-in-Publication Data

Atlas of cutaneous surgery / [edited by] June K. Robinson . . . [et al.].—1st ed.
p. cm.
ISBN 0–7216–5404–5
1. Skin—Surgery—Atlases. I. Robinson, June K.
[DNLM: 1. Skin—surgery—atlases. 2. Skin Transplantation—
methods—
atlases. WR 17 A8818 1996]
RD520.A88   1996   617.4′770022′2—dc20
DNLM/DLC   94–25752

Atlas of Cutaneous Surgery   ISBN 0–7216–5404–5

Printed in the United States of America.

Last digit is the print number: 9   8   7   6   5   4   3   2   1

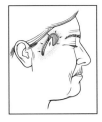

Contributors

ELIZABETH M. BILLINGSLEY, M.D.
Assistant Professor, Pennsylvania State University
College of Medicine, Hershey, Pennsylvania
Considerations in Achieving Hemostasis

DOMINIC A. BRANDY, M.D., B.S.
Clinical Instructor, Department of Dermatology,
University of Pittsburgh Medical Center; Faculty, St.
Francis Central Hospital, Pittsburgh, Pennsylvania
Hair Replacement Surgery

KATHRYN L. BRANDY, R.N.
Head Nurse, Cosmetic Surgery Center, Pittsburgh,
Pennsylvania
Hair Replacement Surgery

ERIC A. BREISCH, PH.D.
Assistant Clinical Professor of Pathology, Department of
Pathology, University of California, San Diego, School
of Medicine, La Jolla, California; Clinical Anatomist,
Department of Pathology Children's Hospital, San
Diego, California
Superficial Cutaneous Anatomy

HAROLD J. BRODY, M.D.
Associate Clinical Professor, Department of
Dermatology, Emory School of Medicine, Atlanta,
Georgia
Chemical Peel

WILLIAM P. COLEMAN, III, M.D.
Clinical Professor of Dermatology, Tulane University of
Medicine, New Orleans, Louisiana
Liposuction; Dermabrasion

PAUL S. COLLINS, M.D.
Guest Lecturer, Stanford Medical School, Stanford,
California
Blepharoplasty; Browlift Surgery

RAFAEL FALABELLA, M.D.
Professor, Universidad del Valle; Professor, Hospital
Universitario del Valle, Cali, Colombia
Surgical Techniques for Repigmentation

JESSICA L. FEWKES, M.D.
Assistant Professor, Harvard University; Associate
Dermatologist, Massachusetts General Hospital, Boston,
Massachusetts
Anesthesia

ROY G. GERONEMUS, M.D.
Clinical Associate Professor of Dermatology, New York
University Medical Center; Director, Laser and Skin
Surgery Center of New York, New York, New York
Laser Treatment of Vascular Lesions

MARTIN B. GIANDONI, M.D.
Chief, Dermatology Service, William Beaumont Army
Medical Center, El Paso, Texas
Surgical Wound Dressing

RICHARD G. GLOGAU, M.D.
Clinical Professor of Dermatology, University of
California, San Francisco, San Francisco, California
*Composite Graft; Chemical Peels; Soft Tissue
Augmentation Techniques*

WILLIAM J. GRABSKI, M.D.
Director, Dermatology Surgery, Brooke Army Medical
Center, Ft. Sam Houston, Texas; Clinical Associate
Professor, Department of Medicine, University of Texas
Health Science Center, San Antonio, Texas
Surgical Wound Dressing

GLORIA F. GRAHAM, M.D.
Clinical Professor, University of North Carolina,
Department of Dermatology, Chapel Hill, North
Carolina; Carteret County Hospital, Morehead City,
North Carolina
Cryosurgery

HUBERT T. GREENWAY, M.D.
Assistant Clinical Professor, University of California,
San Diego, San Diego, California; Head, Mohs Surgery;
Cutaneous Oncology Division of Dermatology and
Cutaneous Surgery; Scripps Clinic and Research
Foundation, La Jolla, California
Superficial Cutaneous Anatomy

ROY C. GREKIN, M.D.
  Associate Clinical Professor, Department of
  Dermatology, University of California, San Francisco,
  San Francisco, California
  *Preoperative Considerations for Antibiotic Prophylaxis
  and Antisepsis; Mohs' Micrographic Surgery*

ANN F. HAAS, M.D.
  Assistant Professor, Department of Dermatology,
  University of California, Davis, Sacramento, California
  *Preoperative Considerations for Antibiotic Prophylaxis
  and Antisepsis; Composite Graft*

GEORGE J. HRUZA, M.D.
  Assistant Professor of Dermatology, Surgery, and
  Otolaryngology, Washington University School of
  Medicine; Director, Cutaneous Surgery Center, Barnes
  Hospital, St. Louis, Missouri
  Laser Surgery for Pigmented Lesions

A. PAUL KELLY, M.D.
  Professor and Chairman, Department of Internal
  Medicine—Chief, Division of Dermatology, Drew
  University of Medicine and Science; Staff Physician,
  King/Drew Medical Center; Associate Professor,
  University of California, Los Angeles, School of
  Medicine, Los Angeles, California
  Keloid Surgery

CLIFFORD M. LAWRENCE, M.D., F.R.C.P.
  Clinical Lecturer, Medical School, Newcastle
  University; Consultant Dermatologist, Royal Victoria
  Infirmary, Newcastle, England
  Common Problems of the Ear

PHILIP E. LEBOIT, M.D.
  Associate Professor of Pathology and Dermatology,
  University of California, San Francisco, San Francisco,
  California
  Biopsy Techniques

DAVID J. LEFFELL, M.D.
  Associate Professor, Dermatology, Plastic Surgery and
  Otolaryngology, Yale School of Medicine; Attending
  Physician, Yale–New Haven Hospital, New Haven,
  Connecticut
  Split-Thickness Skin Grafts

MARY E. MALONEY, M.D.
  Associate Professor, Pennsylvania State College of
  Medicine; Associate Professor and Staff Physician,
  Milton Hershey Medical Center, Pennsylvania State
  College of Medicine, Hershey, Pennsylvania
  Considerations in Achieving Hemostasis

SETH L. MATARASSO, M.D.
  Clinical Assistant Professor of Dermatology, University
  of California, San Francisco, San Francisco, California
  Chemical Peels; Soft Tissue Augmentation Techniques

LAWRENCE S. MOY, M.D.
  Clinical Faculty, University of California, Los Angeles,
  Medical School, Los Angeles, California
  Superficial Chemical Peels with α-Hydroxy Acids

RONALD L. MOY, M.D.
  Assistant Professor, Division of Dermatology,
  University of California, Los Angeles, School of
  Medicine; Director of Dermatologic Surgery, VA–West
  LA Medical Center, Los Angeles, California
  Advancement Flap

SUZANNE OLBRICHT, M.D.
  Instructor, Harvard Medical School; Director of
  Dermatologic Surgery, Beth Israel Hospital, Boston,
  Massachusetts
  Continuous-Wave Lasers

KATIA C. ONGENAE, M.D.
  Research Fellow, Department of Dermatology, Boston
  University School of Medicine, Boston, Massachusetts
  Cultured Epidermal Grafts

TANIA J. PHILLIPS, M.D., F.R.C.P.C.
  Associate Professor, Department of Dermatology,
  Boston University School of Medicine; Attending
  Physician, Boston University Medical Center, Boston
  City Hospital, Boston, Massachusetts
  Cultured Epidermal Grafts

JUNE K. ROBINSON, M.D.
  Professor of Dermatology and Surgery, Departments of
  Dermatology and Surgery, Northwestern University
  Medical School, Chicago, Illinois
  *Biopsy Techniques; Electrosurgery; Considerations in
  Achieving Hemostasis; Technique of Suture Placement;
  Elliptical Incisions and Closures; Advancement Flap;
  Rotation Flap; Transposition Flap; Common Problems
  of the Ear*

RANDALL K. ROENIGK, M.D.
  Associate Professor, Mayo Medical School; Consultant,
  Mayo Clinic and Mayo Foundation, Rochester,
  Minnesota
  Full-Thickness Skin Grafts

STUART J. SALASCHE, M.D.
  Associate Professor—Dermatology, University of
  Arizona Health Science Center, Tucson, Arizona
  Nail Unit Surgery

ROBERT A. WEISS, M.D.
  Assistant Professor of Dermatology, The Johns Hopkins
  University School of Medicine, Baltimore, Maryland
  Sclerotherapy

RONALD G. WHEELAND, M.D.
Professor and Chairman, Department of Dermatology,
University of New Mexico School of Medicine;
Department of Dermatology, University of New Mexico,
Albuquerque, New Mexico
Tattoo Removal

DUANE C. WHITAKER, M.D.
Professor of Dermatology, University of Iowa College
of Medicine; Director of Dermatologic Surgery and
Cutaneous Laser Surgery, University of Iowa Hospitals
and Clinics, Iowa City, Iowa
Rotation Flap

JOHN M. YARBOROUGH, M.D.
Clinical Professor of Dermatology, Department of
Dermatology, Tulane University School of Medicine,
New Orleans, Louisiana
Dermabrasion

MARK J. ZALLA, M.D.
Assistant Professor, Mayo Medical School, Rochester,
Minnesota; Senior Associate Consultant, Mayo Clinic
Scottsdale, Scottsdale, Arizona
Full-Thickness Skin Grafts

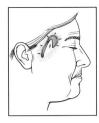

Preface

The *Atlas of Cutaneous Surgery* is an essential part of a multi-volume educational publication effort, *Cutaneous Medicine and Surgery: An Integrated Program in Dermatology*. Knowledge of the basic surgical principles and of advanced surgical techniques is essential in dermatologic training and in the office practice of dermatology. All chapters in this atlas are contributed by authors known for their experience and expertise in defined areas of cutaneous surgery. In almost all instances, these same authors have been part of a multidisciplinary team who have written chapters on related topics in the text *Cutaneous Medicine and Surgery*.

This atlas uses the clinical case model to define the benefits of a particular surgical procedure. Each chapter draws upon the author's clinical knowledge by presenting specialized tables listing indications and contraindications; an explanation of the risks and benefits to the patient; intraoperative needs; postoperative management; and anticipated adverse sequelae of the procedure. The medical artist's illustrations of the basics of anatomy, planning, and performing the range of cutaneous surgical procedures enhance the presentation of the clinical case. The author's vision, transformed and crystallized in the artist's drawings, rapidly communicates the essential information. In the belief that studying our complications is often more illuminating than studying our successes, each chapter presents a section on potential complications of surgery.

The *Atlas of Cutaneous Surgery* is organized into four sections: basic procedures; tissue movement and transfer (flaps and grafts); special anatomic units and techniques; and cosmetic surgery. The usual developmental progression of the cutaneous surgeon is from the acquisition of basic skills to the more difficult techniques of tissue movement and transfer. At that point, the cutaneous surgeon is able to augment the basic procedures with a selection of special techniques, including those of cosmetic cutaneous surgery. Dermatologists have a tradition of outpatient-based surgery and have expanded on the scope of procedures performed in this setting. For the last twenty years, advances in instruments and the techniques of anesthesia and surgery both in the reconstructive and cosmetic aspects of the field have permitted increasingly more complex procedures to be performed as outpatient surgery.

The limits of cutaneous surgery continually expand as primary care physicians and specialists from a variety of disciplines learn from one another and expand the scope of their practices to provide better patient care. The clinical case provides the basis for learning; hence this atlas uses the surgical care of patients as a model for transferring information to the reader. We believe that all readers may benefit from the collective experience of these authors.

JUNE K. ROBINSON
KENNETH A. ARNDT
PHILIP E. LEBOIT
BRUCE U. WINTROUB

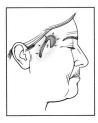

Acknowledgments

We are grateful to the husband and wives of the editors for their love and support. The artistry of Lauren Shavell transformed surgical concepts to a beautiful reality. We thankfully acknowledge the assistance of our colleagues, nurses, and secretaries at our respective institutions, and Judith Fletcher and Dolores Meloni of the W.B. Saunders Company.

JUNE K. ROBINSON
KENNETH A. ARNDT
PHILIP E. LEBOIT
BRUCE U. WINTROUB

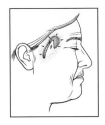

Contents

section one

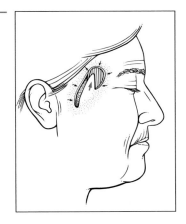

Basic Cutaneous Surgery Concepts

JUNE K. ROBINSON

Fundamental knowledge and technical skills must be acquired and mastered before performing more complex procedures such as skin flaps and grafts, cosmetic procedures (e.g., dermabrasion), or surgery in specialized anatomic units (e.g., nail surgery or ear surgery). In this section, the fundamental information is presented in a manner that reflects its clinical relevance. The technical skills and basic procedures become the building blocks for the next section on tissue movement by flaps and grafts.

In clinical experience, these basic procedures remain among the most commonly performed procedures. Utterly reliable and relatively complication-free results are achieved by experienced dermatologists in office-based surgery with these basic procedures. Since this is the clinical experience of many dermatologists over many decades, it is likely to remain the same in the future. Skin biopsies

by punch biopsy, shave biopsy, or saucerization excision and electrosurgery, cryosurgery, and elliptical excisional surgery will remain commonly practiced procedures despite advances in technology. The dermatologist will choose among the various techniques based on what is needed to treat the disease process, on the patient's needs, and on the surgical skills of the physician.

Dermatologists acquire extensive knowledge about the biology and pathology of the skin and its diseases. This knowledge forms the basis of therapeutic decisions and selection among a range of medical and surgical options. The ability to bring the best of both medical and surgical therapy to the patient is one of the strengths of dermatology, which is both a medical and a surgical specialty. Although individual dermatologists may be more comfortable with either the medical or the surgical aspects, all

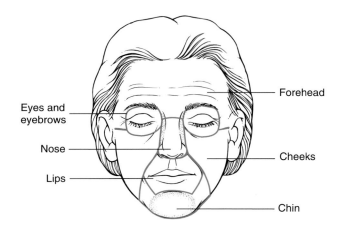

Eyes and eyebrows

Nose

Lips

Forehead

Cheeks

Chin

FIGURE I–1. The boundaries of the cosmetic units of the face are good sites for placement of elective incision lines.

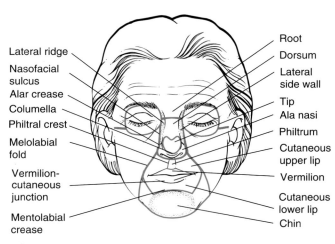

Lateral ridge
Nasofacial sulcus
Alar crease
Columella
Philtral crest
Melolabial fold
Vermilion-cutaneous junction
Mentolabial crease

Root
Dorsum
Lateral side wall
Tip
Ala nasi
Philtrum
Cutaneous upper lip
Vermilion
Cutaneous lower lip
Chin

FIGURE I–2. Boundaries of the cosmetic units of the central face are defined by the contour lines of the nose, lips, and chin.

aspects are encompassed within dermatology. For those individuals whose interest and experience carries them into dermatologic surgery, there seems a natural progression in learning first basic procedures, then tissue movement, and then cosmetic procedures. This atlas is organized with the intent of enhancing that natural evolution in interest and skills.

PLANNING THE PROCEDURE

A basic consideration before starting any type of surgical procedure is camouflage of the scar that will result from the procedure. Certain principles of aesthetic units, contour lines, relaxed skin tension lines of the face, and relaxed skin tension lines and positions of function of the body and limbs will assist in scar camouflage.

The major aesthetic units of the face (the forehead, nose, eyes, lips, cheeks, and chin) (Fig. I–1) are subdivided into units whose skin surface attributes are consistent within the unit (Figs. I–2 through I–5). Surface characteristics such as pigmentation, texture, hair quality, pore size, sebaceous quality, and response to blush and flush stimuli are similar within a single unit. Elasticity and mobility of the skin may vary within a unit. The boundaries of these cosmetic units may provide good places to electively situate inci-

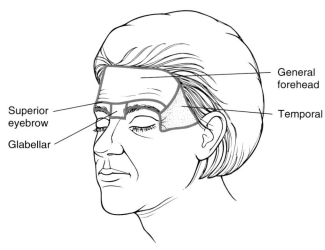

Superior eyebrow

Glabellar

General forehead

Temporal

FIGURE I–3. Four components form the cosmetic unit of the forehead.

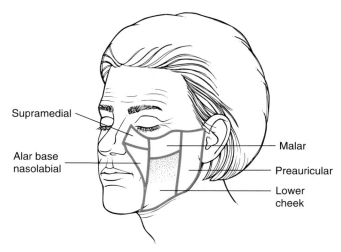

Supramedial

Alar base nasolabial

Malar

Preauricular

Lower cheek

FIGURE I–4. Five components form the cosmetic unit of the cheek.

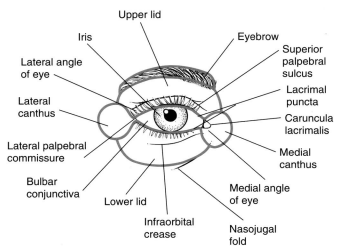

FIGURE I–5. The topographic landmarks and components of the eye area.

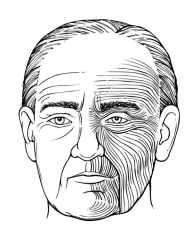

FIGURE I–6. Relaxed skin tension lines of the face at rest with gravitational forces exerted from a seated position. With aging and sun exposure the lines become more pronounced.

sions. For instance, the junction of the pyramid of the nose and medial cheek provides a natural line of definition along which an incision may be placed. The boundaries of the cosmetic units form contour lines (see Figs. I–2 through I–5). Contour lines, existing wrinkles formed by gravity with the patient sitting or formed during expression, help to determine placement of incision lines (Fig. I–6). Age and sun exposure can accentuate the wrinkles that appear along the course of the relaxed skin tension lines. In younger patients the elasticity or resilience of the skin is greater, so there is more opportunity to stretch the skin. In older patients, elastotic changes produce redundancy of the skin with excess folds of tissue or wrinkles.

On the trunk and extremities, wrinkles usually are not prominent and cannot be used to predict skin tension lines. In general, incision lines are circumferential on the trunk and extremities and can be predicted by laxity of the skin that is formed when the underlying muscles contract (Figs. I–7 and I–8). Compressing the skin between the thumb and forefinger in the direction of the relaxed skin tension line results in easy wrinkling (Fig. I–9). If the compression is not in the relaxed skin tension line, few wrinkles appear.

A fundamental knowledge of surface anatomy and underlying structures is necessary in the practice of obtaining local and nerve block anesthesia and for planning place-

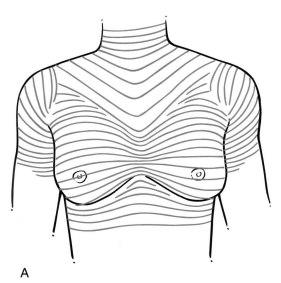

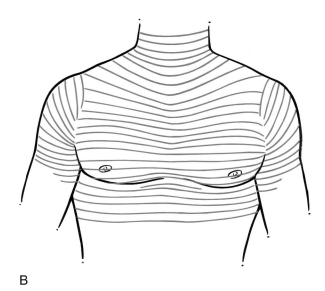

A   B

FIGURE I–7. Relaxed skin tension lines of the body vary slightly in women *(A)* and men *(B)*.

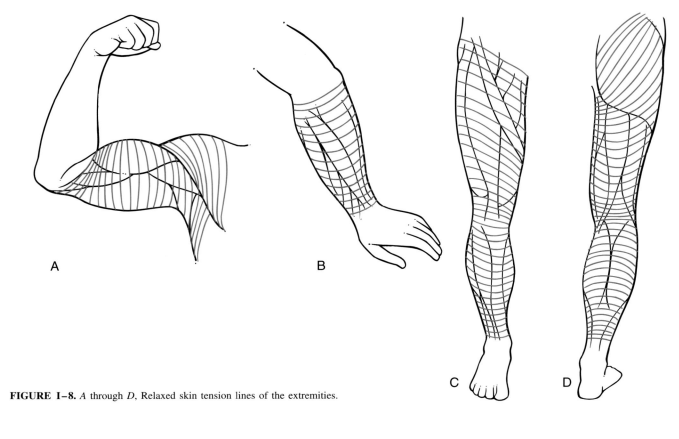

FIGURE I–8. *A* through *D*, Relaxed skin tension lines of the extremities.

FIGURE I–9. The compression test to determine the relaxed skin tension lines. *A*, Compression of the skin between the thumb and forefinger produces wrinkles and defines the placement of incision lines. *B*, Compression produces little wrinkling and convinces the surgeon that this is not the correct orientation for the incision.

ment of incision lines or changes in skin surface resulting from other forms of surgery (e.g., cryosurgery or chemical peeling). Technical skills are honed in the laboratory on inert materials such as foam or cadaver specimens to learn how to handle instruments with ease, tie square knots, place sutures properly, plan tissue movement, and execute the surgical plan. Finally the knowledge and technical skills of the student are brought to the patient and procedures are performed under supervision. It is the hope of all the authors and editors that the information presented in

this atlas will assist the learning process of the student of dermatologic surgery at all phases in the individual's learning curve.

Suggested Reading

1. Gonzalez-Ulloa M, Castillo A, Stevens E, et al. Preliminary study of the total restoration of the facial skin. Plast Reconstr Surg 1954; 13:151–161.

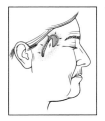

chapter 1

Superficial Cutaneous Anatomy

HUBERT T. GREENWAY and ERIC A. BREISCH

The dermatologic surgeon must have an awareness of the underlying anatomy to accomplish and perform cutaneous surgery. This is critical to "plan" the procedure as well as to "avoid" certain structures where possible and prevent complications. By necessity, one must look at anatomy in a structured, organized fashion; in reality, the anatomy is dynamic and the presentation of life itself.

Certain regions of the body are of particular interest in cutaneous surgery because of the relationship of the surface skin to the underlying structures (Table 1–1; Fig. 1–1). Topographic anatomy or surface landmarks are useful in describing the location of the surgery. Particular regions of the body have special terminology to describe the features that are frequently relevant to the function of the region (Table 1–2).

THE FACE AND SCALP

The surface anatomy of the face is best appreciated by referring to the bony landmarks of the frontal, maxillary, zygomatic, and mandibular bones. Each of these bones has distinctive features that contribute to the features of the face. The fixed bony landmarks can be used as reference points to specifically locate (i.e., measuring in millimeters) overlying cutaneous lesions.

TABLE 1–1. Superficial Anatomy of the Face and Scalp

Surface anatomy of the skull
Muscles of facial expression
Blood vessels of the face and scalp
Lymphatics
The facial nerve
Sensory nerves and innervation
Selected specialized structures

Bony Landmarks

The squamous portion of the *frontal bone* forms the foundation of the forehead. In addition to the overlying periosteum, the cortical bone normally provides a barrier to tumor growth. At times, a portion of the outer table may be removed to evaluate tumor invasion. This procedure leaves the remaining outer table, diploë, and inner table of the frontal bone intact. The distinctive features of the frontal bone that contribute to the face are as follows:

- The superciliary arches, forming the bony ridges underlying the eyebrows.
- The glabella, the smooth elevation of bone in the midline that connects the superciliary arches.
- The nasion, which is a craniometric point located in the midline and indicates the articulation between the frontal bone and the paired nasal bones.
- The supraorbital foramen, which is located approximately 2 cm lateral from the nasion along the superior margin of the orbit and can be palpated and identified during a supraorbital nerve block procedure.

The *maxillary bone* forms the foundation for the midportion of the face. It consists of

- The alveolar process, which lodges the upper dentition.
- The canine eminence, an elevation of bone in the alveolar process created by the canine tooth.
- The canine fossa, a broad depression on the maxilla located immediately lateral to the canine eminence.
- The infraorbital foramen, located in the body of the maxilla approximately 5 mm below the inferior margin of the orbit. The infraorbital nerve exits the foramen and may be blocked. Note that the supraorbital, infraorbital, and mental foramina all lie in a straight vertical line medial to the pupil of the eye when gaze is directed forward.

5

The *zygomatic bone,* malar portion, forms the foundation for the upper cheek region. Whitnall's tubercle is a small bony projection of the zygomatic bone at the lateral margin of the orbit.

The *mandible* forms the lower jaw.

- The mandibular alveolar process lodges the lower dentition.
- The body of the mandible presents a sharp inferior margin that extends posteriorly to the angles of the jaw.
- The mental protuberance forms the tip of the chin.
- The mental foramen is located within the body of the mandible, approximately 1 cm above the inferior margins of the mandible at the interspace of premolars. The mental nerve may be blocked as it exits the mental foramen.
- The ramus of the mandible presents a sharp posterior margin.

The *temporal* and *zygomatic* bones form the zygoma or zygomatic arch.

Muscles of Facial Expression

All of the muscles of the facial expression are innervated by the branches of the facial nerve (see Fig. 1-1; Table 1-3). The loss of function of any of these muscles affects the appearance of the face either in repose or in expressing emotions.

Loss of nerve innervations of central facial muscles can have devastating consequences. The zygomatic branch of the facial nerve provides primary innervation of the orbicularis oculi muscle, and there is a small component of innervation by the temporal branch of the facial nerve. The closure of the eyelids by the orbicularis oculi muscles causes the squeeze effect of blinking that moves tears across the globe. Without this function, the eye becomes dry and clarity of vision can be affected (see Fig. 1-1; Table 1-3).

The muscles associated with upper lip function are primarily innervated by the buccal branch of the facial nerve, with secondary innervation by means of the zygomatic branches of the facial nerve. The muscles of the lower lip, with the exception of the platysma, are innervated primarily by the marginal mandibular branches and secondarily by the buccal branches of the facial nerve (see Fig. 1-1; Table 1-3).

Blood Vessels of the Face and Scalp

Arterial supply is from the external carotid and internal carotid arteries and their branches. This is a high-pressure

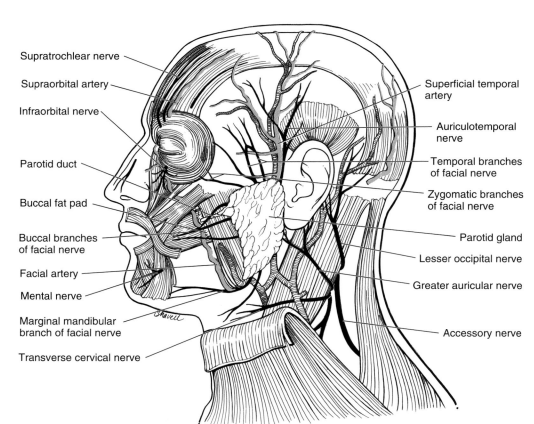

Supratrochlear nerve
Supraorbital artery
Infraorbital nerve
Parotid duct
Buccal fat pad
Buccal branches of facial nerve
Facial artery
Mental nerve
Marginal mandibular branch of facial nerve
Transverse cervical nerve

Superficial temporal artery
Auriculotemporal nerve
Temporal branches of facial nerve
Zygomatic branches of facial nerve
Parotid gland
Lesser occipital nerve
Greater auricular nerve
Accessory nerve

FIGURE 1-1. Superficial anatomy of the head and neck. Arteries are in red.

TABLE 1–3. Muscles of Facial Expression and Their Innervation

Muscle Innervation Branch	Action	Facial Nerve Branch Innervation
Scalp		
Occipitalis	Moves scalp posteriorly	Postauricular
Frontalis	Raises eyebrows	Temporal
Periorbital		
Corrugator supercilli	Pulls eyebrows medially	Temporal
Orbicularis oculi	Closes eyelid	Temporal and zygomatic
Nose		
Procerus	Pulls skin over glabella inferiorly	Temporal
Nasalis	Dilates nares	Buccal
Depressor septi	Pulls columella inferiorly	Buccal
Mouth		
Zygomaticus major and minor	Elevates corner of mouth	Buccal
Levator labii superioris	Elevates upper lip	Buccal
Levator labii superioris alaeque nasi	Lifts upper lip and dilates nares	Buccal
Levator anguli oris	Elevates corner of mouth	Buccal
Risorius	Pulls corner of mouth laterally	Buccal
Depressor anguli oris	Depresses corner of mouth	Buccal and marginal mandibular
Depressor labii inferioris	Depresses lower lip	Marginal mandibular
Mentalis	Protrudes lower lip	Marginal mandibular
Platysma	Pulls corner of mouth inferiorly	Cervical
Buccinator	Flattens cheek	Buccal
Orbicularis	Closes, purses, and protrudes lip	Marginal mandibular

system; thus suture ligation of severed vessels (i.e., superficial temporal and facial arteries) may be indicated. There is adequate crossover flow from the opposite side (see Fig. 1–1).

There are six major arteries supplying the face and scalp:

1. The *facial* artery is palpable as it crosses the mandible (Fig. 1–2). It branches out into the inferior labial (Fig. 1–3), superior labial, and angular (Fig. 1–4) arteries.

2. The *superficial temporal* artery is palpable at the superior pole of parotid gland (see Fig. 1–2). It branches into the transverse facial and frontal arteries (Figs. 1–5 and 1–6).

3. The branches of the *maxillary* artery are infraorbital, buccal, and inferior alveolar (mental artery).

4. The *ophthalmic* artery branches into the supraorbital, supratrochlear, palpebral, dorsal nasal, and lacrimal arteries.

5. *Posterior auricular* artery

6. *Occipital* artery

The venous drainage parallels the arterial supply and consists of the supraorbital, ophthalmic, angular, anterior facial, and superficial temporal veins.

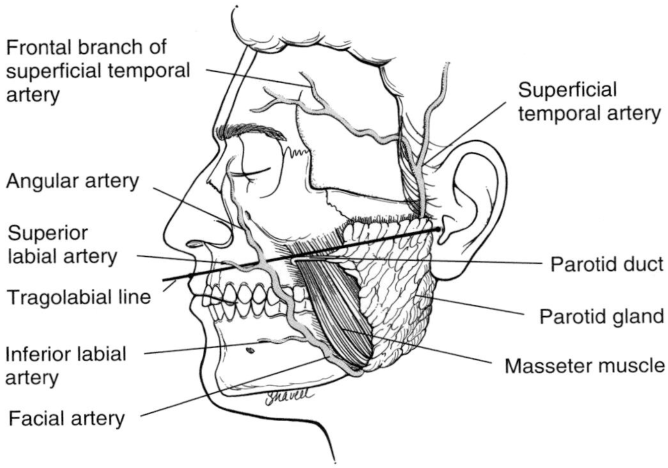

Frontal branch of superficial temporal artery
Angular artery
Superior labial artery
Tragolabial line
Inferior labial artery
Facial artery
Superficial temporal artery
Parotid duct
Parotid gland
Masseter muscle

FIGURE 1–2. Arterial supply of the face in relationship to the masseter muscle and parotid gland. The point where the parotid duct crosses the anterior border of the masseter muscle is plotted along a line connecting the tragus to the middle of the upper lip, the tragolabial line *(black)*.

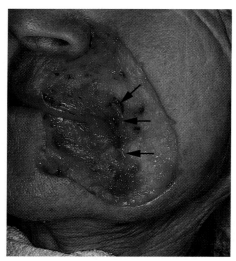

FIGURE 1–3. The facial artery enters the face at the lower border of the jaw, just in front of the anterior border of the masseter muscle. It is possible to palpate the pulsation here. The artery may be exposed during resection of a skin cancer. It takes a diagonal path across the face just lateral to the oral commissure *(arrows)*, then runs adjacent to the nose as the angular artery. (Courtesy of June K. Robinson, M.D.)

Lymphatics

The presence or absence of clinical lymphatic involvement should be documented for neoplasms that have potential for metastatic spread. The following seven regions are commonly checked (Fig. 1–7):

1. The scalp is drained by three regionally positioned nodes: occipital, retroauricular, and superficial parotid nodes.
2. The eyelids drain into two different sets of regional nodes:
    a. Lateral aspects of eyelids — superficial parotid
    b. Medial aspects of eyelids — facial
3. The nasal region drains into the facial nodes.

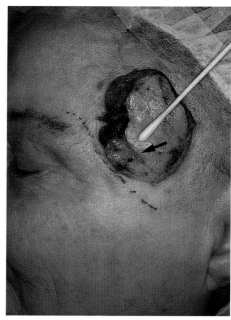

FIGURE 1–5. The frontal branch of the superficial temporal artery is exposed during resection of a tumor *(arrow)*. The temporal branch of the facial nerve remains functional in this case. Before surgery, the potential area for the temporal branches of the facial nerve, described as lying between two diverging lines drawn from the earlobe to the lateral brow (gentian violet seen on the skin surface) and the lateral end of the highest forehead crease, were drawn. In this area, the nerve is immediately subcutaneous and not protected by overlying muscle or parotid. The cotton swab lies on the fascia. (Courtesy of June K. Robinson, M.D.)

4. The masseteric and malar regions of the face drain into the superficial parotid nodes.
5. The infraorbital and buccal regions of the face drain into the facial nodes.

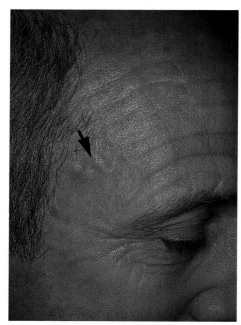

FIGURE 1–6. Tortuous engorged frontal branch of superficial temporal artery is visible on the surface of the skin *(arrow)*. (Courtesy of June K. Robinson, M.D.)

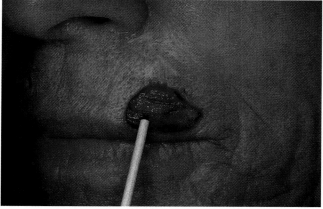

FIGURE 1–4. During resection of a skin cancer of the left upper lip, the superior labial artery is exposed after it branches off the facial artery. The muscle of the orbicularis oris has been resected. The superior labial artery lies behind the muscle. (Courtesy of June K. Robinson, M.D.)

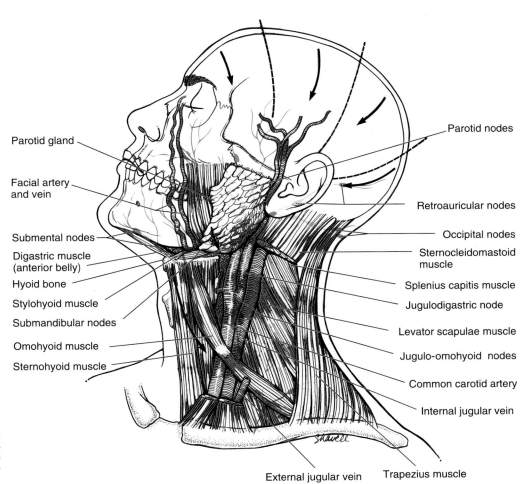

Parotid gland

Facial artery and vein

Submental nodes

Digastric muscle (anterior belly)

Hyoid bone

Stylohyoid muscle

Submandibular nodes

Omohyoid muscle

Sternohyoid muscle

Parotid nodes

Retroauricular nodes

Occipital nodes

Sternocleidomastoid muscle

Splenius capitis muscle

Jugulodigastric node

Levator scapulae muscle

Jugulo-omohyoid nodes

Common carotid artery

Internal jugular vein

External jugular vein **Trapezius muscle**

FIGURE 1–7. Lymphatic system of the head and neck indicated in red. Dotted lines indicate borders between drainage areas; arrows indicate direction of lymph flow.

6. The labial regions drain into two sets of cervical nodes: the submental and submandibular. The middle third of the lower lip will drain into both ipsilateral and contralateral nodes, while the remainder of the lips (both upper and lower) drain only into ipsilateral nodes.

7. The anterolateral aspect of the auricle drains into the superficial parotid nodes. The posteromedial aspect of the ear drains into the retroauricular nodes.

Facial Nerve

The facial nerve is responsible for innervation of all of the muscles of facial expression. It innervates these muscles by penetrating their deep surface, except for the buccinator, which is supplied on its superficial aspect. The facial nerve emerges from the stylomastoid foramen and quickly penetrates the parotid gland. Within the parotid gland the nerve splits into five major branches, which leave the protection of the parotid gland and are named according to the regions of the face they supply (Figs. 1–8 through 1–15). These branches are temporal (Figs. 1–9 through 1–13), zygomatic (see Fig. 1–14), buccal (see Fig. 1–14), marginal mandibular (see Fig. 1–15), and cervical.

Once the facial nerve branches leave the parotid gland they are considered to have safe and danger zones as they

continue to the target muscles. The facial nerve is protected by the parotid gland while within the boundaries of the danger zone, and it is only the extraparotid course of the branches that is of concern. Injury to a nerve branch within its danger zone will result in muscle paralysis and a resulting facial asymmetry. The danger zone of the facial

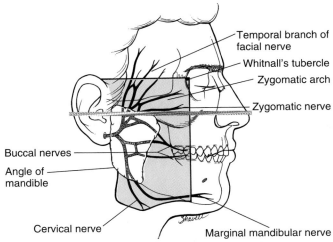

Temporal branch of facial nerve

Whitnall's tubercle

Zygomatic arch

Zygomatic nerve

Buccal nerves

Angle of mandible

Cervical nerve

Marginal mandibular nerve

FIGURE 1–8. Branches of the facial nerve. Pink shaded area represents "nonprotected zone" where branches have emerged from parotid gland and course superficially prior to muscle innervation.

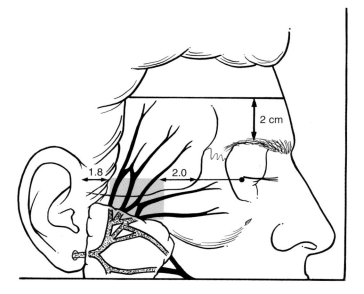

FIGURE 1–9. Landmarks for the temporal branch of the facial nerve. The facial nerve emerges behind the lobe as indicated by the lighter color of the nerve below the lobe and behind the parotid. Pink shaded area represents the "nonprotected zone."

nerve (see Fig. 1–8) is described with the following boundaries:

- Starting at the ear, a horizontal line 1 cm above the zygoma and ending at Whitnall's tubercle. The lateral aspect of the brow is a useful surface landmark for the danger zone.
- A vertical line starting at Whitnall's tubercle and ending at the inferior margin of the mandible
- Starting from the inferior margin of the mandible, a curved line extending 2 cm below the margin of the mandible and ending at the angle of the mandible

In cutaneous surgery the branches of the facial nerve may be anesthetized by local anesthesia with temporary loss of function and resultant facial muscle paralysis. Perineural tumor invasion is rare but may also cause paralysis. Local anesthetic agents or physiologic saline may be injected to elevate overlying tissue (i.e., over the most commonly encountered danger zone over the temporal branch) (see Fig. 1–9) to "lift away" the tissue from the underlying facial nerve. In addition, at certain times, excision and closure may be oriented perpendicular to the normal skin tension lines to parallel the course of the nerve and prevent

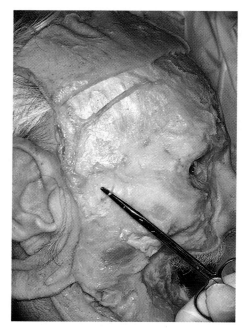

FIGURE 1–10. Cadaver prosection by Drs. June K. Robinson and J. Michael Wentzel illustrates one of the rami of the temporal branch of the facial nerve as it crosses the zygomatic arch. At this point (also illustrated in Figure 1–9) over the zygomatic arch, the nerve is particularly vulnerable as it lies in the superficial musculoaponeurotic system (SMAS) just beneath the subcutaneous fat and over the bony prominence.

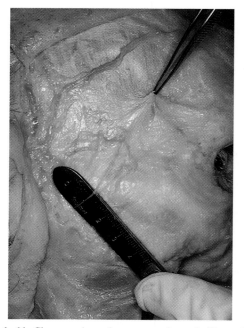

FIGURE 1–11. Close-up view of same area shown in Figure 1–9. The scalpel handle is under the temporal branch of the facial nerve, which has been dissected out of the SMAS at the zygomatic arch. On the forehead, about 2 cm above the brow, the forceps picks up the nerve as it is covered with SMAS. The nerve is clearly visible through the SMAS over the distance between the two surgical instruments. (Courtesy of June K. Robinson, M.D.)

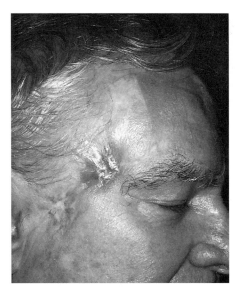

FIGURE 1–12. Two months after surgery, the wound created by resection of a recurrent basal cell carcinoma with Mohs' micrographic surgery is visible as a shiny red area. This area overlies the course of the temporal branch of the facial nerve, which was resected. (Courtesy of June K. Robinson, M.D.)

injury. Nerve identification and avoidance is best at all times (see Figs. 1–9 through 1–15).

Sensory Nerves and Innervation

Forehead and scalp sensation is derived from the branches of the trigeminal (supratrochlear, supraorbital, zygomaticotemporal, and auriculotemporal nerve), cervical plexus (lesser occipital), and the dorsal rami (greater occipital).

On the face, the zones of sensation are as follows:

- *Periorbital:* ophthalmic and maxillary divisions of the trigeminal nerve supply sensation
- *Nose:* terminal branches of ophthalmic and maxillary divisions of the trigeminal nerve supply sensation to various regions of the nose as follows:

  Supratrochlear and infratrochlear: root, bridge, and upper side wall
  Dorsal external nasal via anterior ethmoidal: lower dorsum and tip
  Infraorbital nerve: lateral side wall, ala
  Depressor septi: columella.

- *Cheek:* mandibular and maxillary divisions of the trigeminal nerve supply sensation through the infraorbital, zygomaticofacial, and auriculotemporal branches. Also the greater auricular nerve provides minor input.
- *Lips:* maxillary and mandibular branches of the trigeminal nerve through the infraorbital and mental branches provide sensation.
- *Ears:* sensation is provided by means of the following nerves:

  Auriculotemporal: anterior upper ear including tragus, crus of helix, and also the anterior half of the external canal
  Great auricular: most of the anterior and posterior surface

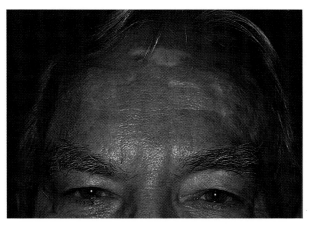

FIGURE 1–13. Ptosis of the right brow 2 months after surgery in same patient shown in Figure 1–12. Note the asymmetry of forehead wrinkles. This case is discussed further in Chapter 30. (Courtesy of June K. Robinson, M.D.)

  Lesser occipital: small area of posterior auricle and mastoid area
  Cranial VII, IX, X (facial, glossopharyngeal, vagus): concha, anthelix, tragus, and posterior half of ear canal

Selected Specialized Structures of the Face

Eye (see Fig. 1–5)

The skin of the eyelid is extremely thin. The eyelashes have great significance. The tarsal plate provides form for the lid but varies in height, with the upper 9 to 11 mm and the lower 4 to 5 mm.

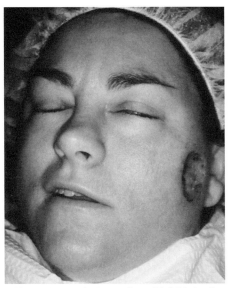

FIGURE 1–14. During surgical resection with Mohs' micrographic surgery of a skin cancer of the left cheek overlying the parotid gland, the buccal and zygomatic branches of the facial nerve are anesthetized, producing temporary motor nerve paralysis. The patient is unable to fully close the left eye and has drooping of the corner of the mouth on the left. Fortunately, nerve function returned as the local anesthesia dissipated. (Courtesy of June K. Robinson, M.D.)

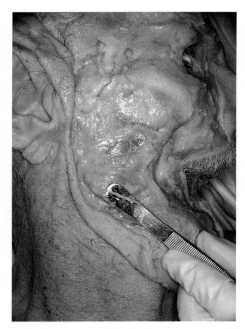

FIGURE 1–15. Cadaver prosection by Drs. June K. Robinson and J. Michael Wentzel demonstrates the marginal mandibular branch of the facial nerve. The nerve is located deep to the platysma until it reaches a point 2 cm lateral to the corner of the mouth. At this point the nerve becomes more superficial and penetrates the facial muscles, which are innervated from below. (Courtesy of June K. Robinson, M.D.)

The lacrimal system consists of the gland that provides primary lubrication and drainage through the upper and lower lacrimal papillae and puncta and duct to the lacrimal sac and then to the nasolacrimal duct to the nasal cavity.

The major clinical considerations in performing surgery of the eyelids are the following:

- To maintain a functional eye—visual acuity
- To use a scleral shield to protect the globe during surgery
- To avoid disruption of the lacrimal system
- To place the patch over the eye in closed position
- To maintain symmetry

Nose (see Fig. I–2)

The skin of the upper nose is mobile and that of the lower nose is adherent and sebaceous. The cartilages that support the skin of the nasal tip are paired lateral nasal, median nasal-septal, and paired greater alar cartilages.

Clinical considerations in performing surgery are as follows:

- To maintain a functional airway
- To remove cartilage or to support tissue, which may require reconstruction with similar tissues
- To treat recurrent and/or aggressive tumors that may spread between cartilages with involvement of cartilage and deeper structures
- To maintain symmetry

Cheek (see Figs. I–1 through I–4)

The skin just lateral to the labial commissure is elevated and is called the modiolus. The modiolus is formed by muscle insertions in this region. Within the cheek the parotid gland protects the facial nerve branches and the parotid duct lies superficial in the mid cheek area. Surgical considerations of the mid cheek area are identification of the parotid duct and avoiding injury to it. If this duct is severed, immediate repair is indicated.

Ear (see Fig. III–1)

The skin of the ear is tightly adherent to the cartilage anteriorly and loosely adherent posteriorly. The lobule lies below the cartilage. The cartilage of the ear is a single plate that provides form and function and a barrier to tumor extension. The fissures of Santorini within the cartilaginous segment of the external auditory canal may allow migration of tumor throughout the cartilage.

Clinical considerations of ear surgery are as follows:

- To maintain a functional ear. The ear canal is protected with a cotton ball during surgery, and hearing is documented before surgery.
- To relieve edema, which under tight anterior skin may cause significant pain
- To keep tumor from spreading through the fissures of Santorini to the parotid gland
- To protect the form of the auricle and to support the eyeglasses
- To maintain normal bacterial flora, which may include gram-negative as well as gram-positive organisms

Lips

The skin of the lips is characterized by the following:

- Multiple creases
- Vermilion border (transition zone)
- Vermilion zone (free red margins; devoid of hair follicles, sweat glands, and sebaceous glands)
- Stratified squamous nonkeratinized layer of epithelium covers inner lip.

The oral cavity is divided into the vestibule and the oral cavity proper.

Skin Tension Lines (see Fig. I–6)

Relaxed or resisting skin tension lines help describe characteristic facial wrinkle lines. Generally, they are *perpendicular* to underlying muscles of facial expression. Asking the patient to make exaggerated facial grimaces can help demonstrate these lines.

Superficial Anatomy of the Neck (see Figs. 1–1, 1–16, and 1–17)

The neck is divided into anterior and posterior triangles by the sternocleidomastoid muscle. Lesions may be localized as to their exact location in the appropriate triangle. Dermatologic surgical procedures in the anterior triangle are for the most part located superiorly where attention should be focused on branches of the facial nerve. Procedures in the posterior triangle should include an awareness of the spinal accessory nerve not covered or protected by the muscle (Figs. 1–16 and 1–17).

Anterior and Posterior Triangles of the Neck

The bony and cartilaginous landmarks of the anterior and posterior triangles of the neck are as follows:

- Mastoid process
- Hyoid bone
- Thyroid cartilage
- Cricoid cartilage
- Trachea

The boundaries of the cervical triangles (Fig. 1–16) are as follows:

- *Anterior cervical triangle*

  Mastoid process
  Mental protuberance
  Jugular notch
  Anterior edge of the sternocleidomastoid muscle
  Inferior margin of the mandible
  Midline extending from the mental protuberance to the jugular notch

- *Posterior cervical triangle*

  Mastoid process
  Posterior edge of the sternocleidomastoid muscle
  Clavicle
  Anterior edge of the trapezius muscle

Muscles

The platysma is a paper-thin muscle that overlies the ventral aspect of the neck. Originating from the fascia of the upper pectoral region, it continues upward into the neck, sweeping across the inferior margin of the mandible to finally insert into the skin of the lower face near the labial commissures. This muscle is innervated by the cervical branch of facial nerve.

Blood Vessels

The arterial supply is through direct penetrating branches from the facial (submental branch), superior thyroid, and transverse cervical arteries. Venous drainage is through the external and anterior jugular veins. Lymphatic drainage is into scattered nodes that drain into the deep cervical lymphatic chain associated with the internal jugular vein. Knowledge of the lymphatic areas and the primary basin they drain is important to document the presence or absence of nodal disease before tumor removal.

Nerves

Motor nerves that may be encountered during cutaneous surgical procedures are the mandibular and cervical branches of the facial nerve and the spinal accessory nerve. The marginal mandibular branch of the facial nerve may be located more superficially in the neck in older patients and is at risk since it may not arborize as early as other branches. Cervical branches of the facial nerve are at risk when a plane of cleavage deep to the platysma is opened

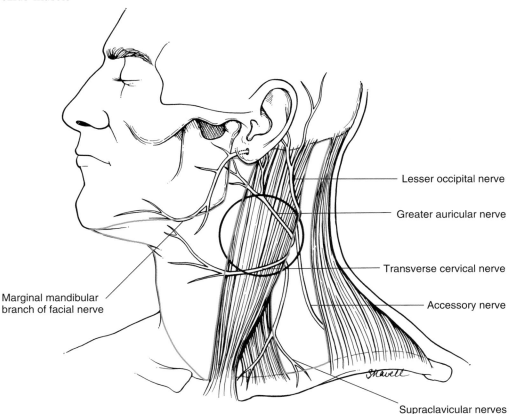

FIGURE 1–16. Triangles of the neck are outlined in red. The danger zone of the neck is centered about a point in the middle of the sterno-cleidomastoid muscle about 6.5 cm below the caudal edge of the external auditory canal. A radius of 3 cm around this point encompasses the emergence over the muscle of the accessory nerve, the greater auricular and lesser occipital nerves, and the transverse cervical nerve *(black circle)*. The nerve emerges below the earlobe as indicated by the dotted line in this area.

Marginal mandibular branch of facial nerve

Lesser occipital nerve

Greater auricular nerve

Transverse cervical nerve

Accessory nerve

Supraclavicular nerves

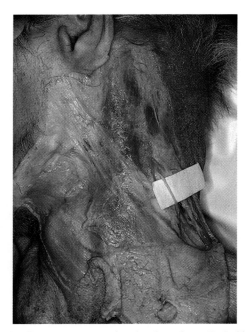

FIGURE 1–17. Cadaver prosection by Drs. June K. Robinson and J. Michael Wentzel demonstrates the spinal accessory nerve as it courses obliquely across the neck just deep to the superficial cervical fascia. (Courtesy of June K. Robinson, M.D.)

near the angle of the jaw. The spinal accessory nerve is encountered within the confines of the posterior cervical triangle. The nerve exits the posterior edge of the sterno-cleidomastoid muscle at the junction of the upper and middle thirds of this muscle (see Figs. 1–16 and 1–17). The spinal accessory nerve courses obliquely across the neck just deep to the superficial cervical fascia to innervate the trapezius muscle. Damage to this nerve may result in the inability to elevate the shoulder on the affected side. It may be of benefit to periodically have the patient elevate the shoulder when performing the procedures over the spinal accessory nerve, in addition to identifying the nerve.

Cutaneous nerve supply to the neck is from branches of the cervical plexus. These branches that enter the neck at the posterior edge of the sternocleidomastoid muscle near its midpoint are the lesser occipital nerve, greater auricular nerve, transverse cervical nerve, and supraclavicular nerve. Local nerve block at this midpoint can provide anesthesia to the lateral neck as well as a portion of the ear.

SUPERFICIAL ANATOMY OF THE HAND

Skin and Fascia

The dorsal skin and fascia are loose except in full flexion. Deeper structures are often visible or palpable through this hair-bearing skin.

Palmar skin and fascia are thicker and inelastic with flexion creases (Fig. 1–18). The skin is well vascularized from below. Fibrous tissue of the palmar fascia separates the subcutaneous tissue from the deeper structures of the hand.

Blood Vessels

Superficial and deep palmar arterial arches arise from radial and ulnar arteries. Common digital arteries arise from the superficial arch. Digital vessels lie dorsal to digital nerves, with Cleland's ligament dorsally and Grayson's ligament volarly maintaining the digital neurovascular bundle.

Nerves

Sensory innervation is through branches of the median, radial, and ulnar nerves. The dorsal surface is innervated by the superficial (sensory) branch of the radial nerve, which is vulnerable to injury because of its superficial location, and by the dorsal (sensory) branch of the ulnar nerve. The palmar surface is innervated by the median and the ulnar nerves.

Clinical Considerations of Hand Surgery

- Epinephrine in a local anesthetic may cause vasospasm and digital ischemia and is contraindicated in digital nerve blocks.
- Palmar incisions should parallel flexion creases or cross high-tension areas at a 45-degree angle.
- Dorsal incisions are commonly transverse but avoid nerves. Curvilinear lazy "S" incisions are better over joints of digits.

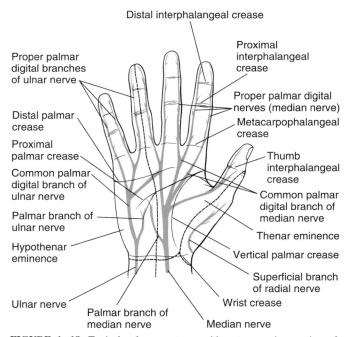

FIGURE 1–18. Topical palmar anatomy with cutaneous innervation of the hand in red. Black dotted lines indicate boundaries of innervation of palmar surface: three and one-half digits by median nerve, one and one-half digits by ulnar nerve.

ANKLE AND FOOT

Surface Anatomy

Lesions may be localized related to underlying bones (Fig. 1–19) or tendons (Figs. 1–20 and 1–21), as listed:

- *Bones:*

  Tibia (medial malleolus)
  Fibula (lateral malleolus)

- *Tendons:*

  Calcaneal tendon (Achilles)
  Peroneus longus and brevis
  Tibialis anterior, extensor halluces longus, extensor digitorum longus and brevis
  Tibialis posterior, flexor digitorum longus, flexor hallucis longus (see Figs. 1–20 and 1–21)

Blood Vessels

The arteries are the anterior tibial artery (anterior medial and lateral malleolar, medial and lateral tarsal, dorsalis pedis, arcuate) and the posterior tibial artery (medial plantar, lateral plantar, peroneal) (see Fig. 1–19). The veins are the dorsal venous arch, greater saphenous vein, and lesser saphenous vein. There are no lymph nodes found in the foot or ankle region. Lymph flows from deep to superficial through web spaces and parallels the saphenous venous system.

Nerves

The cutaneous nerves of the foot and ankle include the following:

- Saphenous nerve
- Superficial peroneal nerve
- Deep peroneal nerve
- Lateral sural cutaneous nerve
- Medial sural cutaneous nerve
- Sural nerve
- Medial plantar nerve
- Lateral plantar nerve

Clinical Considerations of Foot and Ankle Surgery

The dorsal skin is loose. Structures are visible and palpable beneath the skin. It is possible to do longitudinal

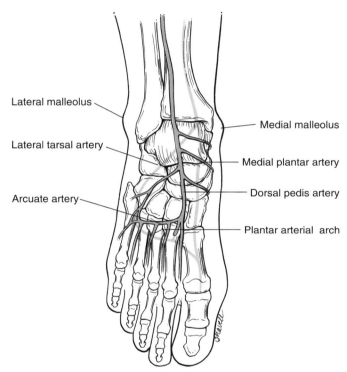

Lateral malleolus

Lateral tarsal artery

Arcuate artery

Medial malleolus

Medial plantar artery

Dorsal pedis artery

Plantar arterial arch

FIGURE 1–19. Relationship of arteries and bones to surface anatomy. The pink color indicates the arteries on the plantar aspect of the foot, and the red color the arteries on the dorsal aspect.

FIGURE 1–20. Medial surface of the foot and ankle and underlying tendons and palpable artery. Pink indicates tendon sheath. The nerve is solid black, and the artery is striated.

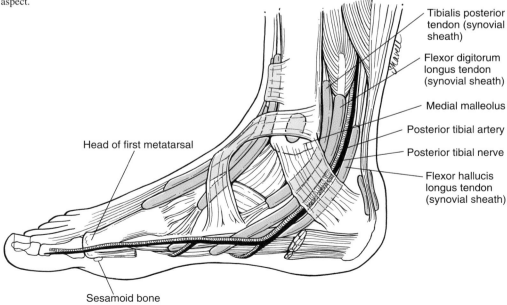

Head of first metatarsal

Tibialis posterior tendon (synovial sheath)

Flexor digitorum longus tendon (synovial sheath)

Medial malleolus

Posterior tibial artery

Posterior tibial nerve

Flexor hallucis longus tendon (synovial sheath)

Sesamoid bone

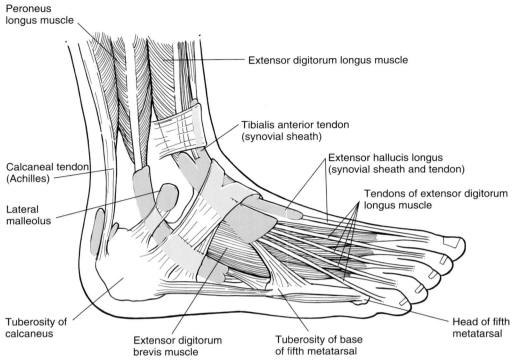

Peroneus
longus muscle

Extensor digitorum longus muscle

Tibialis anterior tendon
(synovial sheath)

Extensor hallucis longus
(synovial sheath and tendon)

Calcaneal tendon
(Achilles)

Tendons of extensor digitorum
longus muscle

Lateral
malleolus

Tuberosity of
calcaneus

Head of fifth
metatarsal

Extensor digitorum
brevis muscle

Tuberosity of base
of fifth metatarsal

FIGURE 1–21. Lateral surface of the foot and ankle and underlying tendons. Pink indicates tendon sheath.

incision and excision (perpendicular to relaxed skin tension lines) to avoid damaging the underlying structures. The plantar skin is adherent to deeper structures. In the Achilles area the tendon is easily outlined and the tendon should not be transected.

Anesthesia: Ankle Block (see Chapter 3)

Useful ankle blocks include the following:

- Posterior tibial nerve block (posterior to artery)
- Peroneal nerve block (at bifurcation of tibialis anterior and extensor hallucis longus tendons)
- Sural nerve block (midway between apex of lateral malleolus and Achilles tendon)
- Ring block, excluding Achilles tendon area

Postoperative care requires the use of bulky dressings and avoidance of weight bearing.

NAILS

The horn plate is rectangular on the distal dorsal segment of the fingers and toes (Fig. 1–22). Terminology useful for nail surgery is listed below:

- Nail plate: cornified epithelial cells
- Nail bed: vascular, semitransparent, pink, adherent to nail plate; no granular layer; longitudinal parallel dermal ridges

- Nail matrix and lunula: forms nail plate
- Proximal nail fold and groove
- Lateral nail fold and groove
- Hyponychium: free edge of distal nail
- Vascular supply: lateral digital vessels with proximal and distal arches
- Nerve supply: digital sensory nerve endings

THE PERINEUM

The perineum, a region of the lower trunk including the skin, subcutaneous tissue, and deeper structures, is located between the thighs, the pubic symphysis, and the tip of the coccyx. The perineum is divided into two triangles by a transverse line joining the ischial tuberosities: anteriorly, the urogenital triangle; posteriorly, the anal triangle (Fig. 1–23). The urogenital triangle, bounded anteriorly by the pubic symphysis and laterally by the ischiopubic rami and ischial tuberosities, contains the structures of the male and the female urogenital triangles.

Structures of the Male Urogenital Triangle

The external genitalia are composed of the following:

- *Scrotum:* a cutaneous sac containing the testis. The skin of the scrotum is thin and pigmented with hair and associated glands. The dartos is a layer of superficial fascia endowed with smooth muscle.
- *Penis:* attached to the linea alba and pubic symphysis by fundiform and suspensory ligaments. It consists of

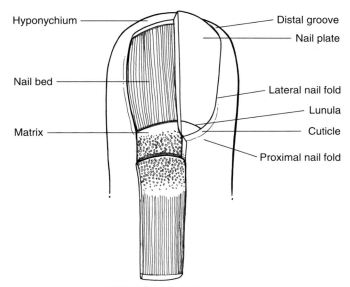

FIGURE 1–22. Nail anatomy.

a root and a body. The body is formed by the union of the corpora cavernosa and the corpus spongiosum (Fig. 1–24). The two corpora cavernosa are bounded by a thick fascia called the tunica albuginea. Buck's fascia, a tough fascial layer, binds all three components with septa separating the corpora cavernosa from the corpus spongiosum. The skin surrounding the body of the penis is very loose and becomes redundant at the prepuce (foreskin), but it is particularly immobile over the corona and glans (Fig. 1–25).

The vessels and nerves are as follows:

- *Arteries:* from the internal pudendal artery—perineal arteries (supplies skin of the urogenital triangle); deep artery of the penis; dorsal artery of the penis; artery of bulb and urethra. Several small superficial arteries arising from the external pudendal artery by means of the femoral artery help to supply the skin of the urogenital triangle.
- *Veins:* deep dorsal veins of the penis receive the drainage of the erectile tissue and drain primarily into the prostatic venous plexus. Superficial veins of the penis and scrotum drain into the external pudendal veins that tend to drain into the proximal segment of the greater saphenous vein.
- *Lymphatics:* lymphatics of the male perineum tend to drain into the superficial inguinal nodes, with some deep portions of the penis draining into the prostatic nodes of the internal iliac nodal system
- *Nerves:*
  - Pudendal nerve—arises within pelvis, exits through the greater sciatic foramen, curls around ischial spine, and passes through the lesser sciatic foramen to enter the perineum within the pudendal canal; perineal branches (supplies the posterior, lateral, and anteroinferior skin of the scrotum), dorsal nerves of the penis (innervate skin of the penis)
  - Posterior femoral cutaneous nerve—perineal branches (innervate skin of the lateral scrotum)
  - Ilioinguinal nerve—anterior scrotal branches (runs through the superficial inguinal ring; innervates skin

of the dorsum and sides of the base of penis and anterosuperior skin of the scrotum
- Genitofemoral nerve—genital branch (passes through the superficial inguinal ring to supply the lateral and superior skin of the scrotum).

Structures of the Female Urogenital Triangle

The external genitalia are as follows:

- *Mons pubis:* skin and subcutaneous tissue overlying the pubic symphysis (Fig. 1–26)
- *Labia majora:* prominent longitudinal folds of skin, supported by underlying fat. They are the homologue to the male scrotum and extend caudally from the mons. The skin overlying the outer aspect is pigmented and well endowed with hair. The space between the labia is called the pudendal cleft. The labia are united anteriorly and posteriorly at the commissures.
- *Labia minora:* smaller folds of skin within the pudendal cleft, surrounding the vaginal vestibule. Posteriorly the labia minora unite as the frenulum of the labia (fourchette). Anteriorly, the labia split into superior (lateral) and inferior (medial) portions: the superior portions pass above the clitoris to form the prepuce, the inferior portions pass below the clitoris, forming the frenulum of the clitoris.
- *Vestibule:* space between the labia minora. Several openings include the external urethral, vaginal, and ducts of major vestibular glands.
- *Clitoris:* homologue of the male penis; formed by the two corpora and a body but not transversed by the urethra
- *Vestibular bulbs:* two masses of erectile tissue buried within the labia minora

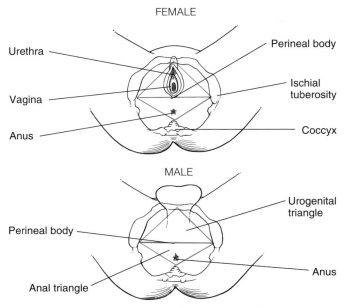

FIGURE 1–23. Anal and urogenital triangles.

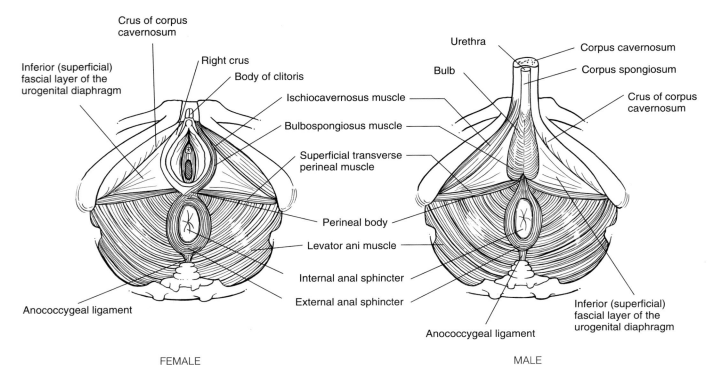

FEMALE   MALE

FIGURE 1–24. The perineum—comparative structures in the male and female.

- *Greater vestibular glands (Bartholin's):* positioned lateral to the lower end of the vagina and behind the vestibular bulbs. The ducts open into the vestibule just above the fourchette.

The vessels and nerves are the

- *Arteries:* correspond to those found in the male. The pudendal artery yields the posterior labial artery to the vestibular bulb and the deep artery of the clitoris.

- *Veins:* parallel the arteries except the deep vein of the clitoris, which enters the pelvis directly to drain into the vesical plexus of veins surrounding the bladder
- *Lymphatics:* drain primarily from the vulva into the superficial inguinal nodes with some joining the deep inguinal nodes.
- *Nerves:* the pudendal nerve arises within the pelvis as described for the male. The skin of the labia majora and minora is supplied posteriorly by the perineal

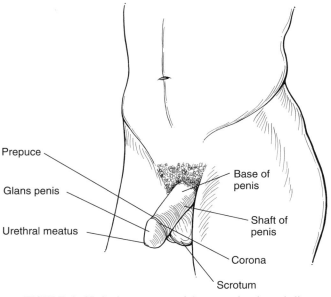

FIGURE 1–25. Surface anatomy of the external male genitalia.

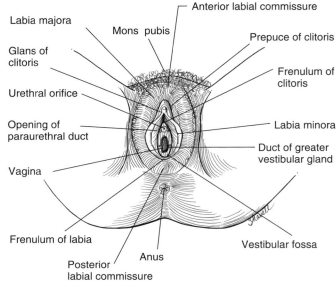

FIGURE 1–26. Surface anatomy of the female perineum.

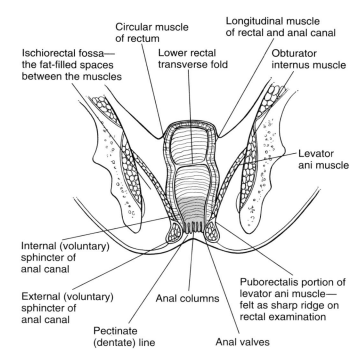

Circular muscle
of rectum

Longitudinal muscle
of rectal and anal canal

Ischiorectal fossa—
the fat-filled spaces
between the muscles

Lower rectal
transverse fold

Obturator
internus muscle

Levator
ani muscle

Internal (voluntary)
sphincter of
anal canal

Puborectalis portion of
levator ani muscle—
felt as sharp ridge on
rectal examination

External (voluntary)
sphincter of
anal canal

Anal columns

Pectinate
(dentate) line

Anal valves

FIGURE 1–27. Coronal views of the rectum and anus. The area in red is below the line of peritoneal reflection at the middle of the rectal valve, about 11 cm from the anal margin. Above this area great caution must be exercised in performing procedures to avoid perforation of the rectal wall. In passing through the anus, the line of demarcation (the pectinate line) that marks the end of the ectodermal anal canal also marks the end of painful sensation. Spasm and distention are felt in the rectum but not pain. The pectinate line separates the lymphatic (ascends above versus drains to superficial inguinal nodes below), vascular (internal above versus external hemorrhoids below) veins, and afferent nerve (visceral above versus somatic below) supply of the anal canal.

branches of the pudendal nerve; anteriorly, the labia and mons are supplied by the ilioinguinal and genito-femoral nerves. The clitoris is supplied by the dorsal nerve of the clitoris.

Anal Triangle

The anal triangle is bounded posteriorly by the tip of the coccyx and laterally by the sacrotuberous ligaments and ischial tuberosities. This relatively simple region contains the terminal portion of the anal canal, the anus (Fig. 1–27). The vessels and nerves include the following:

- *Arteries:* the internal pudendal artery provides the inferior rectal artery, which supplies the skin and musculature surrounding the anus; the perineal branch supplies the remainder of anal triangle.
- *Veins:* inferior rectal veins drain into the internal pudendal veins.
- *Nerves:* the skin of perianal region is innervated through the inferior rectal nerves from the pudendal nerve with some overlap posteriorly from the small perineal branches of the fourth sacral nerve.

- *Lymphatics:* the skin of the perianal region drains into the superficial inguinal nodes; the anal canal below the pectinate line drains into the inguinal lymph nodes, which drain into the pelvic lymph nodes.

Suggested Readings

1. Breisch EA, Greenway HT. Cutaneous Surgical Anatomy of the Head and Neck. New York: Churchill Livingstone, 1992.
2. Clemente CD. Gray's Anatomy, 30th American ed. Philadelphia: Lea & Febiger, 1985.
3. Goldberg S. Clinical Anatomy Made Ridiculously Simple. N. Miami Beach, FL: MedMaster, 1984.
4. Hiatt JL, Gartner LP. Textbook of Head and Neck Anatomy. East Norwalk, CT: Appleton-Century-Crofts, 1982.
5. Hollingshead WH. Anatomy for Surgeons: The Head and Neck, 3rd ed, vol 1. New York: Harper & Row, 1982.
6. Mack GR. Superficial Anatomy and Cutaneous Surgery of the Hand. In: Advances in Dermatology, vol 7. St. Louis: Mosby–Year Book, 1992:315–351.
7. McMinn RMH, Hutchings RT, Logan BH. Color Atlas of Foot and Ankle Anatomy. London: Wolfe Medical Publishers, 1982.
8. Rohen JW, Yokochi C. Color Atlas of Anatomy: A Photographic Study of the Human Body, 3rd ed. New York: Igaku-Shoin, 1993.
9. Salasche SJ, Bernstein G, Senkarik M. Surgical Anatomy of the Skin. Norwalk, CT: Appleton & Lange, 1988.
10. Williams PL, Warwick R, Dyson M, Bannister LH, eds. Gray's Anatomy, 37th ed. New York: Churchill Livingstone, 1989.

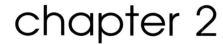

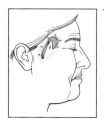

chapter 2

Preoperative Considerations for Antibiotic Prophylaxis and Antisepsis

Antibiotic Prophylaxis

Ann F. Haas and Roy C. Grekin

The specific indications in dermatologic surgery for antibiotic prophylaxis to prevent either wound infection or endocarditis remain ill defined. The relative indications for prophylaxis of wound infections as well as the controversies surrounding the use of antibiotic prophylaxis to prevent endocarditis are addressed here and recommendations based on extensive literature review are offered as guidelines for the dermatologic surgeon.

ANTIBIOTIC PROPHYLAXIS FOR WOUND INFECTION

For the purposes of classification of contamination, wounds are placed into four categories:

1. Class I. *Clean* wounds are created in noncontaminated skin using sterile surgical technique. Such procedures might include excision of noninflamed cysts or excision of benign or malignant tumors, and they have an infection rate of less than 5%.

2. Class II. *Clean-contaminated* wounds include those in contaminated areas (e.g., the oral cavity, respiratory tract, axillae, or perineum) and include breaks in aseptic technique. The infection rate averages around 10%. Most dermatologic surgery procedures result in either class I or class II wounds.

3. Class III. *Contaminated* wounds consist of trauma, have major breaks in sterile technique, or are wounds in which acute, nonpurulent inflammation is encountered, including such entities as intact, inflamed cysts or tumors with clinical inflammation. This class carries a 20% to 30% infection rate.

4. Class IV. *Infected* wounds are grossly contaminated with foreign bodies or devitalized tissue (ruptured cysts, hidradenitis, tumors with purulent or necrotic material). This class carries a 30% to 40% infection rate.

The guidelines proposed by the Centers for Disease Control and Prevention suggest that prophylaxis is most useful for operations associated with a moderate level of contamination.[1] For class I wounds, antibiotics appear to be of no benefit in preventing wound infections.[2–4] Antibiotics are probably helpful in certain types of class II wounds, although there is some uncertainty.[1] Although clean-contaminated head and neck surgical procedures suggest giving antibiotics when the procedure involves incision through oral or pharyngeal mucosa, it remains unclear whether infection rates in uncontaminated head and neck surgery are high enough to justify this prophylaxis. Antibiotics are considered therapeutic, not prophylactic, in class III and IV wounds.

Aside from the level of wound contamination, there are other factors that can contribute to the risk of wound infections. Factors relating to the surgical site, the nature and length of the procedure, and overall patient health status may need to be considered in some circumstances.[5] Combinations of risk factors may increase the risk of wound infection, and therefore possible benefit might be achieved by giving antibiotics before a surgical procedure.

As has been noted, most dermatologic surgery procedures fall into the clean or clean-contaminated category with a low overall incidence of infection in dermatologic surgery units (e.g., <1% annual wound infection rate at the University of California, San Francisco[5]). This means that prophylaxis is probably not routinely needed. However, certain circumstances may make antibiotic prophylaxis for wound infections prudent. Patients undergoing dermatologic surgery procedures involving the oronasal areas that invade mucosa, gastrointestinal and genitourinary areas, and the axillae probably should receive antibiotic prophylaxis (Table 2–1).[5] The specific antibiotic choices given are discussed in a later section.

The generally accepted indications for antibiotic prophylaxis for wound infections include conduct of a clean-contaminated operation and procedures involving insertion of a prosthesis. Less well-accepted indications include clean operations in patients with impaired host defenses or in patients for whom the consequences of infection may have a significant morbidity (the usual rationale for antibiotic prophylaxis in "clean" cases such as cardiac and neurosurgery or ophthalmology). Although the "wound infection risk factors" both in the environment and in the host are acknowledged to a variable degree, there are currently no standard recommendations for antibiotic prophylaxis by risk categories of patients who may develop wound infections. Given the low rate of surgical wound infections in clean or clean-contaminated surgery, studies of such infections associated with this surgery would require large numbers to gain sufficient statistical power to detect any significant differences attributable to an intervention. This problem (i.e., the lack of studies to define the at-risk patient as well as the at-risk procedure and prophylaxis) renders it difficult to uniformly recommend antibiotic prophylaxis for "at-risk" patients. Peterson states that, even in "clean" surgery, "patients who have severe host defense compromise may require the use of prophylactic antibiotics" and believes that the decision to use antibiotics should be made "when the surgeon feels that the insult of the surgical procedure will result in significant bacterial contamination or that the patient's host defenses are inadequate to resist a bacterial insult of any size."[6] Despite being classified as clean-contaminated surgery, most dermatologic surgery procedures are of short duration and associated with a very low risk of significant infection. In most situations, unless the patient is at risk for significant morbidity from an infection that might occur from a selected dermatologic surgical procedure, antibiotic prophylaxis is probably not warranted for the patient who is not "at risk." Each patient's situation is considered on a case-by-case basis, and consultation with a specific subspecialist, when indicated, should be undertaken.

The selection of an appropriate antibiotic both for prevention of wound infection and for endocarditis prophylaxis is made based on the most likely causal organism. The normal resident skin flora varies somewhat with body site. Transient flora lies free on the skin surface without attachment. *Staphylococcus epidermidis*, although making up over 50% of the resident staphylococci, rarely causes wound infection, but it can be a pathogen for prosthetic valve endocarditis and vascular grafts. *Staphylococcus aureus*, which is not a member of resident flora, is found

TABLE 2-1. Antibiotic Recommendations for Prevention of Wound Infections*

Antibiotic	1 Hour Before Surgery	6 Hours Later
Skin (Staphylococcus aureus)		
First-generation cephalosporin	1 g PO	500 mg PO
Dicloxacillin	1 g PO	500 mg PO
Clindamycin†	300 g PO	150 mg PO
Vancomycin†	500 mg IV	250 mg IV
Oral (Streptococcus viridans)		
First-generation cephalosporin	1 g PO	500 mg PO
Amoxicillin	3 g PO	1.5 g PO
Erythromycin†	1 g PO	500 mg PO
Clindamycin†	300 mg PO	150 mg PO
Gastrointestinal / Genitourinary (Escherichia coli)		
First-generation cephalosporin	1 g PO	500 mg PO
Trimethoprim-sulfamethoxazole† (double strength)	1 tablet PO	Can repeat q12h
Ciprofloxacin†	500 mg PO	Can repeat q12h
Gastrointestinal / Genitourinary (Enterococcus)		
Vancomycin†	500 mg IV	250 mg IV

* Choice of antibiotic is based on organism most likely to cause infection. We recommend use of only a single preoperative dose in most cases. For prolonged cases in "contaminated areas," we would consider adding the postoperative dose if dealing with a significant risk of infection.

† Antibiotic alternatives for penicillin-allergic patients.

‡ Use vancomycin if there is reason to believe *Staphylococcus epidermidis* is pathologic and not merely a contaminant.

From Haas AF, Grekin RC. Antibiotic prophylaxis in dermatologic surgery. J Am Acad Dermatol, 1995;32:155–176.

in the perineum and nasal passages of 20% to 40% of normal adults. *Streptococcus viridans* is commonly found in the oral cavity, and both enterococcus and *Escherichia coli* are found in and around the gastrointestinal and genitourinary tracts. Fortunately, enterococcus, which is difficult to treat, is not a common cause of wound infection.

The cephalosporins are a common choice for antibiotic prophylaxis because they have broad-spectrum activity, good tissue penetration, and relative safety. The first-generation cephalosporins are active against most gram-positive cocci, *E. coli, Klebsiella,* and *Proteus mirabilis* but not against enterococci, methicillin-resistant *S. aureus,* other *Proteus* subspecies, *Pseudomonas,* and *S. epidermidis.* Dicloxacillin is a semisynthetic penicillinase-resistant penicillin effective against *Staphylococcus* (although not *S. epidermidis*) and *Streptococcus.* Since neither dicloxacillin nor the cephalosporins are effective against methicillin-resistant *S. aureus, S. epidermidis,* or enterococcus, if these are of potential concern, then intravenous vancomycin should be considered. Erythromycin has been recommended as the drug of choice by the American Heart Association for penicillin-allergic patients. Although it may be a good choice for oral and upper respiratory tract procedures when *S. viridans* is of concern, for dermatologic procedures, *S. aureus* is a more likely pathogen. In general, 65% to 75% of *S. aureus* organisms are inhibited by erythromycin; however, clindamycin is 90% active and vancomycin is 100% active against *S. aureus.* Thus, these drugs appear useful for *S. aureus* prophylaxis in the penicillin-allergic patient. Vancomycin, although difficult to work with in an outpatient setting given its intravenous form, is, perhaps, unfortunately, gaining an increasing role in dermatologic surgery prophylaxis as the result of the evolution of certain drug resistances. Vancomycin is the drug of choice when *S. epidermidis* is considered a pathogen for patients who have had prosthetic cardiac valves placed for fewer than 60 days, for methicillin-resistant *S. aureus,* and for enterococcus. Enterococcus is cephalosporin and nafcillin resistant, and high-level gentamicin resistance is now being seen. It is certainly possible to use vancomycin infusions in the outpatient setting, since it is fairly easy to prepare; however, the special precautions with the use of vancomycin, such as the need for a slower infusion rate and the appropriate dose for age and renal function, should be observed.[5]

Although the fact that any antibiotic prophylaxis needs to be employed before wounding has been well established,[7,8] the duration of that prophylaxis is much less clear. The *Medical Letter on Drugs and Therapeutics* states that "a single dose of a parenteral antimicrobial given within 30 minutes of an operation usually provides adequate tissue concentrations throughout the procedure; . . . when surgery is delayed or prolonged, a second dose is advisable. Postoperative administration of prophylactic drugs is usually unnecessary and may be harmful."[9,10] Studies vary, with some investigators suggesting that a single preoperative antibiotic dose provides optimal prophylaxis and that postoperative doses yield no further benefit.[11–13] However, other investigators believe that a single preoperative dose can be followed by a second dose several hours later for prolonged procedures, for up to a 24-hour course of treatment.[4,14,15] The guidelines for the

timing and duration of antibiotic prophylaxis for prevention of wound infection as seen in Table 2–1 are based on the features of both these approaches.[5] In most cases, the use of a single preoperative dose should be adequate. The exceptions might include prolonged cases, such as a long Mohs' micrographic surgical procedure or a large wound left to heal by second intention (large curettage and electrodesiccation site or large shave biopsy site) in an area of the body where the risk of infection is considered significant. It is probably unnecessary to extend antibiotic coverage beyond 24 hours.

ENDOCARDITIS PROPHYLAXIS

The current American Heart Association guidelines for endocarditis prophylaxis often serve as the standard of care but unfortunately do not specifically address skin surgery. There is much controversy about any recommendations for endocarditis prophylaxis, acknowledged even by the American Heart Association. There have been no adequate, controlled clinical trials of antibiotic regimens to document that antibiotic therapy is effective in preventing development of endocarditis in the presence of bacteria (nor is it likely any such studies will be carried out, since they would require very large numbers of patients and there is the ethical question surrounding the control group). The precise risk of endocarditis is unknown for any specific cardiac lesion and for any traumatic procedure. In addition, it may be the case that many cases of endocarditis may not be preventable with antimicrobial prophylaxis.

Streptococci and staphylococci account for 80% to 90% of the cases of infective endocarditis, but other organisms have also been implicated. The mitral valve is most commonly involved in infective endocarditis. Prosthetic valve endocarditis is a serious complication of valve replacement surgery and is classified as "early" when onset is within 60 days of valve placement and "late" when onset is later than 60 days of valve placement. There is a difference in bacterial etiology between early and late prosthetic valve endocarditis, with *S. epidermidis* being the most common cause of early endocarditis and a higher incidence of non–group D streptococci being seen in late endocarditis (Table 2–2). Aerobic gram-negative bacilli and fungi are also important causes of prosthetic valve endocarditis, which are uncommon in native valve endocarditis. It has been suggested that the pathogenesis of late prosthetic valve endocarditis may be similar to that of native valve endocarditis.

Mitral valve prolapse is a common cardiac diagnosis, but the absolute risk of developing endocarditis if a patient has mitral valve prolapse is small. Using a risk–benefit analysis for penicillin prophylaxis in patients with mitral valve prolapse, Kaye[16] determined that penicillin prophylaxis is warranted only for patients with mitral valve prolapse with a holosystolic murmur; it is optional for late systolic murmur and contraindicated for patients with mitral valve prolapse without murmur. The American Heart Association recommends standard endocarditis antibiotic prophylaxis for patients with mitral valve prolapse and valvular regurgitation.[17–19]

TABLE 2–2. Microorganisms Responsible for Infective Endocarditis: Native vs. Prosthetic Valve

	% Native Valve		% Prosthetic Valve	
	Nonaddicts	*Addicts*	*Early*	*Late*
Streptococci	50–70	20	5–10	25–30
Enterococci	10	8	< 1	5–10
Staphylococci	25	60	45–50	30–40
S. aureus	90	99	15–20	10–12
S. epidermidis	10	1	25–30	23–28
Gram-negative bacilli	< 1	10	20	10–12
Fungi	< 1	5	10–12	5–8
Diphtheroids	< 1	2	5–10	4–5
Culture negative	5–10	10–20	5–10	5–10

From Korzeniowski O, Kaye D. Endocarditis. In: Gorbach SL, Bartlett JA, Blacklow NR, eds. Infectious Diseases. Philadelphia: WB Saunders Co., 1992:548–557.

Bacteremia is an event that must occur before development of endocarditis. It is well known that random bacteremias occur commonly, including bacteremias from toothbrushing, dental flossing, use of wooden cleansing devices, chewing paraffin, and normal mastication, as well as defecation.[20–22] In addition, in several studies about half the patients who develop endocarditis do not have a recognized predisposing cardiac lesion for which prophylaxis would be considered.[21,23–26] Patients with underlying heart disease (assuming that they can be identified in every case) may be continually at some risk of developing endocarditis, and it may not be possible to determine with certainty which one of many bacteremias, including iatrogenic ones, may be responsible for a given episode of endocarditis. Data exist on the incidence of transient bacteremia following certain iatrogenic procedures, but the incidence of bacteremia varies widely between studies. For example, although invasive dental procedures undoubtedly cause bacteremia, it appears that dentist-induced bacteremias are usually low grade in intensity and transient in duration, with blood becoming sterile in 15 to 30 minutes after cessation of the procedure.[11,22] Although one retrospective study suggested that dentist-induced bacteremias are responsible for 90% of infective endocarditis,[27] there is evidence to suggest that the correlation is much lower. Several investigators have concluded that dentist-induced bacteremias and infective endocarditis may be associated in less than 4% of cases.[23,24,28]

In addition to the unknown risk of bacteremias following procedures, there have been many studies suggesting that antibiotic prophylaxis is not very effective in preventing endocarditis. In one report, of 52 cases of endocarditis prophylaxis failure, in 12% the patients had received currently recommended American Heart Association regimens.[27] Only about two thirds of cases of endocarditis are caused by streptococci or other organisms against which the recommended prophylactic regimens are likely to be active.[26]

The incidence of infective endocarditis in a general population has not changed since the advent of antibiotic prophylaxis.[25,29] This suggests that we still do not know which patients are at risk. The majority of endocarditis occurs in patients without known risk factors, except for the population of intravenous drug abusers.[25] Also we do not know the true incidence of endocarditis occurring after various types of bacteremias, which procedures should be covered, or which antibiotic regimens are most effective. It may also be the case that antibiotic prophylaxis does not work. Despite all of the controversy, the American Heart Associ-

TABLE 2–3. American Heart Association Guidelines for Endocarditis Prophylaxis: Cardiac Conditions*

Endocarditis Prophylaxis Recommended
  Prosthetic cardiac valves, including bioprosthetic and homograft valves
  Previous bacterial endocarditis, even in the absence of heart disease
  Most congenital cardiac malformations
  Rheumatic and other acquired valvular dysfunction, even after valvular surgery
  Hypertrophic cardiomyopathy
  Mitral valve prolapse with valvular regurgitation

Endocarditis Prophylaxis Not Recommended
  Isolated secundum atrial septal defect
  Surgical repair without residua beyond 6 months of secundum atrial septal defect, ventricular septal defect, or patent ductus arteriosus
  Previous coronary artery bypass graft surgery
  Mitral valve prolapse without valvular regurgitation†
  Physiologic, functional, or innocent heart murmurs
  Previous Kawasaki disease without valvular dysfunction
  Previous rheumatic fever without valvular dysfunction
  Cardiac pacemakers and implanted defibrillators

* This table lists selected conditions but is not meant to be all inclusive.

† Individuals who have a mitral valve prolapse associated with thickening and/or redundancy of the valve leaflets may be at increased risk for bacterial endocarditis, particularly men who are 45 years of age or older.

From Schulman ST, Amren DP, Bisno AL, et al. Prevention of bacterial endocarditis: American Heart Association committee report. Circulation 1984;70:1123A–1127A.

ation has established guidelines for endocarditis prophylaxis for certain cardiac conditions (Table 2–3) and for certain dental and surgical procedures (Table 2–4).

The "risk" of various dermatologic surgical procedures for causing potential endocarditis has never been adequately documented, and it is only recently that attempts have been made to quantitate bacteremia resulting from skin surgery. It has been shown that manipulation of clinically infected skin is associated with a high incidence (>35%) of bacteremia with organisms known to cause endocarditis.[30–32] For surgery on clinically uninfected skin, the incidence of bacteremia is virtually unknown. Sabetta and Zitelli[33] studied 35 patients undergoing surgery on eroded but not clinically infected lesions and 15 patients who underwent surgery on cutaneous neoplasms with intact skin surfaces. One patient in the eroded group developed a transient bacteremia (2.5%) based on blood cultures, and the responsible organism was *S. aureus*. None of the patients with intact skin lesions developed bacteremia. The organisms most frequently colonizing eroded, cutaneous tumors were *S. aureus,* coagulase-negative staphylococci, diphtheroids, and streptococci, all organisms that are common causes of prosthetic valve endocarditis. Sabetta and Zitelli concluded that, in their small sample, the incidence of bacteremia during simple excisional surgery on eroded but not infected cutaneous neoplasms is less than 8.4% and recommended prophylactic antibiotics only for those patients with eroded cutaneous tumors and prosthetic valves. Wilson and colleagues[34] found a 2.1% incidence of bacteremia in 240 healthy patients who had random blood cultures performed (the predominant organism was *S. epidermidis*). Zack and associates[35] studied blood cultures from 21 patients undergoing scalpel excision or curettage and electrodesiccation of eroded, clinically noninfected, or intact skin lesions. All blood samples, drawn 30 minutes after start of the surgical procedure, were culture negative at 14 days. Halpern and coworkers[36] studied 45 patients undergoing Mohs' micrographic surgery, hair transplants, repairs of Mohs' defects, dermabrasion, skin grafting, cyst excision, scar revision, and wart excision. Six of the cutaneous neoplasms were ulcerated but not clinically infected. Three patients (7%) had positive blood culture samples drawn 15 minutes after initiating the procedure, and the organisms were *Propionibacterium acnes* and *Staphylococcus hominis*.

From these few, small studies it would appear that the incidence of bacteremia after surgical manipulation of intact skin must be very small and may not warrant antibiotic prophylaxis in all high-risk individuals. The question of bacteremia from eroded skin needs to be investigated further, as does bacteremia occurring after procedures involving more heavily colonized areas such as the axillae, groin, and feet. The question remains, even if transient bacteremias are found in these instances, are they "sufficient" to cause endocarditis in those "at risk"?

RECOMMENDATIONS

For the purposes of the guidelines in Tables 2–5 and 2–6,[5] "high risk" patients are those whom the American

TABLE 2–4. American Heart Association Guidelines for Endocarditis Prophylaxis: Dental or Surgical Procedures*

Endocarditis Prophylaxis Recommended

Dental procedures known to induce gingival or mucosal bleeding, including professional cleaning
Tonsillectomy and/or adenoidectomy
Surgical operations that involve intestinal or respiratory mucosa
Bronchoscopy with a rigid bronchoscope
Sclerotherapy for esophageal varices
Esophageal dilatation
Gallbladder surgery
Cytoscopy
Urethral dilatation
Urethral catheterization if urinary tract infection present
Urinary tract surgery if urinary tract infection present†
Prostatic surgery
Incision and drainage of infected tissue†
Vaginal hysterectomy
Vaginal delivery in the presence of infection†

Endocarditis Prophylaxis Not Recommended‡

Dental procedures not likely to induce gingival bleeding, such as simple adjustment of orthodontic appliances or fillings above the gum line
Injection of local intraoral anesthetic (except intraligamentary injections)
Shedding of primary teeth
Tympanostomy tube insertion
Endotracheal intubation
Bronchoscopy with a flexible bronchoscope, with or without biopsy
Cardiac catheterization
Endoscopy with or without gastrointestinal biopsy
Cesarean section
In the absence of infection, for urethral catheterization, dilatation and curettage, uncomplicated vaginal delivery, therapeutic abortion, sterilization procedures, or insertion/removal of intrauterine devices

* This table lists selected procedures and is not meant to be all inclusive.
† In addition to a prophylactic regimen for genitourinary procedures, antibiotic therapy should be directed against the most likely bacterial pathogen.
‡ In patients who have prosthetic heart valves, a previous history of endocarditis, or surgically constructed systemic-pulmonary shunts or conduits, physicians may choose to administer prophylactic antibiotics even for low-risk procedures that involve the lower respiratory, genitourinary, or gastrointestinal tract.
From Schulman ST, Amren DP, Bisno AL, et al. Prevention of bacterial endocarditis: American Heart Association committee report. Circulation 1984;70:1123A–1127A.

Heart Association also considers "high risk" (see Table 2–3). The apparent incidence of bacteremia after surgical manipulation of intact skin is very low, and for that reason there is no group of individuals "at risk" for intact skin procedures, nor should it be necessary to give routine prophylaxis to "high risk" patients undergoing manipulation of intact skin for such things as biopsies, small procedures, and simple excisions that can be closed within a short period of time. There may be certain situations in which it might be appropriate to give antibiotic prophylaxis to "high risk" patients for intact skin procedures. For instance, it would not be necessary to give a patient with a prosthetic heart valve antibiotics for punch biopsies or for small surgical procedures in noncontaminated areas that could easily be closed within a short period of time. How-

TABLE 2-5. Recommendations for Endocarditis Prophylaxis in Dermatologic Surgery

Procedure	Persons at Risk	Prophylaxis
Surgical manipulation of intact skin	None	No (see text)
Surgical manipulation of eroded, noninfected skin	American Heart Association ``high risk''	Yes
Surgical manipulation of infected/abscessed skin; presence of distant skin infection	American Heart Assocation ``high risk'' Ortho prostheses Ventriculoatrial/peritoneal shunts	Yes

ever, it would be prudent to give antibiotic prophylaxis to a patient with a prosthetic valve for large excisions that may require more than 20 minutes to close or for procedures performed on areas of the skin considered ``contaminated.'' Consideration may be given to the addition of one or two postoperative doses of antibiotics (in addition to the preoperative dose) to ``high risk'' patients having large wounds allowed to heal by second intention or undergoing Mohs' micrographic surgery that may involve several hours before the wound is closed.

Since the risk of bacteremia even in surgical manipulation of eroded skin is low, whether to use antibiotic prophylaxis in any of these instances may be left to physician discretion. This decision is based on the nature of the procedure, the risk of the antibiotics, and the consequences of either infection of the device or subsequent endocarditis. Relatively little is known about the risks of previously implanted prosthetic devices becoming infected after certain procedures that may cause transient bacteremia or even if the presence of those devices, if infected, can be caus-

ally related to endocarditis. Because patients who have orthopedic prostheses and ventriculoatrial or peritoneal shunts who undergo surgical manipulation of infected or abscessed skin or in the presence of distant skin infections may be at significant risk for morbidity after infection, antibiotic prophylaxis should be strongly considered.[5]

These guidelines for antibiotic prophylaxis for prevention of wound infection and for endocarditis prophylaxis are based on an extensive review of the surgical literature and the dermatologic literature, and on the recommendations of the American Heart Association. Since there are no standard accepted guidelines specific for skin surgery, it is necessary that any decision to employ antibiotic prophylaxis must ultimately rest on the physician and his or her assessment of the procedure, the particular patient, and the information obtained from subspecialist consultations. Moreover, as we better understand the mechanisms of endocarditis and their relationship to transient bacteremia, we can better define the risks of bacteremia after skin surgery and modify the American Heart Association's guidelines.

TABLE 2-6. Endocarditis Prophylaxis Regimen for Dermatologic Surgery

Antibiotic	1 Hour Before Surgery	6 Hours Later
Contaminated Skin (Staphylococcus aureus)		
First-generation cephalosporin	1 g PO	500 mg PO
Dicloxacillin	1 g PO	500 mg PO
Clindamycin*	300 mg PO	150 mg PO
Vancomycin (*Staphylococcus epidermidis*)†	500 mg IV	250 mg IV
Gastrointestinal/Genitourinary (Enterococcus)		
Low risk		
Amoxicillin	3 g PO	1.5 g PO
High risk		
Ampicillin	2 g plus	
Gentamicin	1.5 mg/kg IV/IM	
Amoxicillin		1.5 g PO
Or, alternatively,		
Vancomycin plus	1.0 g IV	
gentamicin	1.5 mg/kg IV/IM‡	
Oral (Streptococcus viridans)		
Amoxicillin	3 g PO	1.5 g PO
Erythromycin*	1 g PO	500 mg PO
Clindamycin*	300 mg PO	150 mg PO

* Antibiotic alternatives for penicillin-allergic patients.
† Parenteral vancomycin hydrochloride will need to be added if dealing with methicillin-resistant *S. aureus* and for patients with prosthetic cardiac valves.
‡ Can repeat dose in 8 hours.
From Haas AF, Grekin RC. Antibiotic prophylaxis in dermatologic surgery. J Am Acad Dermatol, 1995;32:155–176.

Antisepsis

Ann F. Haas

Antisepsis is the prevention of sepsis by the inhibition or destruction of the causative organism. Techniques of antisepsis are directed against potentially pathogenic microbes and include such practices as prepping the skin preoperatively with a disinfectant or preoperative handwashing with an antibacterial agent. Aseptic technique includes measures to prevent the entrance of microbes into wounds, such as using sterile gowns, gloves, masks, drapes, and instruments (Table 2–7).

The normal flora of the skin is usually divided into residents and transients. The goal of presurgical preparation of the skin is to remove the transient (pathogenic) bacteria and to decrease the resident flora to the lowest possible level. The resident flora is composed of specific bacteria that tend to be nonpathogenic and, although usually superficial, can be found in the deeper layers of skin, especially in the pilosebaceous units. The normal flora of the skin varies somewhat with body site.[37] *Staphylococcus epidermidis* constitutes more than 50% of the resident staphylococci and colonizes the upper part of the body. *Staphylococcus aureus,* which is not a common member of the resident flora, is found in the perineum of up to 20% of persons and in the nasal passages of 20% to 40% of normal adults. Transient bacteria survive on the skin surface without being able to multiply. It is the transient organisms that are usually involved in wound infections. The most important is probably group A β-hemolytic *Streptococcus.* Large studies of surgical wound infection have shown that microorganisms introduced into the wound at the time of operation are responsible for the vast majority of postoperative wound infections.[38–40] In dermatologic

surgery, exogenous sources such as the patient's nose and skin are more commonly found to be sources for clean surgical infections.[41,42] One study, using "clean technique," showed that aerobic bacterial counts of the surgical field at three separate intervals during the surgical procedure for both short and long Mohs' micrographic surgical procedures were less than 100,000 colony-forming units/cm^2.[43] This suggests that at least the microbiologic component of wound infections for this group of patients is adequately reduced by "clean technique."

PREPARATION OF THE SURGICAL FIELD

Hair Removal

If hair must be removed before the surgical procedure, it is best done by clipping rather than by shaving. Shaving traumatizes the skin surface and enhances bacterial growth.[38] Although hair can be a source of *S. aureus,* not shaving or clipping the hair results in the lowest wound infection rates.[38]

Preoperative Skin Preparation

Although it is impossible to completely sterilize the skin,[44] it is possible to remove the transient and pathogenic bacteria and to decrease the resident flora to the lowest possible level by using a mechanical scrub and an effective antiseptic agent.[45] The detergent scrub (such as a combination of water and chlorhexidine or an iodophor surgical scrub) to remove bacteria and loosen dirt is followed by an antiseptic applied just before the procedure.[45] There are many variations of skin preparation, including using a 2-second wipe with a 70% isopropyl alcohol pad and then a 10-second skin preparation with a povidone-iodine (Betadine) swab.[43] Iodophors and chlorhexidine are probably the agents of choice for sustained antimicrobial activity and the least risk of systemic toxicity.

Chlorhexidine (Hibiclens) appears to have greater advantages over the other agents in most circumstances. Chlorhexidine is effective against both gram-positive and gram-negative organisms, has a rapid onset of activity, and has sustained residual activity. Chlorhexidine produces greater immediate decreases in resident flora when compared with hexachlorophene (pHisoHex) and povidone-iodine.[46] Further decreases in transient flora have occurred with repetitive use of chlorhexidine but not povidone-iodine or hexachlorophene. The *Medical Letter on Drugs and Therapeutics,* in a review of skin antimicrobial agents,

TABLE 2–7. Potential Causes of Wound Infection

Factors Related to Surgical Technique
Meticulous surgical technique (suture and tissue technique, eliminating dead space)
Adequate hemostasis
Judgment of surgeon

Local Wound Factors
Wound classification
Wound location and vascular supply
Oxygenation
Need for use of drains

Patient Factors
Dressings and wound care
Age and overall health (malnutrition, diabetes, obesity, immunologic status)
Presence of remote infection
Drugs

stated that chlorhexidine "combines the broad spectrum antibacterial action of alcohol and the iodophors with the prolonged action of hexachlorophene."[47] Unlike hexachlorophene, chlorhexidine is not absorbed through the skin. Although chlorhexidine is safe for oral mucosa, it should be kept away from the eyes, since it can cause irritation (secondary to the detergent base) and away from the middle ear, since it can be toxic to the inner ear.

Hexachlorophene is effective against gram-positive organisms, but it is less effective against gram-negative organisms and fungi. The maximum antibacterial effect is achieved after successive days of use, so it is not ideally suited as a preoperative scrub. It can be absorbed through the skin, and percutaneous absorption has caused neurotoxicity in infants and possible teratogenicity in adults who are regularly exposed.

Iodophors (povidone-iodine, poloxamer-iodine) are effective against a wide range of bacteria and some fungal spores. They do not leave a reliable residuum on the skin surface. Skin reactions can occur in iodine-sensitive persons; and if applied to a large area of mucosa or denuded skin, the iodophors can be systemically absorbed and can cause toxicity. Iodophors can be used safely around the eyes.

Alcohol has been effectively used for years as a skin disinfectant. Two studies have confirmed that either 70% ethyl alcohol or alcohol and green soap were adequate for preoperative skin preparation.[38,48] Isopropyl alcohol has a broader range of antibacterial activity and is less volatile than ethyl alcohol. Alcohol may be more effective as an antiseptic agent when combined with other antiseptic agents.[49]

Benzalkonium chloride (Zephiran) is a quaternary ammonium that is little used today because the solution was more prone to contamination than other antiseptics. It is commercially available in single-use pledget form, which minimizes contamination. It does not irritate mucous membranes and can safely be used around the eye.

Technique of Preparing the Field

Antiseptics should be applied from the center of the operative field to the periphery, using a circular motion, and include an area sufficient to result in a completely prepped surgical field once the drapes have been placed. Antiseptics are meant to be used for disinfection of intact skin and should not be used *in* the wound. The use of antiseptics on clean or contaminated wounds has been shown to interfere with wound healing. The deleterious effects of antiseptics on clean or contaminated wounds include leukocyte toxicity,[50] increasing the intensity of inflammation,[50] and directly impairing wound contraction and re-epithelialization.[51] Surgical drapes protect the wound from contamination by nearby organisms during the surgical procedure and help prevent sutures, instruments, and other materials from being contaminated by the surrounding skin. Surgical drapes made of cloth are the easiest to apply and will stay in place better than some of the disposable drapes. When procedures are performed around the face, cloth drapes are more comfortable for the patient. If

cloth drapes are used, they should be made of a very densely woven cotton and preferably chemically treated to provide some degree of moisture barrier. Because bacteria are drawn through a wet cloth, the cloth drape (or gown) loses its property as an aseptic barrier when it becomes wet.[52] Holes (either from wear or by repetitive use of surgical towel clips) permit the passage of bacteria. Heat-sealed patches made of the same base material should be used for mending reusable fabrics, and towel clips should be used only at the very edges of the fabric.

There are now many single-use, disposable fabrics available for both surgical drapes and gowns, and they are commonly found in office-based surgical settings. Drapes are made either as single sheets or with fenestrations. They are impermeable to moisture, and some are designed with either a layer of plastic between two layers of paper or plastic under the layer of paper. These drapes often do not remain in contact with the surgical site, and because they slide, fluid can leak underneath them. Some drapes also have adhesive along the edge or around the fenestration that helps them remain in place. Plastic does not "breathe" well, and patients can find this type of drape warm, especially if used for a facial procedure.

A difference has been observed between cotton and the newer, nonwoven "disposable" fabrics in their capacity to prevent penetration by bacteria, seemingly in favor of the nonwoven fabrics.[53] The nonwoven material offered greater protection in lengthy operations.[54] A study comparing an all-cotton clothing and drape system to a polypropylene coverall and laminated gown and drape system in open-heart surgery concluded that the noncotton system significantly reduced both particle and bacterial contamination of the air and bacterial sedimentation during cardiac operations.[55] Another study, involving over 2000 clean and clean-contaminated general surgical procedures, compared infection rates between cases in which a disposable gown and drape system was used (spun-lace fabric) and cases using a 280-thread count cotton system.[56] The risk of developing a wound infection was two and one-half times higher for a cotton system than for the spun-lace fiber gown and drape system. European studies have shown similar results, with one study noting that the greatest reduction in wound infection rates with the single-use, disposable gown and drape system was seen for clean wounds.[57,58] Although there has been convincing evidence as to the effectiveness of nonwoven surgical drapes in preventing wound infections, for short procedures, such as those in dermatologic surgery, it may be reasonable to use high thread count cotton drapes that have been treated with some agent to make them relatively impermeable.

BARRIER PROTECTION OF HEALTH CARE PERSONNEL

The use of surgical masks by operating room personnel is based on the hope that the patient can be protected against microbes discharged from the mouth and upper respiratory tracts of surgical personnel. There has been some controversy over the effectiveness of face masks in protecting the patient. Face masks may simply alter the direction of the flow of bacteria out the sides of the masks, and by rubbing the skin on the face they may dislodge skin scales that are a known source of *S. aureus*.[59] One study reported that the incidence of wound infection in a hospital surgical room for a 6-month period was not altered by discontinuing the use of face masks.[60] Although the use of masks to prevent contamination of the patient is controversial, there may be indications for their use in the cases of surgical personnel with active upper respiratory tract infections to minimize shedding from the nasopharynx, and possibly if the surgeon is a known carrier of hepatitis B virus.[61] Certainly the mask does serve a protective function in terms of protecting the surgical personnel from contamination by saliva droplets or blood from the patient, and wearing of masks is recommended by the Centers for Disease Control and Protection.[62]

The purpose of surgical clothing today includes not only protection of the patient from bacteria that can be transmitted from surgical personnel but also protection of surgical personnel from infectious agents in the blood of the patient. When gowns become wet, bacteria can be drawn toward the surgeon or toward the patient; therefore, disposable gowns that are waterproof can help to protect surgical personnel from blood-borne contaminants as well as decrease the bacterial count. For dermatologic surgery, the gown is more commonly used for the protection of the surgeon and clothing during procedures in which splash, spray, or aerosol is possible (e.g., dermabrasion or incision of large cysts). Disposable paper gowns are probably the easiest to use; but if a complete moisture barrier is desired, then the waterproof disposable gown would be preferred. From investigations of both gown materials and ''strike through'' come some straightforward recommendations by Quebbeman and coworkers[63] that may be relevant for dermatologic surgery:

> For procedures where it is anticipated that there may be blood loss greater than 100 mL, where the procedure may be lengthy or where the patient is a known carrier of a blood-borne infectious agent, it might be prudent to wear a covergown of a fabric which is impenetrable to both bacteria and blood. In certain cases, it might be prudent to have a few gowns on hand with reinforcement at the upper chest and sleeves. For cases of short duration with anticipated minimal blood loss, a single layer gown of a disposable fabric might be considered.

Although plain bar soap removes the majority of contaminating organisms from the hands by mechanical means, the use of antiseptics, such as chlorhexidine or povidone-iodine, may be preferable because of the broad spectrum of de-germing activity and rapid onset of action. The bacterial count on the skin surface of the hands should be kept as low as possible, because it increases with the length of time that the occlusive, sterile gloves are on during the surgical procedure.

Studies that have compared various lengths of preoperative surgical hand scrubs with various antiseptics, with and without the use of a brush, concluded that the shorter, no-brush scrub procedure with a standard antiseptic was as effective as the longer, two-brush method.[64]

The use of gloves is to be advocated in all outpatient surgical situations because wearing gloves protects physicians and patients from possible hepatitis B virus and the human immunodeficiency virus that causes the acquired immunodeficiency syndrome.[62,65] In cases in which sterility is not absolutely necessary, one can use nonsterile examination gloves for various minor procedures.

DEVICES THAT ENTER THE SURGICAL FIELD

Electrocoagulation Equipment

There are several methods of handling electrocoagulation equipment during surgery while trying to maintain a sterile field. Depending on the type of equipment available, a sterile Bovie-type handpiece with a sterile cord can be placed into the sterile field and the plug handed off to the assistant, who is ungloved. For those with office Birtcher wall or portable units, a sterile Penrose sleeve, a sterile surgical glove, or a commercially available sterile sheath device can be slipped over the handpiece, which is then carefully placed at the edge of the sterile field. A sterile disposable tip can then be inserted through the sheath (or at the end of the Penrose sleeve) into the handpiece.

Another technique enlists the aid of an ungloved assistant. A bleeding point is grasped with a sterile hemostat or small sterile forceps. The ungloved assistant can take the electrosurgical handle and place the sterile disposable electrode in contact with the sterile metallic instrument. The power is then conducted from the electrode through the sterile instrument to the surgery site. For procedures requiring electrocautery without need to maintain a sterile field, there are nonsterile sheath protectors for handpieces (or nonsterile gloves).

There is some controversy regarding the use of reusable electrodes between patients after electrodesiccation or electrocautery. Studies have shown that both hepatitis B virus and herpes simplex virus have survived electrodesiccation in laboratory experiments.[66,67] A study by Bennett and Kraffert[68] demonstrated the ability to contaminate sterile needle electrode tips with bacteria from inoculated tissue during electrodesiccation but not during electrocoagulation, suggesting that electrocoagulation current is more bactericidal than is electrodesiccation current.[68] The amount of bacterial killing is apparently dependent on the dose of current used. Although not a universal recommendation, both to protect patients and surgeons, some clinicians have advocated changing electrosurgical instrument tips between patients to avoid the possibility of transfer of infectious agents.[68]

Dermabrasion Equipment

Sterile sheath devices can be placed over the handpiece of a hand engine for the purposes of dermabrasion or harvesting hair transplant plugs. If there is no need to maintain a sterile field, a nonsterile glove or a condom can be used as a sheath to protect the instrument from contamination.

Suction Equipment

Both sterile and nonsterile tubing is available commercially. Either commercially available presterilized plastic tips or resterilizable metal tips can be used. Alternatively, a presterilized glass medicine dropper can be added to the surgical tray and easily fits most commercially available suction tubing.

References

1. Centers for Disease Control. Guidelines for Prevention of Surgical Wound Infections, 1985. Atlanta: US Department of Health and Human Services, 1985.
2. Johnson JT, Wagner RL. Infection following uncontaminated head and neck surgery. Arch Otolaryngol Head Neck Surg 1987;113:368–369.
3. Weber RS, Callender DL. Antibiotic prophylaxis in clean-contaminated head and neck oncologic surgery. Ann Otol Rhinol Laryngol 1992;101:16–20.
4. Nichols RL. Use of prophylactic antibiotics in surgical practice. Am J Med 1981;70:686–692.
5. Haas AF, Grekin RC. Antibiotic prophylaxis in dermatologic surgery. J Am Acad Dermatol, in press.
6. Peterson LJ. Antibiotic prophylaxis against wound infections in oral and maxillofacial surgery. J Oral Maxillofac Surg 1990;48:617–620.
7. Burke JF. The effective period of preventive antibiotic action in experimental incisions and dermal lesions. Surgery 1961;50:161–168.
8. Burke JF. Preventing bacterial infection by coordinating antibiotic and host activity: A time-dependent relationship. South Med J 1977;70:24–26.
9. Antimicrobial prophylaxis for surgery. Med Lett Drugs Ther 1985;27(703):105–108.
10. Antibiotic prophylaxis in surgery. Med Lett Drugs Ther 1989;31:105–108.
11. Hirschmann JV. Controversies in antimicrobial prophylaxis. Chemotherapia 1987;6:202–207.
12. Scher KS, Wroczynski AF, Jones CW. Duration of antibiotic prophylaxis: An experimental study. Am J Surg 1986;151:209–212.
13. Nichols RS. Surgical wound infection. Am J Med 1991;91:545–645.
14. DiPiro JT, Record KE, Schanzenback KS, et al. Antibiotic prophylaxis in surgery: II. Am J Hosp Pharm 1981;38:487–494.
15. Sebben JE. Prophylactic antibiotics in cutaneous surgery. J Dermatol Surg Oncol 1985;11:901–906.
16. Kaye D. Prophylaxis for infective endocarditis: An update. Ann Intern Med 1986;104:419–423.
17. Dajani AS, Bisno AL, Chung KJ, et al. Prevention of bacterial endocarditis. JAMA 1990;264:2919–2922.
18. Schulman ST, Amren DP, Bisno AL, et al. Prevention of bacterial endocarditis. Am J Dis Child 1985;139:323–325.
19. Schulman ST, Amren DP, Bisno AL, et al. Prevention of bacterial endocarditis: American Heart Association committee report. Circulation 1984;70:1123A–1127A.
20. Pallach TJ. A critical appraisal of antibiotic prophylaxis. Int Dent J 1989;39:183–196.
21. Von Reyn CF, Levy BS, Arbeit RD, et al. Infective endocarditis: An analysis based on strict case definitions. Ann Intern Med 1981;94:505–518.
22. Everett DE, Hirschman JV. Transient bacteremia and endocarditis prophylaxis: A review. Medicine 1977;56:61–77.
23. Bayliss R, Clarke C, Oakley CM, et al. The bowel, the genitourinary tract and infective endocarditis. Br Heart J 1984;51:339–345.
24. Tzukert AA, Leviner E, Benoliel R, et al. Analysis of the American Heart Association's recommendations for the prevention of infective endocarditis. Oral Surg Oral Med Oral Pathol 1986;62:383.
25. Bayliss R, Clarke C, Oakley C, et al. The teeth and infective endocarditis. Br Heart J 1983;50:506–512.
26. Kaye D. Prophylaxis against bacterial endocarditis: A dilemma. In: Kaplan EL, Taranta AV, eds. Monograph No. 52. Dallas: American Heart Association, 1977:67–69.
27. Durack DT, Kaplan EL, Bisno AL. Apparent failures of endocarditis prophylaxis. JAMA 1983;250:2318–2322.
28. Gunteroth WG. How important are dental procedures as a case of infective endocarditis? Am J Cardiol 1984;54:797–801.
29. Tzukert AA, Leviner E, Sela M. Prevention of infective endocarditis: Not by antibiotics alone. Oral Surg Oral Med Oral Pathol 1986;62:383.
30. Richards JH. Bacteremia following irritation of foci of infection. JAMA 1932;99:1496–1497.
31. Fine BC, Sheckman PR, Bartlett JC. Incision and drainage of soft tissue abscesses and bacteremia. Ann Intern Med 1985;103:645.
32. Glenchur H, Patel BX, Pathmarajah C. Transient bacteremia associated with debridement of decubitus ulcers. Milit Med 1981;146:432–433.
33. Sabetta JB, Zitelli JA. The incidence of bacteremia during skin surgery. Arch Dermatol 1987;123:213–215.
34. Wilson WR, Van Scoy RE, Washington JA. Incidence of bacteremia in adults without infection. J Clin Microbiol 1975;2:94–95.
35. Zack L, Remlinger K, Thompson K, et al. The incidence of bacteremia after skin surgery. J Infect Dis 1989;159:148–150.
36. Halpern AC, Leyden JJ, Dzubow LM, et al. The incidence of bacteremia in skin surgery of the head and neck. J Am Acad Dermatol 1988;19:112–116.
37. Roth RR, James WD. Microbiology of the skin: Resident flora, ecology, infection. J Am Acad Dermatol 1989;20:367.
38. Cruse PJE, Foord R. The epidemiology of wound infection: A ten-year prospective study of 62,939 wounds. Surg Clin North Am 1980;60:27.
39. Ritter MA, Eitzen H, French ML, et al. The operating room environment as affected by people and the surgical face mask. Clin Orthop 1975;111:147.
40. Jepsen OB. Contamination of the wound during operation and postoperative wound infection. Ann Surg 1973;177:178.
41. Kune GA. Postoperative wound infections: A study of bacteriology and pathogenesis. Aust NZ J Surg 1983;53:245.
42. Postlethwait R. Principles of operative surgery: Antisepsis, technique, sutures and drains. In: Sabiston DC, ed. Textbook of Surgery: The Biological Basis of Modern Surgical Practice, 12th ed. Philadelphia: WB Saunders Co., 1981:317.
43. Takegami KT, Siegle RJ, Ayers LW. Microbiologic counts during outpatient office-based cutaneous surgery. J Am Acad Dermatol 1990;23:1149.
44. Dzubow LM, Halpern AC, Leyden JJ, et al. Comparison of preoperative skin preparations for the face. J Am Acad Dermatol 1988;19:737.
45. Sebben JE. Sterile technique and the prevention of wound infection in office surgery: II. J Dermatol Surg Oncol 1989;15:38.
46. Peterson AF. Comparative evaluation of surgical scrub preparations. Surg Gynecol Obstet 1978;146:63.
47. Chlorhexidine and other antiseptics. Met Lett Drugs Ther 1976;18(21):85–86.
48. Davies J, Babb JR, Ayliffe GA, et al. Disinfection of the skin of the abdomen. Br J Surg 1978;65:855.
49. Sebben JE. Sterile technique and the prevention of wound infection in the office surgery: I. J Dermatol Surg Oncol 1988;14:1364.
50. Viljanto J. Disinfection of surgical wounds without inhibition of normal healing. Arch Surg 1980;115:253.
51. Botton L, Olenlacz B, Constantine BO, et al. Repair and antibacterial effects of topical antiseptic agents in vivo. In: Maibach H, Lowe N, eds. Models in Dermatology, vol 2. Basel: Karger, 1985:145–158.
52. Beck WC, Collette TS. False faith in the surgeon's gown and drape. Am J Surg 1952;83:125.
53. Nagai I, Katoda M, Takechi M, et al. Studies on the bacterial permeability of non-woven fabrics and cotton fabrics. J Hosp Infect 1988;7:261.
54. Treggiari M, Benevento A, Caronno R, et al. The evaluation of the efficacy reducing the incidence of postoperative wound infections. Min Chir 1992;47:49.
55. Verkkala K, Makela P, Ojajarvi J, et al. Air contamination in open heart surgery with disposable coveralls, gowns, and drapes. Ann Thorac Surg 1990;50;757.
56. Moylan JA, Fitzpatrick KT, Davenport KE. Reducing wound infections. Arch Surg 1987;122:152.
57. Muller W, Jiru P, Mach R, et al. The use of disposable draping materials in the operating room and its effect on the postoperative wound infection rate. Wien Klin Wochenschr 1989;101:837.
58. Werner HP, Horlborn J, Schon K, et al. Influence of drape permeability on wound contamination during mastectomy. Eur J Surg 1991;57:379.

59. Bennett RG. Fundamentals of Cutaneous Surgery. St. Louis: CV Mosby, 1988.
60. Orr NW. Is a mask necessary in the operating theatre? Ann R Coll Surg Engl 1981;63:390.
61. Gaja AZ. Hepatitis and the dentist. Mayo Clin Proc 1983;58:550.
62. Centers for Disease Control. Acquired immune deficiency syndrome (AIDS): Precautions for clinical and laboratory staffs. MMWR 1982;31:577.
63. Quebbeman EJ, Telford GL, Hubbard S, et al. In-use evaluation of surgical gowns. Surg Gynecol Obstet 1992;174:369.
64. Galle PC, Homeslely HD, Rhyne AL. Reassessment of the surgical scrub. Surg Gynecol Obstet 1978;147(2):215–218.
65. Rimland D, Parkin WE, Miller GB, et al. Hepatitis B outbreak traced to an oral surgeon. N Engl J Med 1977;296:953.
66. Sheretz EF, Davis GL, Rice RW, et al. Transfer of hepatitis B virus by contaminated reusable needle electrodes after electrodesiccation in simulated use. J Am Acad Dermatol 1986;15:1242.
67. Colver GB, Peutherer JF. Herpes simplex virus dispersed by hyfrecator electrodes. Br J Dermatol 1987;117:627–629.
68. Bennett RG, Kraffert CA. Bacterial transference during electrodesiccation and electrocoagulation. Arch Dermatol 1990;126:751–755.

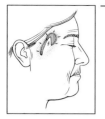

chapter 3

Anesthesia

JESSICA L. FEWKES

Anesthesia is a necessary first step in any surgical procedure. Whether it is done by hypnosis, cryogenics, injectable lipids, or acupuncture, each surgeon must have a method that ensures patient comfort throughout a proposed procedure. Otherwise, both surgeon and patient will be tense and surgery becomes an unnecessarily unpleasant experience. The patient then takes that negative attitude to each future surgical encounter and may transfer it to the relationship with the surgeon.

Local anesthesia, the reversible loss of sensation in a relatively small or circumscribed area of the body, can be achieved by topical application or injection of agents. Regional anesthesia involves either large areas of subcutaneous tissue or larger peripheral nerves.

TOPICAL ANESTHETICS

The variety of topical agents that have been used to blunt the sting of injection include 2% to 20% topical lidocaine preparation as jellies or sprays on open wounds or on mucous membranes; sprays of freon, ethyl chloride, or liquid nitrogen as short-acting agents; ice; and iontophoresis of lidocaine.

A short spray of liquid nitrogen has been used to quickly anesthetize the skin to allow introduction of a needle and infiltration of a very small area. However, sometimes the spray scares patients, it is slightly uncomfortable, and it can be used for only a limited area.

A topical anesthetic that has been in use in Sweden for almost 10 years is EMLA (eutectic mixture of local anesthetics). It is a combination of lidocaine and prilocaine each at a 25-mg/mL concentration. Its specific compounding as an oil-in-water emulsion increases the absorption of the actual drug over previous topical formulations. The success of this cream in Europe in reducing the pain of

venipuncture in children has led it to be used as a standard preparation for such procedures.

EMLA, which comes as a cream, is applied in a thick layer to the proposed surgical site and covered with a tightly occlusive dressing such as plastic wrap. The patient may apply EMLA and the dressing before coming to the office. The thinness of the skin determines the length of time of the application. Thin skin needs less time to achieve anesthesia. If anesthesia on the face is required, about 1 hour is sufficient; but anesthesia of areas of the trunk and extremities requires 2 hours and anesthesia of mucous membranes takes 15 minutes. Palms and soles show either little or no response to EMLA.

After the dressing is removed and the cream is wiped off with alcohol, the majority of patients will have significant blanching from vasoconstriction of the application area. The duration and depth of anesthesia are highly variable but may range from 15 minutes to 2 hours.

EMLA has provided effective local anesthesia for curettage, dermabrasion, epilation, injection, laser surgery for vascular and pigmented lesions and tattoos, mucosal anesthesia, shave excision, split-thickness skin graft donor sites, and ulcer debridement. The current recommendation for its use from the manufacturer is to apply 2.5 g over 25 cm² of skin for minor procedures and 2.0 g per 10 cm² for more painful ones. It is available in a 5-g tube that is marketed with two occlusive dressings. Metabolites of prilocaine form methemoglobin, which can be a problem in infants; thus, EMLA should not be used on infants younger than 3 months old.

Lidocaine comes in a topical form (as a 2% or 5% jelly or ointment). It is very useful on mucosal surfaces, and is relatively ineffective on intact skin. Other mucosal surface drugs are tetracaine or proparacaine for the eyes. These anesthetics are ester linked and are therefore contraindicated in patients with allergies to topical anesthetics, hair dyes, p-aminobenzoic acid, and sulfonamides.

INJECTABLE ANESTHETICS

Injectable anesthetics are used for local anesthesia, which is defined as the blockage of nerve conduction in a circumscribed area. The goal of local anesthesia is the elimination of pain caused by the surgery. Pain is mainly carried by small C and larger A delta nerve fibers, which are the most sensitive to local anesthetic infiltration. Other fibers, which carry temperature, touch, and pressure sensations, will be variably blocked. Because not all nerve fiber conduction is totally blocked, it is helpful to inform the patient that he or she may feel pressure or pulling during the procedure even though the area is completely anesthetized. In this way, the patient will not become anxious if he or she continues to have some sensations other than pain during the procedure.

The ideal anesthetic should have the characteristics listed in Table 3–1. Many different ones have been used throughout history, but the introduction of cocaine in 1884 began the modern era of local anesthesia. The group used most widely today are compounds related to cocaine. They fall into two categories: esters or amides (Table 3–2).

The addition of epinephrine is fairly routine in many solutions to counteract the vasodilatory effect of the anesthetic. Epinephrine also provides hemostasis at the site of surgery and prolongs the duration of the anesthetic at the site. The very long-acting anesthetics are often marketed without epinephrine because it adds little to their duration. In general, epinephrine use is contraindicated on the penis or digits. Some of the relative contraindications are listed in Table 3–3.

The adverse effects of these anesthetics are shown in Table 3–4. These are usually dose related. The recommended dosages for lidocaine with and without epinephrine are shown in Table 3–5. Lidocaine may be used for local excisions during pregnancy. During lactation, even though lidocaine is excreted in small amounts, there are no safety concerns for the infant.

If the patient states he or she has an allergy to the anesthetic and it is not to the ester group, which has a higher incidence of allergic reaction (i.e., sensitivity to p-aminobenzoic acid or sulfur derivatives or pseudocholinesterase deficiency), the epinephrine, or the additives (such as methylparabens), then alternative injectable agents that can be used are promethazine (Phenergan), diphenhydramine (Benadryl), and normal saline.

TABLE 3-1. Characteristics of an Ideal Injectable Anesthetic

Nonirritating
Nonallergenic
No permanent nerve damage
Low systemic toxicity
Short onset
Long duration

TABLE 3-2. Some Commonly Used Local Anesthetics

Esters
Cocaine
Procaine
Tetracaine
Chloroprocaine
Amides
Lidocaine
Mepivacaine
Bupivacaine
Etidocaine
Prilocaine

TABLE 3-3. Contraindications to the Use of Epinephrine in Injectable Anesthetic Solutions

Medications
Monoamine oxidase inhibitors
Tricyclic antidepressants
Phenothiazines
Propranolol
Some antihypertensive agents
Amphetamines
Digitalis
Medical States
Peripheral vascular disease
Acute angle glaucoma
Hyperthyroidism
Unstable mental status
Pregnancy
Severe hypertension or cardiovascular disease

TABLE 3-4. Adverse Effects of Injectable Anesthetics

Central Nervous System
Light-headedness
Tinnitus
Perioral tingling
Metallic taste
Tremors
Slurred speech
Seizures
Cardiovascular
Myocardial depression

TABLE 3-5. Recommended Maximum Dosage of Lidocaine in 70-kg Adult

With epinephrine: 7.0 mg/kg (500 mg total)
Without epinephrine: 4.5 mg/kg (300 mg total)

TABLE 3–6. Characteristics of Commonly Used Local Anesthetics Without Epinephrine

Agent	Onset	Duration
Procaine	Fast	Short
Tetracaine	Slow	Very long
Lidocaine	Fast	Long
Mepivacaine	Fast	Long
Bupivacaine	Slow	Very long
Etidocaine	Fast	Very long

TECHNIQUE

The anesthetic is chosen that best fits the procedure planned (long and short duration, local infiltration, or nerve block) (Table 3–6). It is drawn up into a syringe that will contain enough anesthetic to numb the entire area in question (Table 3–7). Any large-bore needle can be used to make this step proceed quickly. The smaller 30-gauge needle is then attached to the syringe. This very slender needle causes less pain on injection. The length of the needle used is relative to the size of the area to be injected. The larger the area, the longer the needle. As with any invasive procedures, gloves must be worn and universal precaution guidelines should be followed.

Many techniques have been suggested for decreasing the pain of injection. Buffered solutions (Table 3–8) of anesthetics, freshly mixed solutions, warming the solution, and using a topical anesthetic first (e.g., liquid nitrogen or EMLA) have all been described and work well. Nothing seems to be more effective, however, than the following:

1. Preparing the patient for the injection.
2. Talking to the patient during infiltration of the anesthetic.
3. Pinching the skin at the site or elsewhere during injection.
4. Injecting the anesthetic into the deep dermis.
5. *Very slowly* infiltrating the skin with the anesthetic.

The needle should be placed at one end of the lesion to be treated. It is not necessary to insert the needle at different sites throughout the entire area to be anesthetized. The anesthetic will diffuse. Therefore, only one or two punctures are necessary unless the lesion is very large (Fig. 3–1). If it is necessary to reintroduce the needle, it should be done within the area that is already numb.

The ideal placement of the tip of the needle is in the dermis. Then the infiltration will lead to a gentle elevation

TABLE 3–7. Equipment Needed for Injection of Anesthetic Agents

Alcohol wipes
Luer-Lok syringes (1, 3, 5 mL)
30-gauge needles ($\frac{1}{2}$ and 1 inch)
22-gauge needles

TABLE 3–8. Buffered Lidocaine

Sodium bicarbonate (8.4% solution): 1 part
Lidocaine with epinephrine: 9 parts

of the whole area. If needle placement is too superficial, an accentuation of all the follicles is seen and a more painful injection results (Fig. 3–2). If needle placement is too deep, no elevation occurs in the tissue, a risk is run of injecting anesthetic directly into a vessel and creating higher systemic doses with their associated toxicity, and the anesthetic effect wears away much more rapidly.

VARIATIONS ON LOCAL INFILTRATION

A ring or field block infiltrates the area around a surgical site usually so as not to distort it. The area ringed might be the lesion itself. An example would be infiltrating around a cyst that was to be excised or an anatomic location better served with a ring block. Examples of field blocks are the nose, the digits, the penis, and the ear (Figs. 3–3 through 3–6). However, depending on the distance from the lesion that the anesthetic is placed, there will be no hemostasis at the surgical site from the epinephrine. This should be taken into consideration when this method is chosen. A longer 1-inch needle is usually chosen for blocks.

Nerve block is used to block the nerve before it reaches the operative site. Less anesthetic is used, and yet a greater area is anesthetized. This anesthetic is placed at a deeper level (i.e., subcutaneous) than the field block. Because of this, the anesthetic may diffuse more rapidly, shortening its duration at the site and taking longer to achieve anesthesia.

Detailed knowledge of anatomy is a prerequisite to performing nerve blocks. Once the nerve trunk has been lo-

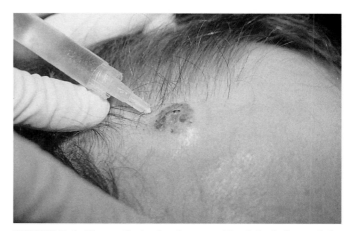

FIGURE 3–1. The needle is placed at one side of the lesion, and the anesthetic is slowly infiltrated into the deep dermis and allowed to diffuse. Without removing the needle, it is slowly advanced while injecting the anesthetic to the other side of the lesion. The entire lesion is elevated as the anesthetic is correctly placed in the dermis.

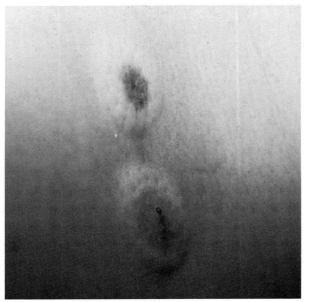

FIGURE 3–2. The peau d'orange look occurs when the anesthetic is placed very high in the dermis. The distention of the skin causes added discomfort to the patient.

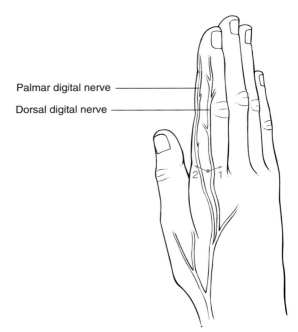

FIGURE 3–4. Digital ring block. The needle is placed midway between the dorsal and palmar surfaces. It is advanced first dorsally and then withdrawn but not pulled out and then advanced toward the palm. This is then repeated on the opposite side. Care must be taken not to inject too much volume of anesthetic and constrict blood flow into the digit.

calized, care must be taken to (1) avoid nicking the nerve, which may cause permanent loss of sensation; (2) not inject into a foramen, thereby compressing the nerve; (3) not inject into a vessel, thus increasing the toxicity of the anesthetic agent; and (4) avoid eliciting paresthesia.

Sensory innervation to the face is demonstrated in Figure 3–7. To locate the three major nerves for the midface, draw a line from the midline of the pupil vertically up to the forehead and down to the chin. This line should cross the supraorbital foramen, the infraorbital foramen, and the mental foramen. By depositing, subcutaneously, 1 to 2 mL of a long-acting anesthetic without epinephrine *near* the foramen, anesthesia should be achieved.

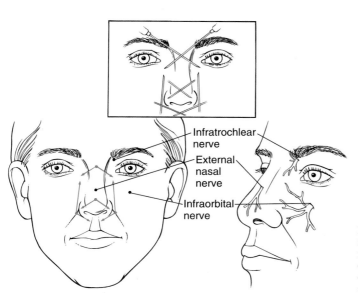

FIGURE 3–3. Field block of nose. The sites of needle insertion and the line of infiltration of anesthesia *(red)* are shown in relation to the sensory nerves of the nose.

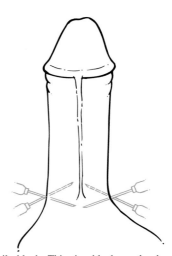

FIGURE 3–5. Penile block. This ring block can be done with only two injection sites. It is advisable to use plain lidocaine to reduce the risk of necrosis. Similarly, the total volume of injected anesthesia should not exceed 10 mL. Excessive anesthetic placed around the base of the penis can constrict the blood supply and result in necrosis. Hemorrhage into the shaft of the penis can be avoided by the use of a 30-gauge needle. When anesthesia of the prepuce is necessary, a penile block is preferable because injection of large amounts of anesthesia into the prepuce can result in sloughing.

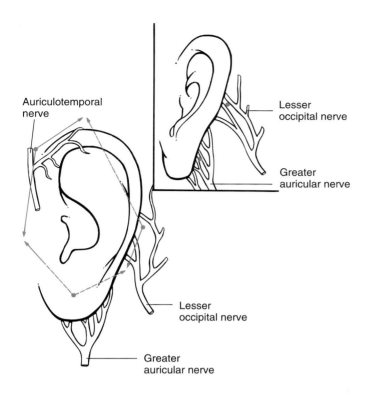

Auriculotemporal nerve

Lesser occipital nerve

Greater auricular nerve

Lesser occipital nerve

Greater auricular nerve

FIGURE 3–6. Ear block. This field block will not numb the concha and the ear canal. The red circles are the sites of needle placement, and a suggested trajectory for the needle *(red arrows)* is shown for placing the anesthetic in relation to the major nerves that innervate the ear. The red lines are broken to indicate that the injection is behind the ear.

Other useful nerve blocks are done for the foot (Figs. 3–8 and 3–9).

Ankle blocks can be used for many types of foot surgery. It is not always necessary to block all five nerves. Depending on the operative site, it may be necessary to block only the sural nerve (see Fig. 3–8). If deep structures are involved, then the tibial nerve (see Fig. 3–8) and the deep peroneal nerves (see Fig. 3–9) are blocked beneath the fascia.

At the ankle the tibial nerve runs deep to the posterior tibial artery and medial to the Achilles tendon (see Fig. 3–8A). After palpating the artery below the malleolus, insert the needle behind it and penetrate the deep fascia until contact with the bone is felt. Inject 3 to 5 mL of local anesthetic. The tibial nerve supplies the deep structures of the foot and most of the skin of the sole of the foot and plantar surfaces on the toes (see Fig. 3–8B). Terminal branches also supply the dorsal surfaces of the distal parts of the toes, including the toenails.

Also approached from the posterior position, the sural nerve is in the superficial fascia and may be blocked by subcutaneous infiltration between the lateral malleolus and the Achilles tendon (see Fig. 3–8A). The sural nerve supplies the lateral border of the foot and the small toe (see Fig. 3–8B).

Anterior ankle blocks of the superficial peroneal nerve and the deep peroneal nerve are also performed at two different depths. The superficial peroneal nerve (see Fig. 3–9A) is blocked by a ring of subcutaneous infiltration of 5 mL of anesthesia at the level of the lateral malleolus. It supplies the skin of the dorsum of the foot (see Fig. 3–9B). The deep peroneal nerve (see Fig. 3–9A) runs with the artery that becomes the dorsalis pedis artery and is

under the extensor retinaculum. The needle is inserted closer to the artery than the tendon and penetrates the fascia to contact the bone. It supplies the deep structures and a small area between the great and second toes (see Fig. 3–9B).

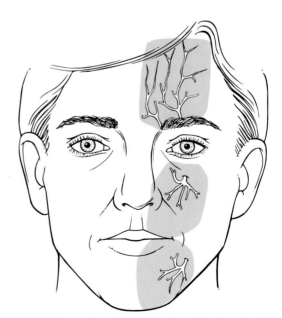

FIGURE 3–7. Sensory innervation of the face. The foramina of the three major nerves of the midface (supraorbital, infraorbital, and mental) are in a line that extends vertically from the pupil up to the forehead and down to the chin. This line is approximately 2.5 cm lateral to the midline. The nerves and their corresponding areas of innervation are shown in red.

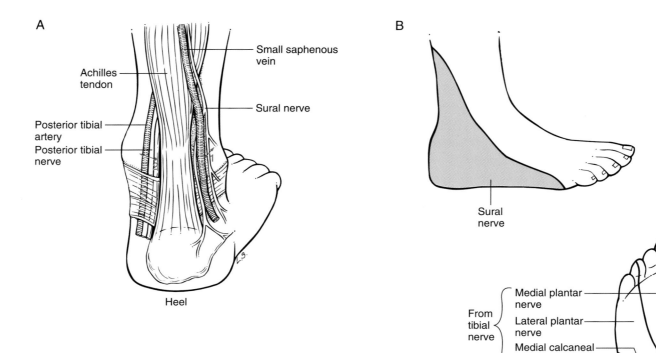

A

Achilles tendon

Posterior tibial artery

Posterior tibial nerve

Small saphenous vein

Sural nerve

Heel

B

Sural nerve

From tibial nerve

Medial plantar nerve

Lateral plantar nerve

Medial calcaneal branch

Sural nerve

FIGURE 3–8. Posterior ankle block is performed with the patient prone. *A,* Injection point 1, between the Achilles tendon and the lateral malleolus, blocks the sural nerve. Injection point 2 is just posterior and lateral to the palpable posterior tibial artery at the level of the medial malleolus and blocks the tibial nerve. *B,* The surface area of the foot anesthetized by a posterior ankle block of the sural nerve *(red).* The rest of the sole of the foot is supplied by the tibial nerve.

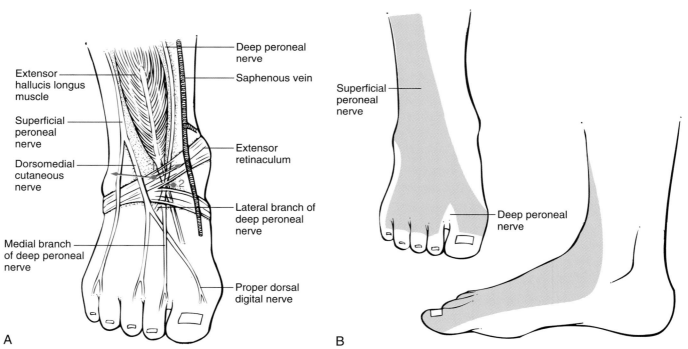

A

Extensor hallucis longus muscle

Superficial peroneal nerve

Dorsomedial cutaneous nerve

Medial branch of deep peroneal nerve

Deep peroneal nerve

Saphenous vein

Extensor retinaculum

Lateral branch of deep peroneal nerve

Proper dorsal digital nerve

B

Superficial peroneal nerve

Deep peroneal nerve

FIGURE 3–9. Anterior ankle block. *A,* Injection point 1 is just lateral to the extensor hallucis longus at the upper extent of the lateral malleolus. This will anesthetize the dorsum of the foot with the exception of the first web space. With injection at point 2 the deep peroneal nerve supplying the first web space is also anesthetized. *B,* Surface area of foot anesthetized by an anterior ankle block of the superficial peroneal nerve and deep peroneal nerve.

Because of the small size of these nerves that are being blocked, intraneural injection can cause damage even with small volumes of anesthesia. If paresthesias occur on placement of the needle, the needle should be withdrawn and re-sited before making an injection. If arterial puncture occurs, a hematoma may form and reduce peripheral blood flow. Care in performing nerve blocks is recommended for patients with peripheral vascular disease.

Suggested Readings

1. Arndt KA, Burton C, Noe JM. Minimizing the pain of local anesthesia. Plast Reconstr Surg 1983;72:676.
2. Auletta MJ, Grekin RC. Local Anesthesia for Dermatologic Surgery. New York: Churchill Livingstone, 1991.
3. Bennett RG. Anesthesia. In: Bennett RG. Fundamentals of Cutaneous Surgery. St. Louis: CV Mosby, 1988;194–239.
4. Bezzant JL, Stephen RI, Petelenz TJ, et al. Painless cauterization of spider veins with the use of iontophoretic local anesthesia. J Am Acad Dermatol 1988;19:869–875.
5. Chandler MS, Grammer LC, Patterson R. Provocative challenge with local anesthesia in patients with a prior history of reaction. J Allergy Clin Immunol 1987;79:883.
6. Cohen SJ, Roenigk RK. Nerve blocks for cutaneous surgery on the foot. J Dermatol Surg Oncol 1991;17:527–534.
7. Cooper CM, Gerrish SP, Hardyick M, Kay R. EMLA cream reduces the pain of venipuncture in children. Eur J Anaesth 1987;4:3–12.
8. deJong RH, Heavner JE. Diazepam prevents local anesthetic seizures. Anesthesiology 1971;34:523.
9. deWaard-vander Spek FB, Oranje AP, Lilliaborg S, et al. Treatment of molluscum contagiosum using a lidocaine/prilocaine cream (EMLA) for analgesia. J Am Acad Dermatol 1990;23:685–688.
10. Fisher DA. Local anesthesia in dermatologic surgery (letter). J Am Acad Dermatol 1990;22:139–141.
11. Foster CA, Aston SJ. Propranolol–epinephrine interaction: A potential disaster. Plast Reconstr Surg 1983;72:74–78.
12. Hallen B, Carlsson P, Uppfeldt A. Clinical study of a lidocaine/prilocaine cream to relieve the pain of venipuncture. Br J Anaesth 1985;57:326–328.
13. Lippman M, Rumley W. Medical emergencies. In: Dunagan WC, Ridner ML, eds. Manual of Medical Therapeutics. Boston: Little, Brown & Co, 1989:484–489.
14. Lycka BAS. EMLA: A new and effective topical anesthetic. J Dermatol Surg Oncol 1992;18:859–862.
15. Reynolds F. Adverse effects of local anesthetics. Br J Anaesth 1987;59:78–95.
16. Ritchie JM, Greene NM. Local anesthetics. In: Gilman AG, Goodman LS, Rall TW, Murad F, eds. Goodman and Gilman's The Pharmaceutical Basis of Therapeutics, 7th ed. New York: Macmillan, 1985:302–321.
17. Stewart JH, Cole GW, Klein JA. Neutralized lidocaine with epinephrine for local anesthesia. J Dermatol Surg Oncol 1988;14:41–54.
18. Van der Burght M, et al. Duration of analgesia following application of eutectic mixture of local anaesthetics (EMLA) on genital mucosa. Acta Derm Venereol 1993;73:456–458.
19. Winton GB. Anesthesia for dermatologic surgery. J Dermatol Surg Oncol 1988;14:41–54.

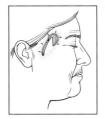

chapter 4

Biopsy Techniques

JUNE K. ROBINSON and PHILIP E. LeBOIT

SELECTION OF BIOPSY SITE AND TYPE OF BIOPSY

Biopsies are performed to establish a diagnosis, to remove a neoplasm and check its margins to ensure complete excision, and to assess the effectiveness of a therapeutic procedure on a previously diagnosed condition. The biopsy procedure results in a specimen, the histopathologic examination of which can aid the clinician. Even among trained dermatologists, clinical accuracy is not always sufficient,[1] and support for a clinical diagnosis from histopathologic examination of tissue is frequently necessary. The manner in which the biopsy is performed depends on the anticipated depth of the disease process and the potential consequences of placement of a scar from the biopsy procedure.

The area that is most representative of the disease process and is uncomplicated by changes unique to the anatomic region should be selected.[2] For instance, when a drug eruption is suspected and areas of the trunk and extremities are involved, the biopsy specimen should be taken from a fully developed lesion on the trunk rather than from a similar lesion on the lower leg. In general, biopsy specimens of the lower leg, even in young persons, show stasis vascular changes that complicate the interpretation of the histologic presentation and heal very slowly. Similarly, obtaining a biopsy sample from the palm and sole should be avoided whenever possible. For a generalized eruption, the trunk, arm, and upper leg are the more favorable biopsy sites. The elbows and knees are subjected to pressure and friction in everyday life, and sampling from these areas should be avoided.

Once having decided that a biopsy is necessary, the physician must choose among various modalities: punch biopsy, shave or saucerization biopsy, scissors removal, and elliptical excisional or incisional biopsy. In time, physicians develop individual preferences for the type of biopsy based on their skills and the suspected disease process. A superficial disease process such as a seborrheic keratosis, solar keratosis, or a wart, in which the pathologic changes are largely limited to the epidermis, is easily sampled by the shave technique with an acceptable cosmetic result. A deep-seated lesion such as eosinophilic fasciitis or a sampling of skin and muscle together, as is performed to evaluate patients in whom dermatomyositis is suspected, is best approached by an incisional technique with a scalpel, using sterile technique and a three-layer closure of muscle, fascia, and subcutaneous tissue.[3] Eruptions with actively progressing borders usually assume a circular or circinate shape. A fusiform incisional biopsy bridging the area from normal skin, crossing the active border, and including the central portion is best. Similarly, in skin lesions characterized by atrophy or sclerosis, an elliptical incisional biopsy is most desirable. This should bridge the area of normal and diseased skin and be of sufficient depth to include the entire thickness of the dermis and most of the subcutaneous fat. It is of particular importance not to bevel the edges of the biopsy specimen inward when trying to demonstrate the atrophic dermis of atrophoderma of Passini and Pierini. Each of the principal biopsy techniques and its particular advantages and disadvantages are presented in Table 4–1.[4–12]

Whenever possible the biopsy specimen should include subcutaneous fat because in many dermatoses, characteristic histologic features are found in the lower dermis or subcutaneous fat. Punch biopsies that are 3 or 4 mm in diameter are the usual procedure for obtaining specimens for histopathologic examination. Since it may not be possible to obtain adequate amounts of subcutaneous tissue by punch biopsy, elliptical incisional biopsies are often advisable for the study of subcutaneous lesions or panniculitis. In patients with panniculitis who would be likely to have problems with wound healing, the skin can be pinched between the thumb and forefinger before insertion of the punch, resulting in a larger sampling of the subcutis,[13] but the preferred biopsy technique is elliptical incision.

In the case of pigmented lesions that are clinically suspected of being malignant and of fungating or nodular processes, an incisional biopsy that extends beneath the deepest part of the lesion and includes as much of the lesion as possible should be performed. This is especially important in the evaluation of cutaneous lymphoid infiltrates, in which the density of involvement of the dermis and subcutis (i.e., "top heavy" vs. "bottom heavy") can be important.

TABLE 4-1. Selected Examples of Diseases Correlated with Type of Biopsy Most Likely to Assist in Diagnosis

Disease	Punch	Shave	Excision by Saucerization	Excision or Incision with Ellipse
Pigmented lesion suggestive of malignancy[4,5]	Yes as a sampling technique	No	Yes	Yes
Fungating or nodular process	No	No	Yes	Yes
Basal cell carcinoma	Yes	Yes	Yes	Yes
Keratoacanthoma, squamous cell carcinoma	No	No	Yes	Yes
Wart	No	Yes	No	No
Seborrheic or solar keratosis[6]	Yes if need to rule out malignancy	Yes	No	No
Inflammatory processes[7]	Yes	No	Yes	Yes
Panniculitis, scleroderma, morphea, atrophic diseases, erythema nodosum	No	No	No	Yes
Alopecia areata[8]	Yes, transversely sectioned	No	No	No
Blistering disorders	Yes	No	No	No
Hypertrophic lichen planus	No	No	Yes	Yes
Oral lesions[9-12] Persistent ulcerations Leukoplakia Vesicular lesions Pigmented lesions	Yes	No	No	Nodular lesions Leukoplakia Pigmented lesions

Punch Biopsy

Depending on the size of lesion involved and the instrument used, the punch biopsy may be either incisional, resulting in partial removal of the lesion together with a section of normal skin, or excisional, resulting in removal of the entire lesion. Punch biopsy is performed with a circular cutting instrument or punch, which is commonly available in sizes ranging from 1.5 mm to 6 mm. The sizes most frequently used are 3 and 4 mm. Although the disposable punch is lightweight and may not feel evenly balanced in the hand of the physician, it is sharp every time, and because it is disposable it eliminates the work of cleaning the instruments and the possible infection of health care workers.

The biopsy site is cleansed gently with alcohol, leaving scales and vesicles intact. If the demarcation of a lesion is subtle, such as is the case with urticaria, the boundaries of a lesion can be outlined with a pen before anesthetic is injected. The site is injected with a local anesthetic by raising a skin wheal with 0.2 to 0.5 mL of anesthetic injected into the deep dermis. When the circular incision with the punch has been carried to the subcutaneous fat, the punch is removed. Shallow punch biopsy specimens are easily misinterpreted, require more manipulation to extract, and do not give the patient the complete benefit of the procedure. At this stage, there may be considerable oozing of blood. An assistant should apply firm pressure around the perimeter of the defect so that adequate visualization of the base can be obtained. The small cylinder of tissue is gently lifted, and the base is transected at the level of the subcutaneous tissue with a small scissors, such as an iris

scissors. When the punch is removed, an oval defect is left (Fig. 4-1).

Hemostasis can be obtained by applying direct pressure with a chemical agent such as Monsel's solution (ferric subsulfate solution), or aluminum chloride 25% in isopropyl alcohol 50%, for 5 to 10 minutes. Also a Gelform pledget may be placed into the base of the wound and pressure applied. If a suture is to be used to oppose the edges, no chemical hemostatic agent is placed in the wound. Proper suture placement will usually stop the bleeding. If an artery is transected by the punch, the two ends will retract under the edges of the wound. This makes it difficult to gain enough exposure through a 3-mm circular defect to be able to place two clamps on the severed artery. When a lesion is located on the face over arteries that may be superficial enough to be injured by a punch biopsy (e.g., temporal artery lateral to the eyebrow, the angular artery at nasolabial fold junction with the ala, and the supraorbital artery at the medial end of the brow), another type of biopsy should be planned.

One of the disadvantages of the punch biopsy is that the small size of the specimen may lead to difficulty in histopathologic interpretation. Sampling error can be minimized by care in deciding which portion of a lesion to biopsy (Table 4-2). When a fresh blister is to be sampled, a topical refrigerant such as ethyl chloride spray can be used to freeze the blister in place while the punch biopsy is done. This eliminates the shearing effect of the punch, which may cause loss of the blister roof. If there is an attempt to obtain more tissue, it should be done by using a larger punch to perform the biopsy rather than by ringing the lesion with multiple smaller biopsy sites. This creates

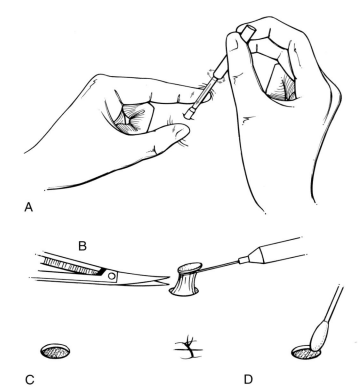

FIGURE 4–1. Punch biopsy. *A,* After the area to be biopsied is anesthetized, the skin around the area infiltrated with anesthesia and is drawn taut with the thumb and forefinger of the physician's free hand. *B,* The orifice of the punch is applied firmly to the skin surface with the handle held perpendicular to the skin. A gentle, but firm, downward pressure is exerted at the same time that the handle is rotated between the thumb and forefinger. This motion will carry the punch through the subcutaneous fat.

Care is required in removing the specimen made with a punch. If a toothed forceps is used, there is a tendency to crush the tissue as it is being lifted from its bed. This produces an artifact that may interfere with the pathologist's ability to make an accurate diagnosis. This artifact may be avoided by a simple maneuver. Downward pressure on the skin around the cylinder will cause it to pop up. The cylinder can then be lifted with the tip of the needle that was used to administer the anesthesia. *C,* The direction of tension should be along the line of elective incision. This force will cause the eventual defect to be oval rather than round. *D,* The incision can be closed with a single suture, resulting in a closure as close to a linear one as possible; or a hemostatic agent is applied with a cotton swab and the area heals by second intention.

an unsightly ring or target appearance when the biopsy sites heal. In inflammatory conditions, the 4-mm punch is generally preferable. Removal of a specimen smaller than 4 mm in diameter may allow histologic confirmation of a tumor but is often inadequate for diagnosis of inflammatory processes.

The punch biopsy is usually inadequate to diagnose diseases of adipose tissue (e.g., morphea, panniculitis, erythema nodosum). When the primary pathologic process is in the panniculus, the punch biopsy fails to yield sufficient quantity of fat for histopathologic diagnosis. In these instances, an incisional elliptical biopsy is more likely to yield a sufficient quantity of tissue for diagnosis. Similarly, in pigmented lesions suspected of being a melanoma, an elliptical biopsy that encompasses the entire lesion with a border of 1 to 2 mm and is carried through the fat is preferable.[4] The rim of nonpigmented skin enables the histopathologist to determine whether a lesion is well or poorly circumscribed. Often, the most peripheral cells of melanocytic neoplasms are amelanotic and may be transected if the biopsy incision is flush with the clinically perceived border of the lesion. Smaller pigmented lesions may be encompassed by a 3- to 6-mm punch biopsy; however, if the lateral extent of the lesion cannot be obtained within this size, then the elliptical excision should be performed. Another indication for elliptical excision rather than the punch biopsy technique is with very thickened, hypertrophic skin such as hypertrophic lichen planus or blastomycosis. In dermatologic conditions with thickening of the horny layer or anatomic locations with a thick horny layer such as the callused sole of the foot, punch

biopsy may not be sufficient to get deep enough into the dermis and adipose tissue to see the site of the primary pathology (see Table 4–1).

TABLE 4–2. Selection of Biopsy Sites for Direct Immunofluorescent Microscopy

Disease	Biopsy Site
Bullous pemphigoid and pemphigus	Multiple 3-mm perilesional biopsy in erythematous areas of early pinpoint vesicles.
Dermatitis herpetiformis	3-mm perilesional biopsy and 3-mm biopsy of normal skin. If only one biopsy specimen is obtainable, normal skin is preferred.
Discoid lupus erythematosus	3-mm biopsy of an erythematous area of the lesion
Systemic lupus erythematosus	3-mm biopsy of an erythematous area of the lesion and 3-mm biopsy of normal, sun-exposed forearm skin, when biopsy specimen is needed for diagnosis. In selected patients, 3-mm biopsy specimen of normal (light-protected) buttock skin can be useful for prognosis.

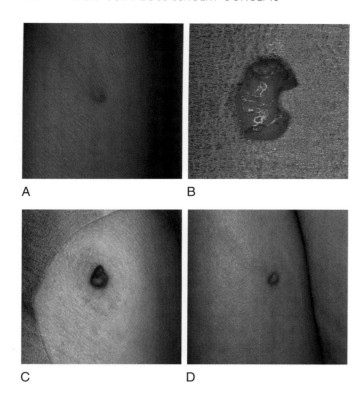

A   B

C   D

CASE 1

FIGURE 4–2. *A,* A 6-mm, firm, slightly tender lesion of the forearm is removed with a 6-mm punch biopsy carried through to fat depth. Before the anesthetic is injected, the biopsy site is marked with gentian violet. *B,* The specimen obtained with the punch biopsy is a core of tissue. There is a slight taper from the epidermis *(top)* to the dermis. *C,* The bleeding is stopped with electrocautery, and the defect heals by second intention. At the superior margin of the biopsy site, gentian violet remains on the skin surface. Blood stains the surrounding skin. *D,* One year after punch biopsy of the dermatofibroma the biopsy site remains hyperpigmented. The size of the scar could have been made smaller if a suture had been placed.

A round cosmetic defect may result from using a large (5- or 6-mm) punch (Case 1, Fig. 4–2). This cosmetic result usually cannot compare with that of an elliptical excision. In some cases the removal for cosmetic reasons of a 2- or 3-mm circular lesion by the punch technique with suture closure of the wound yields a result as good as that with elliptical excision and is much faster to perform. When closing defects created by the 4-mm punch and ones larger in size, dog-ears commonly result and may be revised at the time of the procedure.

Shave Biopsy and Saucerization Biopsy

The difference between a shave biopsy (Fig. 4–3) and a saucerization biopsy (Fig. 4–4) is the depth achieved in excising the specimen. Shave biopsy removes the portion of the skin elevated above the plane of surrounding tissue either because of the exophytic nature of the process, the manner of injection of local anesthetic, or the manner of stabilizing the skin by pinching it between the thumb and forefinger (Case 2, Fig. 4–5). Saucerization biopsy excises below the surface of the surrounding skin (in a circular manner around the lesion) down into the level of the subcutaneous fat (Case 3, Fig. 4–6; Case 4, Fig. 4–7). The decision to perform a saucerization or shave biopsy requires good judgment and an accurate clinical impression of the preoperative diagnosis.

Shave biopsy is an appropriate technique for superficial exophytic conditions such as seborrheic keratoses, solar keratoses, and warts and for cosmetic removal of some melanocytic nevi (see Case 2, Fig 4–5).[6] Broad shave biopsies are especially useful in obtaining a wide expanse of epidermis within which to look for the changes of

mycosis fungoides when the patch stage of that disease is suspected. Even in this setting, a shave biopsy should either supplement or follow a punch biopsy. In conditions for which shave biopsies are appropriate, the characteristic histologic changes are expected to be present in the epidermis or papillary dermis. In such cases, a biopsy specimen may be taken in a horizontal plane parallel to the surface of the skin. The shave is made at a depth between the deep papillary dermis and the midreticular dermis (see Fig. 4–3). This procedure produces a cosmetically acceptable result (see Case 2, Fig. 4–5). Because it leaves the lower portion of the dermis intact, it also gives maximum flexibility in selecting a postbiopsy treatment plan for basal cell carcinoma. This is important if the biopsied tumor will be subsequently treated by curettage and electrosurgery. The ''hammock'' of dermal connective tissue remains intact to scrape against. A dermal defect would allow the curette to slip into the subcutis where it would flounder around, thus interfering with defining the deep extension of the skin cancer with the curette.[4]

Shave biopsies are not suitable for inflammatory skin diseases in general,[7] for neoplasms that clinically appear to infiltrate the dermis, or for pigmented lesions in which there is even a faint clinical suspicion of melanoma. For such lesions, fusiform incisional biopsy through the ''heart'' of the lesion to muscle (in the case of dermatomyositis) or the deep subcutis is recommended. Whenever possible, excisional biopsy of pigmented lesions that may be melanomas is recommended.[6] Accurate measurement of the deepest penetration of the melanoma cells in serial sections of a histopathologic specimen guides the assessment of prognosis, and indeed too superficial a biopsy can compromise the pathologist's ability to make a correct diagnosis by rendering it impossible to assess maturation of

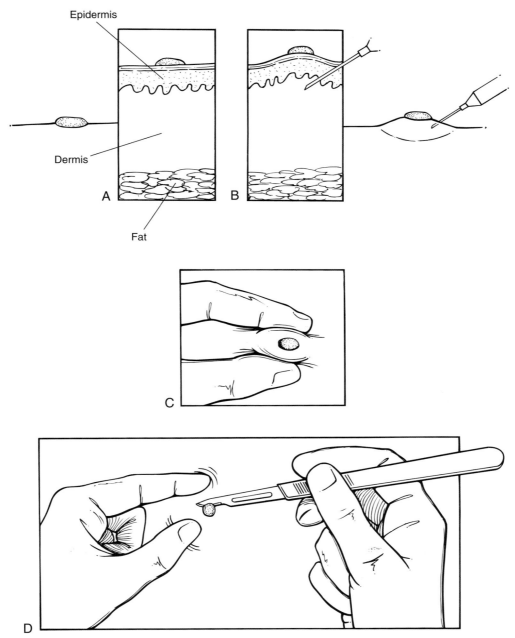

FIGURE 4–3. Shave biopsy. *A* and *B*, The epidermal process is elevated above the surrounding tissue by injecting local anesthesia or *(C)* by pinching the skin between the thumb and forefinger. *D*, If the skin is elevated by the bleb of anesthesia and a biopsy at the papillary dermis is required, then the skin can be made taut and the blade moves under the lesion in a horizontal plane parallel to the skin surface.

melanocytes or the presence of a second population of residual benign nevus cells at the base of the lesion. Shave biopsies that fail to encompass the entire breadth of a lesion compromise the evaluation of such key features as width, circumscription, and symmetry.[5] Shave biopsy may fail to distinguish between solar keratosis, invasive squamous cell carcinoma, and keratoacanthoma.

Since a saucerization biopsy (see Fig. 4–4) is essentially a circular excision to the depth of fat, it can be performed for lesions that involve the dermis (e.g., atypical nevi,

melanoma, or squamous cell carcinoma). In choosing to perform this type of biopsy, the location must be selected to provide good second intention wound healing (see Case 4, Fig. 4–7). A hypopigmented, hyperpigmented, or hypertrophic scar may result (see Case 3, Fig. 4–6 and Case 5, Fig. 4–8).

The instruments used to perform both shave and saucerization biopsies are a scalpel and a toothed forceps. For shave biopsies, some experienced physicians prefer to use a hand-held razor blade.[14] This is a matter of personal

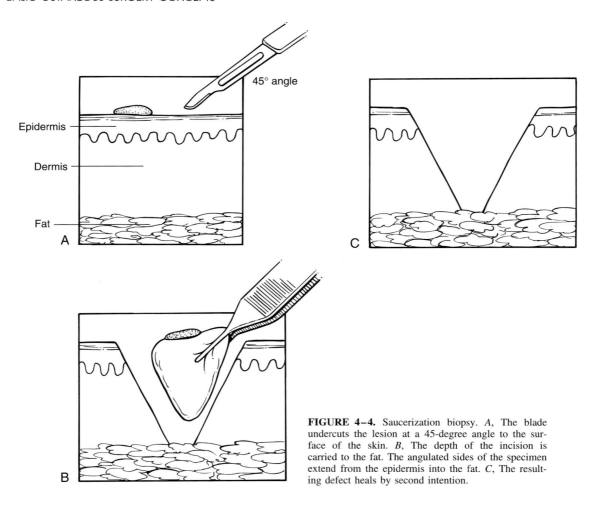

FIGURE 4–4. Saucerization biopsy. *A*, The blade undercuts the lesion at a 45-degree angle to the surface of the skin. *B*, The depth of the incision is carried to the fat. The angulated sides of the specimen extend from the epidermis into the fat. *C*, The resulting defect heals by second intention.

preference. The razor blade is bent into an arc between the forefinger and thumb of the surgeon's hand. The arc of the blade moves through the tissue and conforms to the depth of tissue one desires to remove. If utmost skill in applying pressure to the blade is not used, it is possible to remove a central trough under the lesion with the U-shaped blade. If the surgeon loses his or her grip, the blade's own released tensile strength may cause it to spring upward and inadvertently remove too superficial a specimen. Control of the double-edged razor blade by those who are skilled in its use yields a fine cosmetic result with smooth edges and fine tapering of the cut.

Flexibility in contouring of curved surfaces of the body is obtained by using local anesthesia to elevate the lesion above the surrounding skin surface (see Fig. 4–3). With the operator's hand resting firmly in contact with a solid anatomic flat surface of the patient, the blade is lightly applied to the junction of normal-appearing skin and slightly raised lesion. When saucerization is performed around a lesion suspected of being an atypical or dysplastic nevus, it is important not to transect the most peripheral cells, which are often nonpigmented. One way of ensuring this is to score the surface of the skin around the periphery of the lesions, allowing a 2-mm margin of normal-appearing skin before beginning the procedure. In using a No. 15

blade, this initial cut is best made with the tip of the blade. The tip of the blade is always pointed slightly up to prevent going unnecessarily deep into the deeper dermis. When using a No. 10 blade to remove lesions larger than 1.0 cm in diameter, lead with the broad, flat cutting surface of the belly of the blade. The scalpel handle is held like a butter knife. This broader cutting surface lessens the opportunity of producing a jagged surface on the wound caused by ''sawing across'' the surface with two or three strokes of a No. 15 blade.

In performing shave biopsy, the operator's thumb and forefinger roll the skin, which has been infiltrated with anesthesia, in such a manner as to create a flat cutting surface for the scalpel blade and to provide a tamponade effect on the blood vessels in surrounding skin. If a margin of tissue surrounding and below the lesion is desired, the shave should be done immediately after injecting the anesthetic while the tissue is maximally elevated by the fluid. If less depth is required, it is necessary to inject less anesthetic and wait a few minutes until swelling subsides. A single, steady, sweeping motion of the blade over the junction of normal skin surface and the lesion and parallel to it will remove the elevated lesion (see Fig. 4–3). Sometimes the last attachment to the skin is more easily severed with elevation of the specimen with a forceps.

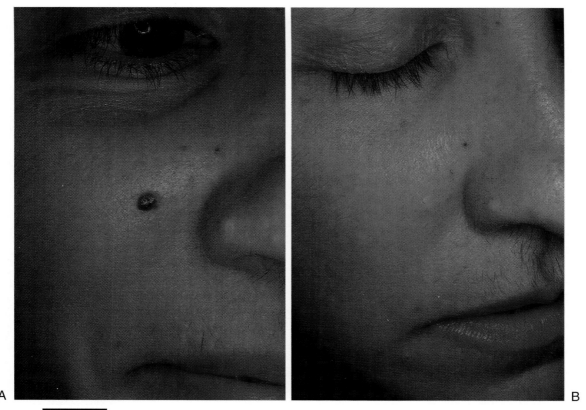

A

B

CASE 2

FIGURE 4-5. *A,* This woman desired removal of the facial seborrheic keratosis that was unchanged and that had been present for more than 10 years. She also wished the smallest possible scar. *B,* Three years after biopsy and removal of the seborrheic keratosis by shave biopsy there is a barely perceptible area of hypopigmentation. Shave biopsy at dermal depth should not leave a depression. This is a good result.

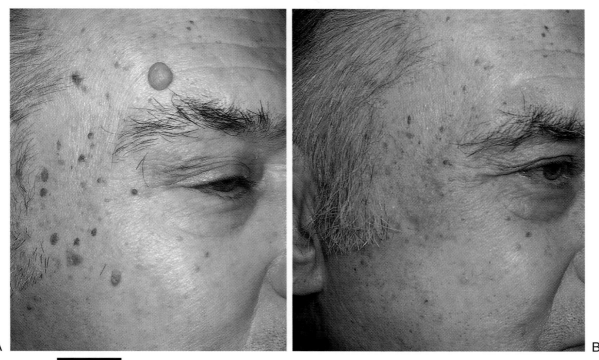

A

B

CASE 3

FIGURE 4-6. *A,* The appearance before saucerization biopsy and removal of a neurofibroma over the right eyebrow. *B,* One year after removal of the large facial lesion by saucerization technique, the appearance is enhanced and visible scarring is limited to a slightly depressed hypopigmented area.

47

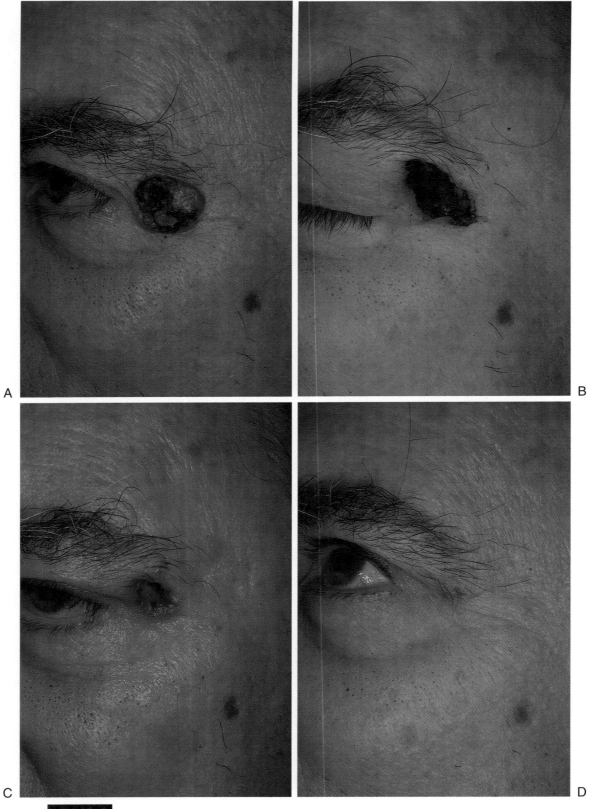

A

B

C

D

FIGURE 4–7. *A,* This elderly man reported rapid growth of this 2.0-cm lesion. Because the eyelid and lateral canthal areas are favorable areas to allow healing by second intention, a saucerization biopsy down to fascia over muscle was done. *B,* Appearance of the defect after the deep saucerization removal of the fat underlying the lesion. The bleeding was stopped with Monsel's solution and pressure. *C,* One week after removal of the lesion, which proved to be a keratoacanthoma, there is very little inflammation. *D,* Six months after the saucerization removal of the keratoacanthoma there is no return of the process and the area has healed without distortion of the lid or canthus. The lateral and medial canthal areas of the eye are extremely favorable locations for healing larger wounds by second intention.

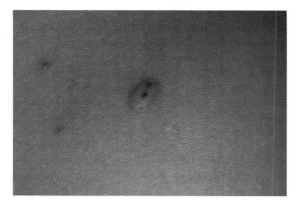

FIGURE 4–8. This 13-year-old girl with dark hair and eyes had a nevus removed from the anterior chest by shave biopsy 4 months previously. Now she has return of pigment centrally and a hypertrophic scar. Since the biopsy of the nevus was benign, the hypertrophic scar was treated with intralesional corticosteroid injections. This patient is predisposed to hypertrophic scar formation by her age and the location of the biopsy site on the anterior chest.

Bleeding can be stopped with application of a styptic such as aluminum chloride (35% in 50% isopropyl alcohol). If there is a slightly raised lip, this can be beveled down with the use of light electrodesiccation followed by the use of a 1-mm curette around the rim and light abrasion of this rim with a gauze pad.

The simplicity of shave biopsy is favored for multiple biopsies, and the ease of the procedure allows pathologic examination of tissue obtained under adverse conditions in children and hesitant adults. Although the technique is easily acquired and gives a fine cosmetic result, it must be noted that nevi removed in this manner may return with central pigmentation (Case 5, Fig. 4–8).[15] This is especially common in patients younger than age 30 who have nevi removed and who have dark hair and eyes and skin that is more deeply pigmented. If this happens and the pigmented area is sampled again, it must be noted on the form that is submitted to the pathologist, since recurrent nevi can feature pagetoid spread of melanocytes within the epidermis. A pathologist who is not aware of the prior removal of the nevus may misinterpret these findings as melanoma.

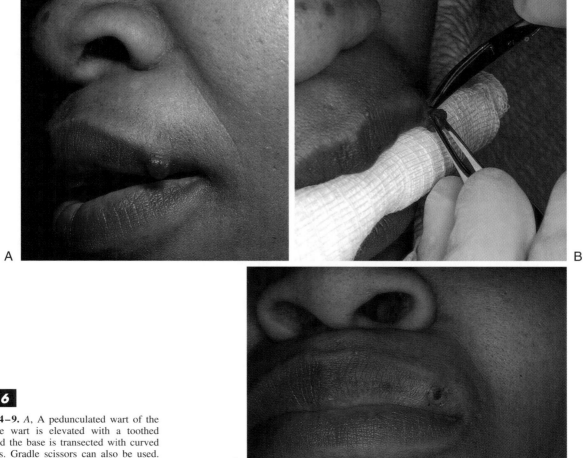

FIGURE 4–9. *A*, A pedunculated wart of the lip. *B*, The wart is elevated with a toothed forceps, and the base is transected with curved iris scissors. Gradle scissors can also be used. *C*, Pinpoint electrocautery controls bleeding.

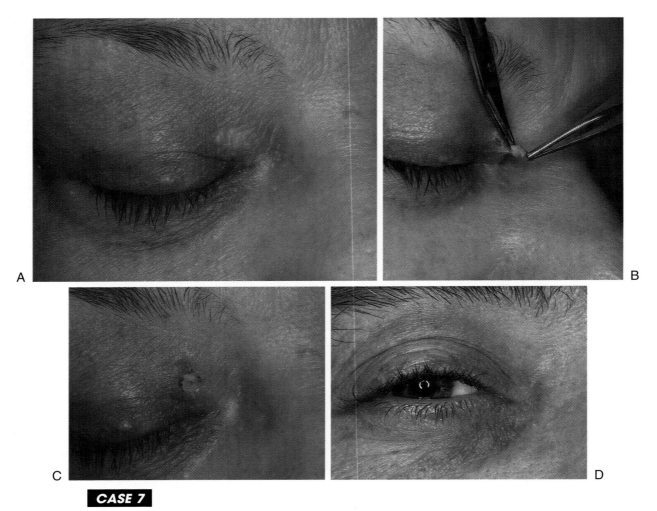

CASE 7

FIGURE 4–10. *A*, Xanthelasma of the upper eyelid is well defined by its yellow color. *B*, The skin surface over the xanthelasma is held with a forceps, and the Gradle scissors is used to gently dissect the base of the lesion. *C*, Bleeding is controlled with pinpoint cautery. The area heals by second intention. *D*, One year after scissors removal of the xanthelasma there is cosmetic improvement.

Scissors Removal

The technique of scissors removal is reserved for benign pedunculated lesions (Case 6, Fig. 4–9). This is a simple effective method for conditions such as filiform warts, skin tags, and polypoid nevi. It does not result in scarring because of the superficiality of the excision and is particularly effective when pedunculated lesions extend above the surface of glabrous skin (e.g., penis, eyelid, or sides of the neck) (Case 7, Fig. 4–10). In some instances, the blades of small scissors such as iris or Gradle scissors are slipped under the tag and it is snipped off without the injection of local anesthetic. The base is transected with a snip of the scissors. Bleeding is controlled by application of 35% aluminum chloride solution. No bandage is required.

Elliptical Incisional and Excisional Biopsy

None of the preceding biopsy techniques requires as much time, advance preparation of instruments and the surgical field, or skill as the elliptical biopsy. This type of biopsy also involves slightly more risk and discomfort to the patient. Nonetheless, use of the elliptical (fusiform) technique is absolutely essential when larger or deep specimens must be taken. Neither shave nor punch biopsy can effectively take such a specimen (see Table 4–1). Situations in which such a specimen is indicated are diseases with significant changes in the deep dermis extending to the fascia (e.g., dermatomyositis, scleroderma, eosinophilic fasciitis, panniculitis, or mesenchymal neoplasms). In these examples, the specimen is removed from the most indurated portion of the skin. Another type of condition in which elliptical incisional specimens are necessary is when the specimen for microscopic examination must include either a continuum from uninvolved normal skin through an indurated or inflammatory border into a necrotic central shallow ulcer or a thickened area of skin or when the pathologic process may have skipped areas of normal skin between areas of active disease. Similarly, a specimen containing a continuum from normal to affected skin allows assessment of surgical margins and simplifies diagnosis of disease processes such as pyoderma gangrenosum, keratoacanthoma, and verrucous carcinoma. A final class of cases requiring this technique involves pigmented lesions that may be melanomas. If total excision for diagnosis is not possible, then the darkest area of the growth and/or the elevated portion is chosen for the site of incisional biopsy. It is essential that if the elevated portion of a melanocytic neoplasm is incised, the incision should be deep enough to encompass the deepest melanocyte in that area. The sections of a histopathologic specimen produced by such an excisional biopsy guide subsequent therapeutic surgical removal of the surrounding skin. Details on planning and performing elliptical surgical procedures are discussed in Chapter 9.

BIOPSY OF THE ORAL CAVITY

Vermilion of the lip, buccal, gingiva, and the anterior two thirds of the tongue can be exposed in a cooperative patient and bleeding controlled with the use of local anesthesia. The specialized nature of presentation of diseases in the mouth[9-11] and need to close the wound with sutures mean that punch or elliptical biopsies are performed more than any other type.[12] Inside the oral cavity and on the portion of the lip that contacts the other lip, the suture of choice is silk because of its supple qualities when moist. To protect the suture line from accidental trauma in eating, benzocaine (Orabase) can be applied to cover the sutures.

Biopsy of buccal mucosa is assisted by the use of a modified chalazion clamp that applies pressure to control bleeding (Case 8, Fig. 4–11).[16] The silk suture that closes the defect is placed before removing the clamp.

After applying topical viscous anesthesia, the extended tongue is grasped with a gauze pad and local anesthetic is infiltrated into the biopsy site on the tongue. The tongue may be stabilized by placing a single suture into the tip. This suture is pulled forward and held by a clamp by the assistant while the biopsy is performed. Immobilization of the tongue is necessary to perform a biopsy of the tongue because the patient cannot hold out the tongue on his or her own. The stabilizing suture is removed at the end of the procedure.[17]

A silver nitrate stick or electrocautery may suffice to control bleeding. If one elects to place a suture, it is useful to place a deep and wide loop under the biopsy site before biopsy. It is much easier to tie the suture after biopsy than to try to place a suture in a bloody field.

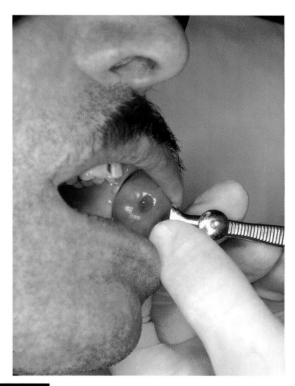

CASE 8

FIGURE 4–11. The chalazion clamp stabilizes the buccal mucosa and provides hemostasis for performing a punch biopsy of an area of leukoplakia. To protect the deeper structures of the cheek from inadvertent injury, the local anesthetic is injected in sufficient volume to "balloon" up the overlying buccal mucosa. The downward pressure on the punch biopsy ceases once the pop through the dermis is felt. A silk suture will be placed before releasing the clamp. The silk suture is removed in 5 to 7 days.

References

1. Lighthouse AG, Kopf AW, Garfinkel L. Diagnostic accuracy: A new approach to its evaluation. Arch Dermatol 1965;91:497–502.
2. Pinkus H, Mehregan AH. A Guide to Dermatohistopathology. New York: Appleton-Century-Crofts, 1981.
3. Robinson JK. Surgical gems: Biopsy to and including muscle. J Dermatol Surg Oncol 1979;5:595.
4. Bart RS, Kopf AW. Techniques of biopsy of cutaneous neoplasms. J Dermatol Surg Oncol 1979;5:979–987.
5. Macy-Roberts E, Ackerman AB. A critique of techniques for biopsy of clinically suspected malignant melanomas. Am J Dermatopathol 1982;4:391–398.
6. Kopf AW, Popkin GL. Shave biopsies for cutaneous lesions. Arch Dermatol 1974;110:637.
7. Ackerman AB. Shave biopsies: The good and the bad, the right and the wrong. Am J Dermatopathol 1983;5:211–212.
8. Headington JT. Transverse microscopic anatomy of the human scalp: A basis for morphometric approach to disorders of the hair follicle. Arch Dermatol 1984;120:449–456.
9. Jorizzo JL, Salisbury PL, Rogers RS, et al. Oral lesions in systemic lupus erythematosus. J Am Acad Dermatol 1992;27:389–394.
10. Mashberg A. Erythroplasia vs leukoplakia in the diagnosis of early asymptomatic oral squamous carcinoma. N Engl J Med 1977;297:109–110.
11. Chimenti S, Calvieri S, Ribuffo M. Malignant melanoma of the oral cavity. J Dermatol Surg Oncol 1981;7:220–224.
12. Frim SP. Biopsy of lesions in the mouth. J Dermatol Surg Oncol 1981;7:985–987.
13. Crollick JS, Klein LE. Punch biopsy diagnostic technique (letter). J Dermatol Surg Oncol 1987;13:839.
14. Shelley WB. The razor blade in dermatologic practice. Cutis 1975;16:843–845.
15. Porter JM, Treasure J. Excision of benign pigmented skin tumors by deep shaving. Br J Plast Surg 1993;46:255–257.
16. Roth RJ. An instrument and technique to facilitate biopsies of lesions of the structures of the mouth and within the oral cavity. J Dermatol Surg Oncol 1981;7:862–863.
17. Harahap M. How to biopsy oral lesions. J Dermatol Surg Oncol 1989;15:1077–1080.

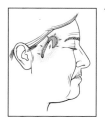

chapter 5

Cryosurgery

GLORIA F. GRAHAM

Cryosurgery is one of the most commonly performed techniques for the treatment of benign and premalignant disorders of the skin (Tables 5–1 through 5–4). It is also being used more frequently for the treatment of malignant skin tumors. Because benign lesions require less duration and depth of freeze than do malignant lesions, it is possible to achieve good-to-excellent cosmetic results.

TABLE 5–1. Cryosurgery: Indications, Contraindications, Limitations

Indications

Benign
  Warts
  Seborrheic keratosis
  Lentigines
  Keratoacanthoma
  Keloids
  Chondrodermatitis
  Sebaceous hyperplasia
Premalignant
  Actinic keratosis
  Lentigo maligna
Malignant
  Basal cell carcinoma
  Squamous cell carcinoma
  Kaposi's sarcoma

Contraindications

Tumors without definable margins
Abnormal cold intolerance
Lack of skill of the operator

Limitations

Final cosmetic result may be hypopigmentation or peripheral hyperpigmentation.
Hypertrophic scars are rare but may occur if combined with shave excisions, although freezing reduces tendency for hypertrophic scarring.
Atrophy is rare.
Temporary neuropathy resolves in 3 to 6 months.

Cryosurgery is the method of therapy using freezing temperatures to destroy tissue by probe, spray, or cotton swab. Tissue temperatures in the freezing range are produced. The cotton swab or dipstick method affords less adequate control. There is inadequate depth of freeze owing to the less efficient heat sink. The repeated dipping of the cotton swab into liquid nitrogen is time consuming and has the disadvantage of possible viral contamination of the liquid nitrogen. The cryospray method involves the application of an intermittent spray directed toward the center of the lesion for a specified number of seconds or minutes (Table 5–5). The cryoprobe technique involves selection of a probe size and type suitable for the lesion diameter. The cryoprobe is precooled to prevent cryoadhesion. Then it is applied to the lesion with pressure for a specified period of seconds or minutes.

The treated lesion is characterized by circumscribed necrosis. Although melanocytes and osteocytes are easily de-

TABLE 5–2. Cryosurgery: Patient Preoperative Discussion

1. Healing of benign lesions takes 10 to 14 days. Healing of malignant lesions takes 4 to 6 weeks.
2. No bandages are necessary, but a clean, dry bandage may be used if the area is unsightly or easily traumatized.
3. For the first week there is a blister that turns into a scab or crust. This will separate and come off in approximately 2 weeks for benign lesions and 4 weeks for malignant lesions.
4. Cleanse the area in the shower with soap and water daily.
5. There are no limitations on physical activity unless the wound is on the lower leg. Elevation of the leg is helpful to prevent swelling and to promote more rapid healing.
6. After the crust comes off, the wound is first pink and then often lighter than the surrounding skin.
7. Sunscreen should be used to protect the new skin.

TABLE 5–3. Cryosurgery: Operative Issues

Preoperative Evaluation

History
  Abnormal cold intolerance
  Bleeding diathesis
  Hepatitis, human immunodeficiency virus infection
  Immunosuppression
  Prosthesis, artificial valves
  Telangiectasia
Examine previous scars
Consider degree of pigment

Preoperative Equipment Needs

Hand-held instrument with various-sized tips or blunt-type needles
Cotton swabs
25- to 35-L Dewar (insulated thermos) with withdrawal device
Luer-Lok adaptor
Cryoprobes
Otoscope cones or Neoprene filter adaptor cones
Eyeshield, Jaeger lid retractor or spoons (plastic) or tongue blades for protecting the eye from cold conduction
Depth-dose measurement devices

Intraoperative Needs

Depth-dose measurement; watch to measure time; rule to measure lateral spread freeze; pyrometer to determine temperature under tumor; thermocouple (esp. for malignant lesions)

TABLE 5–4. Cryosurgery: Postoperative Care

Pain Management

Pain is not frequent, except for warts treated on the hands and feet and tumors over the temple area.
Acetaminophen may be used for headache if site is on the temporal area.
Acetaminophen with codeine may be needed for warts on the plantar surface of the foot.

Dressings

None on smaller sites <1 cm in diameter.
A dry, sterile dressing may be used if the area is unsightly.
If the original eschar separates and is removed prematurely or due to a traumatic incident, Duoderm or similar dressing may be used.

Complications

Hyperpigmentation may be lessened by using sunscreen.
Delayed bleeding may occur when the tumor involves a vessel, but this is rare.
Pseudoepitheliomatous hyperplasia for 4 to 6 weeks to 3 to 6 months is self-limited.
Hypertrophic scars (uncommon) may be treated by massage or intralesional steroid.
Infection is rare and is treated with appropriate antibiotic or antiviral systemic medication.
Periorbital edema may be lessened by pretreatment with systemic steroids.
Slow healing wounds, especially on the lower legs, can be treated with Duoderm or similar dressing.

vitalized, squamous cells are more resistant. Cellular tissue sloughs quickly, but fibrous stroma, large arteries, nerves, and cartilage resist change. Bone, while devitalized with extended freezing, resists sloughing, and the matrix is a framework for repair.

The commonly used cryogens are carbon dioxide (solid, $-78.5°C$), nitrous oxide (liquid, $-89.5°C$), and liquid nitrogen ($-195.8°C$), the most efficient heat sink. To maximize tissue destruction, the following considerations are important: fast freeze to a lethal temperature of $-50°C$, thaw slowly and completely, provide a short thawed interval between cycles, and repeat the freeze–thaw cycle.

Cryosurgery may be combined with curettage and may follow shave excision, especially in the treatment of carcinomas (Figs. 5–1 through 5–7). In these cases, a preoperative local anesthetic is necessary and is helpful in elevating the lesion away from cartilage or bone, thus facilitating the freezing process.

Text continued on page 59

TABLE 5–5. Cryosurgery: Treatment Chart

Type of Lesion	Treatment	Tip*	Time† (seconds)	Target (mm)	Technique	Thermocouple‡	Result
Hypertrophic actinic keratosis	Choice	B	F = 20–30 T = 30–40	2	Cryospray (1 cryocycle)	No	Excellent to good
Seborrheic keratosis	Alternate or adjunct	B	F = 10–20 T = 20–30	2.5	Cryospray (1 cryocycle)	No	Good to fair
Dermatofibroma	Choice or alternate	Probe	F = 20–30 T = 30–40	3–4	Cryospray or cryoprobe (1 cryocycle)	No	Good to fair
Basal cell carcinoma	Choice or alternate	>1 cm = A <1 cm = B	F = 60–120 T = 60–180	3–4	Cryospray or cryoprobe (2–3 cryocycles)	Yes	Good to fair
Lentigo maligna	Choice	A or B	F = 60–120 T = 90–180	3–4	Cryospray or cryoprobe (2–3 cryocycles)	Yes	Excellent to good

*Tip size for the Brymill Cry Ac unit: A = largest diameter, 0.040 inch; B = medium diameter, 0.0312 inch.
†F, freezing; T, thawing. These times based on using B tip.
‡Thermocouple use important while learning technique, when treating tumors around the eye or other difficult locations, and to prevent overfreezing.

FIGURE 5–1. After the tumor is debulked by shave excision and curettage, the exposed surface of the tumor is sprayed. The lateral spread of freeze extends 0.5 cm beyond the exposed surface of the tumor; however, if the tumor is clinically believed to be deeper than 0.5 cm, then the lateral spread of freeze should be greater than 0.5 cm. The lateral spread of freeze should be equivalent to the tumor depth.

The thermocouple needle is placed under the deepest penetration of the tumor. Thermocouple monitoring ensures that the tumor destructive temperature of −50°C is achieved at the base of the tumor. When using a Cryac unit to treat a basal cell carcinoma, freeze time is usually approximately 60 seconds, halo thaw time is 90 seconds, and complete thaw time is 2 to 5 minutes.

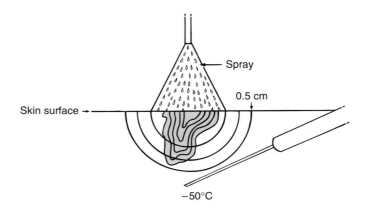

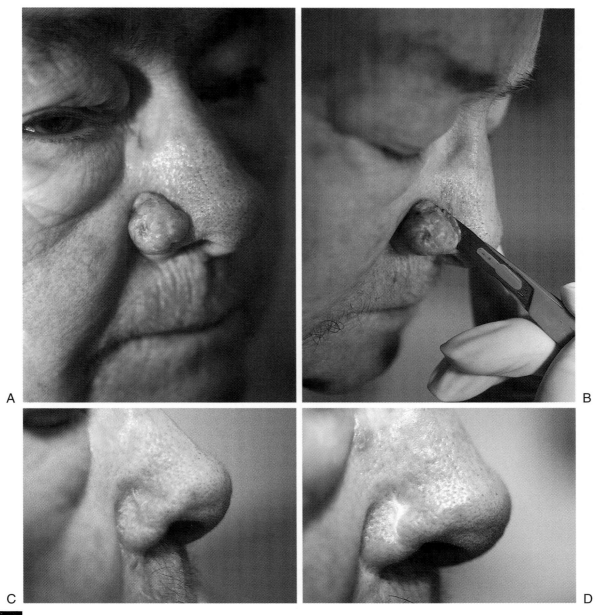

CASE 1

FIGURE 5–2. *A,* Appearance of 2.0-cm nodular basal cell carcinoma of right ala before surgery. *B,* Shave removal of exophytic portion to provide a specimen for biopsy and to debulk the tumor before cryosurgery. *C,* At the 2-month follow-up there is a slightly hypertrophic area in the treatment site and minimal elevation of the alar rim. *D,* One year later there is no clinically apparent recurrence. The treatment site has a hypopigmented scar.

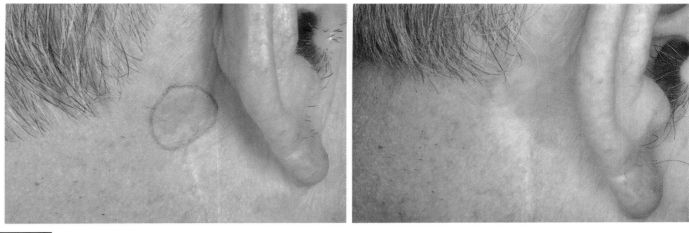

A

CASE 2

FIGURE 5–3. *A*, Preoperative appearance of a morphea-type basal cell carcinoma with the clinically apparent margins marked. *B*, The result at 1 year shows the anticipated flat, hypopigmented treatment site. There is some central erythema. This is an acceptable result for cryosurgical treatment that required a double freeze–thaw cycle.

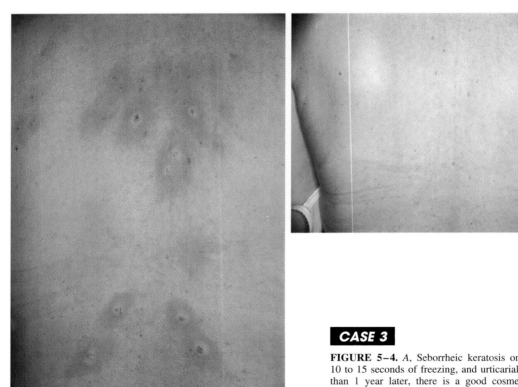

B

CASE 3

FIGURE 5–4. *A*, Seborrheic keratosis on the back was treated with 10 to 15 seconds of freezing, and urticarial wheals developed. *B*, More than 1 year later, there is a good cosmetic result with no apparent change on the skin surface. (From Graham G. Cryosurgery. Clin Plast Surg 1993;20:81–147.)

A

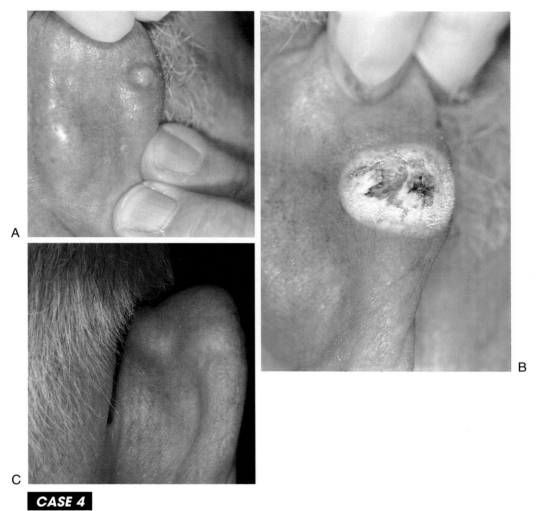

CASE 4

FIGURE 5–5. *A,* Preoperative appearance of a nodular basal cell carcinoma of the helical rim of the ear. *B,* The tumor margins are defined by curettage and then treated with cryosurgery. The lateral spread of freezing is well defined. *C,* One year later there is no loss of contour of the rim of the ear and an acceptable cosmetic result.

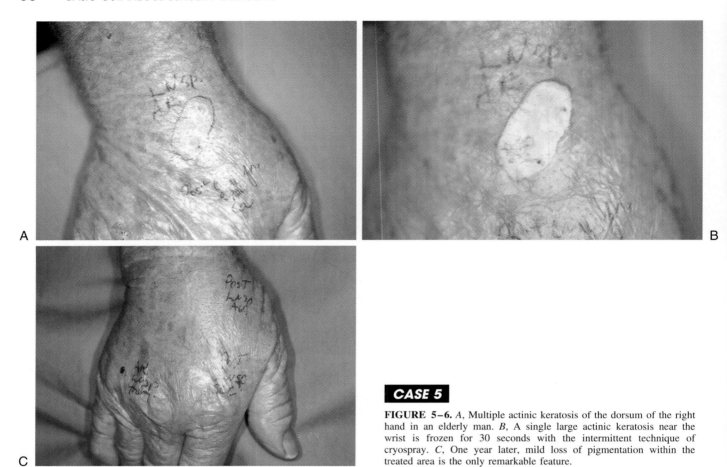

CASE 5

FIGURE 5–6. *A*, Multiple actinic keratosis of the dorsum of the right hand in an elderly man. *B*, A single large actinic keratosis near the wrist is frozen for 30 seconds with the intermittent technique of cryospray. *C*, One year later, mild loss of pigmentation within the treated area is the only remarkable feature.

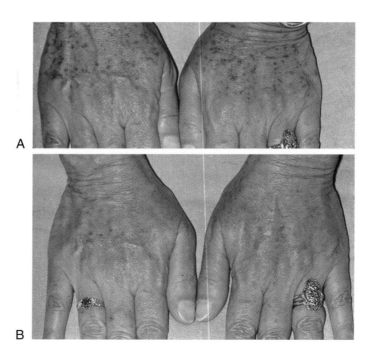

CASE 6

FIGURE 5–7. *A*, The dorsa of both hands have multiple lentigines. *B*, Three weeks after treatment with cryosurgery, there is no change in the background pigmentation and the lentigines are gone. Nitrous oxide was used as the cryogen, producing an excellent result. (Courtesy of León Neumann, M.D.)

Suggested Readings

1. Allington HD. Liquid nitrogen in the treatment of skin disease. Calif Med 1950;72:153.
2. Elton RF. Complications of cutaneous cryosurgery. J Am Acad Dermatol 1983;8:513.
3. Gage AA, Kuflik EG. Cryosurgical equipment. In: Cryosurgical Treatment for Skin Cancer. New York: Igaku-Shoin, 1990:53.
4. Graham GF. Cryosurgery. Clin Plast Surg 1993;20:131.
5. Graham GF. Cryosurgery. In: Wheeland R, ed. Cutaneous Surgery. Philadelphia: WB Saunders Co., 1993.
6. Graham GF, Stewart R. Cryosurgery for unusual cutaneous neoplasms. J Dermatol Surg Oncol 1977;3:437.
7. Kuflik EG, Gage AA. The five-year cure rate achieved by cryosurgery for skin cancer. J Am Acad Dermatol 1991;24:1002.
8. Kuflik EG, Webb W: Effects of systemic corticosteroids on postcryosurgical edema and other manifestations of the inflammatory response. J Dermatol Surg Oncol 1985;11:464.
9. Lubritz RR. Cryosurgery of benign and premalignant cutaneous lesions. In: Zacarian SA, ed. Cryosurgical Advances in Dermatology and Tumors of the Head and Neck. Springfield, IL: Charles C Thomas, 1977:55.
10. Spiller WF, Spiller RF. Cryosurgery in dermatology office practice. South Med J 1975;68:157.
11. Stewart RS, Graham GF. A complication of cryosurgery in a patient with cryofibrinogenemia. J Dermatol Surg Oncol 1978;4:10.
12. Torre D: Cryosurgery. In: Newcomer VD, Young EM, eds. Geriatric Dermatology. New York: Igaku-Shoin, 1988:55.
13. Torre D. Cryosurgical instrumentation and depth dose monitoring. In: Breitbart E, Dachow-Siwiec E, eds. Clinics in Dermatology: Advances in Cryosurgery. New York: Elsevier, 1990:48.
14. Zacarian SA. Cryosurgery for cancer of the skin. In: Zacarian SA, ed. Cryosurgery for Skin Cancer and Cutaneous Disorders. St. Louis: CV Mosby, 1985:96.
15. Zacarian SA. Cryosurgery of lentigo maligna. In: Zacarian SA, ed. Cryosurgery for Skin Cancer and Cutaneous Disorders. St. Louis, CV Mosby, 1985:1992.

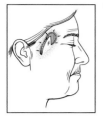

chapter 6

Electrosurgery

JUNE K. ROBINSON

In electrosurgery tissue is either cut or destroyed by heat generated by an electrosurgical apparatus. The actual extent of tissue destruction goes beyond the visible charred area produced at the time of surgery. Electrosurgery is fast, easy, efficient, and relatively inexpensive to perform (Tables 6–1 through 6–4). Electrosurgery equipment in contact with blood should be either disposable or sterilized for each patient in the same way as all other surgical equipment contaminated by contact with blood.

ELECTROCAUTERY

Metal is heated by electric current and directly applied to tissue that is either desiccated, coagulated, or necrosed. No electric current passes to the patient. The instrument may be either battery powered or dependent on an electrical outlet. In either case, the tip of the unit is made of wire with a high resistance, such as platinum alloy. When the current flows through the wire its temperature increases and the wire starts to glow red. As it gets hotter it turns white.

Since the penetration of this heat is limited to the papillary dermis, some practitioners prefer the use of this instrument for the treatment of superficial exophytic growths such as seborrheic keratosis, molluscum, and flat warts. In this method the glowing needle tip lightly touches the surface of the lesion, which bubbles and then carbonizes. In using the instrument, the tip is maintained at a fairly acute angle to the skin to avoid touching an area of the patient's skin that is not anesthetized. The crusted lesion is shed later. Lesions that are entirely intraepidermal may be removed without scarring by this method.

The advantages of electrocautery are that it can be used to produce coagulation in patients with pacemakers and can produce hemostasis in a bloody field when electrodesiccating currents are relatively ineffective. The chief disadvantage is that removal of large tumors or use in deeper lesions with greater bleeding is very time consuming.

HIGH-FREQUENCY ELECTROSURGICAL APPARATUS

The alternating-current frequency must be rapid enough not to induce neuromuscular response. High-frequency current is conducted from the treatment electrode to the tissue. The tip of the electrode does not produce heat or become hot as it conducts the oscillating electrical energy in a highly concentrated fashion to the tissue. The tissue offers a high degree of resistance to the electrical current, and the vibrating energy causes mechanical disruption of the cells and heat.

This current may be delivered by either monoterminal or biterminal equipment. In the biterminal mode, the patient is grounded by a relatively large "indifferent" terminal (electrode) that is in even contact with the skin surface. This indifferent electrode disperses the current harmlessly over an area of about 20 square inches while the treatment electrode concentrates the same energy at a small point in the tissue. Incorporating the patient as part of the circuit allows the production of more intense current with a lower voltage.

In monoterminal operation, the patient is not incorporated directly into the circuit. The patient sheds electrons to the air, floor, and so on. A much higher voltage is needed to produce destruction about the needle tip of the treatment electrode. This effectively minimizes the heat produced in the tissues and results in less destruction of tissue.

Electrocoagulation destroys tissue by heat that is generated by the resistance of tissue within the high-frequency electrical field. The patient is always incorporated into the biterminal circuit, which uses a lower voltage. The flow of electricity is enhanced by the use of the indifferent electrode to complete the circuit. The tissue is "boiled," with loss of cellular architecture extending some distance beyond the field. Rapid clotting of blood is achieved, but the electrosurgical current cannot stop bleeding once blood is present. Hemorrhage must be controlled by direct pres-

TABLE 6-1. Electrosurgery: Indications, Contraindications, Risks, Limitations

Indications

Electrofulguration or Electrodesiccation of Benign Epidermal Processes

Epidermal nevi
Dermatosis papulosa nigra
Molluscum contagiosum
Seborrheic keratosis
Sebaceous hyperplasia
Skin tags
Syringoma
Warts

Electrocoagulation

Benign lesions
   Angioma
   Pyogenic granuloma
   Telangiectasia
   Venous lake
   Hirsutism
Precancerous lesions
   Actinic keratosis
   Keratoacanthoma
Malignant lesions
   Superficial and nodular basal cell carcinoma

Electrosection (Benign Lesions)

Acne keloidalis nuchae
Condyloma acuminatum
Hidradenitis suppurativa
Rhinophyma

Contraindications/Risks

Impaired wound healing
Demand pacemakers and interference with cardiac monitoring devices for high-frequency electrosurgical apparatus
Burns of patient's skin from improper contact with indifferent electrode for high-frequency electrosurgical apparatus
For electrocautery:
   Use near paper drapes
   Ignition of skin preparations: alcohol, chlorhexidine (Hibistat)

Limitations

Some bleeding in early postoperative period
Some tenderness and erythema in area around treatment site
Sloughing of necrotic tissue
Eschar formation
Permanent postoperative complications:
   Hypopigmentation or hyperpigmentation
Hypertrophic scar, especially of the upper lip, deltoid-sternal areas
Atrophic scar

Factors Influencing Final Result

Type of current (coagulation, cutting)
Type of current application (monoterminal or biterminal)
Current intensity, power setting
Length of application
Size of electrode (ball, loop, needle tip)
Density and moisture content of the tissue

TABLE 6-2. Electrosurgery: Patient Preoperative Discussion

1. Healing should take 2 weeks.
2. No bandages are necessary.
3. Cleanse the area in the shower with soap and water daily.
4. A scab or crust will form. It will fall off in approximately 2 weeks.
5. There are no limitations on physical activity except if the wound is on the lower leg. If that is the case, elevate the leg when resting.
6. When the wound is healing, it will first be pink, then it will become darker or lighter than the surrounding skin.

TABLE 6-3. Electrosurgery: Operative Issues

Preoperative Evaluation

History
   Bleeding diathesis
   Hepatitis, human immunodeficiency virus infection
   Immunosuppression
   Prosthesis, artificial valves
   Demand pacemaker
   Examine other scars for healing

Preoperative Equipment Needs

Electrocautery with sterile tip or high-frequency electrosurgical apparatus
Barrier protection, including mask and eye protection and gloves
Topical antibacterial preparation
Local anesthesia

Intraoperative Needs

Labeled specimen bottle
No paper drapes with electrocautery
No alcohol or chlorhexidine in the field
Smoke evacuator for extensive electrosurgery

TABLE 6-4. Electrosurgery: Postoperative Care

Pain Management

Acetaminophen for headache if site is on the temporal area
Tylenol with codeine for weight-bearing extremities with a large surface area

Dressings

None on smaller sites <1 cm in diameter
Cover larger areas with a Telfa pad and antibacterial ointment.

Complications

A hypertrophic scar forms 4 to 6 weeks after surgery. Treat the scar by having the patient massage it for 15 minutes a day for 4 months. It should resolve spontaneously in 6 months. If it does not resolve, intralesional corticosteroid injections are indicated.
Treat infections with appropriate antibiotic or antiviral systemic medication.

sure, hemostat, or suction. When bleeding has momentarily stopped, final sealing of capillaries or vessels can be accomplished by short application of electrocoagulation current. The current is delivered to the hemostat or to a forceps that grasps the tissue. Electrocoagulation current delivered in this manner causes less adjacent tissue damage by limiting current flow to the small area between the two tips of the forceps. In general, arteries large enough to be named should be ligated instead of just applying electrocoagulation by means of the hemostat.

Electrofulguration (sparking) dehydrates and produces superficial destruction of tissue with the patient not being part of the circuit (monoterminal). The needle does not directly contact the tissue, but the current is transmitted by an electrical arc or spark. Minimal heat is produced in the tissue. Electrodesiccation (drying) is the same as fulguration, but the needle is held in contact with the tissue. If the current is great enough, then coagulation by heat also occurs.

When used in the cutting current mode for electrosection (biterminal), the waveform differs from the other uses, cells are exploded about the electrode, and there is little coagulation or carbonization of tissue. In practice, the lesion is scooped off with a wire loop electrode. Facility in use of the cutting current is acquired by practicing the depth of the cut and speed at which the electrode is moved. This biterminal cutting current and wire loop or hockey stick electrode are used to debulk protuberant masses such as neurofibroma, rhinophyma, or condyloma (Case 1, Fig. 6–1) before coagulating the base. Slow speed increases the thickness of the coagulum. Tissue adheres to

the electrode when insufficient current is used. The odor of the smoke plume generated by electrosurgical operations is offensive to many individuals and may require the use of a smoke evacuation system. The cutting current offers no real advantage over conventional surgery, and there is somewhat slower wound healing.

In cosmetic removal of an epidermal process (seborrheic keratosis, warts), electrofulguration may follow shave removal, follow or precede curettage, or be used alone with removal of coagulum by rubbing a piece of gauze across the treatment site. Light fulguration produces little destruction of tissue. One should use the briefest possible application of current while keeping the electrode in slow motion without actually touching the skin lesion. The lesion will lighten and shrink. At the end of treatment, hair follicles remain intact.

Small telangiectasias of the face are treated either by inserting a sterile epilating needle into the vessel and electrocoagulating it at the lowest wattage or placing the nee-

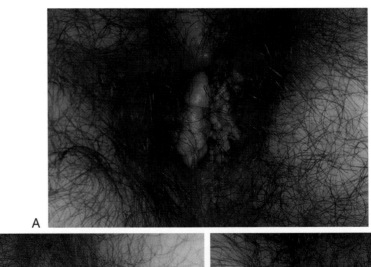

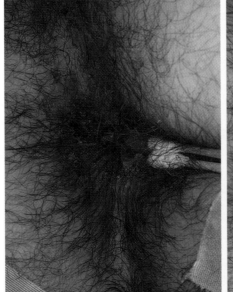

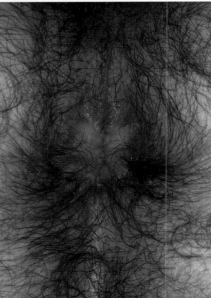

CASE 1

FIGURE 6–1. *A*, Condylomata acuminata of the rectal area should be prepared for electrosurgery by local anesthesia and clipping the hair. *B*, After removal of the external lesions with the cutting current and the wire loop electrode, pinpoint electrocoagulation of the base is performed. An anuscope is then used to examine the internal mucous membranes. Electrosurgery may also be used to remove these lesions. *C*, Two weeks after surgery the area has healed. New condylomata are apparent at the margins of the treated areas. These are less protuberant and may respond to 20% podophyllin in tincture of benzoin. Removal of the exophytic mass provided relief to the patient, who was bleeding during defecation.

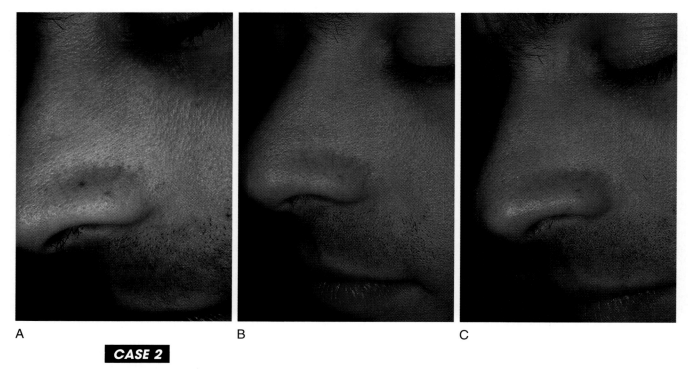

A   B   C

CASE 2

FIGURE 6–2. *A*, Telangiectasia about the alae of a 24-year-old man before treatment by grounded bipolar electrocautery delivered by piercing the skin with an epilating needle. *B*, Six months after treatment, the treated telangiectases are lightened. *C*, Two years after treatment, the patient returns for treatment of a new area of the alar rim.

dle on the skin surface over the vessel and electrocoagulating it (Case 2, Fig. 6–2). If care is not exercised to limit the destruction, then pitted scars may result. Telangiectases on the lower extremities are more likely to scar, hyperpigment, or form depressed tracts. Sclerotherapy seems preferable on the legs.

The majority of early small, nodular, and superficial basal cell carcinomas can be treated with curettage followed by electrocautery, biterminal electrocoagulation, or monoterminal electrodesiccation. After the area is carefully anesthetized, a medium-sized curette is used to scoop out the gelatinous carcinoma (Fig. 6–3). Then the bleeding at

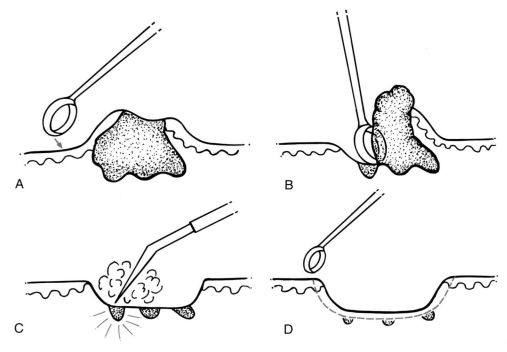

A

B

C

D

FIGURE 6–3. Curettage and electro-desiccation. *A*, Curette in position to remove the basal cell carcinoma. *B*, Curette scooping out the gelatinous material. Islands of tumor remain at the base of the wound in three areas. *C*, Electrodesiccation with needle tip in contact with the tissue. Smoke is created. Tissue damage extends into the dermis and along the epidermis. *D*, A smaller curette is used to explore the margins and base of the lesion for pockets of tumor and charred material down to a firm base.

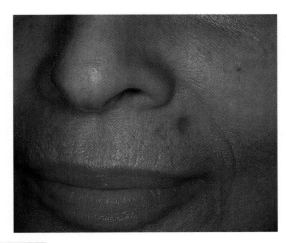

CASE 3

FIGURE 6-4. Electrosurgery complication. Eight weeks after electrosurgery of a basal cell carcinoma of the upper lip, the area is both hyperpigmented and hypertrophic. Intralesional corticosteroids were injected at 3-week intervals over four sessions to flatten the lesion. The upper lip is particularly prone to hypertrophic scar development.

the base is controlled with either electrocautery or electrodesiccation and a 1- to 2-mm perimeter of tissue is destroyed after each curettage. Then a small curette is used to explore the margins and base of the lesion in at least three different directions. The carbonized tissue is removed, and the base has a gritty feel. The commonly used method employs two or three cycles of curettage followed by electrodesiccation. Healing occurs over 10 to 14 days and in some areas may be hypertrophic (Case 3, Fig. 6-4).

Suggested Readings

1. Batting CG. Electrosurgical burn injuries and their prevention. JAMA 1968;204:91-95.
2. Burdick KH. Electrosurgical Apparatus and Their Application in Dermatology. Springfield, IL: Charles C Thomas, 1966.
3. Krull EA, Pickard SD, Hall JC. Effects of electrosurgery on cardiac pacemakers. J Dermatol Surg 1975;1:45.
4. Sheretz EF, Davis GL, Rice RW, et al. Transfer of hepatitis B virus by contaminated reusable needle electrodes after electrodesiccation in simulated use. J Am Acad Dermatol 1986;15:1242-1246.

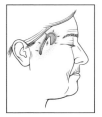

chapter 7

Considerations in Achieving Hemostasis

Hemostatic Techniques in Dermatologic Surgery

Elizabeth M. Billingsley and Mary E. Maloney

Hemostasis is vitally important in all surgical procedures. Adequate control of bleeding without unnecessary tissue destruction is the goal in any procedure. The dermatologic surgeon needs to be familiar with all available methods of obtaining hemostasis and be able to choose the best method for each situation. It is also important to understand the risk factors for excessive bleeding and how to manage any of the complications of bleeding during the postoperative course.

CHEMICAL AGENTS

Several chemical agents are available for use in dermatologic surgery to achieve hemostasis (Table 7–1). These include aluminum chloride, Monsel's solution, silver nitrate, trichloroacetic acid, and phenol (Fig. 7–1). These agents work through protein precipitation and are applied with light pressure in a rolling motion (Fig. 7–2). The field should be dry before their application, since blood will interfere with the tissue reaction.

Aluminum chloride (20%–50%) may be mixed in water, alcohol, ether, or glycerol. Lower concentrations are commercially available as Drysol. This agent is applied to a superficial wound with a swab using light pressure and a twisting motion. The method of action may be related to protein precipitation by the aluminum ion and the acidic nature of the solution. Tissue coagulation and damage along with vasoconstriction lead to activation of the extrinsic pathway of coagulation. The advantages include low

cost, availability, ease of storage and handling, and lack of tissue necrosis. Also, using aluminum chloride in a wound does not increase the diameter of the wound, as it will not damage intact stratified squamous epithelium. However, it is caustic and caution must be used when it is applied near the eyes, since it can irritate or even cause corneal abrasion or erosion. It should not be used in deep wounds because it can delay healing and increase scarring. It does not leave a "tattoo" of pigment but may induce a histiocytic reaction.

Monsel's solution is 20% ferric subsulfate. It is swabbed onto the bleeding surface, and light pressure is applied. Ferric ions denature and agglutinate protein, including fibrinogen. Its low pH and subsulfate group denature protein, which occludes blood vessels. Advantages include reasonable cost, availability, and ease of storage and handling. Its disadvantages are that it is caustic and may destroy connective tissue. It should not be used in wounds that are to be closed with sutures. There is also a small risk of tattooing, which is believed to be due to iron deposition or stimulation of melanocytes.

Silver nitrate is available as a solution (20% to 50%) or on preapplied applicators. It is applied to bleeding surfaces with light pressure. The silver ions combine with tissue protein to form insoluble precipitates that physically block open vessels. Advantages include its reasonable cost, its availability, its germicidal action, and its ease of storage and handling. Its disadvantages are that it is slow working, has a variable response, and is caustic. Although the eschar usually prevents deep penetration, it can be difficult to control the depth of tissue destruction. It may also "tattoo" by leaving silver in the dermis.

TABLE 7-1. Comparison of Methods of Hemostasis

Method of Hemostasis	Indications	Advantages	Disadvantages
Chemical	Superficial wounds	Inexpensive Readily available Easy to use	Caustic Tattooing Can enlarge wound
Electrosurgery (electro-desiccation with mono-terminal and biterminal instruments)	Vessels < 1 mm	Effective Quick	Risk of burn Necrosis Caution with pacemakers Chance of rebleeding
Suture	Vessels > 1 mm	Effective Strong Readily available	Chance of slipping Foreign body reaction to suture Necrosis if too much surrounding tissue is tied
Physical agents (e.g., gelatin sponge)	Superficial or deep wounds Oozing wounds	Easy to use Convenient	Foreign body reaction Can potentiate infection Expensive (some)

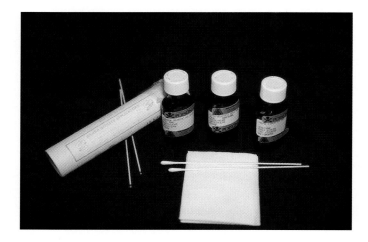

FIGURE 7-1. Several examples of topical hemostatic agents, including *(left to right)* silver nitrate sticks, aluminum chloride, trichloroacetic acid, and phenol.

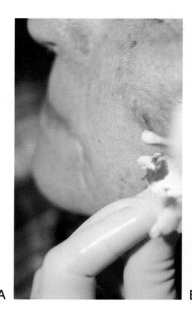

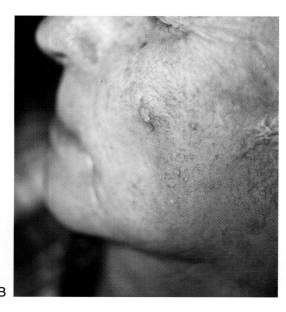

FIGURE 7-2. Use of aluminum chloride demonstrating *(A)* application to a dry wound bed and *(B)* final result.

A

B

Trichloroacetic acid and dichloroacetic acid are available in strengths of 30% to 50% in alcohol. These are excellent hemostatic agents that are readily available and easy to use but will enlarge the original wound as they coagulate surrounding epithelium.

Phenol in strengths of 50% to 100% is readily available and effective. However, it is seldom used because of its potent ability to coagulate intact epidermis.

ELECTROSURGERY

The term *electrosurgery* includes electrocautery and high-frequency electrosurgery. Possible mechanisms of hemostasis include shrinkage of vessel walls, welding of vessel walls, or intravascular thrombic occlusion.

Electrocautery passes no current to the patient. Heated metal is brought into contact with tissue, and heat only is transferred, resulting in tissue desiccation, coagulation, or necrosis. The tip of the electrocautery unit (usually platinum) is heated to a bright red color (white is too destructive) and is applied directly to the vessel. Since no current passes through the patient, electrocautery is safe to use in patients with pacemakers. It is also effective in a bloody surgical field. (See Chapter 6 for further discussion of electrosurgery.)

High-frequency electrosurgery uses alternating current to destroy, cut, or coagulate tissue. Alternating current actually passes through the patient, generates heat through tissue resistance, and can be used to coagulate blood vessels (Fig. 7–3). Coaptive vessel coagulation (biterminal electrocoagulation) involves use of a hemostat or forceps to isolate the vessel and compress it. The active electrode is touched to the instrument, conducting its current to its tips and then to the vessel, where heat is produced and the vessel is sealed. Appropriate heat application results in tissue retraction and white color change, whereas excess heat results in a popping sound and ultimately necrosis. Minimal tissue should be grabbed by the instrument. With monoterminal electrodesiccation, the active electrode touches the vessel itself and uses much lower current. For both monoterminal and biterminal electrosurgery the wound bed should be dry and free of blood for electrosurgical current to flow effectively. Cotton swabs can be quite helpful in drying the field (see Table 7–1).

Theoretically, high-frequency electrosurgical devices can interfere with cardiac pacemakers. There are two types of pacemakers: fixed rate (continuous and asynchronous) and demand (noncontinuous and synchronous). The fixed rate pacemakers emit impulses, even if the patient has a physiologic heartbeat. They are resistant to electromagnetic radiation and relatively safe to use with electrosurgery. Demand pacemakers are either triggered or inhibited by heartbeats. The sensing function can pick up electromagnetic radiation from the electrosurgical apparatus and therefore interfere with proper function. Firing may be inhibited because of sensed electromagnetic radiation. Bradycardia or asystole may result if electrical interference is prolonged or potential reprogramming of the pacemaker's rate could occur. The electromagnetic radiation from electrosurgical units usually does not cause a problem because most pacemakers have a metallic covering to

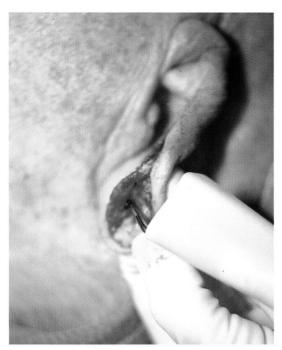

FIGURE 7–3. Electrosurgery used to achieve hemostasis by coagulation of blood vessels.

shield out any stray electromagnetic radiation. Recommendations for patients who have pacemakers include the following:

1. Avoid electrosurgery, if possible. Instead, use electrocautery.
2. Consult with the patient's cardiologist.
3. Place the indifferent electrode as far from the heart but as close to the active electrode as possible.
4. Use short bursts (less than 5 seconds).
5. Do not use the active electrosurgical electrode in skin overlying the heart of a pacemaker patient or in skin overlying the pacemaker power source.

The carbon dioxide or any of the visible light lasers (e.g., argon, copper, krypton) may also be used for hemostasis. Lasers act by delivering intense thermal energy to coagulate and seal small vessels and capillaries (up to 0.5 mm in diameter). They are not effective on larger vessels and are slow. The thermal energy may damage surrounding epithelium if it is not focused directly on the bleeding site. Lasers are expensive, cumbersome, and not readily available, and strict safety measures must be followed when they are used.

MECHANICAL/PHYSICAL AGENTS

Suture material may be used to tie off a bleeding vessel (Case 1, Fig. 7–4A). This is not often required for dermatologic procedures, but for some large vessels there is an increased chance of rebleeding after electrocoagulation. Often bleeding is not readily apparent because of the epinephrine effect of anesthesia and the natural vasoconstric-

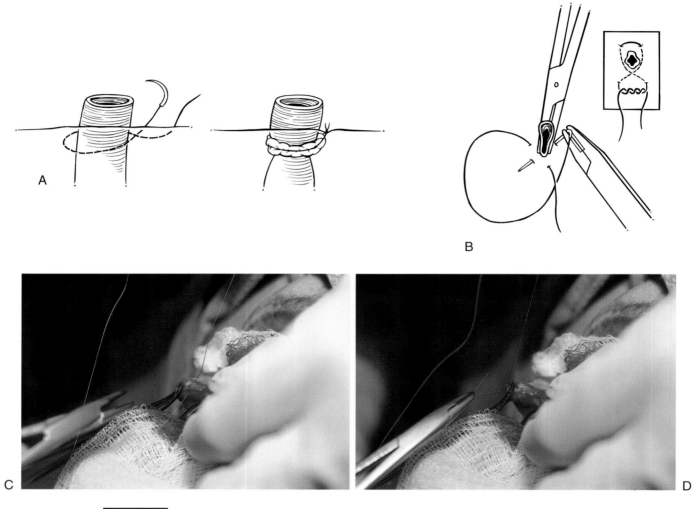

FIGURE 7–4. The use of hemostatic sutures. *A,* A simple vessel tie places a pursestring suture around the vessel and includes a small amount of tissue to keep the suture from slipping off the vessels. *B,* The figure-of-eight suture encircles the vessel with two passes of the needle and applies pressure as it is tied down. *C,* After isolating and clamping the labial artery using a hemostat, a suture is placed beneath the artery to include a small amount of supporting tissue. *D,* The suture is tied around the labial artery.

tion in an injured vessel. A common recommendation is that if a vessel is large enough to be readily identified (usually > 1 mm), it should be ligated (see Table 7–1). The vessel should be visualized and grasped with a hemostat, using care not to crush the surrounding tissue. The vessel is tied using the figure-of-eight stitch, and a small amount of supporting tissue may be included in this stitch (Case 1, see Fig. 7–4*B* through *D*). This would help prevent the knot slipping off the vessel but may increase the amount of devitalized tissue. The amount of suture buried should be minimized, but both ends of the severed artery should be tied, since many arteries can have sufficient backflow to cause significant bleeding or hematoma formation. The newer synthetic absorbable sutures are often used since catgut and chromic sutures have less holding time and cause greater tissue reactivity. Occasionally the

surgeon may choose a monofilament nonabsorbable suture to tie larger vessels.

Hemostatic materials include gelatin sponge, oxidized cellulose, microfibrillar collagen, and topical thrombin (see Table 7–1). These provide a matrix to speed coagulation and encourage natural coagulation factors.

Oxidized cellulose (Oxycel, Surgicel), available as pledgets, gauze pads, and strips, is an absorbable fiber prepared from cellulose. It is placed on the bleeding site and held firmly. It initially swells and fills the cavity, providing internal pressure, and also serves as a meshwork for coagulation by blocking blood vessels. Its acidic properties may cause small vessel contraction and local deposition of fibrin. Advantages include its wide availability and antibacterial properties. It is relatively inexpensive and easy to handle and mold. The material is removed from the tissue by liquefaction and phagocytosis. Its disadvantages are that a foreign body reaction may occur if excess amounts are used. Caution should be used in areas where compression can compromise surrounding structure.

Gelatin sponge (Gelfoam) is an absorbable material made from animal skin gelatin. It is rich in proline and glycine. The gelatin sponge is placed into the wound and can absorb many times its own weight within its meshes. It adheres to bleeding surfaces and facilitates blood clotting through release of thromboplastin, and possibly by concentrating clotting factors within it. Clot and then granulation tissue form within the sponge meshes. When it is applied to the skin, it liquefies in 2 to 5 days. If it is implanted in tissues, it is absorbed in 4 to 6 weeks. When used in punch biopsy sites, it is recommended that an exposed portion be left above the skin surface to serve as a wick. Advantages include its convenience and its reasonable cost. It is absorbable and causes little tissue reaction. Its disadvantages are that it can potentiate infection in a wound colonized by bacteria. Lymphocytic reactions, fibrous tissue reactions, and abscesses have been reported. Also, epithelium-coated gelatin foam cysts can occur.

Microfibrillar collagen (Avitene, Collastat) is a fluffy white material made from bovine collagen broken down into fibrils. It is applied to the wound and held firmly in place while it adheres to bleeding surfaces. Hemostasis is based on interaction of platelets with collagen, leading to platelet aggregation and clot formation. Advantages of microfibrillin collagen are that it is absorbed, usually without a foreign body reaction, within 3 months and can be used for superficial or deep hemostasis. Its disadvantages are that it is expensive and may potentiate infection in contaminated wounds. It also firmly adheres to wet gloves and instruments.

Topical thrombin is of bovine origin and is a powder available in 1,000-, 5,000-, and 10,000-unit vials. It works by direct physiologic activation of fibrinogen to form fibrin and clot. Thrombin is used as a solution or as a powder. It can be diluted to the desired concentration (usually 100 units/mL for dermatologic surgery) in isotonic saline. For profuse bleeding, concentrations as high as 1000 to 2000 units/mL may be required. For oozing wounds, the powder (usually the 1000-unit dosage) is dusted directly on the wound. This may be helpful after procedures such as dermabrasion. Its advantages are that it does not injure the underlying wound bed or adversely affect wound healing. There is no increased incidence of infection or granuloma formation. Its disadvantages are that it is expensive and it can be difficult to handle. If thrombin enters any major blood vessel, extensive intravascular clotting can occur.

There are several other useful techniques for achieving hemostasis in dermatologic surgery. Pressure alone can collapse blood vessels, allowing platelet aggregation and clotting to occur. It often can be sufficient to achieve complete hemostasis but may require considerable time. Firm direct pressure on the site of bleeding for 5 minutes can usually control brisk or persistent oozing. Bone wax may be used to control bleeding in bone. It is made of 90% refined beeswax. It is available in stick form and is pressed into the bone at the bleeding site acting as a tamponade. Its advantages are that it is readily available, inexpensive, and easy to store and use. However, foreign

body and inflammatory reactions are possible, and it may be a nidus for infection or interfere with formation of new bone. Acrylates are rapidly polymerizing plastics. They are available in drop or spray and may be used in hemostasis or tissue gluing. They polymerize, adhere to the tissue, and mechanically obstruct bleeding and fluid drainage. They are eventually resorbed. They are relatively inert but are difficult to handle and have been associated with tissue inflammation and toxicity.

PREOPERATIVE ASSESSMENT

A good personal and family history is essential to detect potential problems with hemostasis that might occur during dermatologic surgery. Patients should be asked if they have a history of bleeding problems or an inherited clotting disorder. Patients with severe nutritional deficits or liver disease may be at risk for bleeding because of a lack of factors in the clotting cascade. A history of anticoagulation or use of aspirin or nonsteroidal anti-inflammatory drugs is vital and needs to be asked of each patient. If something in the history suggests a bleeding problem, a screening panel could be considered. This would include a complete blood cell count with platelet count, a bleeding time to check platelet function, a clotting time, and a prothrombin time and partial thromboplastin time (Table 7–2). The patient should provide a list of all medications, including over-the-counter products, because aspirin is contained in many allergy, headache, and cold remedies. The patient should specifically be asked about use of aspirin, ibuprofen, and nonsteroidal agents (Table 7–3), as well as warfarin (Coumadin). It is recommended that the patient avoid alcohol in the perioperative period because it is a potent vasodilator.

Patients on anticoagulants require special attention to prevent bleeding during the perioperative period. Warfarin causes a tendency for late bleeding at the time of clot retraction and organization. The risk of life-threatening bleeding is quite small. Warfarin depletes the reduced form of vitamin K and the activity of vitamin K–dependent coagulation proteins II, VII, IX, and X. Patients who take warfarin can be divided into a high-risk group, meaning those at high risk for thromboembolic complications (e.g., hypercoagulable states and prosthetic heart valves), and a low-risk group, including those patients taking warfarin as treatment for deep venous thrombosis, stroke prevention, atrial fibrillation, or after myocardial infarction.

TABLE 7–2. Hemostasis: Preoperative Assessment

1. Personal or family history of bleeding problems
2. History of liver disease or poor nutritional status
3. Medication history
   a. Aspirin
   b. Nonsteroidal anti-inflammatory agents
   c. Anticoagulants
4. If history is suggestive of bleeding problem, the following laboratory tests should be done:
   a. Complete blood cell count with platelets
   b. Bleeding time
   c. Prothrombin time and partial thromboplastin time

TABLE 7–3. Characteristics of Anticoagulants

Anticoagulant	Site of Effect	When to Expect Bleeding	When to Stop Medication Before Surgery
Aspirin	Platelets (irreversible)	During surgery	10 days
Nonsteroidal anti-inflammatory agents	Platelets (reversible)	During surgery	1 day
Warfarin (Coumadin)	Vitamin K–dependent clotting factors II, VII, IX, and X	After surgery	1 week in high-risk patients 3 days in low-risk patients
Heparin	Antithrombin III	During surgery	4–6 hours

Usually warfarin can be continued without a major risk to the patient, although there is a risk of delayed postoperative bleeding and hematoma formation. In these patients it is important to pay special attention to intraoperative hemostasis. It is also possible to check a prothrombin time 1 to 2 weeks before the surgery and adjust the warfarin dose to the lowest therapeutic dose. In some cases it may be necessary to stop the warfarin, such as with scalp surgery or in a patient with elevated blood pressure. If it is a high-risk patient, the warfarin should be stopped 1 week before surgery. Full-dose subcutaneous heparin should then be instituted. On the day of surgery, low-dose heparin of 5000 units twice daily should be given. After surgery, full-dose heparin may be resumed and warfarin should be restarted. The heparin should be stopped when full anticoagulation from warfarin is achieved. For the low-risk patient, the warfarin may be stopped 3 days before surgery and the regular preoperative dose may be resumed 1 day postoperatively. The patient's primary physician should be consulted before discontinuing or adjusting the warfarin dose.

Aspirin is the single largest cause of operative bleeding in cutaneous surgery. There is no group of high-risk patients in whom life-threatening complications would develop if it were stopped temporarily. Aspirin causes an irreversible inhibition of cyclo-oxygenase and thromboxane synthesis by platelets. Platelet activation and secretion of platelet products are decreased, leading to depressed primary hemostasis by platelet plug formation. The effect of aspirin lasts the life span of the platelet (7 to 10 days). One baby aspirin is sufficient to inhibit all platelet function. The bleeding associated with aspirin use is excessive oozing from all vessels. This is an immediate problem. Once hemostasis has been achieved and the platelet aggregation step passed, there should not be further bleeding unless trauma dislodges the clot (see Table 7–3).

The activity of many nonsteroidal anti-inflammatory drugs is through reversible inhibition of cyclo-oxygenase and thromboxane synthesis, ultimately resulting in a reduction of thromboxane. There is less clinical effect on hemostasis because of the reversibility. The effect occurs only when the nonsteroidal drug is in the circulation and therefore depends on the half-life of the drug.

Recommendations regarding aspirin are to stop all aspirin products 7 to 10 days before surgery. The aspirin can be resumed 1 day after surgery. If possible, acetaminophen should be used for analgesia during the postoperative period. In general, nonsteroidal anti-inflammatory drugs should be stopped 24 hours before surgery and resumed the following day. This may vary with the particular drug. For example, piroxicam has a longer half-life and requires stopping the medication 2 to 4 days before surgery. The primary physician should be consulted if aspirin is being used as a platelet inhibitor.

Several intraoperative techniques should be used to achieve hemostasis and minimize postoperative bleeding. A blood vessel that is cut during surgery will continue to leak if it is only nicked. Complete transection of the vessel is required to allow it to contract and retract. Adequate wound exposure is also necessary to identify all bleeding sites. This is especially important in the scalp where blood vessels may be held open by the rich fibrostroma and retract while they are still bleeding. Suction is quite helpful to visualize bleeding points during cutaneous surgery. Most suction machines consist of flexible disposable tubing with a small tip. An eyedropper can be used as a tip for suction during dermatologic surgery (Fig. 7–5). The tip should be placed into the wound to evacuate blood and help pinpoint specific bleeding vessels. Cotton-tipped swabs and skin hooks can be quite helpful in identifying bleeding sites. The swabs can be used to apply pressure, hold wound edges apart, and absorb blood. Skin hooks help provide visualization beneath undermined margins. In addition, the importance of good lighting cannot be overemphasized. Meticulous hemostasis during the procedure is important to prevent bleeding during and after surgery.

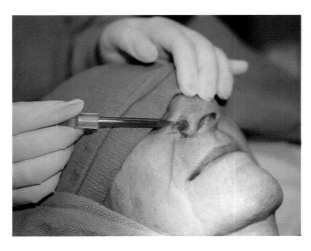

FIGURE 7–5. Suction being used to control bleeding.

POSTOPERATIVE COMPLICATIONS

Postoperative bleeding can occur after dermatologic surgery. The epinephrine used with local anesthesia provides vasoconstriction and helps control bleeding during the procedure. As this effect wears off, the vessels dilate and may bleed. Insecure vessel ligation, clot retraction, or trauma to the wound may also produce bleeding. For these reasons, a pressure dressing is often applied for the first 24 hours after surgery. These consist of multiple layers of dressing, with the lowest layer adherent to underlying tissue. A bulky absorbent layer of gauze, cotton, or sponge is then covered by a stretchable outer layer, often of elastic tape or stretchable gauze (Kerlix). Care must be taken that the bandage is not too constrictive as to cause ischemia. This occurs if the dressing pressure exceeds intravascular hydrostatic pressure. Nonpressure dressings still exert minimal pressure on the wound and may be helpful with postoperative hemostasis. These consist of a nonadherent contact layer (Telfa), an absorbent layer (eye pad, cotton, gauze), and an outer wrap of gauze and paper tape.

A patient having postoperative bleeding should lie down, remove the saturated dressing, and, using a clean dressing, apply steady pressure directly to the wound for 15 to 20 minutes without lifting the dressing to peek at the wound. If the bleeding is not controlled with direct pressure, the surgeon should meet the patient in the surgeon's office or in the emergency room. The patient should be warned preoperatively about the possibility of hemorrhage into the wound and surrounding skin, leading to bruising. This may be especially prominent around the eyes.

Management of Hematomas

June K. Robinson

Hematomas can be either expanding, requiring reoperation with opening the initial incision for evacuation (Case 2, Fig. 7–6), or small and organized, requiring stab incision and drainage or aspiration of the serous material of a more organized hematoma with an 18-gauge needle (Case 3, Fig. 7–7). Most hematomas occur within 24 hours of the procedure, but they can occur many days after the operation. Exertional activity that elevates blood pressure can cause bleeding and should be avoided for the first week after surgery.

Large expanding hematomas are the most common in the immediate postoperative period as the vasoconstriction of the local anesthetic dissipates. Onset is well known to the patient, who experiences sudden and acute pain that is followed by unilateral firm swelling. This pain is usually not responsive to the usual postoperative pain control with acetaminophen with codeine. Failure or delay in evacuating an expanding hematoma risks vascular compromise of the surgical site and eventually of the patient.

After the clot is removed, the wound is irrigated and any bleeding vessels are ligated (see Fig. 7–6F). Since this usually occurs within 24 hours after surgery, the wound edges are closed. Removal of the hematoma results in prompt pain relief. Extensive ecchymosis and prolonged edema generally follow treatment of a hematoma (see Fig. 7–6G). The patient should be warned about this at the time the hematoma is evacuated and reassured that the final result should not be changed by the episode of bleeding. The patient's condition is observed closely until healing is complete.

The more common hematoma, an organized hematoma, formed after surgery is small, is not painful, and is not even evident until the general postoperative swelling subsides in 5 to 7 days after surgery. It appears as an area of firmness or a subcutaneous nodule with slight skin surface irregularity. An effort should be made to evacuate the hematoma by either stab incision with a No. 11 blade away from the incision line or by aspiration when it liquefies at postoperative day 7 to 14 (Case 3, Fig. 7–7). After the fourteenth day, the clot is so fibrotic that removal is not possible (Case 4, Fig. 7–8). Fibrotic organized hematomas can be managed with warm compresses and intralesional injections of very low doses of corticosteroids.

Organized hematomas delay wound healing and predispose the wound to develop infection or dehiscence. If wounds are opened to evacuate organized hematomas after 4 days, then healing proceeds by second intention. A second surgical repair may be performed to improve the appearance of the resulting scar. This second procedure usually is delayed for 10 to 12 months after wound healing; however, if the scar impairs function then a repair can be performed at 4 to 6 months.

A wound that undergoes dehiscence and is not contaminated may be resutured within 24 hours of separation if the base is viable and the wound edges are re-excised. Although the use of prophylactic antibiotics is controversial,

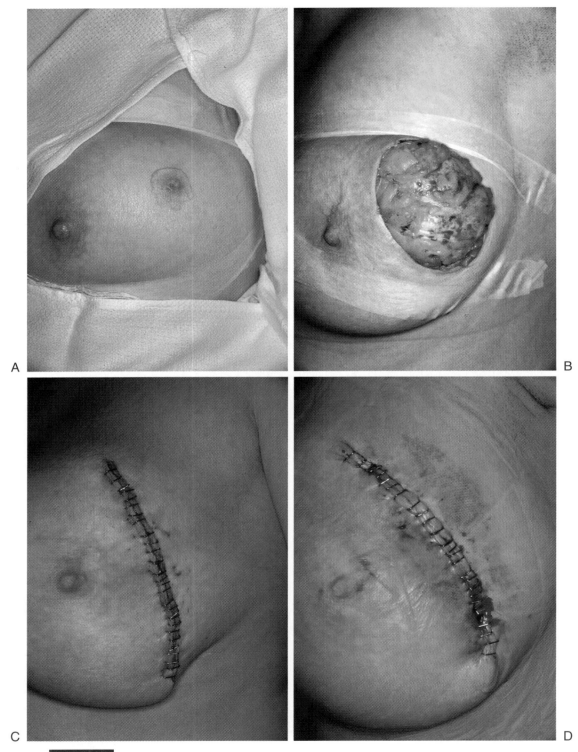

CASE 2

FIGURE 7–6. Complication: expanding hematoma. *A,* Preoperative appearance of a dermatofibrosarcoma protuberans of the left breast. The palpable border is marked with mercurochrome. *B,* After resection with Mohs' micrographic surgery with local anesthesia with 1% lidocaine with epinephrine 1 : 100,000, coagulation of bleeding vessels was achieved with point bipolar grounded electrocoagulation. *C,* The wound was closed with buried sutures and skin staples. *D,* The patient was awakened from sleep within 10 hours after surgery by severe acute pain radiating into her shoulder. The breast was firm and painful to her touch. Blood stained the bandage, and the condition did not improve after she applied 20 minutes of steady pressure. When the dressing was removed under sterile conditions by the surgeon, fresh blood drained from the inferior aspect of the wound.

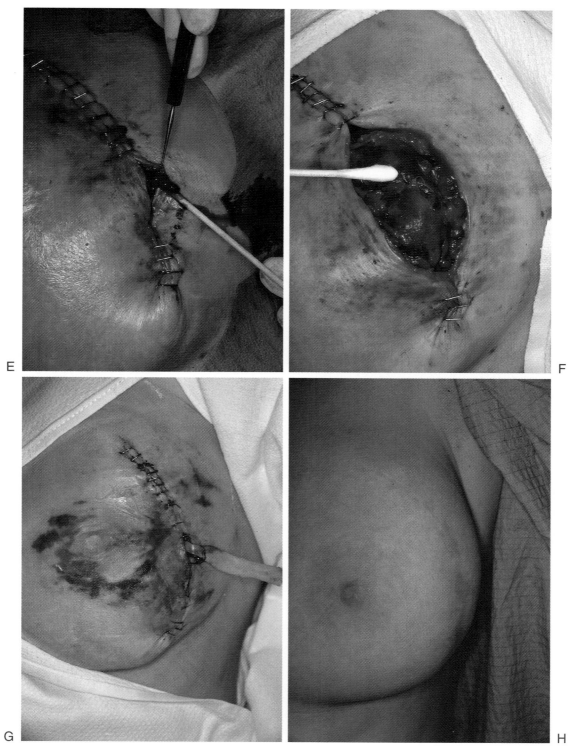

Continued on page 76

◄ **FIGURE 7–6** *Continued E,* With the use of local anesthesia with 1% plain lidocaine, staples overlying the area of draining blood were removed. Gelatinous masses of coagulated blood as well as bright red blood oozed from the wound 12 hours after surgery. *F,* More staples were removed to see the base of the wound, which was irrigated to remove all clots. The bleeding artery was identified, clamped, and ligated. The cotton swab points to the suture ligature. The wound was closed and a drain was placed.

Because the evacuation of the hematoma occurred within 24 hours of the initial surgery, it was not necessary to trim the wound edges. The evacuation procedure was done under sterile conditions.

It is likely that one of the vessels coagulated but not ligated during the initial procedure dilated as the local tissue epinephrine dissipated. The coagulum was dislodged by the force of blood in the dilated artery, and the patient experienced rapid onset of swelling and pain. The breast area is not conducive to postoperative pressure dressings. The patient wore a sports-type bra after surgery to apply pressure but took it off to go to bed. Bleeding apparently started after going to bed since she awakened with pain. *G,* Thirty-six hours after the initial surgery and 24 hours after evacuation of the expanding hematoma, there was no fresh blood draining from the wound. The drain was removed. Drains offer a track for infection from skin organisms to the depth of the wound; thus, they are removed rapidly. Wound healing around the site of the drain proceeded more slowly than the rest of the incision line. Staples and sutures were removed from the rest of the incision 7 days after surgery. *H,* Three years after surgery, the wound is slightly spread at the site of insertion of the drain. There is no recurrence of the tumor and the patient has an excellent final result.

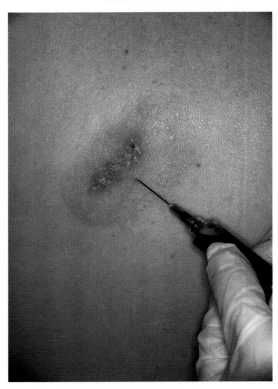

CASE 3

FIGURE 7–7. Liquefied hematoma. Twelve days after excision of a lipoma of the back the liquefied hematoma is aspirated with an 18-gauge needle.

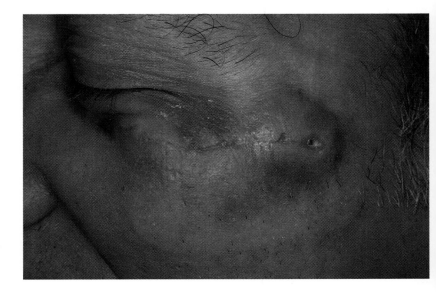

CASE 4

FIGURE 7–8. Fibrotic hematoma. Fourteen days after excisional surgery to remove a nevus of the cheek, the hematoma under both ends of the incision line is organized. An attempt to "milk" the large hematoma from the lateral end of the incision failed.

many physicians will use an antibiotic to cover *Staphylococcus aureus* in wounds with organized hematomas or dehiscence.

Selected Readings

1. Barr RJ, Alpern KS, Jay S. Histiocytic reaction associated with topical aluminum chloride (Drysol reaction). J Dermatol Surg Oncol 1993;19:1017–1021.
2. Bennett RG. Fundamentals of Cutaneous Surgery. St. Louis: CV Mosby, 1988:336–337, 379–382, 564–565, 583.
3. Goldsmith SM, Leshin B, Owen J. Management of patients taking anticoagulants and platelet inhibitors prior to dermatologic surgery. J Dermatol Surg Oncol 1993;19:578–581.
4. Grabski WJ, Salasche SJ. Hemostatic techniques and materials. In: Wheeland RG, ed. Cutaneous Surgery. Philadelphia: WB Saunders Co., 1994:189–198.
5. Insel PA. Analgesic-antipyretics and anti-inflammatory agents. In: Gilman AG, et al., eds. Goodman and Gilman's The Pharmacological Basis of Therapeutics, 8th ed. New York: Pergamon Press, 1990:638–681.
6. Larson PO. Topical hemostatic agents for dermatologic surgery. J Dermatol Surg Oncol 1988;14:623–632.
7. Larson PO. Surgical complications. In: Mikhail GR, ed. Mohs Micrographic Surgery. Philadelphia: WB Saunders Co., 1991:193–196.
8. Maloney ME. Management of surgical complications and suboptimal results. In: Wheeland RG, ed. Cutaneous Surgery. Philadelphia: WB Saunders Co., 1994:921–934.
9. Stegman SJ, Tromovitch TA, Glogau RG. Basics of Dermatologic Surgery. Chicago: Year Book Medical Publishers, 1982:3–6, 32–35.

chapter 8

Technique of Suture Placement

JUNE K. ROBINSON

The goal of skin closure is to create a mature scar that is narrow and level with the surrounding skin and has minimal stitch marks. This can be achieved by careful reapproximation of tissues. The underlying muscles should be reapproximated to muscle, fat to fat, and skin to skin. The closure is done in layers to eliminate dead space. Tension is distributed throughout the wound but especially in the deeper layers to relieve stress on the surface of the skin. Deep sutures should hold the epithelium in approximation with slight eversion of the wound edges. A number of techniques of suture placement are used to achieve this goal.

Suture materials are classified as absorbable and nonabsorbable. The absorbable materials are most often used in the deep layers and are buried. Some commonly used absorbable sutures listed in increasing order of strength and durability before absorption are plain catgut, chromic catgut, Dexon, and coated Vicryl. Permanent sutures for use in the skin are either braided or monofilament materials. Braided materials such as silk lie flat when moist but lack the tensile strength of monofilament sutures such as nylon and Prolene.

Taping the wound after suturing is useful in relieving tension from the sutures and to act as a splint in limiting motion about the area. Use of these wound tapes (e.g., Steri-Strips, Clearon) may be continued for several weeks after sutures are removed.

"NO TOUCH" SUTURING TECHNIQUE

Mounting Needle in the Needle Holder

Needles should be grasped in an area one fourth to one half of the distance from the swaged area to the point (Fig. 8–1). The needle should be placed securely in the tip of

the needle holder and passed to assistants on the needle holder (Fig. 8–2). Once the needle passes through the wound and is contaminated with blood, the gloved nondominant hand of the surgeon can no longer be used to re-mount the needle. Similarly, the nondominant hand of the surgeon should not enter the field to stabilize tissue in placing sutures. This adaptation of previously used common techniques in suturing was necessitated by recognition of the number of inadvertent glove tears and piercings in the forefinger and thumb of the nondominant hand. Use of the "no touch" suture technique is meant to decrease the risk of human immunodeficiency virus infection by accidental needlestick injury. It is both time consuming and awkward to learn and perform for those who are accustomed to re-mounting the needle in the needle holder with the nondominant hand. Given the risks, it would seem prudent to practice this technique of handling sutures and needles.

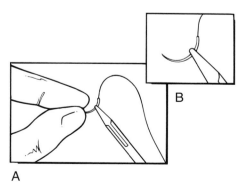

FIGURE 8–1. *A*, Needles are grasped in an area one fourth to one half of the distance from the swaged area to the point. Placement near to or on the swaged area should be avoided. *B*, The needle is placed securely at the tip of the needle holder jaws.

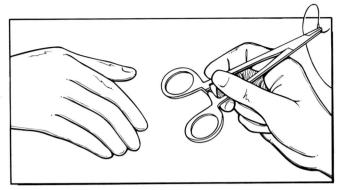

FIGURE 8–2. When the needle holder with the needle is passed to the surgeon, the needle points in the direction in which it will start to be used without need for readjustment. Similarly, needles are returned to the assistant mounted in the jaws of a needle holder.

The nondominant hand of the surgeon holds a smooth-tipped forceps that is used to stabilize the tip of the needle until it can be firmly grasped with the needle holder (Fig. 8–3). The needle holder is then used to pull the suture through. If the tissues are not approximated by buried subcutaneous sutures, then the needle will need to be re-mounted in going from one side of the wound to the other. Re-mounting is done by holding the needle with the smooth-tipped forceps and placing the needle holder at the proper position on the needle (Fig. 8–4).

Instrument Ties

After the suture is in place in the tissue, then the end of the suture with the needle is placed in the field out of the path of the hands and instruments. The non–needle-bearing or free end of the suture is pulled through the wound until it is about 2 cm from the surface of the skin. The needle-

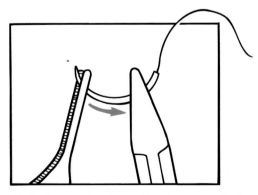

FIGURE 8–4. Re-mounting the needle. If the wound edges are not approximated by buried subcutaneous sutures, then the needle will be exiting at the depth of the wound on one side, and re-mounted in the needle holder to enter the depth of the wound on the opposite side. Avoid using the needle to bridge tissues in suturing. The smooth-tipped forceps holds the needle while the needle holder moves back along the curvature of the needle to the proper location. (*Arrow* indicates the motion of the needle holder along the needle.)

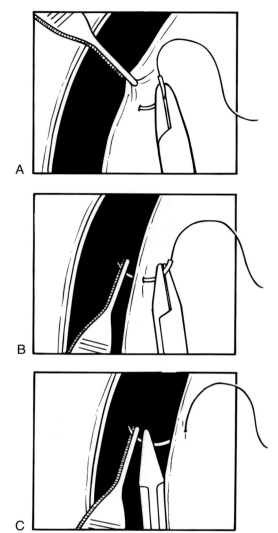

FIGURE 8–3. Passing the needle through the skin using the "no touch" technique. *A*, The needle is inserted at a 90-degree angle to the skin surface for an interrupted suture. The wound edge is stabilized by the forceps that is held in the nondominant hand. In placing the needle in tissue, force is applied in the direction following the curve of the needle. *B*, While using the forceps to grasp the needle coming through the depth of the wound, the needle holder continues the motion. *C*, As the needle emerges farther, release the needle holder and use it to pull through on the needle. Do not damage taper points or cutting edges when using the needle holder to pull the needle out through the tissue. The needle should be grasped as far back as possible.

bearing end of the suture is grasped in the nondominant hand. It is stabilized far away from the needle. The fixed or needle-bearing end is wrapped twice in clockwise revolutions (Fig. 8–5*A*) around the closed but not clamped jaws of the needle holder.

The free end is grasped with the needle holder and pulled through the loop with the instrument (Fig 8–5*B*). The half-hitch is set with the segments uncrossed (Fig. 8–5*C*). Then the mirror-image half-hitch is formed in the same way, but the fixed segment is wrapped counterclockwise around the jaws of the instrument (Fig. 8–5*D*).

The knot is squared by crossing the hands to the opposite side.

BURIED SUBCUTANEOUS SUTURES

Since most wounds are closed under tension, a subcuticular closure is helpful in relieving that tension from the cutaneous sutures. Some locations have a sebaceous quality of the skin that tends to particularly accentuate suture tract marks from interrupted sutures and tends to have inverted wound edges (e.g., chin, upper lip, and lower one third of the nose). Buried sutures force the wound edges into eversion and approximate the wound without stepping of the edges. At the junction of the cosmetic units of the nose and the upper lip, it is possible to close the wound with buried subcutaneous sutures and use minimal or no interrupted sutures, to decrease the chances of suture tract marks.

In areas with a great deal of tension on the incision line, buried sutures cannot prevent later spreading of the scar (e.g., trunk, deltoid area of the arm). Since these buried sutures are left in the underlying tissue for an indefinite period of time until absorbed, the tension on the skin is alleviated for a time beyond when the skin sutures are normally removed, thus preventing "railroad track" marks in addition to spread scars on the trunk. In locations under a great deal of tension, buried sutures may be stacked at different levels (e.g., fat and deep dermis with one loop mostly in the subcutaneous fat with a small portion in the dermis and a second loop mostly in the dermis). A portion of a dermal-subdermal suture needs to be placed in the dermis to give sufficient strength to the closure.

In placing a buried dermal or dermal-subdermal suture the stitch begins deep in the wound and passes to the superficial aspect of one side of the wound (Fig. 8–6, point 1). Then the needle is re-mounted and enters at the superficial aspect of the other side of the wound and exits in the deep part of the wound (see Fig. 8–6, point 2). The suture does not pierce the epidermis. When tied, the knot is buried deep in the wound. Thus the knot is not in the way of placement of epidermal sutures and is less likely to be extruded later ("spitting"). In tying these subcutaneous sutures, it is sometimes necessary to use a gentle rocking motion to get the edges opposed and to tie in the long axis of the depth of the wound and not "up over the edges" of the wound. Placing these sutures requires large "bites" of tissue lateral to the wound edge. The greater the amount of lateral dermal tissue included in the path of the needle, the closer and more everted the wound edges.

Another technique of buried suture placement is to place three to four subcutaneous sutures across the wound and then hold the ends in clamps until all are tied down (Fig. 8–7).

Lastly, a pursestring suture can be used to close dead space in the wound (Fig. 8–8). For instance, after removal of a lipoma, two or more pursestring sutures can be stacked over one another to close the dead space. A half-pursestring–half-vertical buried subcutaneous suture can be used in wounds with unequal thickness of dermis and subcutaneous sutures. For example, insetting a cheek advancement flap under the sill of the nose is achieved by first placing a standard vertical buried subcutaneous suture on the flap and then horizontally rolling in a pursestring under the sill of the nose (Fig. 8–9). This purposeful inequality of the wound heights re-creates the melolabial (nasolabial) fold.

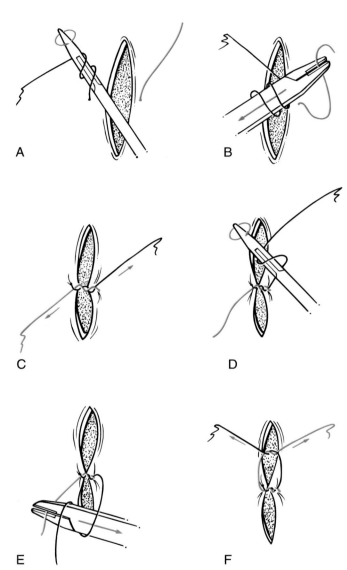

A

B

C

D

E

F

FIGURE 8–5. Instrument tie and square knot. *A,* The needle-bearing end (black suture) is wrapped twice around the needle holder by turning the needle holder. The needle is maintained in the field but out of the motion of the hands. Turning the needle holder rather than wrapping the needle-bearing end of the suture around the needle holder minimizes the free motion of the needle in the field. *B,* The free end of the suture (red suture) is pulled through the loops. *C,* The half-hitch is set with the segments uncrossed. *D,* A counterclockwise turn of the needle holder creates a loop of suture. *E,* The free end is grasped. *F,* The knot is squared by crossing the hands to the opposite side. Red arrows indicate motion of needle holder and tension on the suture.

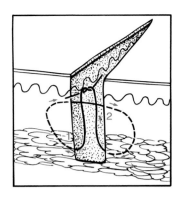

FIGURE 8–6. Buried subcutaneous suture: the vertical dermal-subcutaneous suture. Entry points for the needle are numbered in red. The suture begins in the depth of the wound and rolls toward the surface, reenters the opposite side of the wound in the dermis, and rolls deep. Deep-superficial, superficial-deep is chanted while placing this suture with a buried knot. The knot is tied along the long axis of the incision.

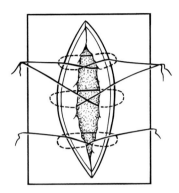

FIGURE 8–7. Multiple, buried subcutaneous sutures may be placed in the depth of a wound under a lot of tension. The free suture ends are held by clamps to keep them from tangling. The sutures are serially tied down rapidly.

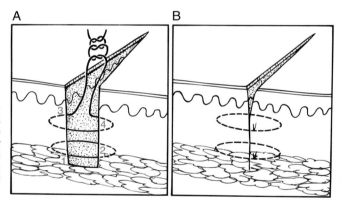

FIGURE 8–8. Buried subcutaneous suture. *A*, Pursestring sutures are stacked over one another or placed singly to close dead space in a wound (e.g., after cyst removal). Needle entry points are indicated by red numbers. *B*, Pursestring sutures are parallel to the skin surface throughout their course.

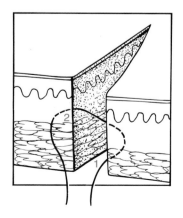

FIGURE 8–9. Buried subcutaneous suture: half vertical–half pursestring. Wound edges of unequal height are created by starting a vertical, buried subcutaneous suture on the thicker side with the greater dermal depth and insetting the thinner side with a horizontally placed pursestring suture. This purposeful inequality of wound heights re-creates the melolabial fold in the cheek advancement flap to reconstruct the upper lip (see Chapter 10). Red numbers indicate entry points of the needle.

INTERRUPTED SUTURE

The proper path of a simple interrupted suture enters the skin at an angle 90 degrees to the skin surface (Fig. 8–10A, point 1) and travels obliquely as it descends into the depth of the wound. The needle exits the wound in the center and is repositioned on the needle holder to reenter the wound on the opposite side (Fig. 8–10A, point 2). The aim is to make the suture loop broader at the base than at the skin surface, thus ensuring eversion of the wound edges. Wound eversion counteracts the eventual scar contraction, which will pull the incision downward toward the depths of the wound (Fig. 8–10B). Knots are positioned to the side of the wound. Knots are also placed away from structures that will be irritated by rubbing against the knot in the process of daily functions (e.g., eyelid, lips, nostril). If possible, knots on the skin surface are not placed in areas with high risk of contamination (e.g., mouth). If a knot is necessary on a weight-bearing surface of the foot or a mucous membrane such as the lining of the eye or mouth, then silk suture is used. The silk suture knot is kept moist with ointment and lies flat without abrading. In the final analysis, knots are placed where it is easiest for the surgeon to tie them but sometimes a variety of locations are available.

If the needle does not exit the wound edge in the middle of the wound before entering the opposite side, there is a good chance that the amount of tissue encompassed by the needle will be more shallow than on the opposite side. This results in uneven skin edges. If the needle becomes bent during suture placement, the surgeon is using too much force to direct the needle into a straight line rather

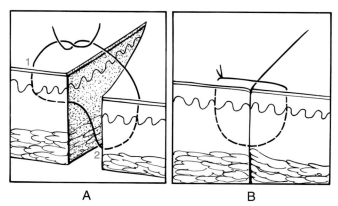

FIGURE 8–11. *A,* Modified interrupted suture for wound of unequal height. Red numbers indicate entry points of the needle. *B,* Shallower depth of suture placed on higher side of the wound and deeper placement on the depressed side of the wound.

than carrying the needle holder by hand and wrist motions through an arc.

When wound edges of unequal height are apposed, a variation of interrupted sutures can equalize the edges. A shallower "bite" is taken on the higher side of the wound, and a deeper bite on the lower side (Fig. 8–11).

The main advantage of the interrupted suture is the ability to adjust wound heights and the tension at each segment of the wound. In general, the more tension on a wound, the closer the sutures should be placed; however, very closely spaced sutures (2 mm apart) result in destruction of tissue at the edge of the wound and decreased wound healing. The spacing between sutures is a function of the tension on the wound edge. In an elliptical (fusiform) excision, the tension is greatest in the center and less at the ends. Spacing of sutures may not have even intervals between sutures along the total length of the incision.

VERTICAL MATTRESS SUTURE

The vertical mattress suture may be placed in wounds under great tension to stretch the skin. It is used as a retention suture, to relieve tension while placing other sutures such as buried subcutaneous sutures and interrupted skin sutures. When used as a retention suture, the vertical mattress suture is removed at the end of surgery.

The vertical mattress suture is placed before simple interrupted sutures. It is not tied so tight as to achieve complete coaptation. The mattress suture produces eversion and approximation of wound edges, but the simple interrupted suture remains the final touch (Fig. 8–12).

Placing this suture requires four steps with resetting the needle in the needle holder each time. The deeper and wider sutures are placed symmetrically on either side of the wound and then the superficial ones that are closer to the incision line are placed.

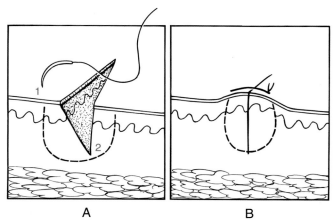

FIGURE 8–10. *A* and *B,* Basic technique: interrupted suture. The needle enters the epidermis (1) and picks up dermis and perhaps some fat depending on the level of undermining. It then enters the opposite of the wound in the depth of the wound at an angle of 90 degrees (2). The exit points on the skin should be equidistant from the incision. The knot is positioned to the side of the wound. The suture loop through the skin is described as flask shaped with a broad base and narrower top. Wound edges are everted to counteract the eventual scar contraction, which will pull the surface downward.

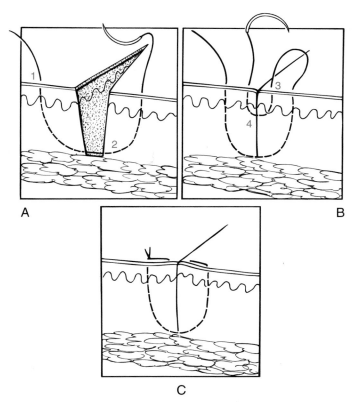

A

B

C

FIGURE 8–12. Vertical mattress suture. *A*, A widely spaced interrupted suture is placed with great depth (1 and 2). *B*, Then the needle is turned back toward the incision line and inserted closer to the incision line with a shallow pass that everts the wound edges. Red numbers indicate entry points of the needle. *C*, The knot lies on one side and cannot be repositioned. Removal of this suture after a week may require insertion of delicate scissor tips below the skin surface to snip one "arm" of the suture.

HORIZONTAL MATTRESS SUTURE

There are four entry points through the skin for this mattress suture, which places pressure parallel to the wound edges (Fig. 8–13). It can be used to enhance hemostasis in wounds with excessive bleeding. Because the suture will cut into the skin, it is padded by placing a bolster of suture packing material between the suture and the skin surface before tying it. This suture is removed as early as is possible.

A modification of this suture is the half-buried horizontal mattress suture that decreases the risk of track marks and is used to even edges of unequal height (Fig. 8–14) and inset the tips of flaps (Fig. 8–15). In flaps such as the A to T, the tip has an acute angle that needs to be made equal in height and apposed to the opposite wound edge (see Chapter 10).

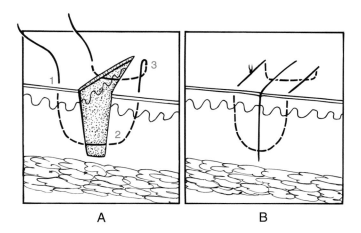

A

B

FIGURE 8–13. Horizontal mattress sutures. *A*, The four needle entry points are numbered in red. *B*, The long arms of the suture are parallel to the incision, putting pressure on the wound edges to control bleeding.

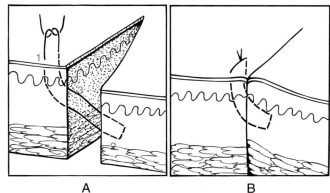

A

B

FIGURE 8–14. Half-buried horizontal mattress suture. *A*, The entry (2) and exit points of the needle on the buried segment of the suture are entirely dermal and parallel to the surface of the skin. *B*, The suture equalizes uneven edges.

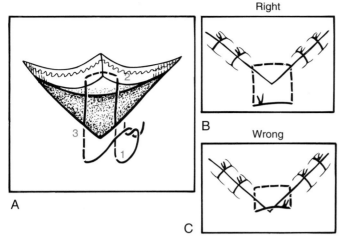

FIGURE 8–15. *A* to *C,* Half-buried horizontal mattress as a tip suture. The suture starts as an interrupted suture (1) and then enters the flap tip at the dermis (2) where it rolls through the dermis parallel to the skin surface and exits in the dermis. It is completed (3) as an interrupted suture.

RUNNING SUBCUTICULAR SUTURE

The running subcuticular (intradermal) suture removes almost all possibility of leaving suture marks; thus, it may remain in place for long periods of time. Some patients have a tendency to pick at sutures (e.g., infirm elderly or pediatric patients). In situations in which the reliability of the patient to return for suture removal or to not manipu-

late sutures is questioned, the running subcuticular suture is ideal.

If wound edges are of equal thickness and have been approximated by subcutaneous sutures to remove all tension from them, the running intradermal or subcuticular pullout suture is a fast suture to place. It lessens the scar potential and may be left in place longer than interrupted sutures. This closure should only be performed with monofilament nylon sutures. Other suture materials will swell so much that they become difficult to remove. It is technically the most difficult to master but offers an excellent cosmetic result in appropriate instances.

After inserting the needle perpendicularly to the skin 3 mm from the tip of the incision, it should be brought out into the center of the incision. Then the needle is mounted in a needle holder in a manner suitable to take small 2- to 4-mm rolling bites of a wound edge in the mid dermis (Fig. 8–16). The wound edge is picked up and everted so that the dermis is visible. The needle moves parallel to the skin surface in the dermis and carries the suture through a 180-degree arc. On emerging from the mid dermis of one wound edge, the needle enters the mid dermis of the other wound edge. The placement of the entrance of the needle on the opposing wound edge is slightly behind the exit of the suture from the other side. This placement forces a bit of extra tissue into the suture line and assists with wound eversion. Sometimes a small gap remains between the wound edges at the completion of the closure, and this should be closed with a superficially placed interrupted suture.

If a continuous running suture is used to close very long wounds, it should be brought out onto the surface of the skin at intervals of 3 to 4 cm to facilitate subsequent removal. The ends are tied over upon themselves in an instrument tie, leaving a small loop (Fig. 8–17; Case 1, Fig. 8–18), or they are taped down to the skin surface. Additional clinical case examples of suture techniques are given in Chapters 9, 10, and 11.

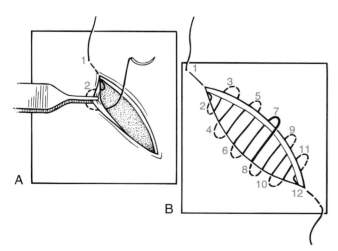

FIGURE 8–16. Running subcuticular suture. *A,* The suture begins as an interrupted one (1). *B,* Then it continues in the manner of a series of small rolling subcutaneous bites of half-buried horizontal mattress sutures (2). If the suture runs longer than 3 cm, it should be brought to the surface with a crossover at the surface. To do this surface crossover, the needle comes up from the dermis (7) through the surface and goes back through the surface to the dermis on the opposite side of the wound (8). Then it begins again on the opposite side of the wound with a series of half-buried mattress sutures and exists at the apex of the incision in the manner of an interrupted suture.

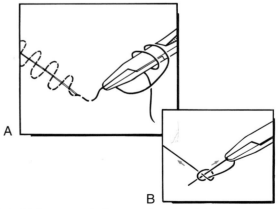

FIGURE 8–17. Instrument tie for a running subcuticular suture. *A,* The long end of the suture is wrapped twice around the needle holder. The needle holder grasps the suture as it emerges from the skin. *B,* The knot slips down the needle holder. Both sides of the knot are tightened by pulling on the loop and the free end. Arrows show motion of pulling. To prevent knot slippage, this maneuver is repeated two more times.

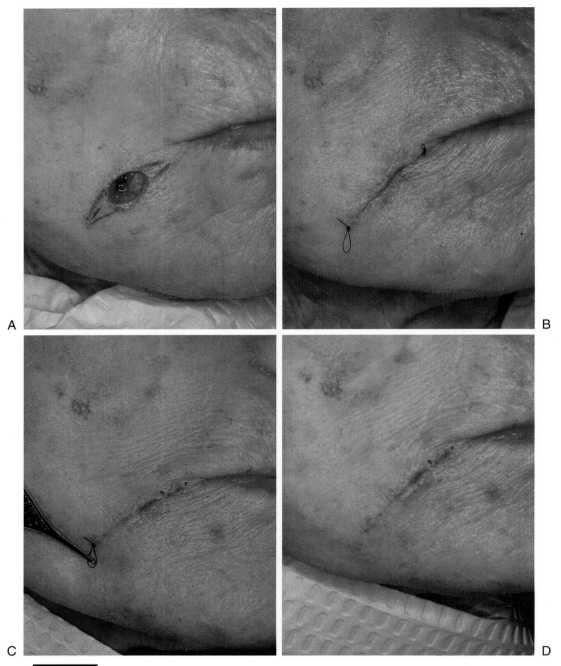

CASE 1

FIGURE 8–18. *A,* A defect of the lower lip and chin and cheek junction is repaired with a closure of unequal lengths to produce a curvilinear incision lying in the wrinkle. *B,* It is closed with three buried subcutaneous sutures and a running subcuticular suture with two small, looped knots. *C,* At suture removal in 1 week, the superior knot is snipped and the lower loop is pulled downward with counterpressure along the incision line. *D,* After suture removal, the wound edges are cleansed daily. Bulky dressings in the postoperative period may cause some drooling at the angle of the mouth. Using this suture allows a minimum of bandages and entry points into the skin and prevents maceration of the wound edges, decreasing the chances of wound infection.

SUTURE REMOVAL

The timing of suture removal is important to the final cosmetic result. If it is done too early, the wound will dehisce; if it is done too late, unsightly stitch marks will result (Table 8–1) (Case 2, Fig. 8–20; Case 4, Fig. 8–22). The surgeon should inspect the wound at appropriate intervals and remove all or alternate sutures. If strangulation of tissue due to excessive swelling is occurring, the suture should be removed (Case 3, Fig. 8–21).

In removing an interrupted suture, the tensile strength of a wound is slight and dehiscence may occur if excessive force is used during suture removal. Fine scissors that cut to the point or a No. 11 blade and a fine, smooth-tipped forceps that grips properly are necessary instruments for this procedure.

First crusted blood is gently cleansed away from the suture with hydrogen peroxide to obtain better visualization of the site. The knot is grasped with the smooth-tipped forceps and the suture is cut with the scissors tip or the cutting tip of a No. 11 scalpel blade as it emerges from the skin on the side of the wound opposite the knot (Fig. 8–19). Gentle pulling with forceps on the knot toward the incision line will free the suture. The portion of the suture that has been exposed on the skin surface is not carried through the depths of the wound. Counterpressure with a finger on the wound site experiencing the tugging may be helpful.

The continuous intradermal (pullout) suture is removed a bit differently (see Fig. 8–18). One end of the loop is cut, and the other is grasped with a straight hemostat or smooth-tipped forceps. A finger of the opposite hand helps to stabilize the incision line, since there is a considerable amount of pressure exerted during suture removal. If the

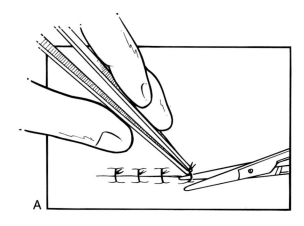

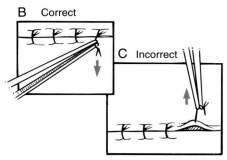

FIGURE 8–19. Suture removal: interrupted suture. *A,* Grasp the knot with a smooth-tipped forceps and slip the scissor tips under the suture. *B,* Pulling the knot across the incision line will remove the suture without placing stress on the incision. *C,* Pulling the suture directly up on the same side of the wound puts tension on the wound.

TABLE 8–1. Guidelines for Suture Removal by Location and Type	
	Number of Days Until Removal
Location	
Eyelid	2–3 days ⎫
Face	5–7 days ⎬ No tension
Neck	5–7 days ⎭
Scalp	7–10 days ⎫
Trunk	10–14 days ⎬ Under tension
Extremities	10–14 days ⎭
Type of Suture	
Interrupted	Remove alternate simple sutures in 5–6 days and all sutures in 7–8 days.
Mattress	Remove the first day that any interrupted suture is taken out.
Continuous or running intradermal	Remove in 7–10 days but may remain 14 days or longer.

suture will not pull out easily, as much pressure as needed is exerted to pull the suture free from the skin and then cut it off as it emerges from the skin. The remaining portion will retract back under the skin. In most instances, monofilament nylon suture material is well tolerated by the body without a visible foreign body reaction. If a problem arises, then open the line of incision and remove the retained suture. Continuous intradermal sutures can be left in the skin for 2 weeks or longer without fear of leaving suture marks on the skin surface.

Wound tapes (e.g., Steri-Strips or Clearon) are removed in a manner that will not place strain on the healing incision. If the patient will be changing these tapes daily, he or she must be taught the proper method of their removal. Each end is picked up and advanced to the center of the tape that lies over the incision. The two ends are held together and then gently lifted up off the incision.

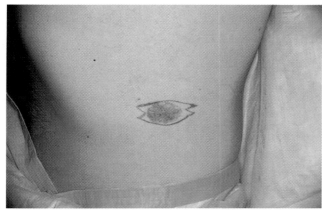
A

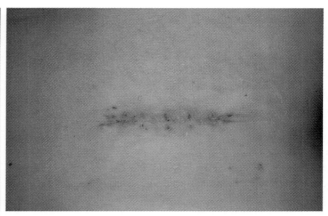
B

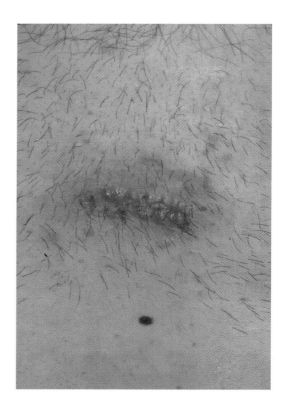

C

CASE 2

FIGURE 8–20. Suture complications. *A*, In planning the excision of a congenital nevus of the left lateral trunk at the waistline of a 13-year-old boy, M-plasties are incorporated to reduce the total length of the incision. *B*, Sutures are removed at 10 days. Small areas of crusting are present around the central sutures that were under a lot of tension. Inflammation of the incision line indicates that necrotic areas along the incision line were produced by too tight sutures. *C*, Tight sutures are the main cause of stitch marks present at 3 months. By local pressure necrosis they actually cut through the skin, thus making incisions that result in crosshatched scars. Another element in stitch marks being created is leaving the stitch in the skin too long. In this case, the rapid healing of this younger person may have allowed suture removal at 7 days even though the wound was on the trunk and under tension. Leaving the stitch in too long will produce epithelium-lined pits and sinus tracts that may become infected.

CASE 3

FIGURE 8–21. Suture complications. A mid-back incision of a 40-year-old man has become macerated under the dressing. Contact dermatitis is present in a square pattern from the tape. The wound edges are edematous and infected. Sutures were placed under excessive tension and at too close intervals and cut through the wound edges. All sutures are removed. Wet to dry dressings to debride the wound are started three times a day for 20 minutes for 24 to 48 hours. A systemic antibiotic for coverage for *Staphylococcus* is chosen, and wound cultures are taken. The wound heals by second intention.

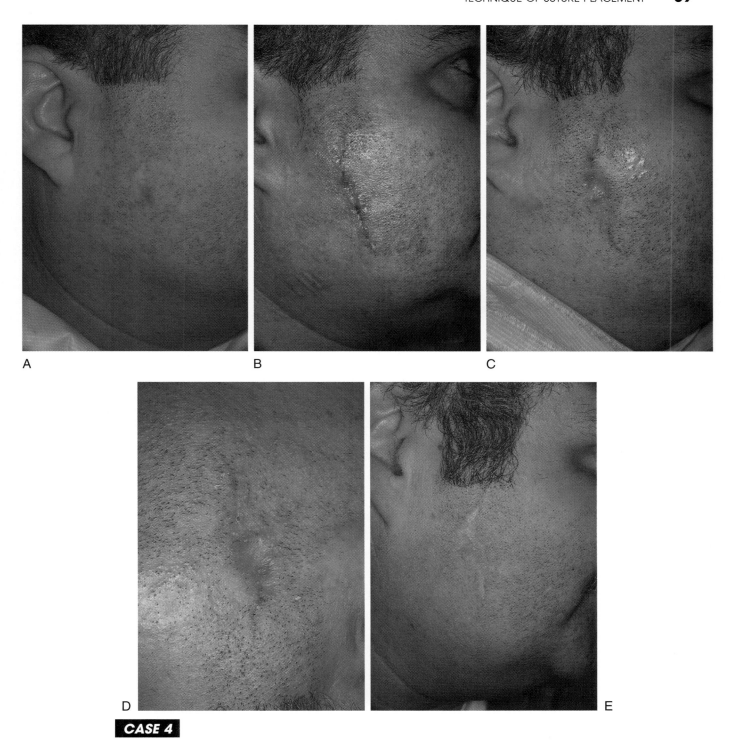

CASE 4

FIGURE 8–22. Suture complications. *A*, Appearance before resection of a basal cell carcinoma of the right preauricular cheek in a 56-year-old man. *B*, One week after surgery, sutures are removed and there is dehiscence over the center of the incision. *C*, One month after surgery, the center of the wound has spread and three areas of punctate erosions appeared within the previously healed incision line. At these three points, suture granulomas from the buried subcutaneous sutures (Vicryl) are present at the area of maximum tension. *D*, In a closer view of the incision, the punctate areas are probed for suture remnants and remaining sutures are removed. *E*, Eight months after surgery the inflamed area has healed and a spread scar exists in the center of the incision.

Suggested Readings

1. Bennett RG. Fundamentals of Cutaneous Surgery. St. Louis: CV Mosby, 1988.
2. Fewkes JL, Cheney ML, Pollack SV. Illustrated Atlas of Cutaneous Surgery. Philadelphia: JB Lippincott, 1992.
3. Gross DJ, Jamison Y, Martin K. Surgical glove perforation in dermatologic surgery. J Dermatol Surg Oncol 1989;15:1226–1228.
4. Mandelbrot DA, Smythe WR, Norman SA. A survey of exposures, practices, and recommendations of surgeons in the care of patients with human immunodeficiency virus. Surg Gynecol Obstet 1990;171:99–106.
5. Robinson JK. Fundamentals of Skin Biopsy. Chicago: Year Book Medical Publishers, 1986.
6. Roenigk RK, Roenigk HH. Dermatologic Surgery: Principles and Practice. New York: Marcel Dekker, 1989.
7. Stegman J, Tromovitch A, Glogau RG. Basics of Dermatologic Surgery. Chicago: Mosby–Year Book, 1982.
8. Swanson NA. Atlas of Cutaneous Surgery. Boston: Little, Brown & Co., 1987.

chapter 9

Elliptical Incisions and Closures

JUNE K. ROBINSON

BASIC ELLIPTICAL INCISION AND EXCISION

Although the name of this incision is a misnomer, it is so ingrained in the language of physicians that it is impossible to change. In geometry the ellipse has no angles and may be conceptualized as a partially flattened circle (Fig. 9–1). In cutaneous surgery, the incision is fusiform or football-shaped with 30-degree angles at the tips. A 3:1 ratio of length to width helps to ensure these favorable 30-degree angles at the apices that allow closure with a minimum of redundancy at the apex. In locations with less tissue laxity or on convex surfaces, this ratio is 4:1 or greater (Tables 9–1 to 9–3).

Using the skin surface topography and relaxed skin tension lines discussed in the introduction to this section, the placement of these lines of excision is drawn onto the patient before injection of anesthetic and before the drape is placed. If it is necessary to clip or shave hair, the hairline is marked with gentian violet before it is difficult to find. The lines are drawn with gentian violet, anesthetic is injected, and then a final cleansing of the skin is patted on before placing the sterile drapes. It is necessary to follow this sequence because swelling produced by infiltration of local anesthetic can distort the surface topography at the operative site (Fig. 9–2). It would be an error to misalign the hair line, lip line, or ends of wrinkles because of failure to mark them before injection of local anesthetic.

At this point in the planning process, it is worthwhile noting that certain sites that have concave surfaces, especially on the face (e.g., temple, inner canthus, nose) and ear, heal secondarily, without suturing, with good functional and cosmetic results. In these cases slow secondary healing maximizes use of surrounding normal tissue and allows time for expansion of it. The advantages of good match of color, contour, and texture as well as absent donor site pain and scarring coupled with simplicity and safety make healing by second intention preferable in cer-

tain locations. The shape of the excision also affects the result. In regions with excessive skin tension on concave surfaces the scar resulting from healing by second intention, without suturing of a round skin defect, may be superior to the healing of a sutured fusiform-shaped defect after excision of a lesion of similar size. Less skin is excised in the circular excision, in fact, approximately half of that removed with a fusiform excision.

PERFORMING THE INCISIONS

In performing the incisions, the skin is pressed down and stretched to enhance hemostasis during the procedure.

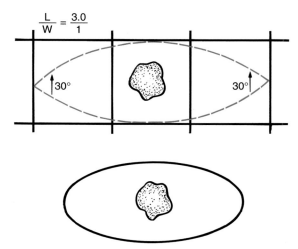

FIGURE 9–1. The shape of an ellipse *(lower figure)* is not truly used in the inaccurately named elliptical incision. The elliptical incision is planned with 30-degree angles at the apices and 3:1 length to width dimensions.

TABLE 9-1. Elliptical Incisions: Indications and Contraindications

Indications

Diseases that are not amenable to electrosurgery or cryosurgery

Facial areas where a fine linear incision can be hidden in the wrinkle lines or boundaries of cosmetic units

Contraindications

Bleeding diathesis

Problems with wound healing

Inability to cease anticoagulants

The scalpel is held perpendicular to the surface of the skin and the surface is incised. The first stroke should carry the blade to the superficial subcutaneous tissue. The incision should be of equal depth throughout its length. The apex of the incision is cut with the tip of the No. 15 scalpel blade and the center of the incision with the belly of the blade. This makes it mechanically easier to avoid overcutting at the apex because the surgeon can see the incision being made with the tip of the blade better than with the belly of it (Fig. 9–3A). Beveling of the wound edges makes it difficult to achieve proper eversion and results in a wider scar. The only site in which beveling is indicated is at the junction of hair-bearing and non–hair-bearing skin (e.g., eyebrow and scalp-face junction). In these locations, the surgeon may attempt to camouflage a scar by undercutting the hair-bearing skin so as not to transect valuable hair

TABLE 9-2. Elliptical Incisions: Patient Preoperative Discussion

1. Decrease or cease smoking and alcohol intake 2 weeks before surgery and for 1 week after surgery.
2. Stop taking aspirin 10 days before surgery.
3. Do not wear cosmetics or moisturizers on the face on the day of surgery. Eat your regular meals and take your other medications.
4. If the surgery is on the arms or legs, there may be restrictions in your daily physical activities during the week after surgery. This will be discussed with you. If surgery is on the foot, special shoes may be needed.
5. Surgery in the region of the mouth may require a change in diet and dental hygiene during the week after surgery.
6. Keep the wound dry until stitches are removed.
7. If the surgery is on the face, sleep with the head elevated. Surgery of the forehead area may cause bruising around the eyes. Surgery of the cheeks may cause bruising in the jaw area.
8. Bruising and swelling may be present for 10 to 14 days after surgery.
9. No strenuous working out or heavy lifting should be done for 7 days after surgery.
10. Stitches are generally removed in 7 to 10 days.
11. After stitches are removed, the incision is covered with Steri-Strips for 2 weeks. Then cosmetics may be used to hide the incision.
12. Further touch-up surgery may be required. This will be discussed with you at your follow-up visit 6 to 8 weeks after surgery.

TABLE 9-3. Elliptical Incisions: Operative Issues

Preoperative Evaluation

History

    Smoking

    Bleeding diathesis

    Impaired wound healing

    Prosthesis

    Demand pacemaker

    Medications

    Hepatitis and human immunodeficiency virus infection

Check other incisions for healing properties

Check for hypertension

Preoperative Equipment Needs

Excision repair tray

Skin marking pen

Sterile field

Intraoperative Needs

Sterile field

Good lighting

Electrosurgical apparatus for hemostasis

Adequate local anesthesia

follicles, which will provide coverage for the scar. The angle of the blade then parallels the direction of hair growth. This is especially important in the eyebrows where even a few millimeters of hair loss is quite noticeable (Fig. 9–4). Beveled incisions have worse results than incisions perpendicular to the skin surface. It is difficult to suture a bevel-edge wound without the thin edge overriding the opposite skin border. After healing, the contraction of the dermal scar tends to have the skin on either side of the incision bulge around the incision.

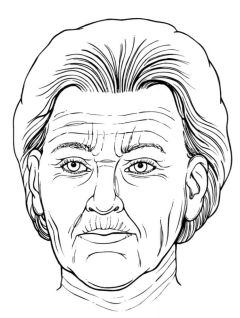

FIGURE 9-2. Placement of elliptical incisions in wrinkles and at junctions of cosmetic units of the face. The outlines of the ellipses are shown in red.

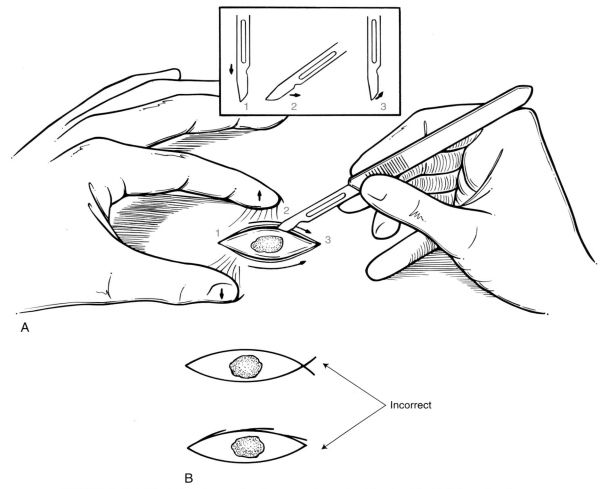

FIGURE 9–3. *A,* The incision is started at the apex under traction. The tip of the blade is used at the apex (1). The blade rocks down to cut with the belly along the midportion of the incision (2) and then rocks up at the opposite apex to cut at the tip (3). *B,* A smooth, steady motion with the blade prevents unnecessary nicks at the apex or along the midportion of the incision.

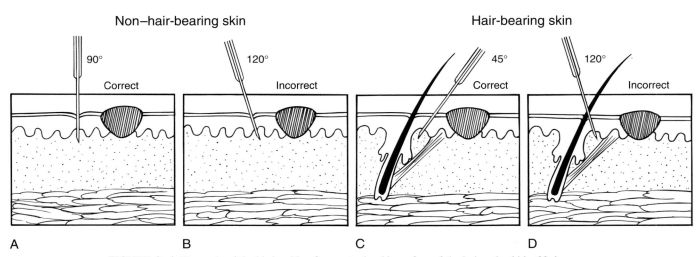

FIGURE 9–4. The angle of the blade with reference to the skin surface of the lesion should be 90 degrees. If this angle is exceeded, then the wound edge is beveled and interferes with wound closure. The only exception is in hair-bearing skin. The blade is then angled to a 45-degree angle with the surface of the skin of the lesion and parallels the path of the hair follicle.

One end of the specimen to be removed is grasped with a toothed forceps, clamp, or skin hook, but the lesion should not be squeezed. Then the ellipse is undercut with either scissors or the blade (Fig. 9–5). Many prefer to start the elevation with a blade and switch to scissors to ensure an even plane throughout the base of the elliptical excision.

The surgeon can check the work by placing the excised specimen on a flat surface. It should be level throughout with 90-degree angles at the borders.

If this step is not mastered and not performed correctly, then mounds of fat will pop up at the edges of the closure sometimes rising when subcutaneous sutures are placed. This makes needlessly large dog-ears and creates boating deformities at the tips that must be revised (Case 1, Fig. 9–6; see also Fig. 9–5D).

UNDERMINING

Local anesthetic must be injected into the full area of the incision, including the area to be undermined. A good general rule is that each side of the incision be undermined by a distance of 2 cm from the excised area. Thus, an excision 2 cm wide and 5 cm long will be undermined by

2 cm on every border including the apices; however, undermining at the apices is frequently less extensive. A proper ring block will encompass a 9 × 8-cm area. Skin hooks or a toothed forceps with no pressure applied is used to elevate the edges of the wound, and the wound edge is rolled backward over the ring finger, which is pushing on the external surface of the skin. In this manner there is excellent exposure of the undersurface of the undermined area. A blunt dissecting scissors is used to undermine the wound edges and apices. The motion used with the scissors in undermining is to insert the closed tips in the appropriate plane and gently spread the tips apart. By repeating this motion, fibrous bands will become evident and these can be cut. Arteries can be seen and clamped before transecting them, and nerves are spared from needless injury (see Case 2, Fig. 9–9).

These fibrous bands connect the underlying muscles and overlying skin. Removing most of these bands around the excision site releases the surface tissue to slide over the underlying tissue. The strengths of these subcutaneous attachments vary in different parts of the body (e.g., weak in the cheeks and neck but fairly strong over the back and shoulders). After undermining, the tissue mobility is limited more by the inherent limited elasticity of the skin than

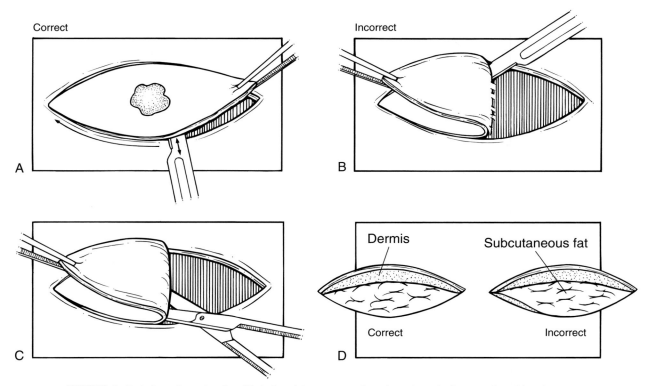

FIGURE 9–5. *A*, In undercutting the elliptical excision an even plane throughout the base can be achieved by using the scalpel in a motion parallel to the skin surface. If the tissue is pulled over the scalpel as the scalpel moves forward with a "sawing" stroke, then excessive depth in the center is avoided. *B*, Elevation of the tissue under tension leads to greater depth in the center of the wound. *C*, Some surgeons prefer to use the flat blades of the scissors resting against the wound base and to elevate the tissue to maintain the plane of removal. *D*, The final goal is even depth across the wound base. If excess fat or dermis is left at the apices of the wound, it elevates the apices and creates "boating" deformities.

by the loose connections that bind the skin to the underlying structures. This undermining process also helps the surrounding tissue to mold itself into more desirable contours to fill the gap created by the excision. Undermining creates a ''plate'' of scar tissue under the surface of the skin that contracts and is remodeled over the next year. This ''plate'' of scar minimizes buckling at the surface and ''pincushioning,'' and may help to reduce spreading of the scar.

The depth of undermining varies with the location: on the face it is just under the dermis, high in the fat above nerves and vessels on the scalp, and under the galea aponeurotica deep to the hair follicles; on the forehead it is below the deep fat; on the nose, upper lip, and neck it is deep to the fat; and on the trunk, arms, and legs it is deep to the subcutaneous tissue above the fascia overlying the muscle (Fig. 9–7). Although the junctions of dermis and fat and of fat and fascia are readily apparent, the galea is often difficult to differentiate from the underlying periosteum. It is helpful to remember that the tough, fibrous galea will move while the underlying gossamer-thin periosteum will not. Once the level of undermining is established, it is important not to stray more deeply since nerves or large vessels may be damaged. When the flap is elevated by pulling upward excessively during undermining, the surgeon may advance more deeply than intended. Proper technique consists of gentle elevation and dissection under direct observation. If the skin is particularly lax, then undermining may be limited to 1 to 2 mm or just enough to allow placement of subcutaneous sutures. In a patient with anticipated problems in coagulation, extensive undermining is not performed since there is a risk of the newly created space filling with blood (Tables 9–4, 9–5).

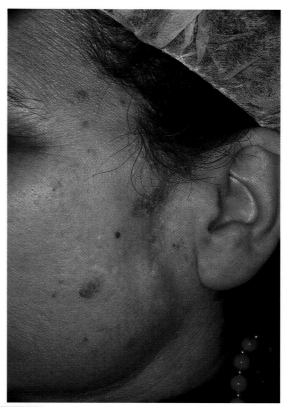

CASE 1

FIGURE 9–6. An example of excessive redundancy at the inferior apex of the incision produced by inadequate removal of fat at the base of the wound, particularly at the inferior aspect of the wound in the preauricular area of the cheek. Although a smaller redundancy may resolve spontaneously over the next 6 months, this large redundancy at the inferior aspect of the incision needs to be revised by excising the excess tissue.

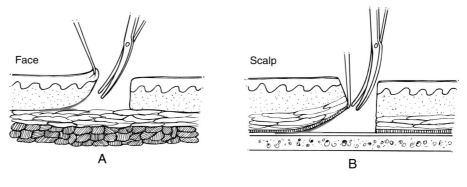

Face

Scalp

A

B

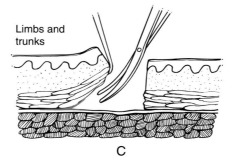

Limbs and trunks

C

FIGURE 9–7. Level of undermining varies with the location on the body. On the face in areas overlying nerves and vessels, the plane of undermining is below the dermis at the junction with the fat. On the scalp, a relatively bloodless plane is below the galea. Trunk and extremities can be undermined deep to the fat and over the fascia. The plane of undermining is indicated in red.

TABLE 9–4. Elliptical Incisions: Postoperative Care

Pain Management

Usually acetaminophen is prescribed for 48 hours.

No aspirin or nonsteroidal anti-inflammatory agents should be taken for 48 hours.

In rare instances, acetaminophen with codeine can be used.

Rest with relative immobility and an ice pack for the first 2 hours after surgery is recommended.

Dressings

Steri-Strips are used over the incision line until suture removal.

Telfa pad and paper tape over the Steri-Strips may be changed daily by the patient if soiled.

A pressure dressing is placed over the Telfa pad for 24 hours when intraoperative bleeding is excessive.

Immediate Postoperative Complications

Hemorrhage: control acute episode (Case 12, Fig. 9–22).

Infection: treat systemically (Case 9, Fig. 9–19).

Dehiscence: debride as necessary (Case 10, Fig. 9–20).

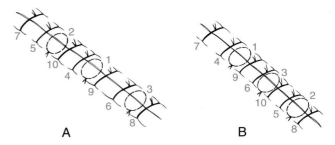

FIGURE 9–8. *A*, A wound with sides of equal length and under no tension is closed with three buried subcutaneous sutures, indicated by broken lines and numbered sequence to the right of the wound. Then interrupted sutures are placed in the sequence numbered to the left of the wound. *B*, If the wound is under tension the initial subcutaneous sutures are placed slightly off the center point of maximal tension. Then the interrupted skin sutures may be placed in the same manner as a wound without tension (as in *A*). If tension remains, the interrupted sutures are placed in a sequence beginning slightly off the center (suture numbers 4 through 10). The sutures are also more closely spaced on the center of the wound than in *A*.

SEQUENCE OF SUTURE PLACEMENT

In a 2- to 4-cm ellipse with equal sides under little tension, the first suture placed is subcutaneous and in the center of the wound. This is followed by two or more subcutaneous sutures closer to the apices (Fig. 9–8*A* sutures 1 through 3). Then interrupted sutures are placed (see

Fig. 9–8*A* sutures 4 through 10). When the wound edges are under tension, a different sequence is used (see Fig. 9–8*B*).

MODIFICATIONS OF THE BASIC ELLIPSE

Wounds of Unequal Length to Produce a Curvilinear Incision

For longer incisions on the face, planning the ellipse with arms of unequal length causes a slight curvature that allows the incision to lie within a wrinkle line. This type of planning does create a slight bowing as the wound contracts. This "bowstring" contracture raises the apices of the wound. When placement of the incision allows this anticipated contracture to conform to facial contours, it may look better than a straight line running across the creases of the face (Case 3, Fig. 9–10; Case 11, Fig. 9–21).

Closure is achieved using the principles of the rule of halves. The first suture (No. 1) is placed halfway between the two ends of the excision (see Fig. 9–10*E*). The next sutures (Nos. 2 and 3) are placed halfway between the first suture and one of the ends. Additional sutures (Nos. 4, 5, 6, and 7) are then placed halfway between the previously placed sutures or between the previously placed sutures and one of the ends of the excision. Each interrupted suture corrects wounds of unequal heights.

S-curve

In locations with complex convex curvatures such as the forearm and lower extremities the incision may be planned to conform to these curvatures around the limb having a relatively small circumference (Case 4, Fig. 9–11).

TABLE 9–5. Examples of Treatment of Permanent Postoperative Changes

Type of Scar	Treatment
Hypertrophic scar	Scar resulted from the region being under tension (deltoid, sternal region). Silastic gel sheeting prior to developing it in these body regions, corticosteroid injections at 2 months
Spread or wide scar (Case 7, Fig. 9–17)	Occurrence in younger patient is unavoidable. Delay re-excision surgery until the patient is older, then consider use of Z-plasty to close wound under less tension
Depressed scar (Case 8, Fig. 9–18)	Scar resulted from depth of tissue lost; thus revision must reapproximate tissues at depths of wound. Collagen injection is beneficial.
One side of scar elevated	Dermabrade.
Pink coloration of scar	Color fades with scar maturation in 1 to 3 years. Camouflage scar with cosmetics or hair style.
White coloration of scar	Use cosmetics or hair style to cover.

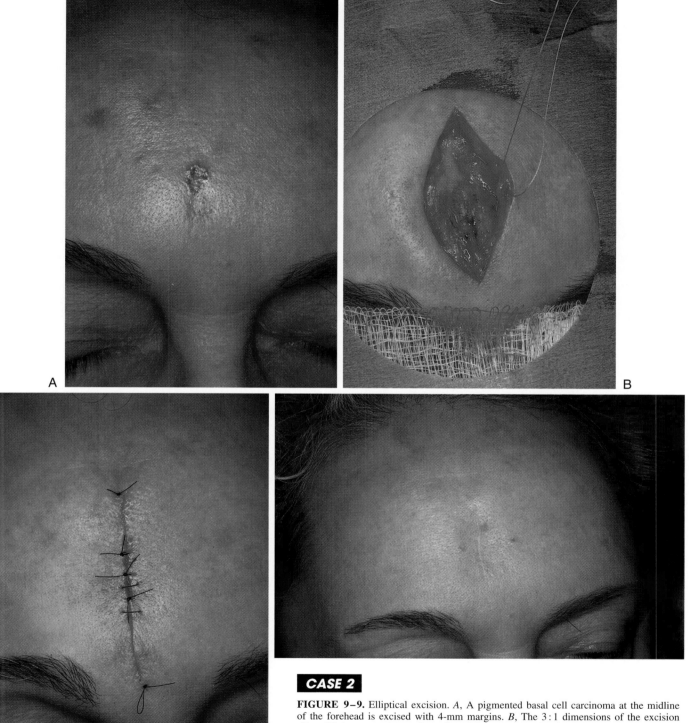

CASE 2

FIGURE 9–9. Elliptical excision. *A,* A pigmented basal cell carcinoma at the midline of the forehead is excised with 4-mm margins. *B,* The 3:1 dimensions of the excision allow 30-degree angles at the apices. The area is undermined readily in this area of relative laxity. The first suture placed is a buried subcutaneous suture in the middle of the incision. *C,* Wound edges are easily approximated with subcutaneous sutures. The running subcuticular suture has incorporated two crossover cutaneous loops. Slight adjustments of the wound edges to produce eversion are made with three interrupted sutures in the center of the incision. *D,* Appearance of forehead 1 year later.

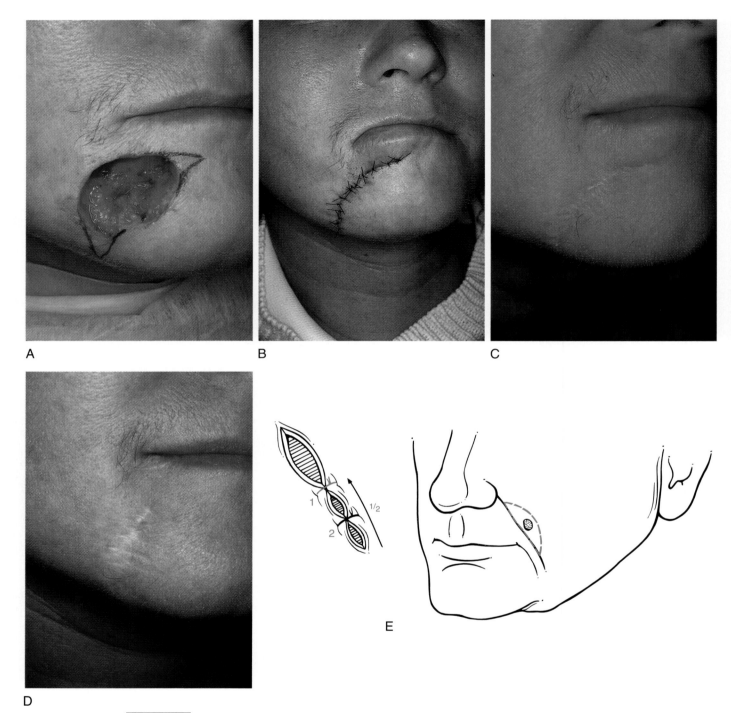

A

B

C

D

E

CASE 3

FIGURE 9–10. Closure by halves. *A,* A morphea-type basal cell carcinoma was resected with Mohs' micrographic surgery with a depth to the level of the fascia. A curvilinear incision is planned at the junction of the mental prominence with the lip. *B,* Closure is achieved by the rule of halves. *C,* Fullness pushes the lower lip up. When the bowstring contraction along the incision occurs, the tip placed in the midline below the middle of the lip will be drawn toward the chin. Thus it is expected that scar contraction will return the lip to its normal position. Local anesthesia may also be accentuating the lip elevation. *D,* Six months later, the incision spread in the middle. The fullness of the lower lip is barely apparent. The whiteness of the incision is noticeable in contrast to the patient's very pink skin tone. *E,* Closure of wounds of unequal length to produce a curvilinear incision is particularly applicable in the nasolabial fold. The first suture (1) is placed halfway between the two ends of the incision. The next suture is placed halfway between the first suture and the end.

M-plasty

If two ellipses are placed side-by-side, M configurations are created at the apices of the incision (Fig. 9–12*B*). The total length of the incision line may be shortened without producing a dog-ear by using two 30-degree angles inset into the tip of the apex of the fusiform incision as an M-plasty. The tip of this triangular flap is minimally advanced and inset with the three-point or half-buried mattress corner suture. By performing an M-plasty at one end of the incision, the length of the scar is shortened by one sixth. Of course an M-plasty can be performed at each end of the incision (double or bilateral M-plasty) to conserve even more tissue. The M-plasty is particularly useful in performing surgery in areas where lines of facial expression radiate out from a single orifice (e.g., crow's feet about the eyes at the temples). Another useful site is in the excision of scalp lesions. The double M-plasty, or use of the M-plasty on each apex of the incision line, can significantly reduce the amount of hair-bearing skin that is lost. Because scalp incisions bleed more heavily than others, the additional advantage offered by the shorter total length of the M-plasty incision is that it results in less bleeding and less surgical time. The hair eventually covers the incision line. The broken lines at the end may look somewhat unnatural if they are not placed into existing wrinkles (Case 5, see Fig. 9–12).

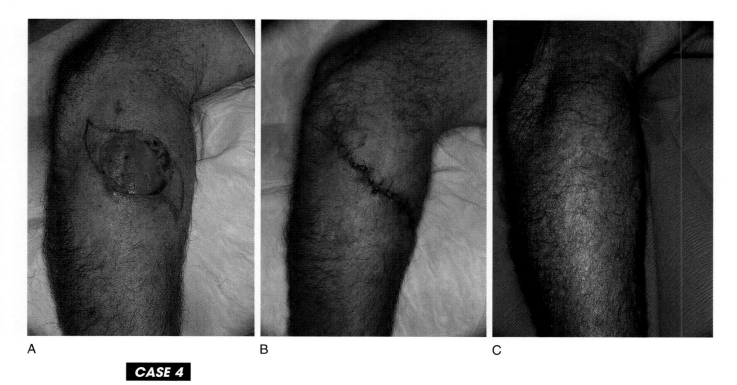

A   B   C

CASE 4

FIGURE 9–11. S-shaped incision. *A*, A squamous cell carcinoma was excised with Mohs' micrographic surgery from the right forearm of an elderly man. Fascia is exposed at the base. The closure is planned with excisions to conform to the curvature of the arm. *B*, An S-shaped incision is formed. The patient's arm was immobilized in a sling for 1 week after surgery. *C*, One year after surgery, the scar has not spread.

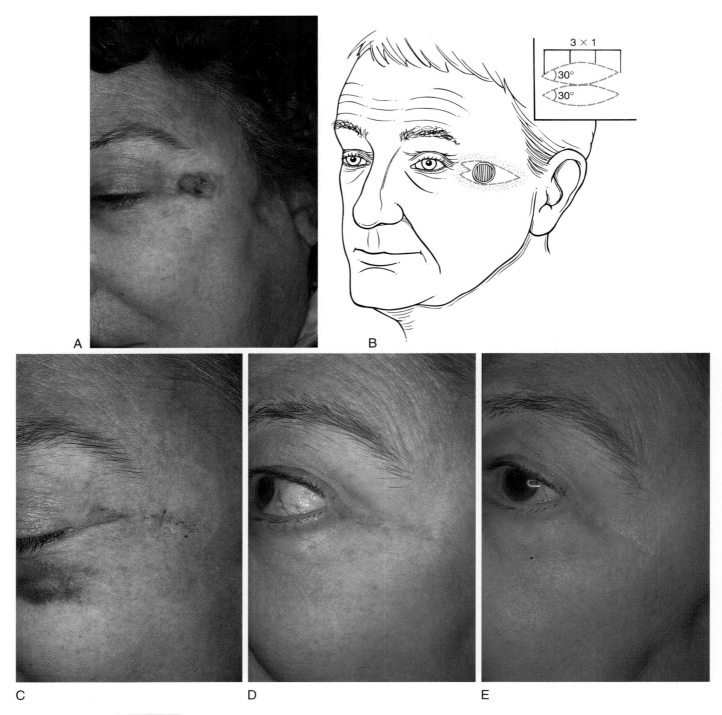

CASE 5

FIGURE 9–12. M-plasty. *A*, Defect created by excision of a basal cell carcinoma with Mohs' micrographic surgery. *B*, M-plasty closure spares extension of the incision into the lateral canthus. The M-plasty may be conceptualized as side-by-side ellipses. Each ellipse has the 30-degree angle at its apex. The tips of the two ellipses form an M. *C*, At suture removal in 1 week there is the expected amount of bruising in the dependent loose tissue of the lower eyelid. *D*, Six months after surgery, the lateral canthus is in proper position. *E*, Three years after surgery, scar contraction has inverted the wound edges and bowstring contracture over the zygoma has elevated the lateral tip of the incision.

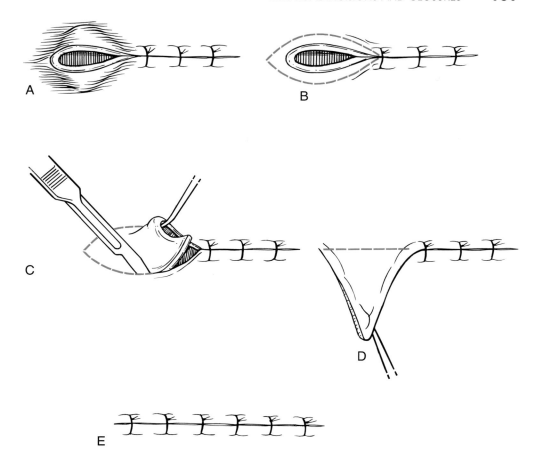

FIGURE 9–13. Dog-ear repair by extension of the line. The excess skin is tented up at the apex of the incision. Equal amounts of tissue on both sides of the wound are excised, thereby extending the original wound dimensions to 3 : 1. The final result is a longer, straight line excision, which is useful for a long horizontal facial line such as the forehead or on the trunk.

Repair of Dog-Ears

Dog-ears, the bunching up of redundant skin formed in closing a wound, may appear when a wound is not properly sutured or when the angle at the apex of a fusiform excision exceeds 30 degrees. In addition to being unaesthetic, the dog-ear pucker at the end of the incision line may hinder closure of a wound by pushing apart the skin borders. If the dog-ear is not too pronounced, it may resolve spontaneously in 6 to 8 weeks after surgery.

To repair a dog-ear, the incision line is selectively lengthened to conform to the ideal 3 : 1 ratio by excising a triangle of skin at any point along the wound where the dog-ear has formed. Although this most commonly is done at the apex of the incision, it may be advantageous to locate the excision of redundant tissue along one of the long incision lines. There are four types of dog-ear revisions commonly performed: (1) extension of the line, (2) hockey-stick revision, (3) T-plasty revision, and (4) M-plasty revision (Figs. 9–13 through 9–16). Because the hockey-stick revision results in a curvilinear incision line, it is usually cosmetically superior to the T or M revision of a dog-ear.

The ellipse and its many variations described in this chapter result in a primary closure. Primary closure uniformly results in a better looking final result than does either a flap or a graft; thus, whenever possible, the primary closure is performed.

Text continued on page 108

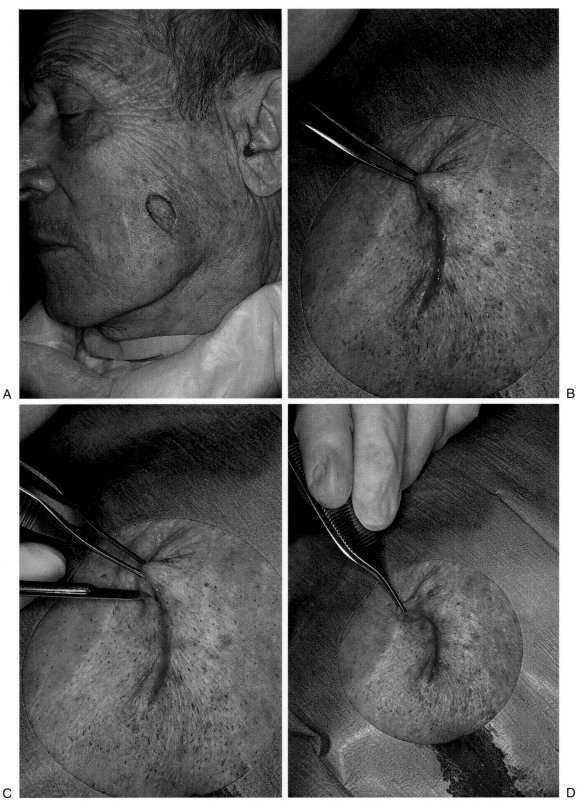

FIGURE 9–14. Dog-ear repair by hockey-stick revision. *A,* After excision of a nodular basal cell carcinoma with 3-mm margins, the defect does not have a 3:1 ratio. The depth of the wound is closed with subcutaneous sutures. *B,* In the hockey-stick revision, the redundant skin is tented up with a skin hook or a toothed forceps. *C,* This is laid over to one side by folding the redundant skin over to the side where it is better to have the incision line curve. The redundant skin is incised at its base at a 45-degree angle to the original incision line. *D,* Then the free margin of the overriding skin is lifted over the remaining skin and an incision line is made.

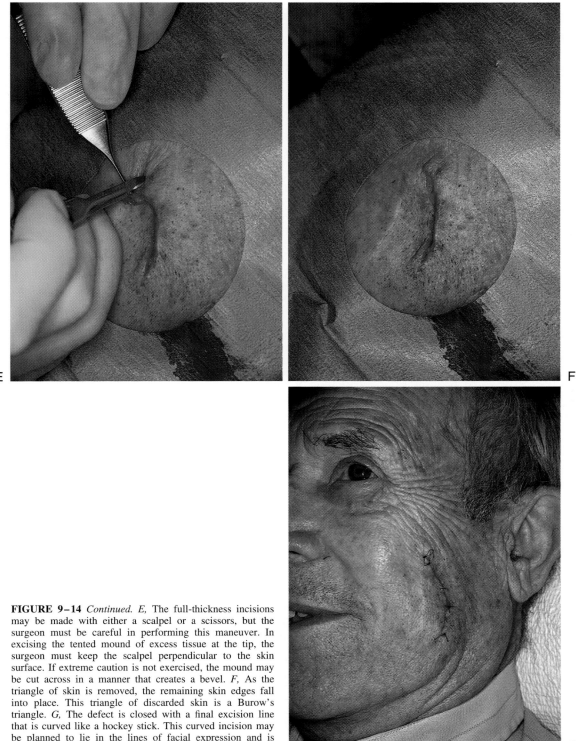

FIGURE 9–14 *Continued. E,* The full-thickness incisions may be made with either a scalpel or a scissors, but the surgeon must be careful in performing this maneuver. In excising the tented mound of excess tissue at the tip, the surgeon must keep the scalpel perpendicular to the skin surface. If extreme caution is not exercised, the mound may be cut across in a manner that creates a bevel. *F,* As the triangle of skin is removed, the remaining skin edges fall into place. This triangle of discarded skin is a Burow's triangle. *G,* The defect is closed with a final excision line that is curved like a hockey stick. This curved incision may be planned to lie in the lines of facial expression and is especially effective in the perioral and periorbital areas.

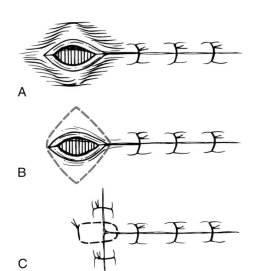

FIGURE 9–15. Dog-ear repair by T-plasty. The redundant skin is bunched up on both sides of the incision. A triangle is excised superior to the wound and another is excised inferior to the wound. A four-point suture secures the center.

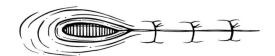

A

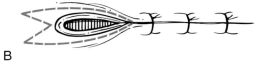

B

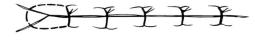

C

FIGURE 9–16. Dog-ear repair by M-plasty. The redundant skin is bunched at the apex with a skin hook, and the mound is subdivided into two separate triangles to be discarded. This revision is particularly appropriate on the face when the broken line can be folded into two intersecting wrinkles.

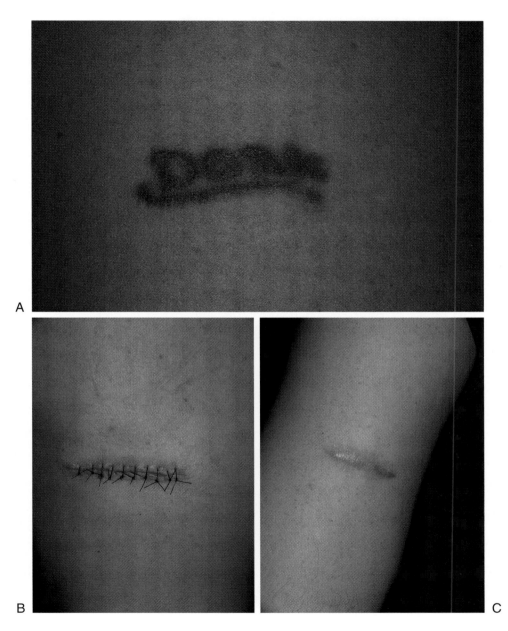

A

B

C

FIGURE 9–17. Complication—spreading of scar. *A*, A 3 × 1-cm tattoo of the left upper arm is excised. *B*, Closure is readily obtained with a double layer of subcutaneous sutures and interrupted skin closure. *C*, After 1 year, the scar has spread. This result is anticipated on the upper arm area and is discussed with the patient before removal of the tattoo.

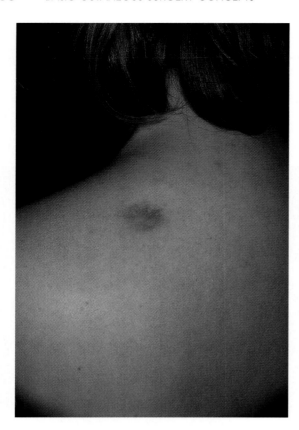

CASE 8

FIGURE 9–18. Complication—depressed area. After resection of a 4.0-cm cyst of the left upper back, a depression results because it was not possible to fill the dead space created by removal of the cyst.

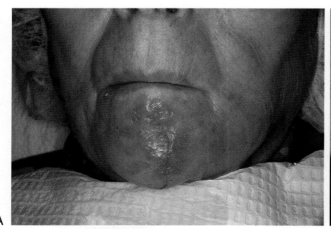 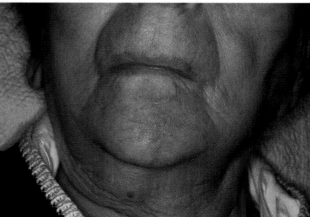

A

B

CASE 9

FIGURE 9–19. Complication—wound infection. *A,* After surgery, the wound was covered with Steri-Strips and a Telfa dressing. Saliva kept saturating the dressing. At the time of suture removal, the area is inflamed and has small pustular lesions. Culture showed *Candida. B,* The patient was treated with topical antifungal preparations. No further dressings were applied. The infection cleared in 2 weeks.

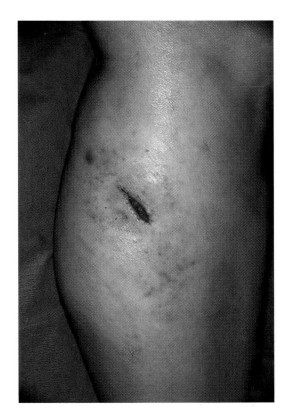

FIGURE 9–20. Complication—dehiscence. After excision of a nevus of the lower leg, the patient did not stop strenuous walking exercises. During her exercises, she felt something "pop." The wound dehisced at 5 days. Now, the wound is cleansed twice a day and will heal by second intention over a period of about 6 weeks.

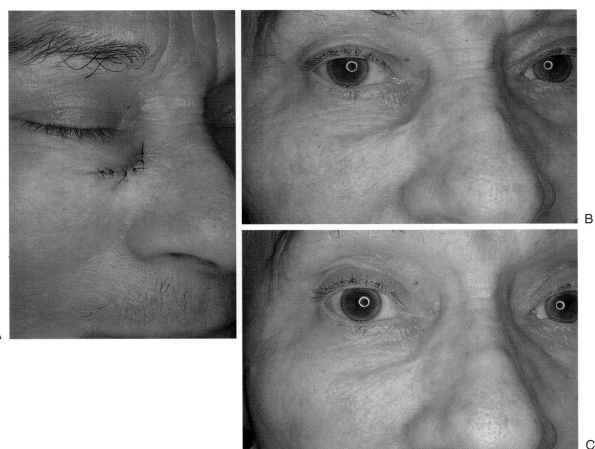

CASE 11

FIGURE 9–21. Complication—bowstring contracture causing webbing. *A,* An incision is placed at the junction of the cheek and eye cosmetic units. *B,* Two months after surgery an epicanthal web forms because of bowstring contracture of the scar. *C,* There is very little change over the next year.

107

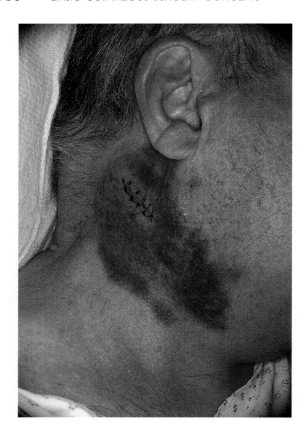

CASE 12

FIGURE 9–22. Complication—hemorrhage. Excisional biopsy of a suspected melanoma in a patient with chronic lymphocytic leukemia resulted in the anticipated ecchymosis 1 week after surgery.

Selected Readings

1. Barnett R, Stranc M. A method of producing improved scar following excision of small lesions of the back. Ann Plast Surg 1979;3:391–394.
2. Cox KW, Larrabee W. A study of skin flap advancement as a function of undermining. Arch Otolaryngol 1982;108:151–155.
3. Goldwyn RM. Value of healing by secondary intention seconded. Ann Plast Surg 1980;4:435.
4. Goldwyn RM, Rueckert F. The value of healing by secondary intention for sizable defects of the face. Arch Surg 1977;112:285–292.
5. Larrabee WF, Sutton D. Variations of skin stress strain curves with undermining. Surg Forum 1981;32:553–555.
6. Robinson JK. Variation in operative technique: the "nip 'n tuck" principle in dermatologic surgery. J Dermatol Surg Oncol 1980; 6:4:282–285.
7. Salasche SJ, Roberts LC. Dog-ear correction by M-plasty. J Dermatol Surg Oncol 1984;10:6:478–482.
8. Stell TM, Green JR. The viability of triangular skin flaps. Br J Plast Surg 1975;28:247–250.
9. Zitelli JA. Wound healing by secondary intention: A cosmetic appraisal. J Am Acad Dermatol 1987;9:407–415.

section two

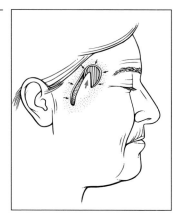

Introduction to Tissue Movement

JUNE K. ROBINSON

Once mastery of the basic techniques of cutaneous surgery is achieved, progression to acquisition of skills of more complicated techniques such as flaps and grafts occurs. By constant handling of human tissues and repetitive exposure to didactic courses, the surgeon gradually evolves his or her techniques and becomes aware of the nuances of flap design, tissue movement, selection of graft donor site, and adaptation to the problem presented by the individual patient. Flaps in real patients are not designed to conform precisely to the picture in a textbook or to the "right" letter of the alphabet for geometric closure but rather to take advantage of an interplay of factors in that particular patient. As each of us progresses in our surgical techniques, the benefits to our patients will be apparent.

A flap is defined as a combination of a unit of skin and subcutaneous tissue bearing its own blood supply that is moved from one location to another. In contrast, a skin graft has no intact blood supply of its own and is moved from a distant site to the recipient site. The graft is more dependent on a favorable recipient site with its own vascu-

lar bed than is a flap which brings its own blood supply with it. Sir Harold Gillies said this in a very succinct manner: "A graft is a piece of detached skin which is dead when you put it on and comes to life later. A flap is a partly attached piece of skin which is alive when you put it on and may die later."

The best choice among the various methods of closing a particular defect includes primary closure, skin grafting, or tissue movement by any one of a variety of flaps. These all require an understanding of the basic dynamics of tissue movement in a particular location as well as the reason for creation of the defect. This careful weighing of many factors, including risk of tumor recurrence, the final cosmetic result, the wishes of the patient, and the type and intensity of postoperative care available, leads the surgeon to a decision of which type of closure seems best in that instance.

In planning a closure, one must take adequate time to evaluate the problem of which closure to choose. Additionally, closure may be delayed until there is assurance of negative margins around the tumor excision. Primary closure frequently gives the best final cosmetic result and should always be considered first on the face. However, the amount of tension created by primary closure may cause loss of function or significant cosmetic distortion (e.g., eversion of a lower eyelid causing exposure of the cornea or distortion of the lid which interferes with normal drainage of tears). In such instances, a flap or graft is necessary. All of the basic techniques of gentle and careful tissue handling remain essential to the eventual survival of the flap or graft.

TERMINOLOGY

Flaps may be defined by their geometry, regional anatomy, name of the person who first described the flap, blood supply, or type of tissue movement involved. The use of terminology based on type of tissue movement leads to the best and easiest understanding of the dynamics of motion of flaps. There are three types of tissue movement: (1) advancement, (2) rotation, and (3) transposition of tissue. These are listed in order of ascending difficulty in mastery.

In this section, the primary tissue movement is described by a red arrow in the diagrams (Fig. II–1). Since motion is hard to convey on the two-dimensional printed page, it may be helpful to consider analogous motions that we make in daily life. A giant step straight forward from standing still is advancement. A pivot with one foot stationary and the other swinging out describes rotation. Leaping into the air and landing in a different place than the launching site describes transposition.

Other definitions are necessary to describe flap design. A *primary defect* is the original wound to be repaired. A *secondary defect* is the defect created by moving tissue from one site to another to close the primary defect.

In addition to the two types of defects created by a flap, there are two types of movement that must be planned in designing the flap. The *primary motion* is the motion of the flap toward the defect. The *secondary motion* is the motion of the tissues surrounding the defect toward the flap. The secondary motion in many cases opposes the primary motion. In many instances, the secondary movement will cover as much of the primary defect as the primary movement. In creating a flap, there is a combination of stresses both primary and secondary that must be anticipated. For example, understanding of the secondary movement about a flap utilizing the lax skin of the lateral canthal area of the lower eyelid will enable one to predict ectropion formation.

Finally there are two essential sutures in flap surgery: the *tension-bearing suture* and the *aligning suture*. As a general principle of tissue movement, the first suture placed bears the greatest tension. Frequently, this suture is temporarily placed until all other sutures are finished. Then this initial tension-bearing suture is removed and replaced with one more able to fine tune the alignment of the flap and wound edges. This initial tension-bearing suture places great stress on the tissue; thus it is wise not to place it into the tip of the flap. The first suture placed may be neces-

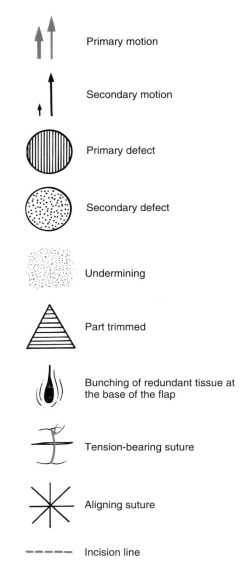

FIGURE II–1. These symbols are used in the diagrams in this atlas. The length of the arrow conforms to the rest of the art presented in an individual case and will change from one drawing to the next. The length of the arrow does not designate the force of the tension. Primary motion is designated by a red arrow, the incision line is shown by a broken red line, and the tension-bearing suture is red.

sary to execute the motion of the flap (e.g., advancement and rotation flaps). In these pulling flaps the first suture placed bears tension and aligns the flap. In the transposition flap, a pushing flap, the first suture placed bears tension and closes the secondary defect but does not align the flap.

Since the initial two or three sutures placed may serve either one or both functions of tension bearing and/or flap alignment, the terminology used in this atlas will be tension bearing (denoted by red in Fig. II–1) or aligning sutures (asterisk in Fig. II–1). We hope that this will clarify the function of the various sutures.

Tension-bearing sutures may either place stress on the flap or relieve stress from the flap. In advancement and rotation flaps, the secondary defect is not created until the primary motion of the flap exposes the secondary defect. For these flaps, the tension-bearing suture executes the motion of the flap, placing stress on the flap, thus creating the secondary defect. In contradistinction, the transposition flap uses the tension-bearing suture to relieve stress on the flap. The transposition flap is moved into its new location and held gently in place with a skin hook, while the initial tension-bearing suture is placed to close the secondary defect. This suture is placed under enormous tension, and once it is in place the transposition flap is prevented from returning to its original location by a solid ''push'' from the tissue closed behind it.

PLANNING A FLAP

In designing flaps, consideration of placement of the secondary defect will place the incision in natural skin lines or along the lines of intersection of cosmetic units of the face to minimize the effect of the scar produced. It will take advantage of available wells of tissue about the face in areas of tissue laxity such as the nasolabial groove, preauricular region, cheek skin, glabellar region, upper eyelid redundant skin, and forehead and neck excess tissue (Fig. II–2). When possible, a flap should match the recipient area in thickness, color, texture, and hair-bearing qualities. It is wise to avoid placing incisions horizontally across the nasal dorsum or oral commissure, crossing the body of the mandible, or excessively utilizing the lax skin of the lower eyelid because wide scars (nasal dorsum, crossing body of mandible) or distortion of important anatomic structures (oral commissure, eyelid ectropion) may

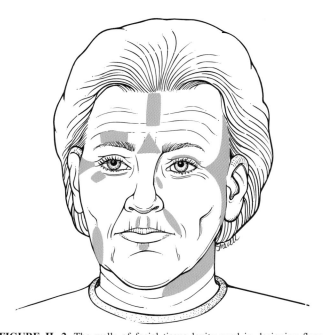

FIGURE II–2. The wells of facial tissue laxity used in designing flaps. Generally the donor site is placed laterally to camouflage it better. Whenever possible, the defect is reconstructed with tissue from the same cosmetic unit of the face. In some rare instances, these sites may also be used as the donor sites for full-thickness skin grafts.

result. As a general principle of facial flap design, the donor site is placed laterally because the medial location is more cosmetically apparent.

The more commonly performed flaps in cutaneous surgery involve movement of tissue adjacent to the defect to cover it and are termed *local flaps*. Local flaps may base their blood supply either on the cutaneous perforating vasculature and subdermal and dermal vascular plexus (random pattern) or on a named artery (axial pattern). The basic cutaneous flaps described in this section are random pattern local flaps.

Standardization of vascular terminology has undergone some changes. This change replaces the term *random* with two new terms depending on the vascular supply. *Reticular* is used for flaps based primarily on epidermal and dermal elements, and *segmental* is used for those based on perforating vessels from the subdermal plexus. *Axial* remains the term for flaps with true subcutaneous vascular pedicle. It will take a while before this change is fully assimilated into the daily usage of surgeons.

The properties of skin elasticity and movability allow tissue movement but vary from one region to another and must be assessed in planning a flap. For example, cheek skin is very elastic (stretchable) and scalp skin is not. Both cheek and scalp skin, after galeotomy, is movable (able to be surgically taken from one site to another); however, scalp skin never becomes as movable as cheek skin. In moving large flaps from one site to another, it may not be possible to close the secondary defect without using a graft. This should be recognized in planning the procedure. Flaps typically provide color, texture, hair-bearing quality of skin, pore size, and thickness of skin, similar to the surrounding skin, but most grafts often do not. Thus in planning the flap there must also be planning of the location of the less cosmetically acceptable graft for the secondary defect. Sensation, sweating, and hair growth are lost immediately after transfer of the flap but may return after an interval of months to years.

In planning a flap, the planned procedure is drawn on the skin using calipers or a ruler. The patient is in an upright position and goes through a range of facial movements. Initially, the flap and surrounding tissues are undermined widely and the elasticity of the skin is tested before incising the skin of the flap. As the flap is rotated, advanced, or transposed into position, bunching of skin about the base of the flap may occur. These ''dog ears'' or standing cones of tissue are excised to allow the flap to move easily into the defect. Burow's triangles can be planned at points of prospective dog-ear problems before the flap is cut. These triangles can then be eliminated or altered in size as the need becomes apparent. In tailoring the removal of Burow's triangles to the specific case, one must not excise them in a manner that narrows the base of the flap, reducing blood supply. The best chance of survival of the tip of the facial flap based on random blood supply from the dermal arcade is one whose design consists of the length not being more than three times the width. Flaps incorporating an artery may be longer than the 3 : 1 ratio. In other locations the length to width ratio varies (e.g., abdomen and chest, 2 : 1; lower extremities, 1 : 1). These classic ratios are based on the specific design requirements and limitations imposed by the location and size of the flap; to a lesser degree they reflect inherent differences in cutaneous circulation.

Equally important to viability of the flap is hemostasis before suturing the flap. Naturally, hemostasis should include atraumatic pinpoint electrocoagulation of bleeding vessels. Irrigation of the field into which the flap is placed will remove clots of blood. Necrotic tissue should be meticulously trimmed away from the bed into which the flap is placed. In testing the mobility of the flap, it may be grasped in the subcutaneous adipose tissue without "crimping" the dermal arcade.

SUTURING THE FLAP

Once the initial tension-bearing suture is placed, the closing tension is distributed along the secondary defect by directed suturing so that the aligning suture or sutures carry very little tension. This distribution of tension helps to prevent tip necrosis. In the advancement flap, the tension-bearing suture also closes the primary defect but tension at the advancing edge of the flap can often be reduced by directed suturing along the sides of the flap. In most transposition flaps, closure of the secondary defect with a tension-bearing suture allows the flap to be pushed easily into the primary defect where it can be sutured with aligning sutures under minimal tension. Once this initial tension-bearing suture is in place, the surgeon knows the flap will reach far enough.

Sometimes even a well-designed flap will not move far enough into the defect. In this instance, a temporary stay suture, a horizontal or vertical mattress suture with a bolster, may be used to place the skin on stretch for 5 to 10 minutes. Putting the skin under a constant stretching force for 2 to 3 minutes several times with a skin hook or a tissue expander may also give a little more coverage for a wound. This phenomenon of "cutaneous creep" is of practical importance. The maximum extensibility of skin is not attained on a first loading. As loading is maintained or repeated several times, the fibers in the dermis become linearly realigned, tissue fluid and ground substance become rearranged, and, in consequence, a greater amount of stretch is obtained. After the natural elasticity of the skin adapts to the increased tension, the stay stitch can then be removed and permanent sutures used to align wound edges. Sutures should not be placed so close to the base of the flap that they reduce the blood supply. If the base is narrow, it may be preferable to use three-point sutures (corner stitches or half-buried sutures) at the base of the flap rather than interrupted ones.

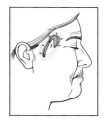

chapter 10

Advancement Flap

Basic Advancement Flap

Ronald L. Moy

The advancement flap is used to repair wounds when the tissue is best moved from either or both sides of the wound. Thus, the best locations for using the advancement flap include wounds on the forehead, helical rim, and upper lip (Case 1, Fig. 10–1). In these locations the adjacent tissue can be advanced into the wound without distorting either the eyebrow or the vermilion border inferior to the wound. The incision lines of the advancement flap can also be hidden in anatomic borders such as the vermilion border or the eyebrow, which leads to better cosmetic results (Fig. 10–2; Tables 10–1 through 10–3).

The planning of the advancement flap must take into account that adequate tissue can be advanced into the wound without excess wound tension. Because the advancement flap creates a large number of incision lines (at least five separate incisions with a double advancement flap) (Case 2, Fig. 10–3; see Variations of the Advancement Flap), it is important to attempt to hide the incision lines within a wrinkle, a cosmetic unit such as the eyebrow, or natural borders such as the helical sulcus. Although not enough tissue may be mobilized with just a single advancement flap, a single advancement flap should be attempted before a double advancement flap since fewer incision lines will be created. Once the flap has been incised, wide undermining is necessary to mobilize the tissue. It is important to decrease wound tension with buried stitches such as 5-0 Vicryl sutures. The most important placement of the initial buried tension-bearing suture is at the point of maximum tension where the advancement flap distal edge is sutured into place.

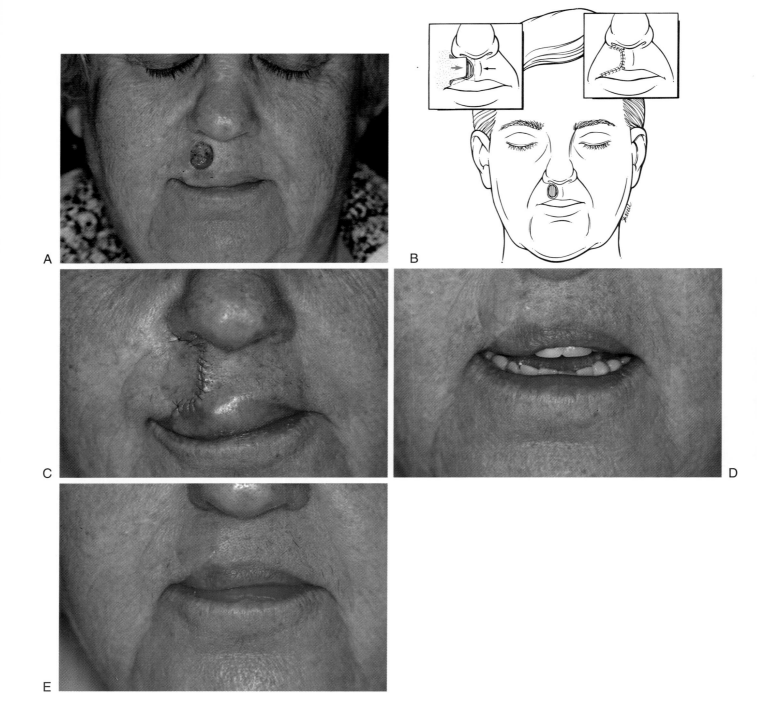

CASE 1

FIGURE 10–1. Single advancement flap. *A,* A woman has a 2.0 × 2.1-cm defect of the right upper lip as a result of resection of a basal cell carcinoma with Mohs' micrographic surgery. *B,* The limbs of the single advancement flap are planned within the boundaries of the cosmetic unit at the sill of the nose and vermilion border. Tissue is removed to allow the incision lines to be placed in these locations. *Inset, top left,* the circular defect is turned into a square to allow the advancing edge of the flap to form the vertical line at the philtrum. The flap is undermined below the hair follicles. *Inset top right,* This very broad-based flap hides the revision of redundant tissue at the base of the flap under the ala of the nose and at the oral commissure. *C,* At the time of surgery the secondary motion about the flap has produced lateral pull of Cupid's bow of the lip. Extension of the incision line along the vermilion border of the lip up to the commissure would allow better mobilization of the lax tissue of the nasolabial fold area. If this had been performed, the midline distortion would be lessened at the time of surgery. *D,* Three months after surgery, much of the midline lateral distortion has resolved. There is a minimal elevation of the lip line at the point of scar contraction along the leading vertical edge of the flap and redundancy of the vermilion of the lip. This lip redundancy can be corrected at this time, thus improving the final result. *E,* After 1 year has elapsed, the lip elevation has improved with softening of the scar. The redundancy is also improving.

TABLE 10-1. Advancement Flap: Indications, Contraindications, Limitation

Indications
Forehead
Upper lip
Extremities
Helix

Contraindications
Cheek
Distal nose

Limitation
May be difficult to hide incision lines

TABLE 10-2. Advancement Flap: Patient Preoperative Discussion

1. Stitches should be removed in 5 to 7 days.
2. The wound area should be kept completely dry for 24 hours, after which a shower, but not soaking, is permissible.
3. Bruising and swelling may be present for first 10 days.
4. The area may need a touch-up surgery (e.g., dermabrasion) in 8 to 12 weeks. The dermabrasion may take at least 10 days to heal.

TABLE 10-3. Advancement Flap: Postoperative Care

Pain Management
Acetaminophen but no aspirin or nonsteroidal anti-inflammatory agents

Dressings
Large pressure bandage consisting of wound closure tape, Mastisol, gauze, and paper tape. Gauze and paper tape are removed in 24 hours while the wound closure tapes are left in place until suture removal.

Complications
Flap necrosis should be allowed to heal by second intention followed by scar revision.
Treat infections with antibiotics.
Scars can be treated with intralesional steroids and dermabrasion.

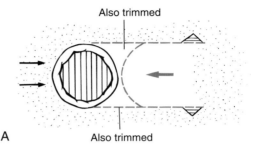

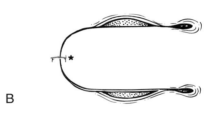

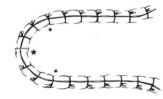

FIGURE 10–2. There are instances when the cosmetic unit of the face is better preserved by rounding the tip of the single advancement flap, thus forming a U-shaped incision. As a general principle of planning advancement flaps, the length of a single advancement flap will be two to three times the length of the defect to be covered. If there is a lot of secondary motion about the flap, then the flap's length may be planned shorter. The flap's dimensions in facial locations should not exceed a length-to-width ratio of 3:1. If a double advancement flap is used, then the length of each flap may be one and one-half to two times the length of the defect. (Courtesy of June K. Robinson, M.D.)

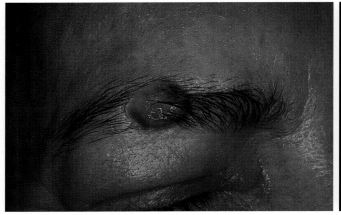

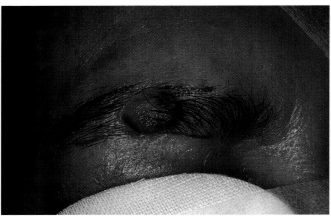

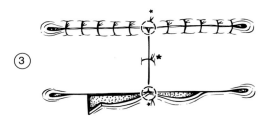

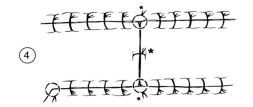

CASE 2

FIGURE 10–3. Bilateral (double advancement flap or H-plasty). *A*, A 1.2-cm defect is created in the middle of the right brow of a 46-year-old woman. *B*, Incision lines are planned within the arched lines of the brow and beveled so that hair follicles are not transected. The flaps are undermined below the hair follicles. In these intraoperative photographs, the eyelid is covered with a white oval eyepad or gauze. *C*, Diagram of the motion of the bilateral (double) advancement flap or H-plasty (*1*). After the tension-bearing suture is placed, the gaping secondary defects appear superior and inferior to the flaps (*2*). Each secondary defect is an elliptical wound with unequal sides. Each secondary defect is closed using the rule of halves. The superior secondary defect is partially closed by a suture at its midpoint (*3*). This single tip stitch (*asterisk*) through the tips of both flaps also aligns the flaps. Because of the arched shape of the incision lines and the laxity of eyelid skin, the larger redundancy (bulging) is inferiorly and laterally placed (*4*). It is revised with a ''hockey stick'' repair.

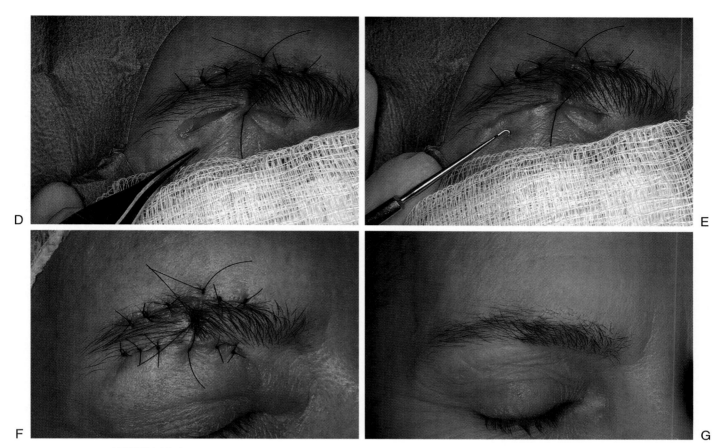

D

E

F

G

FIGURE 10–3 *Continued D*, After the secondary defect above the eyebrow is closed using the principles of closure of a wound of unequal lengths (the "rule of halves"), a single tip stitch aligns the flaps inferiorly. The larger redundancy is demonstrated with the forceps. *E*, "Hockey stick" revision of the redundancy allows opposition of the wound edges. Delicate stabilization of the wound edges by the double-pronged skin hook shows that the lid skin is slightly higher than the flap. The wound edges of unequal height are corrected by suture placement. *F*, All incisions are completely closed with interrupted sutures that correct wounds of unequal height. *G*, Two years after surgery the brow arch is intact and incision lines are imperceptible. With a touch of eyebrow pencil, the arch can be refined further. (*A* to *G* courtesy of June K. Robinson, M.D.)

Variations of the Advancement Flap

June K. Robinson

Other variations of the advancement flap or flaps that have advancement as the primary movement of the flap (Table 10–4) include the A to T (Cases 3 and 4, Figs. 10–4 and 10–5), and the V-Y plasty or the island advancement flaps (Case 5, Fig. 10–6). The A to T flap is a variation that has advantages over the double or bilateral advancement flap because the T creates fewer incision lines that can be more easily hidden than the H created by a double advancement flap. When designed with sufficient arc of rotation, the O to Z is really a double rotation flap rather than an advancement flap (see Chapter 11, Rotation Flap). When designed with inadequate motion of tissue, the advancement flap will undergo necrosis from excessive tension on the flap (Fig. 10–7).

TABLE 10–4. Types and Variations of Advancement Flaps

Single advancement (U-plasty)
Double advancement (H-plasty)
A-T, O-T plasty
V-Y, Y-V plasty, or island advancement

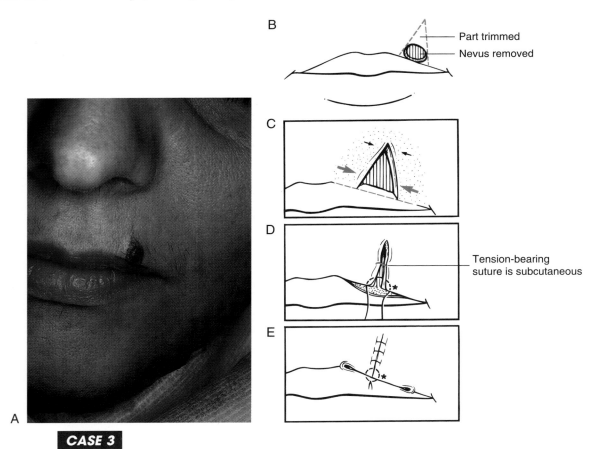

CASE 3

FIGURE 10–4. A-to-T-plasty (a variation of a bilateral advancement flap). *A,* A benign nevus of the left upper lip is a cosmetic concern for this 20-year-old woman. These flaps will be undermined about 1.5 cm from the incision lines. *B,* The circular nevus is converted to a triangular shape whose base lies on the vermilion border. *C,* The horizontal incisions are made along the vermilion, and all aspects of the flaps are undermined. The critical strategy is to mobilize the tissue under the flap by widely undermining (stippled area). The primary motion of the flaps are advancement, but there is a small element of rotation about the apex of the vertical limb of the A-T incision. *D,* The tension-bearing suture is a buried subcutaneous one that is placed first and creates the secondary defect. Then a tip stitch aligns the tips of the flaps.

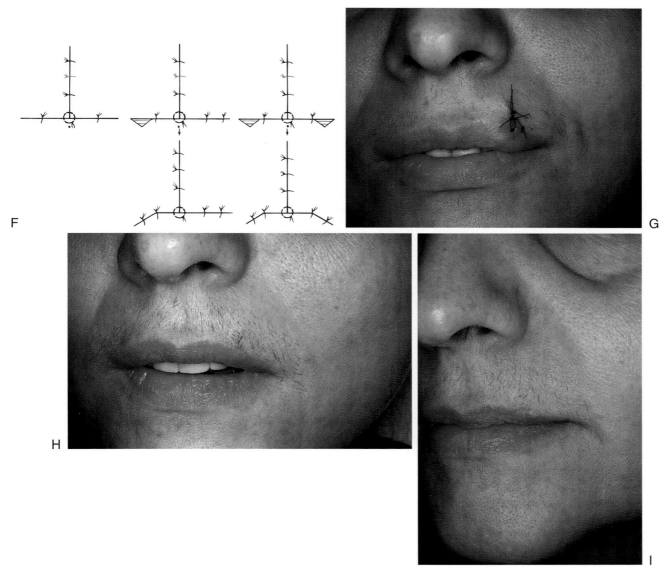

FIGURE 10–4 *Continued E*, Bulging redundancies are created laterally. *F*, Depending on the location and elasticity of the tissue, these redundancies may be revised by correcting wounds of unequal length and height or revising the redundancy on one or both sides. *G*, Immediately after the closure, local anesthetic creates vasoconstriction and edema of the lip. The base or horizontal limb of the A-T incision is placed at the vermilion border. This placement prevents scar contracture across the curvature of the white roll of the lip. *H*, Three months after surgery, the incision is slightly pink and there is a minor redundancy of tissue superiorly at the end of the vertical limb of the A-T incision line. *I*, The minor redundancy of tissue and pinkness of the incision correct themselves with maturation of the incision line 1 year after surgery. The hypopigmented incision line on the vermilion border is what is achieved even in the best of hands. Revision will not improve this result. (*A* to *I* courtesy of June K. Robinson, M.D.)

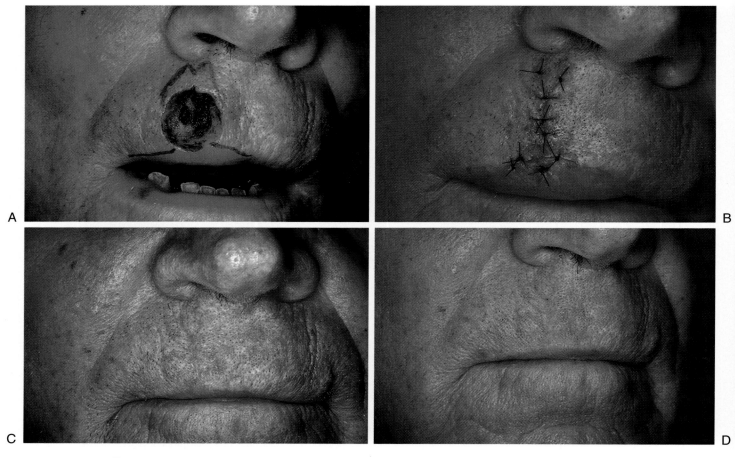

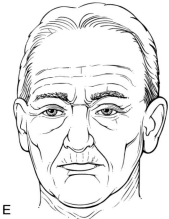

CASE 4

FIGURE 10–5. *A*, A 2.0 × 2.5-cm defect of the right upper lip results from resection of a basal cell carcinoma. The A-T flap is planned with the horizontal limb at the vermilion border and an M-plasty at the tip of the vertical limb. *B*, This M-plasty revises the redundant tissue along the vertical axis of the flap and prevents the lip from being pushed down by the excess tissue. *C*, Six months after surgery, the incisions made for the M-plasty are visible. *D*, One year after surgery, the incision line is less noticeable. Note that this elderly man has thinned lips with no white roll at the border and no Cupid's bow. These are changes associated with aging. This is a good result. *E*, Facial locations that are particularly suitable for the use of A-T plasty. (*A* to *E* courtesy of June K. Robinson, M.D.)

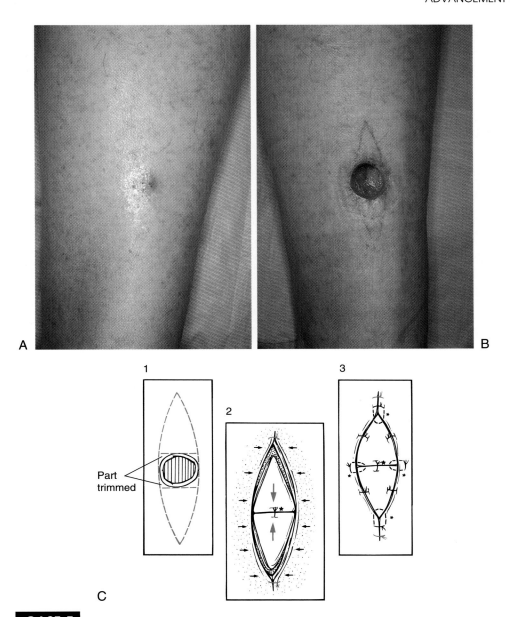

Part
trimmed

CASE 5

FIGURE 10–6. V-Y plasty or island advancement flap. *A,* Preoperative photograph of a basal cell carcinoma of the lower leg that overlies the shin. There is minimal laxity of skin medial and lateral to the wound. *B,* The cancer is excised with 3-mm borders. Even after extensive undermining, apposition of the wound edges would be difficult. The 3 : 1 dimensions of an ellipse are marked on the skin surface with Mercurochrome. *C,* The four rounded tips of the advancing flaps are trimmed, and the 3 : 1 dimensions of the total length of an ellipse are planned (*1*). The V-shaped island of tissue is raised on its narrow pedicle of subcutaneous fat and advanced forward (*2*). The entire flap is dissected from the base until a small central vertical line of tissue is formed from the center of the island. The ability to develop this pedicle depends on the availability of fat in the region. For instance, it is difficult to develop island advancement flaps on a pedicle in the forehead because of the relative dearth of fat but it is easier to develop them on the lip or cheek. The flap is advanced, and with a skin hook holding the flap in place, the tension-bearing sutures close the secondary defects. If in the process of suturing these flaps they turn white, they should be returned to their original position because the blood supply in the pedicle has been kinked or stretched too much and is impaired. The aligning suture is placed into the advancing edges of the two flaps, and tip stitches align the "tails" of the flaps (*3*). Then subcutaneous sutures are placed to close the remaining secondary defects.

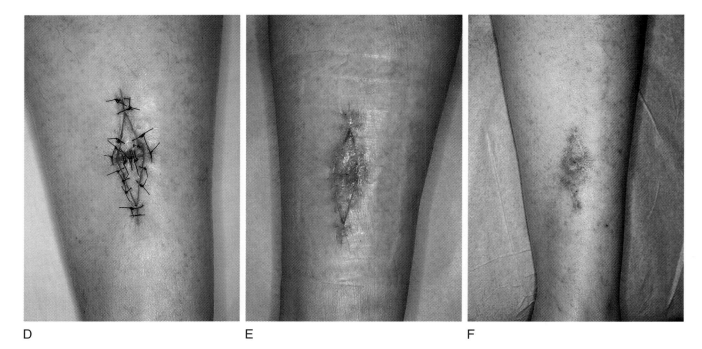

D   E   F

FIGURE 10–6 *Continued D*, After converting the leading edges of both flaps to straight lines, the V incisions to the apices of the ellipse are incised. These islands of tissue are extensively undermined from the apex of the flap to the base until they move forward. Each island on its own pedicle of subcutaneous fat moves forward similar to the motion of the hinge of a door. Then the two areas behind the island are closed. Each is closed in a straight line. These two flaps remain pink; thus, the blood supply is intact and the flaps are viable. *E*, At the time of suture removal in 1 week, the islands are edematous and elevated above the surrounding skin. *F*, Two years after surgery, hyperpigmentation of the incision lines remains as a permanent reminder of the surgery. Hyperpigmentation of wounds of the lower legs is a common occurrence and may remain indefinitely. The elevation of the flaps has subsided. This is a reasonably good result for the lower leg. (*A* to *F* courtesy of June K. Robinson, M.D.)

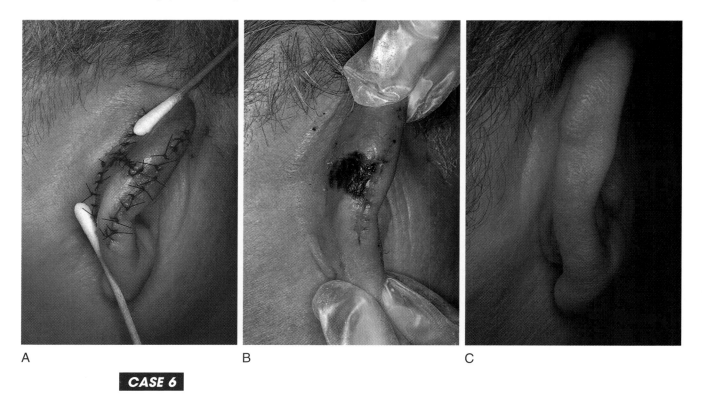

A   B   C

CASE 6

FIGURE 10–7. Advancement flaps: complication. *A*, The posterior aspect of the helical rim of the ear is reconstructed with bilateral advancement flaps under excessive tension. The tips of the flap are white immediately after surgery. To prevent flap necrosis, the timing of the intervention should be in the first 8 hours. Although various vasodilatory agents have been tried, the best way to resuscitate a flap is to replace it in its original position and start again with a design that allows adequate blood supply to the flap. *B*, Necrosis of the tips of the flaps is present at 1 week. The necrotic area separates as an eschar over the next 2 to 3 weeks. *C*, By 3 months, the area heals by second intention and scar remodeling is blending in the area of loss, which is still depressed. (*A* to *C* courtesy of June K. Robinson, M.D.)

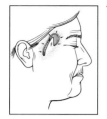

chapter 11

Rotation Flap

Basic Rotation Flap

Duane C. Whitaker

Rotation and advancement of tissue are the two types of movement necessary to close many cutaneous defects. Rotation is often beneficial because it takes advantage of stretch and glide of dermis over subcutaneous tissue (Tables 11–1 to 11–4). It is critical to accurately estimate flap length necessary to close the primary defect. This assessment is made by anatomic location and ease of tissue movement. In the temple and cheek, rotational mobility of skin is often superior to simple advancement. In these sites flap length may be one to four times the diameter of the primary defect. In contrast, a rotation flap may require greater length to close a scalp defect. The surgeon's experience in assessing tissue mobility aids in planning the flap. The donor tissue should be in an adjacent location that permits rotation with the least tension and best placement of dog-ear repair.

A triangular defect is often used to illustrate rotation flap planning. The triangle should be viewed as two radii extending from the center of a circle with the curve of the circle enclosing the third side of the triangle. With this image we can see that the flap will be rotated about a vertex (pivot point). The surgeon will plan both the length and the arc of the flap. When assessing adjacent laxity the surgeon will approximate the degrees of rotation necessary to close the defect (Case 1, Fig. 11–1A). The rotation flap is designed as a tangent to the existing defect. After incision and undermining, the flap is rotated, redundant tissue is excised, and suturing is done as outlined (Case 1, see Fig. 11–1B through J).

TABLE 11-1. Rotation Flap: Indications, Contraindications, Limitations

Indications

Tissue rotates readily
Allows the best donation of adjacent tissue
Places redundant tissue in the best location for repair
Pure advancement will not close the defect

Contraindications

Inadequate movement or rotation
Poorly vascularized tissue

Limitations

Must be applied judiciously
Requires redundant tissue repair usually at both arms of flap
Risk of tip necrosis, especially with back cut

TABLE 11-2. Rotation Flap: Patient Preoperative Discussion

1. The advantage of a rotation flap is repair of surgical defect with similar adjacent tissue.
2. The disadvantage is that a rotation flap requires additional incisions beyond the primary defect.
3. Risks are hematoma, infection, and dehiscence.
4. There is a potential risk of a temporary bulky flap, but risk is less than with a transposition flap.
5. The patient should discontinue or decrease smoking 2 weeks before and 1 week after surgery.
6. It is the patient's responsibility to maintain adequate nutrition, to avoid trauma to the wound site during the first 72 hours, and to care for the wound as instructed.
7. When medically possible the patient will be off all anticoagulants or antiplatelet medications 2 weeks before the procedure.
8. Revision may be advised 6 to 18 months after surgery if scarring complications occur.

TABLE 11-3. Rotation Flap: Operative Issues

Preoperative Evaluation

Bleeding diathesis
Smoking
Impaired wound healing

Preoperative Equipment Needs

Excision repair tray equipped with fine skin hooks or tissue forceps
Skin marking materials, templates if desired
Topical antibacterial skin preparation
Absorbable sutures and monofilament nylon and polypropylene for skin

Intraoperative Needs

Good lighting
Electrosurgical coagulation for hemostasis
Local anesthesia: 1% lidocaine with epinephrine is commonly used
Drains are rarely used.
Meticulous hemostasis before closure is preferred.

CASE 1

FIGURE 11–1. *See legend on opposite page*

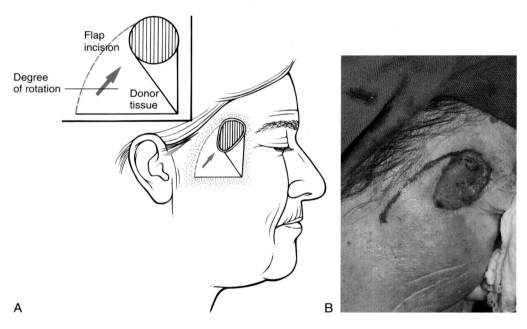

A

B

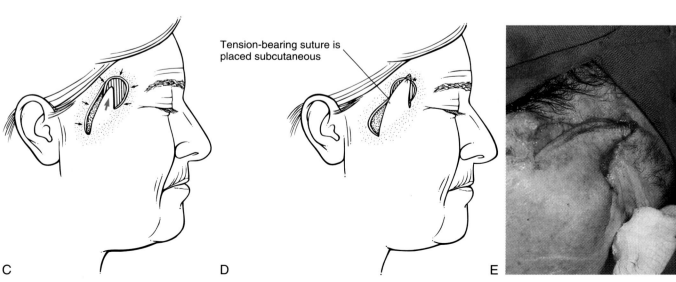

Tension-bearing suture is placed subcutaneous

C

D

E

TABLE 11-4. Rotation Flap:
Postoperative Care

Pain Management

Acetaminophen with codeine is prescribed for the first 48 to 72 hours as needed for pain.

Avoid excessive activity during the first 72 hours.

Protection and minimal movement of the area is required.

Dressings

Wound is dressed with antibacterial ointment, petrolatum, gauze, fluff gauze, and adhesive tape.

Patients are directed to keep the wound clean and dry for 48 hours.

The bandage is removed at home and the wound cleansed twice daily with hydrogen peroxide. Polysporin ointment is applied followed by a dressing.

If there is evidence of swelling, redness, or increased pain, the physician should be called.

Complications

There is the potential for infection, dehiscence, or hematoma, but these are uncommon with proper wound care.

''Trap-dooring'' or hypertrophic scar may occur.

Hypertrophy may be treated with topical or intralesional steroids after 4 weeks have passed.

''Trap-dooring'' or minor scarring is allowed to mature at least 6 months before intervention.

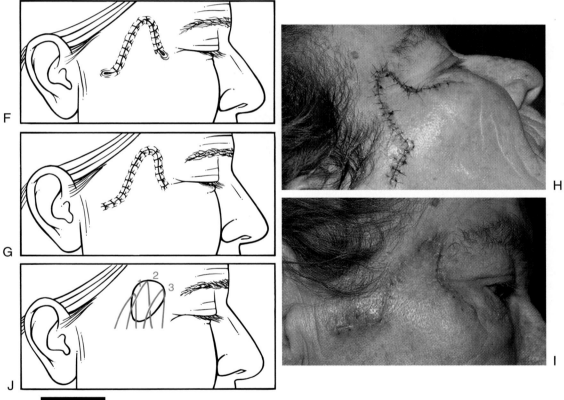

CASE 1

FIGURE 11-1 *Continued A,* Adjacent tissue laxity determines the degrees of rotation through which the flap will move. *B,* The rotation flap is planned. *C,* The flap is undermined and elevated. *D,* The temporary aligning tacking suture is placed. This step is also illustrated in *E. C* and *D* show amount of undermining around the flap, the use of the aligning suture on the tip of the flap, and the closure of the secondary defect by the tension-bearing suture, a subcutaneous one. *F,* The redundancy of tissue over the zygomatic arch of the cheek and in the preauricular area is revised (see also *G*). The redundant tissue forms a larger standing cone in the preauricular area than on the malar cheek. *H,* Revision of dog-ears only slightly lengthens the total incision line. *I,* At the time of suture removal there is no distortion of the lateral canthus. Over the course of a year the result will improve. *J,* Various options are tried before choosing proper tip placement. The tolerance of secondary motion by the surrounding tissue is important in the final outcome. In this example, placement of the tip at position 3 requires the least amount of secondary motion at the lateral canthus. Preserving the position of the lateral canthus is the most important consideration.

Most rotation flaps can be designed freehand with a tissue marking pencil. However, some surgeons may find templates or calipers helpful to ensure that flaps are designed with sufficient length. Fine skin hooks or tissue forceps are required, and good lighting is necessary to achieve hemostasis in undermined tissue. Once the flap has been rotated to a critical point a temporary tacking and aligning suture is often useful for assessing tip placement (Case 1, see Fig. 11–1*D* and 11–1*E*). The tissue adjacent to the remaining defect is then advanced toward the flap to test for the best position of the flap tip (Case 1, see Fig.

11–1*J*). The flap's tip position should be selected according to which placement causes the least distortion of surrounding structures by the secondary motion of the surrounding skin. Absorbable suture material will be used to obtain deep closure, and skin sutures can be used for the remaining closure.

Sites on the face suitable for rotation flap closures include the temples, cheeks, sides and dorsum of the nose, postauricular area, and chin. Rotation flaps can be developed on the extremities (Case 2, Fig. 11–2) and trunk.

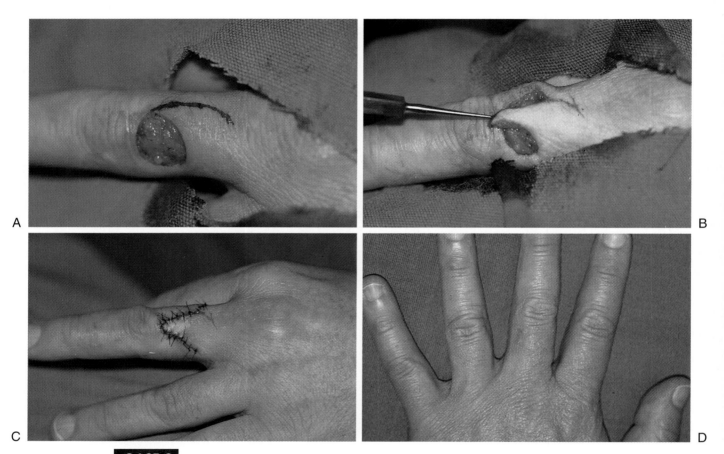

CASE 2

FIGURE 11–2. *A*, Rotation flap is planned to close the defect on the dorsum of the third digit of the hand. *B*, The flap is rotated into position. The tension along the line of maximal tension is demonstrated by the placement of the skin hook. This blanching of the flap shows vascular compromise. *C*, The tip of the flap is white at the completion of surgery. This is a troubling sign that necrosis may result. *D*, Even with slight necrosis of the tip of the flap, the finger has full function at 18 months.

Variations on the Rotation Flap

June K. Robinson

BACK CUT TO RELEASE THE MOTION OF THE FLAP

Each of the variants of the rotation flap (Table 11–5) works very well on convex surfaces such as the malar cheek area or the scalp. In performing rotation flaps, there are times when the lack of tissue mobility may make it impossible to execute the classic design illustrated in Case 1.

In such situations in which sufficient flap rotation is not possible, because of local skin tension or contour of the region, a back cut is necessary to allow the motion of the flap to proceed. With a back cut, an incision is made from the perimeter toward the center of the circle. This allows a defect to open and makes further rotation possible. It also limits the blood supply to the tip of the flap. If the back cut into the base of the flap is made too aggressively, the survival of the flap is endangered (Fig. 11–3).

If the back cut is not made, surrounding tissue (e.g., the lip) may be distorted by secondary motion about the flap (see Case 5, Fig. 11–7).

TABLE 11–5. Rotation Flap Variants

Single rotation
Double rotation (O-Z)
Multiple rotations

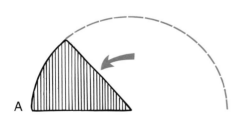
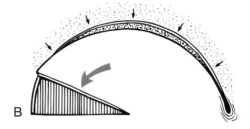
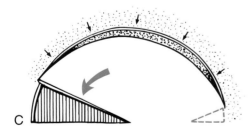
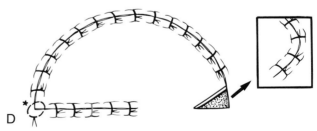

FIGURE 11–3. Back cut to release the motion of the flap. *A,* The flap is planned. *B,* After undermining the area around the flap, the flap is elevated but it is impossible to close the primary defect. *C,* A small back cut into the base of the flap allows the primary motion of the flap rotation to proceed. The primary defect is closed. *D,* The bunching of redundant tissue about the pivot point, seen in *B,* may be used to close the secondary defect by incorporating a Z-plasty (see Chapter 12) or just closed using the principle of halves as shown here.

LENGTHENING THE LEADING EDGE OF THE FLAP

In planning the rotation flap, it is helpful intraoperatively to use a piece of gauze to assess whether the planned flap is able to rotate into the defect (see Fig. 11–3B). The gauze is stabilized on the pivot point of the flap with one of the surgeon's hands. The other hand moves the tightly stretched gauze along the radius of the leading edge of the flap, simulating the motion of the tip of the flap from its original location to its proposed new placement along the line of maximal tension (Fig. 11–4A). If this maneuver shows that there is too much tension, then the circumference of the flap may be increased by lengthening the leading edge of the flap (see Figs. 11–4B and 11–5). Gauze is used to make this measurement rather than a straight ruler because gauze will conform to curvatures in the surface that the flap must drape over. This draping may increase the length of the leading edge of the flap.

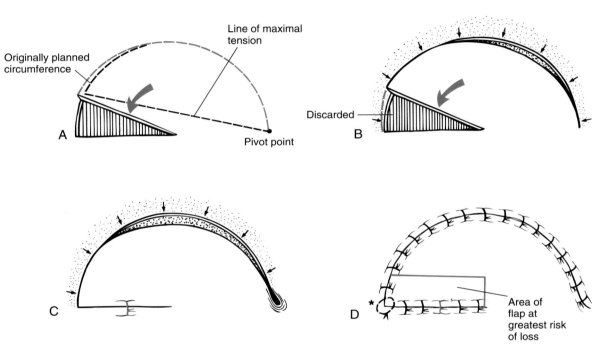

FIGURE 11–4. Lengthening the leading edge of the flap. *A,* After the gauze is stretched from the pivot point along the line of maximal tension and rotated to cover the defect, it is determined that the flap will not cover the defect. The leading edge of the flap is lengthened by extending it beyond the original circumference. *B,* A small portion of skin is excised from the outer edge of the defect, thus allowing the tip of the flap to be inset without undue tension. *C,* After this rotation of the flap is completed by placing the tension-bearing suture at the midpoint of the leading edge of the flap, a bulging of tissue forms about the pivot point. In cases in which a rotation flap is completed without a back cut, the wound has a shorter inner edge and a longer outer edge. The excess of outer skin bulges as a "dog ear." It is revised away from the base of the flap. *D,* The area of the flap at greatest risk of ischemic loss from too much tension or excessive extension of the back cut is at the tip *(area indicated in red).*

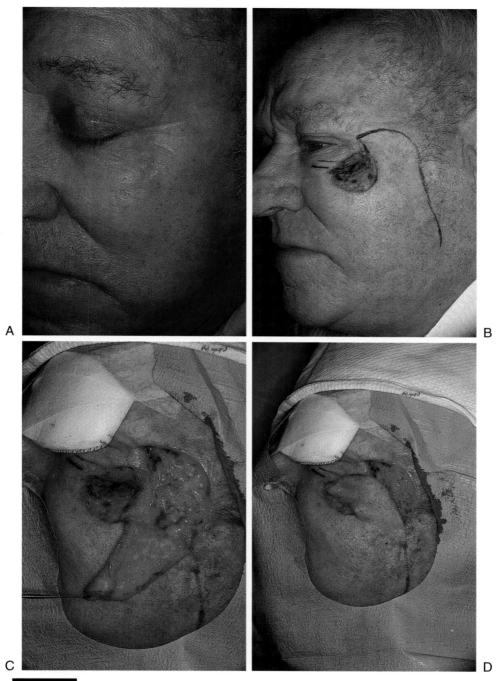

CASE 3

FIGURE 11–5. *A,* Preoperative appearance of a morphea-type basal cell carcinoma of the cheek at the junction with the eye area cosmetic unit. *B,* After excision of the tumor with Mohs' micrographic surgery, a rotation flap is planned to replace the loss of deep tissue and to prevent distortion of the lower lid. The rotation flap uses the well of lax tissue about the temple and preauricular cheek. The incision line follows the junction of the sideburn with the cheek. The leading edge of the flap is lengthened by extending the tip of the flap toward the brow. *C,* The level of undermining of the flap is very superficial in the fat to avoid injury to the temporal and zygomatic branches of the facial nerve. The flap is folded back with a skin hook to demonstrate the level of undermining used in raising the flap. *D,* The flap is placed with a single tension-bearing, buried suture at the middle of the curved incision of the flap as it comes into contact with the skin of the lateral canthus. This suture relieves the tension from the tip and allows delicate optimal placement of the tip with an aligning suture. The placement of the tip of the flap here prevents the eyelid from being everted by the secondary motion of the lower lid about the flap. All secondary motion occurs at the temple and cheek.

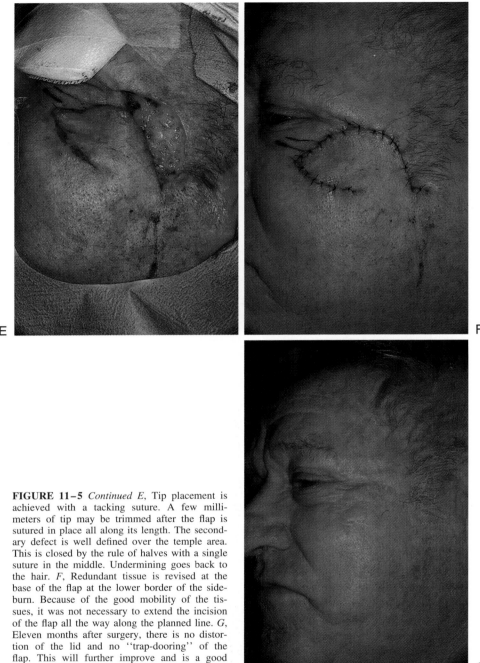

FIGURE 11–5 *Continued E,* Tip placement is achieved with a tacking suture. A few millimeters of tip may be trimmed after the flap is sutured in place all along its length. The secondary defect is well defined over the temple area. This is closed by the rule of halves with a single suture in the middle. Undermining goes back to the hair. *F,* Redundant tissue is revised at the base of the flap at the lower border of the sideburn. Because of the good mobility of the tissues, it was not necessary to extend the incision of the flap all the way along the planned line. *G,* Eleven months after surgery, there is no distortion of the lid and no ''trap-dooring'' of the flap. This will further improve and is a good result.

DOUBLE ROTATION FLAP (O-Z)

The final adaptation in using the rotation flap in skin with limited laxity is to use two or more flaps to cover the defect. This may be particularly effective on the scalp when hair regrowth is expected to cover the pinwheel-shaped scar produced by such flaps. Double rotation flaps may re-create the whorl of hair about the occiput of the scalp.

In planning the double rotation flap, the square defect is divided into two triangular defects. Each defect is then closed with its own rotation flap (Case 4, Fig. 11–6). The tips of the flaps are planned to exceed a 30-degree angle. If the tips become more narrow than this, they do not survive.

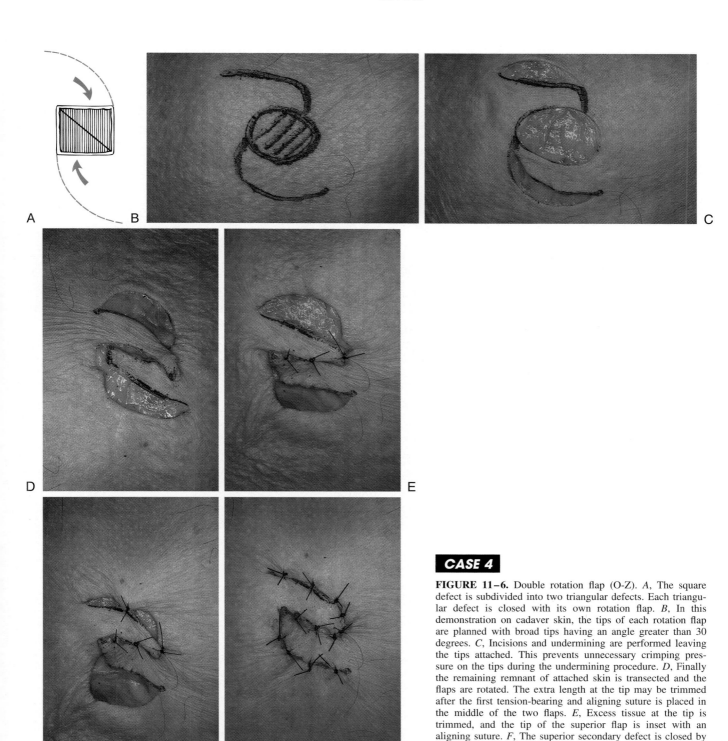

CASE 4

FIGURE 11–6. Double rotation flap (O-Z). *A,* The square defect is subdivided into two triangular defects. Each triangular defect is closed with its own rotation flap. *B,* In this demonstration on cadaver skin, the tips of each rotation flap are planned with broad tips having an angle greater than 30 degrees. *C,* Incisions and undermining are performed leaving the tips attached. This prevents unnecessary crimping pressure on the tips during the undermining procedure. *D,* Finally the remaining remnant of attached skin is transected and the flaps are rotated. The extra length at the tip may be trimmed after the first tension-bearing and aligning suture is placed in the middle of the two flaps. *E,* Excess tissue at the tip is trimmed, and the tip of the superior flap is inset with an aligning suture. *F,* The superior secondary defect is closed by halves. *G,* Both flaps are aligned and secondary defects are closed.

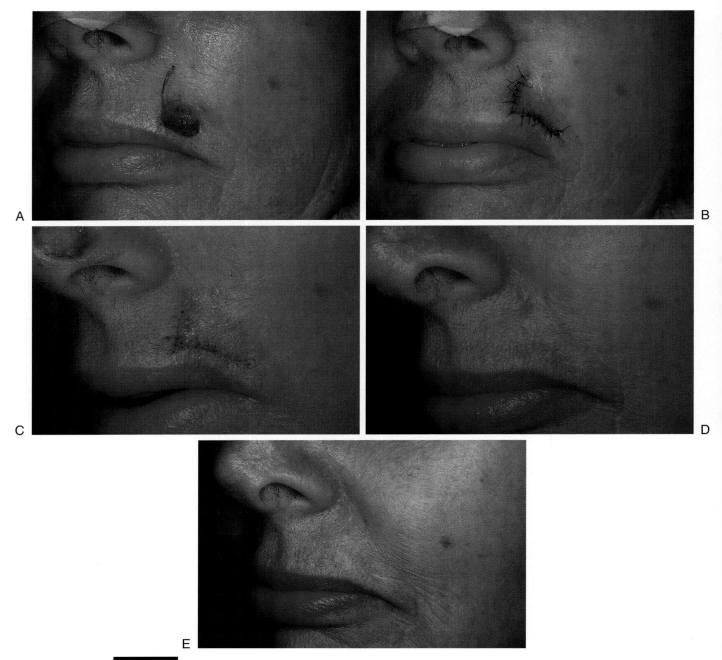

A

B

C

D

E

CASE 5

FIGURE 11–7. Upper lip—complication. *A,* This defect of the upper lip created by resection of a cancer with Mohs' micrographic surgery will be closed with a rotation flap as planned. *B,* In planning the flap, the amount of elevation of the vermilion border produced by secondary motion was not fully considered. Also, by leaving the small bridge of cutaneous skin remaining between the defect and the vermilion border it was not possible to place the incision at the vermilion and to release tissue at the base of the flap by revising the dog-ear at the oral commissure. *C,* At the time of suture removal in 1 week, the flap is somewhat edematous and the lip is elevated. The patient begins to massage the area three times a day for 20 minutes. Massage is a commonly performed postoperative technique thought to be useful. *D,* By 2 months, the flap edema is improved. The lip line is returning toward normal. The patient applies her lipstick a bit inside the vermilion border on this side and a bit beyond the vermilion border on the other side. *E,* At 1 year, the patient is no longer using her lipstick to correct the asymmetry of the vermilion but the unfortunate choice of incision line placement leaves the patient with a white scar across the upper lip.

Suggested Readings

1. Bennett RG. Fundamentals of Cutaneous Surgery. St. Louis: CV Mosby, 1988.
2. Dzubow LM. The dynamics of dog-ear formation and correction. J Dermatol Surg Oncol 1985;11:722–728.
3. Dzubow LM. The dynamics of flap movement: Effect of pivotal restraint on flap rotation and transposition. J Dermatol Surg Oncol 1987;13:1348–1352.
4. Dzubow LM. Facial Flaps: Biomechanics and Regional Application. Norwalk, CT: Appleton & Lange, 1990.
5. Dzubow LM, Zak L. The principles of cosmetic junctions as applied to reconstruction of defects following Mohs surgery. J Dermatol Surg Oncol 1990;16:353–355.
6. Stegman SJ, Tromovitch TA, Glogau RG. Basics of Dermatologic Surgery. Chicago: Year Book Medical Publishers, 1982.
7. Swanson NA. Atlas of Cutaneous Surgery. Boston: Little, Brown & Co, 1987.
8. Tromovitch TA, Stegman SJ, Glogau RG. Flaps and Grafts in Dermatologic Surgery. Chicago: Year Book Medical Publishers, 1989.
9. Whitaker DC, Birkby CS. An approach to cutaneous surgical defects of the forehead and eyebrow following Mohs micrographic surgery. J Dermatol Surg Oncol 1987;13:1312–1317.

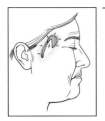

chapter 12

Transposition Flap

JUNE K. ROBINSON

When the motion of the flap carries it over an adjoining piece of skin to be placed in its new recipient site, the flap is a transposition flap. A number of flaps with various geometric patterns (e.g., rhombic) and in many anatomic locations (e.g., forehead) have transposition as their primary motion (Table 12–1). The flap rotates or pivots about a point, the turning point or pivot point, but once the flap is raised it turns through an angle and is elevated over intervening skin. In planning this flap, allowance must be made for the shortening in the length of the flap as it pivots about the turning point (Fig. 12–1). The flap length also shortens as the flap lies over elevations and depressions in contour (Tables 12–2 through 12–5).

The method of using a gauze sponge to determine flap length previously described in planning the rotation flap (see Chapter 11) is especially helpful in estimating the flap length of the transposition flap. The transposition flap buckles as it turns, and the gauze sponge mimics this buckling. In checking the planning of the classic transposition flap, the gauze is held with the thumb of one hand on the turning point (point A) and the other hand at the top of the recipient bed (point C). Then without moving the thumb, the gauze moves to the top of the flap (point B). If the gauze extends beyond the planned tip of the flap, then the flap needs to be lengthened.

In part, the planning of the flap dimensions depends on the secondary motion of the tissue about the flap. In most cases there is relatively little secondary motion. This lack

TABLE 12–1. Types of Transposition Flaps

Single Transposition Flap
Nasolabial flap
Rhombic flap
30-Degree angle transposition flap
Double Transposition Flap
Bilobed flap
Z plasty

TABLE 12–2. Transposition Flap: Indications and Contraindications

Indications
Disperse wound tension and tissue distortion over a wide area
Minimize deformity and helps to prevent scar widening
Contraindications
Long complicated scar that cannot be completely hidden
Pincushioning
Risk of tip necrosis increased by hypertension, diabetes, and smoking
Inability to cease anticoagulants, smoking, and control hypertension

TABLE 12–3. Transposition Flap: Patient Preoperative Discussion

1. Decrease or cease smoking and alcohol intake 2 weeks before surgery and for 1 week after surgery.
2. Stop taking aspirin 10 days before surgery.
3. No cosmetics or moisturizers on the face on the day of surgery. Do eat your regular meals and take your other medications.
4. If the surgery is on the arms or legs, there may be restrictions in your daily physical activities during the week after surgery. This will be discussed with you. If surgery is on the foot, special shoes may be needed.
5. Surgery in the region of the mouth may require a change in diet and dental hygiene during the week after surgery.
6. Keep the wound dry until stitches are removed.
7. If the surgery is on the face, sleep with the head elevated. Surgery of the forehead area may cause bruising around the eyes. Surgery of the cheeks may cause bruising in the jaw area.
8. Bruising and swelling may be present for 10 to 14 days after surgery.
9. No strenuous workouts, heavy lifting (>5 lb) for 14 days.
10. Return for wound check and dressing change by the doctor in 24 hours.
11. Most sutures removed in 7 days, but some may be removed in 10 days.
12. After stitches are removed the incision area is covered with Steri-Strips for 2 to 3 weeks. Then cosmetics may be used to hide the incision.
13. At the time of your visit in 4 to 6 weeks, further refinements to the flap will be discussed with you.

TABLE 12-4. Transposition Flap: Operative Issues

History

Smoking
Bleeding problems
Impaired wound healing
Prosthesis
Medications
Hepatitis or human immunodeficiency virus infection
Demand pacemaker

Physical Examination

Check other incisions for healing
Hypertension, pulse

Preoperative Equipment Needs

Flap repair tray
Skin marking pen
Materials to prepare the sterile field

Intraoperative Needs

Adequate local anesthesia and sedation
Maintain sterile field
Good lighting
Electrosurgical apparatus for hemostasis
In large flaps, suction available
Hemovac suction device available if problems intraoperatively in controlling bleeding

of secondary motion necessitates tapping one of the "wells" of lax tissue to repair the primary defect; thus the flap's width is usually the same as the primary defect. The transposition flap results in a secondary defect at least as great as the primary defect. If possible, the secondary defect is closed side-to-side; however, the donor site may have to be grafted or partially closed and the remainder allowed to heal by second intention. The transposition flap is effectively used for transferring tissue from an area of greater tissue mobility and laxity to an area where tissue is more firmly adherent to underlying structures. The transposition flap pushes tissue into the defect rather than pulling it as the advancement and rotation flaps do.

The classic single transposition flap (see Fig. 12–1) moves in an arc about the turning point. Although it is theoretically possible for the flap to move through an arc of 180 degrees, this is difficult to perform unless the flap is based on an artery. The kink at the base of a random pattern flap moved through 180 degrees decreases the perfusion of the tip. Random pattern transposition flaps commonly do not move through an arc greater than 90 degrees. As the flap moves, a protrusion forms at the base of the flap. The surgeon should resist the temptation to make

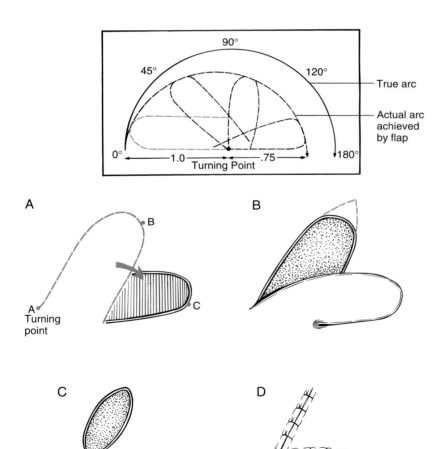

FIGURE 12-1. Transposition flap with 60-degree arc of motion. *A*, Planning the transposition flap requires the ability to predict the length of the flap necessary to cover the primary defect. By recognizing that the flap length depends on the motion about the turning point A; then the distance AC is used to plot AB, the line of maximal tension. As the flap turns through an ever larger arc, the length of the flap shortens. *B*, The area around the secondary defect is undermined widely before placement of the first suture. *C*, The first suture closes the secondary defect and produces bunching at the base of the flap. This redundancy may be revised in a second procedure. The bunching may be somewhat corrected by suturing techniques using wounds of unequal heights. *D*, The final closure results in a lengthy incision line.

back-cuts or remove bunching of skin by dog-ear revisions that may jeopardize the blood supply of the flap. These protrusions can be revised in a second procedure.

After the flap is cut, undermined, and elevated, the first tension-bearing suture placed closes the secondary defect.

The suture pushes the flap forward by pulling together the skin behind it. The flap is commonly used to rebuild defects of the nasal tip and ala by using the well of tissue in the nasolabial fold (Case 1, Fig. 12–2). The inferiorly based nasolabial flap is not based on an artery.

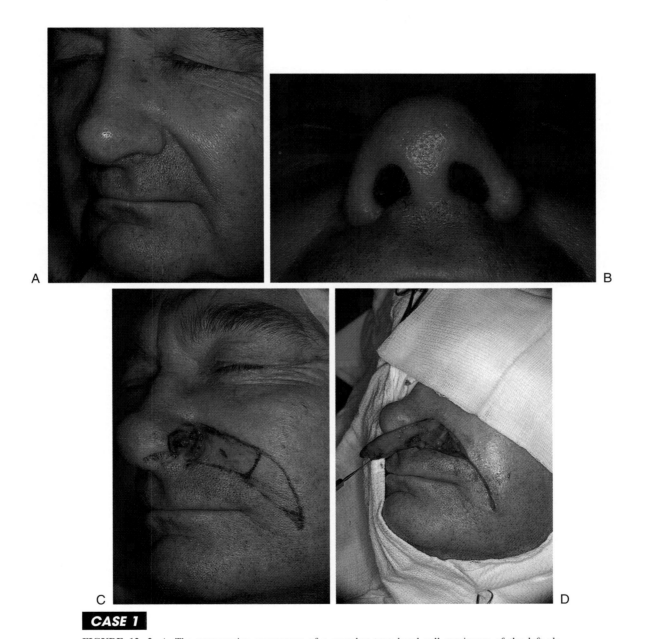

CASE 1

FIGURE 12–2. *A,* The preoperative appearance of a morphea-type basal cell carcinoma of the left ala shows a white, hardened mass extending beyond the central punch biopsy site. *B,* The basilar view shows thickening and infiltration of the ala extending into the nares. *C,* After resection of the cancer with Mohs' micrographic surgery, the loss includes the nasal lining. Pallor of nasal tip is due to epinephrine in the local anesthetic. The ala will be replaced as a cosmetic unit and lining provided by a nasolabial or melolabial flap. The flap design is placed into the nasolabial fold and is extended to include the potentially redundant triangle at the tip with a 30-degree angle. The section of the flap closest to the wound is turned in, and the tip of the flap is thinned excessively beyond the midpoint of the flap marked with gentian violet. This ''in-and-out'' flap folds on itself to create the alar rim. *D,* The secondary defect collapses on itself by a tension-bearing subcutaneous buried suture within the nasolabial (melolabial) fold at the base of the ala. The flap is 6.0 cm in length by 1.5 cm in width. The flap is transposed with a skin hook. The flap is elevated with a bulky base to preserve its blood supply.

Fig. 12–2 continued on following page

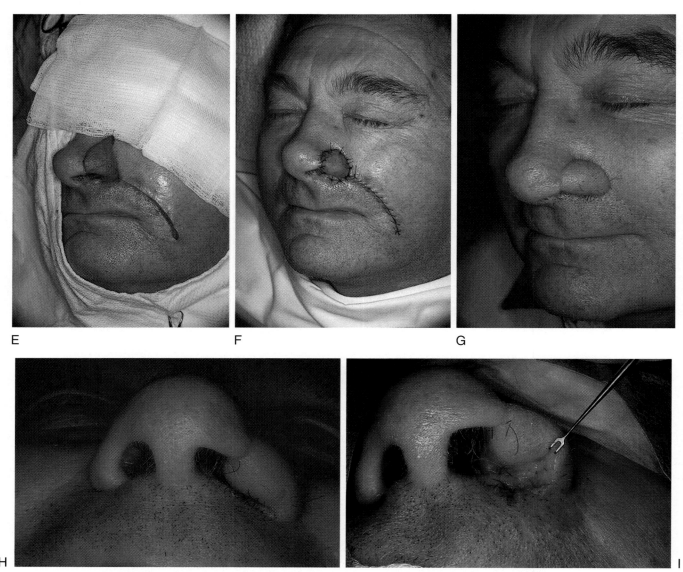

E F G

H I

FIGURE 12–2 *Continued E,* The initial aligning sutures placed into the flap are buried subcutaneous ones that turn the flap to provide the nasal lining. The curl of the alar base and patency of the nasal valve are ensured by a periosteal suture that suspends the weight of the flap from the nasal notch of the maxilla. Since permanent fixation is desired, a nonabsorbable buried suture, such as Prolene, is used for the periosteal suture. The tip of the flap is then folded onto itself to form the alar rim. This portion of the flap will be thinned and the tip trimmed to form the alar crease. *F,* At the conclusion of surgery the flap is a bit dusky but viable. Interrupted sutures were used to approximate wounds of unequal height on the flap. Because the donor site of the nasolabial fold was everted with subcutaneous sutures, a ''baseball'' type over-and-over running suture was used to approximate wound edges. The lip is elevated by the closure of the secondary defect. *G,* This design used the known tendency of the flap to heal with ''pincushioning'' to re-create the bulk of the alae. As expected, 4 months after surgery beard hair is growing on the reconstructed ala. This is plucked or trimmed with scissors. *H,* Basilar view 4 months after surgery shows that the bulkiness of the flap is partially obstructing the nares. This gives the patient a stuffy sensation especially when he is lying flat. *I,* To relieve the stuffy sensation, the flap is debulked with an incision at its base. This is the first revision of the flap and is done at 4 months after surgery to improve function.

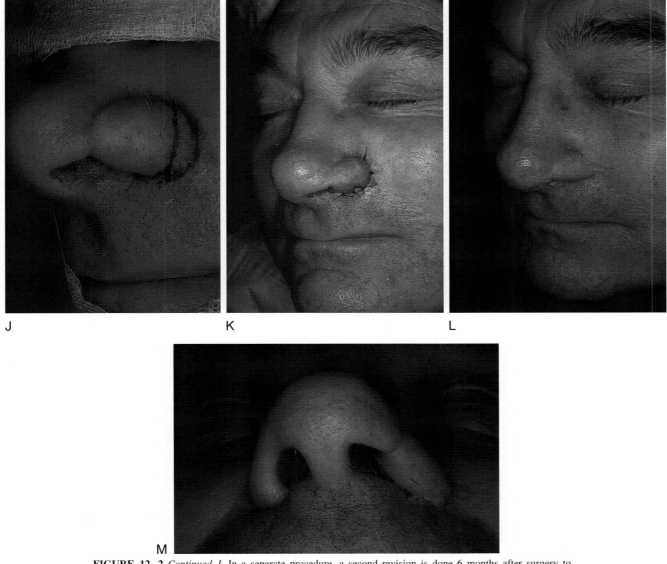

FIGURE 12–2 *Continued J,* In a separate procedure, a second revision is done 6 months after surgery to reposition the flap at its junction of the ala and the cheek. *K,* At the completion of the repositioning procedure, a slight elevation of the lip is present. *L,* One year after surgery, the flap has reconstructed the ala without disturbing the contours of the face. The lip is in normal position. This is an excellent cosmetic and functional result. *M,* From the basilar view, the airway is patent and there is no sensation of stuffiness. Nasolabial transposition flaps are ideal for repairing lateral alar defects.

RHOMBIC (RHOMBOID) FLAP

This single transposition flap is based on the pattern of a rhombus, which has two 60-degree angles and two 120-degree angles. In designing this flap one strives to bring in tissue from areas of laxity. Since the flap may be designed from two of the four potential corners of the rhombus, which is drawn around a circular defect, it is important to analyze (1) the motion of the flap, so that its construction will bring in the most useful tissue, and (2) the secondary motion of tissues surrounding the flap, so that its construction will least distort important landmarks. The most difficult aspect of using the rhombic flap is choosing the proper orientation from the many possibilities. If a surgical defect is round, it can be shaped into a rhombus oriented in any direction—a seemingly infinite set of possibilities. In this situation, the 120-degree angles are placed to point to where the excess of skin lies. If a surgical wound is elongated, the long axis of the rhombus is then established. Still there are four possible flaps that can be constructed off the short axis of the rhombus. Frequently more than one choice will work, but one may be best.

There are two basic criteria for selection of the flap

orientation. First, the flap should be chosen that most easily allows the flap to move into the defect without distortion of surrounding structures (Fig. 12–3D[1], point E moves to point C). Success is ensured if the secondary defect can close with minimal distortion of adjacent structures. Second, inferiorly based flaps will offer better lymphatic drainage and may therefore suffer less from a trapdoor (pincushioning) deformity. On any given rhombus, two of the flaps drawn off the 120-degree angles will usually be inferiorly based and the other two superiorly based.

The flap CDE is designed so that CD is the same length as AB, DE is the same length as BC, and the angle GFE equals the angle ABC, which is 60 degrees. As the flap is elevated, it collapses into the primary defect. The flap plan has changed the direction of tension on the surrounding tissues because in closing the secondary defect by approximating points C and E the forces on the surrounding skin

are 90 degrees to the initial tension of closing points A and C (see Fig. 12–3D[1]) by a primary closure. Thus, dropping the line CD perpendicular to the wide angle (short axis of the rhombus) points to the well of lax tissue (Case 2, see Fig. 12–3C). This line CD will always be perpendicular to the relaxed skin tension lines and cannot be camouflaged, but the long sides of the rhombus are parallel to the relaxed skin tension lines. The final incision line can be visualized in the planning process by holding a finger over lines GH and DE thus mentally erasing them (see Fig. 12–3D[3]).

Once the planning process is completed, the flap is elevated and widely undermined around its base, the donor areas, and the defect. Undermining of recipient sites allows the secondary motion to close the defect when the flap is slightly smaller than the defect. The flap should not be stretched because that will compromise the blood supply. Rather, the flap should drape into position easily.

A

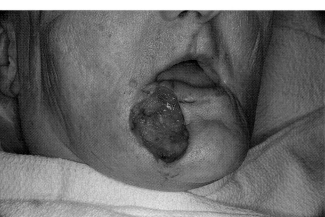

B

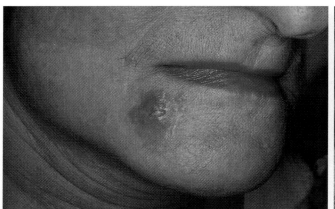

C

CASE 2

FIGURE 12–3. *A,* Preoperative appearance of a basal cell carcinoma with both nodular and morphea components. The tumor extends onto the vermilion of the lip. *B,* At the completion of the resection with Mohs' micrographic surgery, the flap dimensions are planned with the mouth open and shut. The mouth motion increases the dimensions of the flap and must be incorporated into planning the dimensions of the flap. The vermilion border is closed side-to-side before the flap is planned. There is no perforation into the oral cavity at the base of the defect; thus, the flap does not have to provide lining of the mouth. *C,* The dimensions of the rhombus around the primary defect are planned, and the flap dimensions are marked with gentian violet.

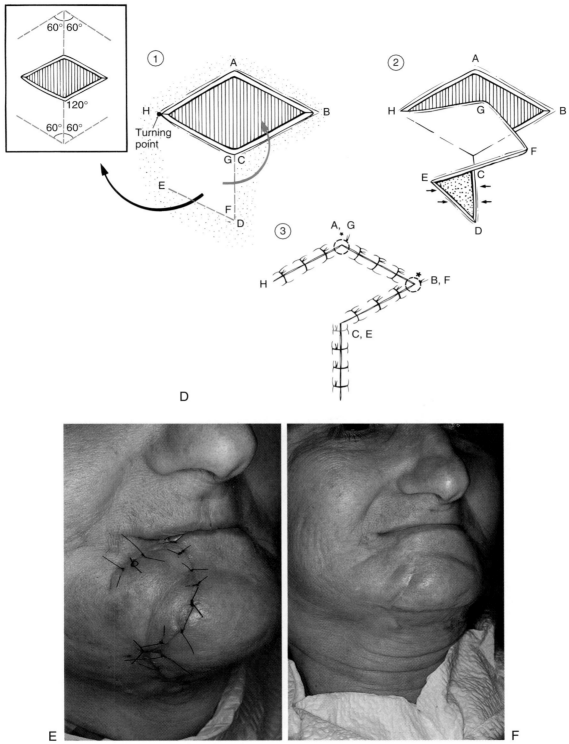

FIGURE 12–3 *Continued D,* Rhombic flap. For any rhombus, there are four different possible flaps to construct off the 120° angle (short axis of the rhombus). To decrease the amount of "pincushioning" it is generally better to try to use a inferiorly based flap. In this clinical example, the lax tissue lies inferior to the rhombus (primary defect) in the neck. *1,* The flap CDE is designed so that CD is the same length as AB and DE is the same as BC. The angle GFE is 60 degrees and fits into the angle ABC. *2,* As the flap is elevated, it collapses into the primary defect. The skin around the secondary defect is extensively undermined. *3,* The tension-bearing suture placed first closes the secondary defect (point CE). *E,* The flap is viable at the wound check in 48 hours, but erythema around the incision line indicates wound infection. A course of oral antibiotics is started. *F,* One year later, the patient has full use of the mouth and a good cosmetic result, considering the size of the defect that was reconstructed.

BILOBED FLAP

This double transposition flap uses two flaps to move the tissue from the area of laxity to the defect. In this maneuver the transposed tissue "walks down a series of steps" to get to the defect. For example the nasal tip defect has very little lax tissue adjacent to it; thus there is practically no secondary motion available. If the choice is to use glabellar lax skin, then it can be "stepped" down the nose by designing the first lobe to be the same size as the defect (Case 3, Fig. 12–4). The first lobe is placed to tap the small well of lax skin in the sidewall of the nose and paranasal cheek. If this well is accessed, then the second lobe from the glabella can be designed slightly smaller than the first because the secondary motion in the paranasal area will allow closure (see Fig. 12–4B).

If the location of the primary defect is in an area such as the cheek that allows secondary motion, then the first lobe can be designed to be smaller than the primary defect. The first lobe can be up to 20% smaller than the original defect. Similarly, if the skin around the first lobe allows secondary motion, then the second lobe can be up to 20% smaller than the primary flap. The second flap is often designed with an elliptical tip to facilitate side-to-side closure of the defect. The tip may be trimmed as needed to cover the defect.

The two lobes are separated by an angle that can vary between 45 and 90 degrees. The greater this angle between the two lobes, the larger the resulting dog-ear. The 45-degree angle appears to be ideal in limiting pincushioning and dog-ears, but the angle is less important than locating the second flap in an area of loose skin (see Fig. 12–4C[1]). Some degree of artistic license is desirable in creation of the bilobed flap, since the needs of the individual case preclude a strictly "by the book" approach. When designing the flaps, it is helpful to envision them pivoting about the central turning point through an arc. Each flap shortens as it turns.

The bilobed flap is particularly suited for reconstruction of the defects up to 1.5 cm in size of the lower third of the nose because of the unique ability of the flap to recruit skin of similar porous texture and preserve function of the nose. The single transposition flap (i.e., rhomboid flap) is more successful on the upper two thirds of the nose. In nasal flaps, adequate thinning of the flap so that no fat remains or deepening the primary defect to remove fat is helpful to prevent flap bulkiness. Widely undermining the skin surrounding the flap and the area beyond the base of the flap is thought to provide a uniform plate of scar contracture in the area, thus limiting the formation of a trap-door defect of the flap (pincushioning).

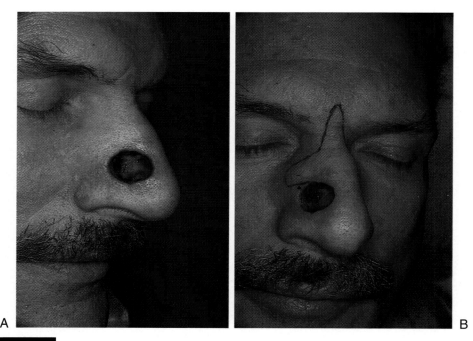

A   B

CASE 3

FIGURE 12–4. Bilobed flap. *A,* A defect of the nasal tip created by resecting a cancer with Mohs' micrographic surgery at the junction of the lateral sidewall of the nose is believed to be too large to repair with a rhombic flap. Rhombic flaps work well to repair smaller defects of the upper two thirds of the nose (the nasal dorsum above the alar crease). *B,* A bilobed flap is planned to use the lax tissue of the glabella. The acute 30-degree angle at the apex of the second lobe from the glabellar area was incorporated with the flap, but this is not shown by the skin surface marking with gentian violet.

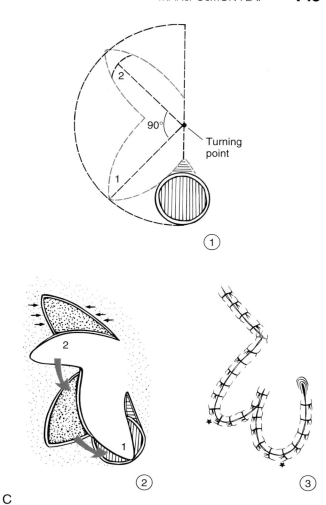

Turning point

①

FIGURE 12–4 *Continued C,* The first lobe forms a 45-degree angle with the defect and is planned to be the same width as the defect *(1).* The second lobe is at a 90-degree angle with the first and incorporates the potentially discarded tip that forms the ideal 30-degree angle for closure at the apex. Both flaps move about the turning point forming an arc. This arc includes the rim of the defect and forms a circle of the motion of the flaps into the defect. The radius of the circle is the length of the lobe of each flap. The second lobe is shorter than the first because secondary motion about the secondary defect will allow closure. A triangle of skin is excised between the defect and the pivot point of the flap before it is moved. The pivot point generally lies about one radius of the defect away from the defect *(2).* As the flaps are elevated, both move together *(3).* The tension-bearing suture placed first closes the secondary defect and pushes the flaps in place. *D,* One week after surgery the area is erythematous owing to recent scrubbing to remove adhesive material. After the first lobe was aligned and the glabellar secondary defect was closed, the second lobe of the flap was a bit too narrow, causing excessive pulling about the medial canthus. *E,* Four months after surgery, the flaps are elevated. The patient massages the area and is reassured that it will improve. *F,* Eighteen months after surgery, the flaps are level with the surrounding skin. The incision line could be improved with dermabrasion to reduce the height of elevation of the flaps. Pulsed-dye laser treatment of nasal telangiectasia would lessen the stark white appearance of the scar.

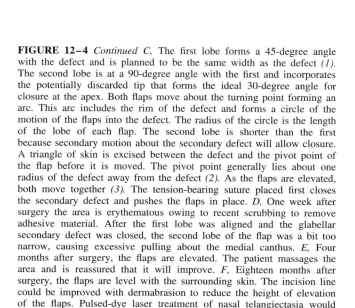

② ③

C

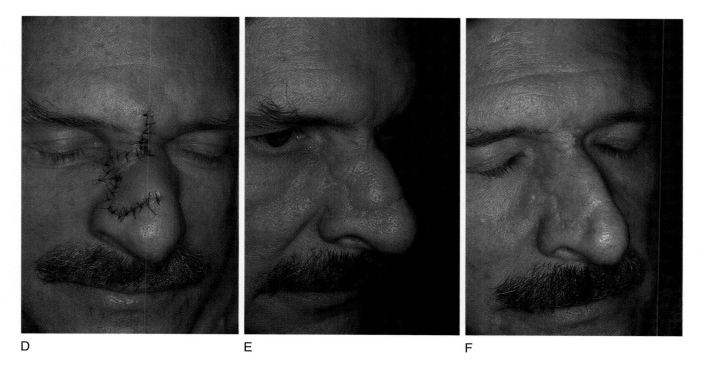

D E F

Z-PLASTY

The next commonly used double transposition flap is the Z-plasty. Although not really used to close a defect, it is often used in adjusting the pulls of closure and directions of final scars. The Z-plasty functions to lengthen the incision line, thus altering the forces of contraction (tension) on the incision lines, and to change the direction of scar lines. In designing the two triangular transposition flaps (Fig. 12–5), the angles of the flaps can be variable. The most gain in lengthening the wound is achieved with 60-degree angles (75% gain), but protrusions will form lateral to the incision. With a 45-degree Z-plasty there is a 50% gain in length, and with a 30-degree Z-plasty there is a 25% gain in length. As the angle becomes more acute, the risk of tip necrosis increases but there is less protrusion laterally.

In the Z-plasty, excess skin located laterally on either side of the line BC is used to lengthen that line; thus, this excess skin partially determines the size of the "Z" (see

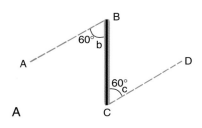

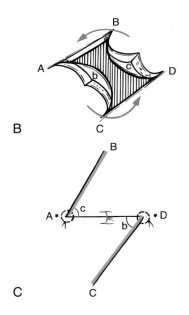

CASE 4

FIGURE 12–5. Z-plasty. *A,* Two triangular flaps each with 60-degree angles are planned with the goal of lengthening the vertical dimension. The 60-degree angles give a 75% gain. This gain can be calculated by AD − BC = gain. *B,* The tips of the flaps are transposed. Points B and C are pushed apart by the flaps. *C,* The closure line.

TABLE 12–5. Transposition Flap: Postoperative Care

Pain Management

Acetaminophen for 48 hours may be sufficient, but often an analgesic such as codeine is necessary

Rest with relative immobility of the area of surgery

If facial surgery, sleep with the head elevated. If an arm was operated on, use a sling to support. If a leg was operated on, elevate the extremity at rest

Dressings

Steri-Strip over the incision line

Nonadherent (Telfa) pad and fluff bulky absorbent dressing with pressure for 24 hours

Dressing change by physician in 24 hours; then just Telfa pad dressing. Check for excessive bleeding and signs of infection at 24 to 48 hours

Complications

Check immediately postoperatively for
  Bleeding
  Infection
  Dehiscence

Permanent Postoperative Changes and Treatment Options

Flap necrosis (Case 7, Fig. 12–9)
In the first week:
  Compress, culture wound; start systemic antibiotics
In the second and third weeks:
  Debride as necessary
  Allow to heal by second intention
By the second month:
  Cover the color change in healed areas with cosmetics
By 1 year:
  Revise contracted areas
Trap-dooring (pincushioning)
  Massage in the first 6 weeks
  Inject corticosteroids at 2 to 3 months
  Debulk at 4 to 6 months
  Break up the curved incision line with Z-plasties
  Dermabrasion

Fig. 12–5*A*). This increase in length will prevent contracture and allow the subsequent scar to conform to surface irregularities such as convexities or concavities. Incorporation of a Z-plasty into a scar may prevent bowstring contracture later. This technique is used to release tight, contracted scars. The less laxity of skin on either side of BC, the greater the need to construct a series of small "Zs" along the scar rather than one or two large "Zs." A series of small "Zs" so constructed will provide the same amount of lengthening along the direction of the original BC cross limb, but the resulting shortening of tissue on either side of line BC will become progressively less as more and smaller Z-plasties are constructed.

It is important to be able to forecast where the transverse limb of the completed "Z" will lie. This can be done by drawing its anticipated position across the scar to be revised. If the Z-plasty is designed to correct a linear

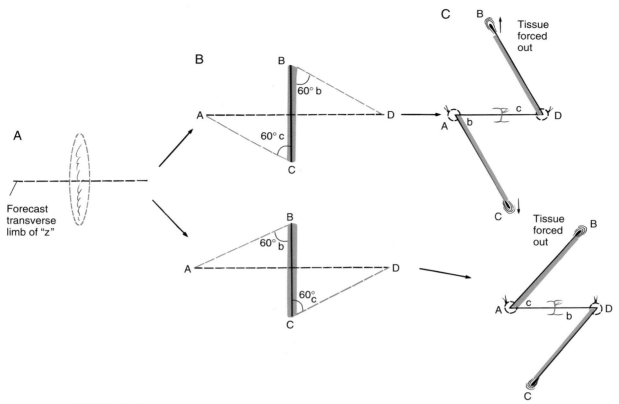

FIGURE 12–6. Forecasting the transverse limb of the Z-plasty. *A,* The scar is excised as an ellipse *(red dotted line represents incision).* The transverse limb will form an angle of 90-degrees to the scar. *B,* The limbs of the Z-plasty can be constructed in two ways. *C,* The final incision line should be planned so that some of the limbs are in the relaxed skin tension lines.

scar, then that scar becomes the central line and is excised through a narrow elliptical excision (Fig. 12–6). Although the axis of the central limb is normally changed 90 degrees, the change may be less or more, depending on the pulls and tensions of surrounding tissues. Note that the lateral incision limbs maintain their initial orientation after transposition. Since there are two different possible orientations for the lateral limbs in any Z-plasty (see Fig. 12–6B), their position should be designed to parallel the relaxed skin tension lines. If designed so that the lateral limbs cross relaxed skin tension lines perpendicularly, those incisions will be visible and may become hypertrophic.

If the flap is used over concave surfaces, the central limb after transposition should not cross the concavity in order to avoid creating a web (Case 5, Fig. 12–7). If the Z-plasty is performed to lengthen a scar or release a web, the scar or web becomes the central line. On the face it is ideal to keep the flaps less than 1 cm in length for ease in concealing the final result.

Although understanding the purpose of transposition flaps is useful, the everyday experience of many dermatologic surgeons is that other repairs may answer the need with fewer complications. The surgeon must always carefully assess the merits of a particular flap procedure and its risks and should choose the technically less difficult and less risky repair that will solve the problem. Once committed to performing a transposition flap, the surgeon proceeds according to the Turkish proverb, "Measure a thousand times and cut once" (Case 6, Fig. 12–8; Case 7, Fig. 12–9).

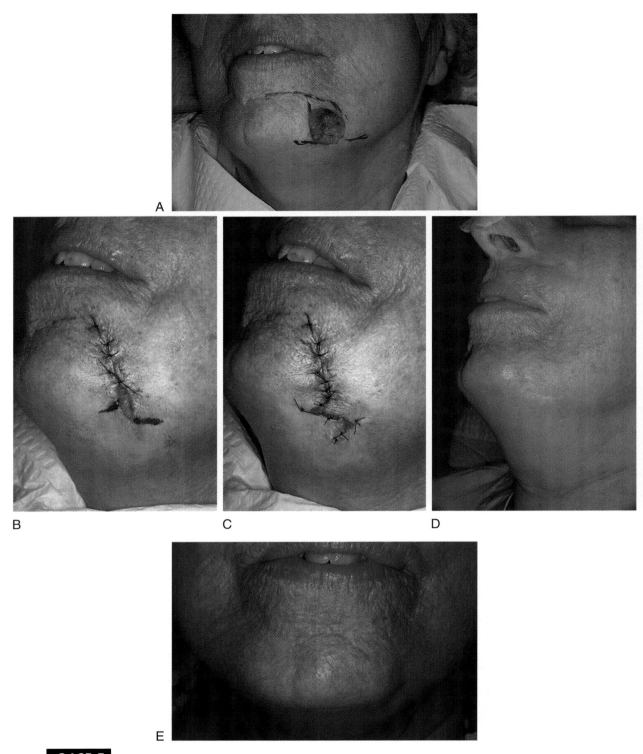

A

B

C

D

E

CASE 5

FIGURE 12–7. Z-plasty. *A,* After excision of a basal cell carcinoma of the chin by Mohs' micrographic surgery the mental crease and mandibular lines are marked. The superior portion of the primary defect is enlarged to allow the closure to lie in the mental crease. *B,* As the side-to-side closure is performed, it is clear that the incision will be carried across the mandibular line. A Z-plasty is planned to allow the incision to lie in the concavity of the neck and provide additional tissue along the mandibular line. The limbs of the Z-plasty are marked with gentian violet. *C,* At the completion of surgery, the flap tips are viable. *D,* One year after surgery, the incision line lies under the mandible. *E,* From the anterior view (1 year after surgery), the scar is hidden at the junction of the lip and the chin. This is an optimal result.

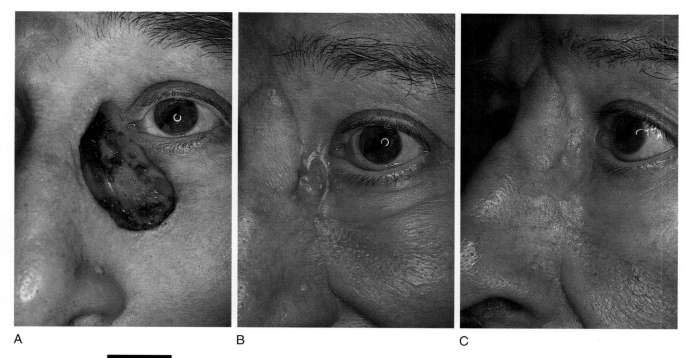

A   B   C

CASE 6

FIGURE 12–8. Transposition flap: complications. *A,* A large defect of the inner canthus and lower lid results from resection of a skin cancer by Mohs' micrographic surgery. Reconstruction was planned with a combination of two flaps: a lower lid advancement flap and a transposition flap from the glabella to the inner canthus. *B,* Insufficient length was planned for the transposition flap as it moved over the hump of the nose. When the leading edge of the transposition flap failed to reach the advancement flap, a full-thickness skin graft from a retroauricular site was used to provide coverage of the remaining defect. At 4 months after surgery, the wound edges around the graft are elevated and the graft is depressed. There is a slight ectropion of the lower lid that is symptomatic. The patient notes a tearing problem with tears spilling over at the medial canthus. *C,* Over the next year, scar maturation and softening did correct the ectropion and no revisions were necessary. Triamcinolone (Kenalog) injections into the area of contraction under the graft were also given.

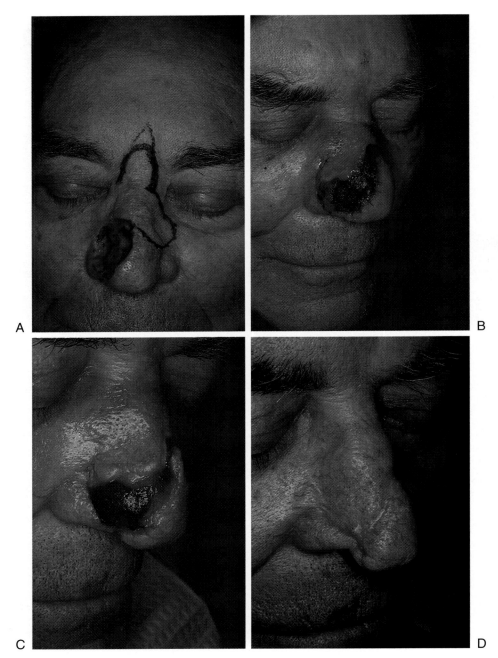

FIGURE 12–9. Transposition flap: complications. *A,* A bilobed flap is planned to replace a large defect of the right ala and nasal tip resulting from Mohs' micrographic surgical resection of a basal cell carcinoma. The base of the wound does not have any perforations into the nares. The patient is hypertensive and smokes two packs of cigarettes a day. *B,* Seven days after surgery, there is extensive necrosis of the tips of both flaps. The patient resumed smoking after surgery by going to his unheated garage in the middle of subfreezing winter temperatures in Chicago. He did not wish his wife to know he was smoking. The flap was doomed by anoxia from cold exposure and cigarette smoking, and the patient was at risk for bleeding problems because of his hypertension. Wet compresses and systemic antibiotics were started. *C,* Three weeks after surgery, the extent of the tissue loss is clear and debridement can be performed without excessive removal of viable tissue. *D,* Six months after surgery, it is surprising how much of the flap survived. There is elevation of the alar rim in the area of greatest contraction owing to loss of the tip of the flap. Improvement of this result will be very difficult because the bilobed flap has already used the patient's available well of tissue and his underlying medical condition puts any surgical procedure at risk of failure.

Suggested Readings

1. Davidson TM, Webster RC, Gordon BR. The Principles and Dynamics of Local Skin Flaps. Chicago: American Academy of Otolaryngology Head and Neck Surgery Foundation, 1983.
2. Hynes B, Boyd JB. The nasolabial flap: Axial or random? Arch Otolaryngol Head Neck Surg 1988;114:1389–1391.
3. Jackson IT. Local Flaps in Head and Neck Reconstruction. St. Louis: CV Mosby, 1985.
4. McGregor JC, Soutar DS. A critical assessment of the bilobed flap. Br J Plast Surg 1981;34:197–199.
5. Riefkohl R, Wolfe JA, Cox ER, et al. Association between cutaneous occlusive vascular disease, cigarette smoking and skin slough after rhytidectomy. Plast Reconstr Surg 1986;77:592–595.
6. Siana JE, Rex S, Gottrup F. The effect of cigarette smoking on wound healing. Scand J Plast Reconstr Surg 1989;23:207–209.
7. Sutton AE, Quatela VC. Bilobed flap reconstruction of the temporal forehead. Arch Otolaryngol Head Neck Surg 1992;118:978–982.
8. Yanai A. Flexible rhombic flap. Plast Reconstr Surg 1986;78:228–235.
9. Yanai A. The Z in Z-plasty must have a long trunk. Br J Plast Surg 1986;39:390–394.
10. Zitelli JA. The bilobed flap for nasal reconstruction. Arch Dermatol 1989;125:957–959.

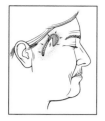

chapter 13

Split-Thickness Skin Grafts

DAVID J. LEFFELL

Split-thickness skin grafting is a technique for the reconstruction of wounds when final cosmesis is not paramount.[1] By definition a split-thickness skin graft contains epidermis and a variable amount of dermis (Fig. 13–1). The amount of dermis present determines the thickness of the graft and therefore its "take rate" or chance of survival. In general, the thinner the graft, the higher the rate of survival but the less optimal will be the cosmetic result.[2] Although factors such as local anesthesia may affect survival of full-thickness skin grafts, this has not been demonstrated for split-thickness skin grafts.[3]

Split-thickness skin grafting may be used to cover large areas, and this must be considered the primary indication (Table 13–1). Because the cosmetic result (usually from graft contraction due to deficient dermis[5]) is often suboptimal, the split-thickness skin graft should only be used in regions and in patients in whom the cosmetic result is not of greatest concern.

DONOR SITES

The donor site must be selected with consideration given to visibility of final donor scar (which will be a broad, hypopigmented patch), ease of harvesting, ease of wound care, and risk of secondary infection. The method of harvesting will also be influenced by location (Fig. 13–2; Tables 13–2 and 13–3).

DONOR SITE PREPARATION

The donor site, selected for ease of graft harvesting and ease of patient care, should be prepped with an antiseptic such as Phisoderm and draped with sterile towels. A small amount of lubricant such as K-Y Jelly or petrolatum should be applied in a very thin layer to facilitate dermatome passage. The donor site should then be treated with 20% aluminum chloride (Drysol) to control bleeding from dermal vessels and dressed as described in Table 13–4.

TABLE 13–1. Split-Thickness Skin Grafts: Indications, Contraindications, Limitation

Indications
Large full-thickness wound
Temporary coverage
Compromised wounds (to hasten healing and minimize infection)[4]
Observation for cancer recurrence

Contraindications
A wound small enough to be repaired by flap or full-thickness graft
Donor defect is created.

Limitation
Cosmetic result may be suboptimal.

TABLE 13–2. Split-Thickness Skin Grafts: Instrumentation

Site	Preferred Method	Limitations
Anterior, lateral and medial thigh	Brown, Padgett, Storz, Davol	Should be used only for large grafts
	Weck, free-hand	Possible irregular specimen
Buttocks	Same	Same
Abdomen	Same	Not an ideal location

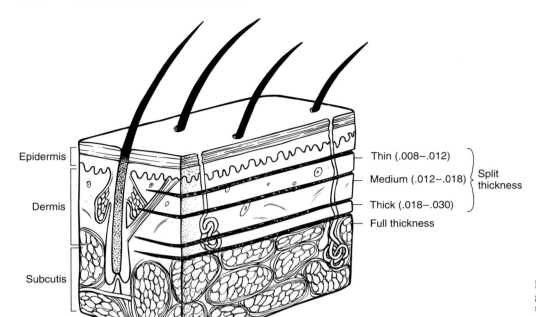

Epidermis

Dermis

Subcutis

Thin (.008–.012)

Medium (.012–.018) } Split thickness

Thick (.018–.030)

Full thickness

FIGURE 13–1. Split-thickness skin grafts may be thin (0.008–0.012 mm), medium (0.012–0.018 mm), or thick (0.018–0.030 mm). Note corresponding anatomic landmarks.

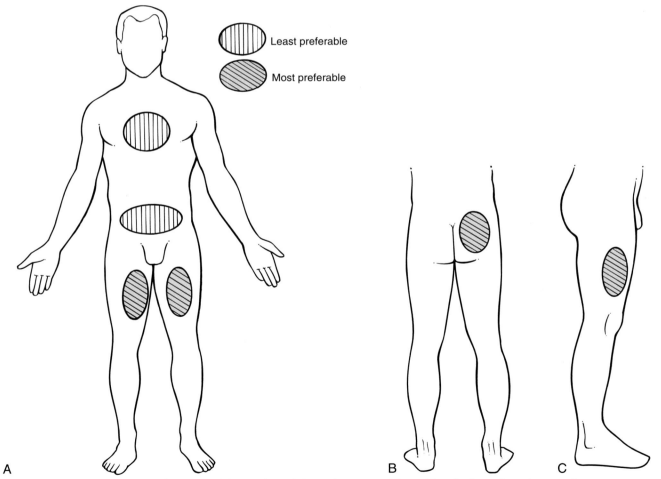

Least preferable

Most preferable

A

B

C

FIGURE 13–2. *A,* Split-thickness skin graft donor sites are noted here with optimal area for patient wound care identified by pink shading. *B* and *C,* When cosmesis of the donor site is a concern, buttock skin should be harvested. Sites are more preferable because of the ability to get a firm, flat area. This makes it easier to harvest the split-thickness skin graft.

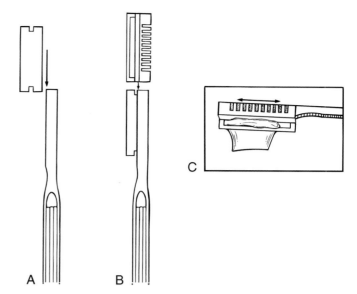

FIGURE 13–3. Assembly of the Weck knife requires two steps. *A*, The blade is inserted into the slot in the handle. *B*, The spacer slides over the shaft of the handle and leaves a defined space between the blade and the spacer. This determines the thickness of the split-thickness skin graft. *C*, The motion *(arrow)* of the handle is a to-and-fro one, like sawing or slicing, that carries the blade forward into the skin. The skin graft comes up between the blade and the spacer.

GRAFT HARVESTING AND APPLICATION[8]

After the defect has been measured and the required graft size determined, the surgeon outlines with gentian violet or an indelible marker (Sharpie pen) a rectangle that subsumes the required graft area. The area is anesthetized in a ring distribution using lidocaine with epinephrine, except when epinephrine is contraindicated. Alternatively, if enough notice is given, topical anesthetic cream (EMLA, eutectic mixture of local anesthetic—lidocaine 2.5% and prilocaine 2.5%, Astra Pharmaceuticals), applied under occlusion for 2 hours provides excellent anesthesia and should be considered for graft harvesting from a large area. Regardless of the graft device used (Figs. 13–3 through 13–5), the skin must be held taut with the aid of an assistant (Figs. 13–6 and 13–7). The harvesting motion should be smooth to prevent uneven graft thickness (Fig. 13–8).[9] The harvested graft is placed in sterile saline until it is needed.

TABLE 13–3. Split-Thickness Skin Grafts: Methods of Graft Harvesting

Type	Advantage	Disadvantage
Freehand with razor blade or No. 15 blade	Rapid, good for small grafts such as pinch grafts	No depth control
Freehand with Weck knife (see Fig. 13–3)	Rapid, can control thickness with spacer	Depth control depends to some degree on pressure applied; saw-toothed graft edges
Davol & Storz dermatomes Davol: battery/Storz: AC (see Fig. 13–4)	Easy to use	Sterility; width of graft (may have to harvest in sections)
Padgett dermatome Brown dermatome (see Fig. 13–5)	Ideal for large grafts	Hesitation in graft harvesting may yield adverse donor scar result

TABLE 13–4. Split-Thickness Skin Grafts: Dressings for Donor Site

Dressing[6]	Method	Comments
Duoderm[7]	Apply directly over wound with at least 1-inch border; apply gauze followed by an Ace bandage (if site is on limb), to absorb oozing. *Alternative:* cover wound with regular hydrocolloid dressing (Duoderm), then put a much larger patch of thin Duoderm for a margin beyond wound of 2 inches.	Many patients complain about oozing; may use this for first 5 days, then change to antibiotic salve and nonadherent (Telfa) pad; patient may have to change Duoderm daily.
Tegaderm Opsite Biocclusive (similar product also marketed under different brand names)	Apply same as above	Oozing also a problem, but this and above method minimize pain; use for 2 weeks, if possible changing every 3 days
Antibiotic ointment and nonadherent dressing	Apply daily	Caution patient not to allow wound to dry.

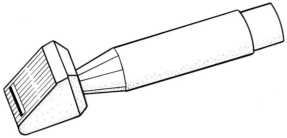

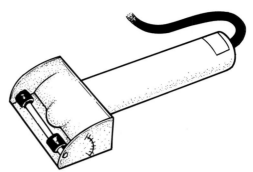

FIGURE 13–4. The Davol dermatome uses a disposable head with a preset width and thickness for the graft. A rechargeable battery handle is the power source.

FIGURE 13–5. The Padgett dermatome has a scale on the side to set the thickness of the graft. It is plugged directly into the electrical outlet.

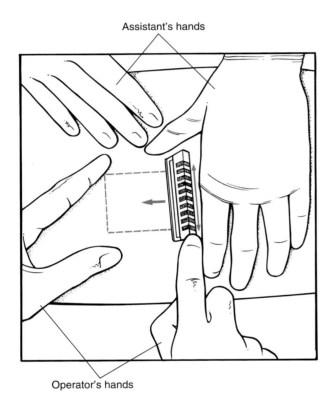

Assistant's hands

Operator's hands

FIGURE 13–6. The skin is held taut with the aid of an assistant as the operator harvests the graft using a Weck knife. The surgeon's motion is like sawing or slicing (*red arrows* indicate the motion).

FIGURE 13–7. *A* and *B*, The surgeon's motion with any dermatome that uses a power supply is similar to a plane landing and taking off. The skin being harvested is elevated by the assistant so it does not bunch up in the well of the dermatome. A Brown dermatome is shown. Failure to move smoothly across the skin at any stage may result in unnecessary donor site scarring.

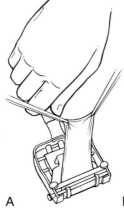

A

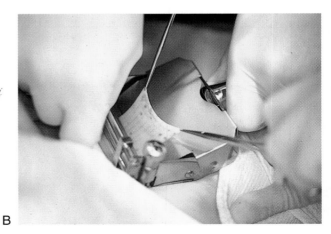

B

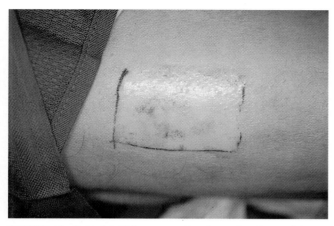

FIGURE 13–8. Partial-thickness wound at donor site after graft harvesting. Note pinpoint bleeding in region of dermal papillae. This confirms superficial nature of graft harvesting. The use of epinephrine in the local anesthetic prevents more vigorous capillary bleeding.

The graft should be draped over the defect (see Fig. 13–10), previously cleansed with antiseptic and rinsed with sterile saline. Especially over concavities one must be certain that the graft has draped completely and no tenting is present[10] (Figs. 13–11 and 13–12). Failure to take into account the additional surface area required for concavities results in harvesting an inadequate graft. The graft may be secured in place with *any* of the methods described in Table 13–5.

GRAFT DRESSINGS[11]

The purpose of the graft dressing is to optimize contact of the graft with the wound bed. Within 3 to 5 days angiogenesis establishes communications with the transplanted skin so that any disruption of those new vessels by shearing forces should be minimized.[12] The options in Table 13–6 are available to be used as a bolus tie over dressing (Fig. 13–9) or secured by taping.

TABLE 13–5. Split-Thickness Skin Grafts: Graft Suturing

Ligature	Method	Comment
6-0 fast absorbing gut	Running suture	No need for suture removal; may not be strong enough in areas of mobility
5-0 or 6-0 nylon or Prolene	Running suture	Requires suture removal at 7–10 days when manipulation may disrupt graft edges
5-0 or 6-0 nylon or Prolene	Interrupted suture with extended tails for bolster	Bolster is helpful where it is otherwise difficult to apply pressure dressing
Steel staples	Space 5 to 7 mm apart depending on region	Ease and speed in application; no staple marks if removed by 5 days

TABLE 13–6. Split-Thickness Skin Grafts: Dressings for Graft Site

Dressing	Application	Comment
Tegapore + iodoform gauze + cotton balls	Tegapore (nonadherent mesh bandage on graft), iodoform gauze applied over this and molded to graft topography, then cotton balls to support graft secured with overlying 4 × 4-inch gauze	Leave in place for 1 week; if bandage is very bloody at second day wound check, may remove iodoform without affecting graft or Tegapore
Tegapore + cotton bolster	Apply Tegapore cut to 5 mm beyond graft size; place petrolatum gauze, wrap around cotton, and secure with bolster method	Some moisten gauze to conform to wound bed, but this may increase risk of infection; and when gauze dries out, it frequently adheres to graft or rest of bandage; avoid unprotected cotton balls since fibers can become enmeshed in graft edges.
Nonadherent dressing + antibiotic ointment + gauze and elasticized tape	Apply ointment daily and replace nonadherent dressing at the same time	This is the least desirable method because it results in too much graft manipulation.

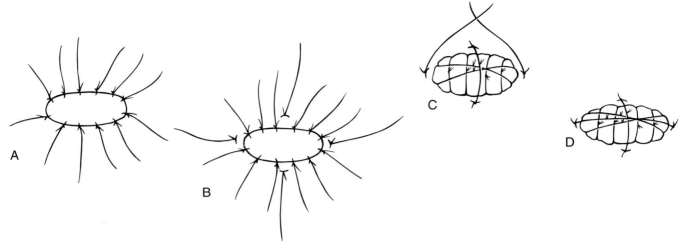

FIGURE 13–9. *A*, Sutures for the bolster are placed into the graft and wound margin like a regular interrupted suture, but one tail is left long enough to tie over the dressing. A hemostat should be available to temporarily hold all ends together so they do not get in the way of placing the next suture. *B*, Some surgeons also place four sutures into the skin away from the graft. *C*, At least four pairs (eight sutures total) should be used, and each should be tied to its corresponding suture on the other side of the bolster. Always tie the sutures that are 180 degrees away from each other rather than going in sequence around the bolster. *D*, If the surgeon chooses to use tie-over sutures distant from the graft, then these sutures are tied last.

TABLE 13–7. Split-Thickness Skin Grafts: Complication and Pitfalls

Complication	Cause	Remedy (if any)
Early		
Misplaced graft	Failure to correctly identify dermal surface by glistening quality	Graft failure; leave in place until it sloughs; wound will heal by second intention
Sheared graft	Inadequate attachment; should always consider basting sutures when graft movement is a possibility	Some of the graft will likely take; must explain problem to patient so he or she knows what to expect
Hematoma Seroma[13]	Patient on anticoagulants or has used aspirin-type compounds; postoperative activity by patient	Prepare large grafts with small, 5-mm incisions to permit drainage of hematoma or seroma; make sure optimal pressure dressing is in place
Infection	Cover all patients prophylactically with 1 week of antibiotics; in ear graft, consider ciprofloxacin to cover *Pseudomonas* when cartilage is exposed	Antibiotics
Late		
Color mismatch[14]	Donor site not from same body region	If major concern, use cosmetics to cover. If erythematous, consider pulsed dye laser
Texture mismatch	Dark scaly appearance due to absence of adnexal structures and accumulation of keratin debris; mismatch may also be due to poor site selection	Clean graft aggressively
Crenulated graft (see Fig. 13–12)	Thin dermis and mobile graft site	Regraft with full-thickness skin graft
Graft failure	See above	Explain to patient that wound will heal by second intention and revision can be considered at a future date

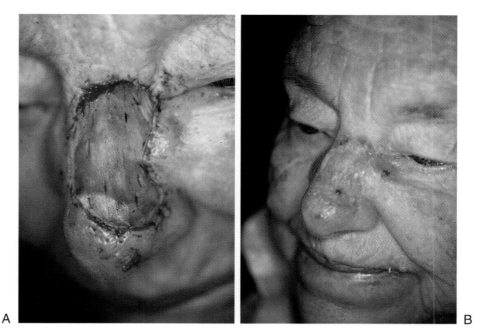

FIGURE 13–10. *A,* Split-thickness skin graft in place over dorsum of nose. This site could have been repaired with a full-thickness skin graft, which may have been preferable for color and texture match. Small incisions have been made to prevent accumulation of blood and wound fluid. *B,* Split-thickness skin graft at 2 weeks demonstrating early blood supply and increasing adherence at graft edges.

A

B

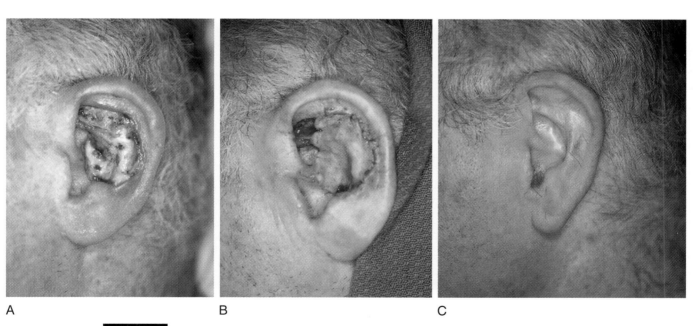

A

B

C

FIGURE 13–11. *A,* Anthelix and conchal bowl defect after excision of recurrent squamous cell carcinoma with Mohs' micrographic surgery. To monitor for tumor recurrence a split-thickness skin graft was chosen. *B,* Split-thickness skin graft sutured in place with 6-0 fast absorbing gut suture, which will not have to be removed. This graft is so thin that it is almost translucent. The poor blood supply of the exposed cartilage of the base necessitated a very thin graft. The portion of the graft at the crus of the anthelix remains to be stretched out to cover the wound. *C,* Follow-up at 1 year after surgery shows that the area of the graft is white and the architecture of the ear is preserved.

**TABLE 13–8. Split-Thickness Skin Grafts:
Patient Postoperative Instructions**

1. A split-thickness skin graft has been selected to speed up the healing of the wound and make wound care as easy as possible.
2. No special care of the graft is required, but it is important to take it easy. This means no sports, heavy lifting, or garden work.
3. In 1 week the pressure bandage will be removed, and since the graft will have attached, normal activity may be resumed. Steri-Strips may be put on the graft at that time and can be removed in 5 days.
4. The donor site requires more attention. A special dressing has been put on to speed the healing by bathing the wound in its natural wound fluids. Often so much wound fluid collects that it drips out and has the appearance of blood. Do not be alarmed, but also be prepared for this dripping since it may soil clothes.
5. After 5 to 7 days, you may discontinue the gelatin- or Saran wrap–type dressing and apply antibiotic ointment twice a day after cleaning the area with soapy water. Do not use hydrogen peroxide. DO NOT LET THE AIR GET TO THE WOUND since it will dry out, and this may cause more pain and delay healing.
6. Your skin graft should heal within 2 weeks, but your wound at the donor site may take 2 to 3 weeks to heal over. After that it will be red for 6 months to a year, but eventually it will approach the color of the skin around it. Hair should grow in the area as before since the hair follicles were not taken with the graft.

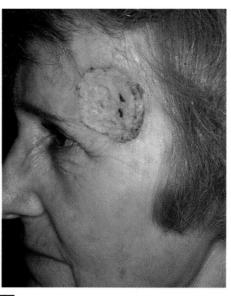

CASE 3

FIGURE 13–12. Sequelae of split-thickness skin grafts. Early postoperative picture of split-thickness skin graft of temple in a woman in her 50s. Note early crenulation. This will likely smooth with time so assurance is necessary. It is also helpful to explain to the patient that revision is a possibility in the future. (Courtesy of Neil A. Swanson, M.D.)

References

1. Swanson NA, Tromovitch TA, Stegman SJ, Glogau RG. Skin grafting: The split-thickness graft in 1980. J Dermatol Surg Oncol 1980;6:524–526.
2. Keswani RK, Goel NK. Contraction and relaxation in split skin autografts: A human study. Indian J Plast Surg 1974;7:46.
3. Wolfort S, Rohrich RJ, Handren J, May JW Jr. The effect of epinephrine in local anesthesia on the survival of full- and split-thickness skin grafts: An experimental study. Plast Reconstr Surg 1990;86:535–540.
4. Van Den Hoogenband HM. Treatment of leg ulcers with split-thickness skin grafts. J Dermatol Surg Oncol 1984;10:605–608.
5. Brown D, Garner W, Young VL. Skin grafting: Dermal components in inhibition of wound contraction. South Med J 1990;83:789–795.
6. Feldman DL. Which dressing for split-thickness skin graft donor sites? Ann Plast Surg 1991;27:288–291.
7. Porter JM. A comparative investigation of re-epithelialization of split thickness skin graft donor areas after application of hydrocolloid and alginate dressings. Br J Plast Surg 1991;44:333–337.
8. Skouge JW. Techniques for split-thickness skin grafting. J Dermatol Surg Oncol 1987;13:841–849.
9. Vecchione TR. A technique for obtaining uniform split thickness skin grafts. Arch Surg 1974;109:837.
10. Polk HC. Adherence of thin skin grafts. Surg Forum 1966;7:487.
11. James MI. Alteration of split skin graft contraction with a synthetic dressing. Eur J Plast Surg 1990;13:97–100.
12. Clemmesen T. The early circulation in split-skin grafts: Restoration of blood supply to split-skin autografts. Acta Chir Scand 1964;127:1.
13. Littlewood AHM. Seroma: An unrecognized cause of failure of split-thickness skin grafts. Br J Plast Surg 1960;3:42.
14. Lopez-Mas J, Ortiz-Monasterio F, Viale De Gonzales M, Olmedo A. Skin graft pigmentation: A new approach to prevention. Plast Reconstr Surg 1972;49:18.

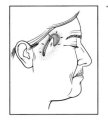

chapter 14

Full-Thickness Skin Grafts

RANDALL K. ROENIGK and MARK J. ZALLA

In a dermatologic surgical practice, there are two common indications for full-thickness skin grafting: hair transplantation and reconstruction of defects that result from excision of malignancy.[1,2] This discussion will be limited to the use of this type of grafting for reconstruction.

When making a decision to reconstruct with a full-thickness skin graft, other options such as primary closure, flap closure, split-thickness skin grafting, or second intention healing are considered. Primary closure and flaps have obvious advantages because the superior blood supply enhances survival of the flap and wound healing. We believe a split-thickness skin graft should rarely be used except perhaps for burn wounds, large defects off the face, or locations with a poor vascular bed such as leg ulcers (Table 14–1). Second intention healing is cosmetically and functionally at least as good if not better than split-thickness skin grafting for most smaller defects.

When the relative immobility or scarcity of tissue adjacent to the defect makes a flap impractical, transplantation of skin from a distant site is the only alternative. If adjacent tissue is severely photodamaged or of poor quality due to prior radiation therapy, distant tissue may be preferable.

In our experience, most full-thickness skin grafts are performed on the head and neck, especially the nasal tip and helical rim.[3] Other favorable sites are the forehead, upper lip, eyelid, and digits. The amount of adjacent tissue laxity is often limited on the forehead and digits, and flaps for large lip defects distort the face. Additional considerations are the surgical difficulty or risks of creating a flap. For example, a two-staged midline forehead pedicle flap to repair a nasal tip defect is significant surgery for a defect that would be more simply repaired by a single procedure with a full-thickness graft. Patients at risk of hemorrhage, who might require extensive undermining to repair large defects with a flap, may also be good candidates for full-thickness skin grafting. In addition, because full-thickness skin grafting provides better protection due to graft thickness than second intention healing or split-thickness skin grafts, a full-thickness skin graft from a donor site on the trunk is a reasonable option for traumatized areas such as the digits or dorsum of the hands, where donor site match is less important (Table 14–2).

Once the decision to perform a full-thickness skin graft has been made, the most important clinical consideration is

TABLE 14-1. Comparison of Skin Grafts

	Full-Thickness	**Split-Thickness**	**Composite**
Nutritional requirements	High	Low	High
Color	Good	Poor	Good
Contraction	Low	High	Low
Durability	Fair	Poor	Fair
Sensation	Good	Fair	Fair
Appendageal functions (hair, eccrine, sebaceous)	Excellent	Poor	Good

Reprinted from Wheeland RG. Skin grafts. In: Roenigk RK, Roenigk HH, Jr, eds. Dermatologic Surgery: Principles and Practice. New York: Marcel Dekker, 1989:324. By courtesy of Marcel Dekker, Inc.

the donor site and the concept of donor dominance. Transplanted tissue retains the character and texture of the site from which it came. Choice of a donor site that matches the skin adjacent to the defect in color, character of the skin appendages, and thickness is critical to the cosmetic outcome.

Traditionally, the retroauricular and supraclavicular areas are common donor sites for facial full-thickness skin grafts so that the donor scar is hidden. The preauricular and submandibular sites provide other options. These donor sites are satisfactory for large defects on the forehead or helical rim but poor choices for a site such as the nasal tip. A less commonly used but very acceptable donor site is the nasolabial fold, which provides a very good match for nasal skin.[4,5] Although the donor scar is in the central facial region, it is easily camouflaged in the crease and heals very well. The upper and lower eyelids are also excellent donor sites for repair of lid defects in patients with excess lid tissue. The inguinal and axillary folds and antecubital fossae are good donor sites for nonfacial defects (Fig. 14–1).

Absolute contraindications for small full-thickness skin grafts are few. Grafts will not take well on avascular beds such as denuded cartilage or bone. In such cases, burr holes through the helical cartilage or outer table of the skull may be helpful. Delayed grafting to allow granulation tissue to develop is another option. Grafting onto fat or tendon poses similar problems. Uncontrollable hemorrhage or persistent oozing is also a contraindication since development of a hematoma below a graft will compromise its survival. Immediate grafting may be contraindicated in patients with multiply recurrent aggressive tumors when observation after excision is desired to detect early recurrence (see Table 14–2).

TABLE 14–2. Full-Thickness Skin Grafts: Indications, Contraindications, Limitations

Indications

Lack of tissue excess
Avoidance of distortion
Poor adjacent tissue quality
Need for single-staged repair
Avoidance of large flap procedures
Sites of trauma

Contraindications

Avascular defect beds
Uncontrolled bleeding
Observation for recurrence

Limitations

Availability of matching donor skin
Large size
Avoidance of trauma
Donor site scar

Limitations to full-thickness skin grafting are likewise few and relate primarily to the availability of well-matched donor skin. Although there are no absolute size limitations for repair with full-thickness skin grafting, very large grafts (>5 cm) may not receive adequate nutrition centrally to allow complete viability. However, even large grafts on well-vascularized beds usually survive. Adequate graft adhesion and neovascularization require immobility of the graft particularly during the first 1 to 2 weeks postoperatively; the decision to graft may be limited by the patient's ability to avoid trauma during this time. The procedure to obtain the graft causes a scar, but donor sites are chosen in

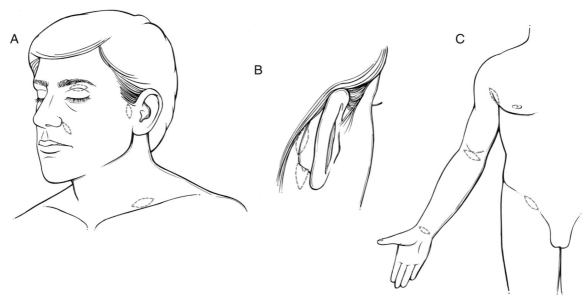

FIGURE 14–1. *A* through *C*, Available donor sites for full-thickness skin grafts. Preauricular and nasolabial fold donor sites are more easily used in women than men whose beard hair follicles can be transplanted. In men, displacement of the sideburn can occur in the preauricular donor site.

part because those scars can be hidden (see Table 14–2). Morbidity is minimal for the donor site since this is usually a simple excision.

PREOPERATIVE EVALUATION

The preoperative history does not differ from that obtained for other cutaneous surgery (Table 14–3). However, attention is paid to the use of anticoagulants, the need for antibiotic prophylaxis, and allergies. If possible, patients taking aspirin-containing medications are requested to discontinue use at least 1 week before surgery, and those taking warfarin (Coumadin), 2 to 3 days before surgery. However, full-thickness skin grafting is a good alternative to an extensive flap when these medications cannot be avoided.

At the time of surgery, the defect to be repaired is shown to the patient. All of the options for closure are considered. Available donor sites are reviewed with particular attention to obtaining good color, texture, and thickness match and the ability to hide the donor site scar. Choice of the donor site is discussed with the patient. Some considerations when choosing the donor site are a previous history of radiation therapy and the presence of other lesions or scars.

PROCEDURE

The equipment required includes routine local anesthesia, antibacterial skin preparations, sterile draping, and a

TABLE 14–3. Full-Thickness Skin Grafts: Operative Issues

Preoperative Evaluation

History
  Bleeding diatheses
  Infections, esp. hepatitis, human immunodeficiency virus
  Medications, esp. aspirin, anticoagulants, immunosuppressive agents
  Antibiotic prophylaxis: prostheses, valvular disease
  Allergies
  Prior radiation theapy
  Consideration of postoperative dermabrasion

Preoperative Equipment Needs

Local anesthesia
Topical antibacterial preparation
Sterile drapes
Standard surgical tray
Gentian violet or marking pen

Intraoperative Needs

Template material optional
Sterile saline solution
Antibiotic ointment
Nonadherent (Telfa) pad
Sterile dental roll or gauze
Bolster suture, 4-0 or 5-0 nylon

standard surgical tray (e.g., scalpel, forceps, needle holder, scissors, suture) (see Table 14–3). Some surgeons use a template of the defect to outline and harvest the graft and secondarily convert the donor site to an ellipse. Aluminum foil in the suture pack works well as a template. We usually harvest the graft directly as an ellipse after measuring to ensure adequate width and length. The graft can be stretched slightly, and the tissue adjacent to the defect can be undermined if necessary to achieve better graft fit. The donor site may be left open until graft placement and then closed routinely. If the graft is not to be placed immediately, it may be kept in sterile saline until needed.

Before placement, the undersurface of the graft should be defatted (Fig. 14–2A), and the dermis may be trimmed as needed to contour to the defect depth.[6] An important consideration is whether the graft has hair. If a graft with hair is being transplanted into a non–hair-bearing area, the follicle bulbs need to be trimmed or destroyed on the undersurface.

When placing the graft an absorbable tacking suture is helpful (usually 5-0 Vicryl on the face) (Fig. 14–2B). This prevents a potential dead space from forming as a result of bleeding and provides stability after removal of the bolster. This suture should not be placed too near the epidermis or slight scarring may be noted after healing. Once the graft is tacked in place, the skin edges are approximated with 6-0 nylon interrupted skin sutures. If harvested as an ellipse, several stabilizing sutures are placed, skin edges are trimmed as necessary, and then the remainder of the interrupted sutures are placed (Fig. 14–2C). For most smaller grafts there is seldom need for drains or fenestrations; however, some surgeons believe that making incisions in the graft helps granulation tissue reach the upper layers of grafted skin to improve survival. We have not found this necessary for most small grafts. After the graft is sutured in place, a bolster dressing is applied over antibiotic ointment and nonadherent gauze (Fig. 14–2D). Sterile dental rolls work well as bolsters for small grafts, or fluffed gauze is used for larger grafts (see Table 14–3). The graft should be immobilized with this dressing for at least a week on the face and 2 weeks off the face. Even minor trauma such as scratching at the skin can loosen the graft enough to cause dehiscence. A protective dressing of gauze and tape is then applied over the bolster.

CASE EXAMPLES

Case 1 occurred in a patient with a nasal tip defect (Fig. 14–3). A full-thickness skin graft from the nasolabial fold is a very reasonable alternative to more complicated options such as a large flap from the nasal dorsum and sidewall or a pedicle flap from the forehead. Note how well the graft matches adjacent tissue when it is taken from the nasolabial fold and how well hidden the scars are postoperatively (Fig. 14–3E). Case 2 demonstrates a patient with radiation dermatitis and a large basal cell carcinoma on the upper lip and cheek (Fig. 14–4). Matching this skin was difficult, but an excision was performed

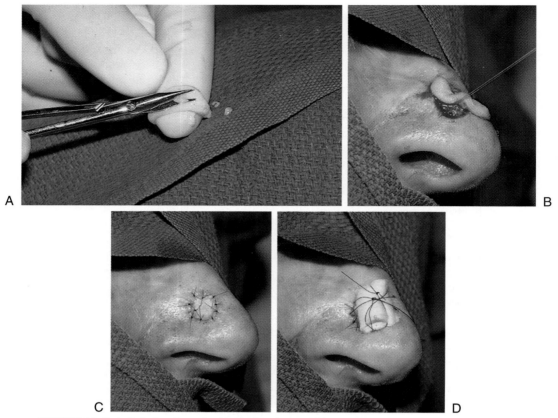

FIGURE 14–2. *A*, Defatting the graft with Gradle scissors. White dermal tissue remains on the graft, which is draped over the surgeon's left index finger. *B*, Placement of a central absorbable tacking suture. *C*, Graft sutured in place. *D*, Dental roll bolster dressing sutured in place.

under the neck in the submandibular area where there was comparably damaged tissue. Rather than using one large graft, the elongated donor site was divided into three grafts that were pieced together like a jigsaw puzzle, attempting to re-create the nasolabial fold. The donor site for case 3 was the antecubital fossa (Fig. 14–5). Full-thickness skin grafts take quite well on the subcutaneous fat of the digits and provide better durability than a split-thickness skin graft. An extensive flap (possibly two stages) is avoided as well. Despite decreased cutaneous circulation in this site, our experience and that of others is that full-thickness skin grafts up to several centimeters in diameter take well.[7]

WOUND CARE

Patients are informed that after the graft is placed a bolster dressing will be sutured over it to provide pressure and stability and that the dressing and graft must stay dry until suture removal. No wound care will be required at the graft site; however, twice-daily cleansing with hydrogen peroxide and application of antibiotic ointment is suggested for the donor site (Table 14–4). On the night of surgery,

the patient is requested to sleep propped on two or three pillows. Wound care to the donor site begins the following morning and will continue until sutures are removed from both graft and donor sites in 7 days. During this time, patients are asked to refrain from vigorous exercise, heavy lifting, or bending over. After removal of the bolster, routine wound care is continued on the graft for an additional 2 to 3 days or until complete healing has taken place, in the event of epidermal or dermal slough. Patients are informed that the surgical sites, especially that of the graft, will remain pink and perhaps itchy for 2 to 3 months and that any firmness or scarring at either site normally softens over the ensuing 6 to 12 months. The possibility of postoperative dermabrasion at 6 to 8 weeks is discussed preoperatively and at follow-up for cosmetically important areas but is usually not necessary.

COMPLICATIONS

Complications after full-thickness skin grafting for small defects are rare (see Table 14–4). It is uncommon that grafts are painful. Infection is rare but may require appro-

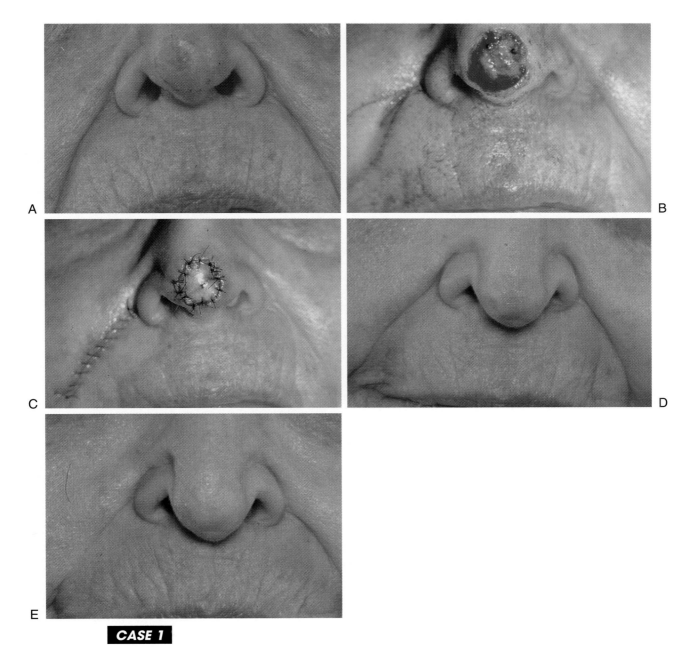

CASE 1

FIGURE 14–3. *A*, Basal cell carcinoma on the nasal tip outlined with gentian violet. *B*, Defect after Mohs' micrographic surgery exposing the perichondrium overlying the nasal tip cartilages. *C*, Appearance immediately after placing a full-thickness skin graft harvested from the right nasolabial fold. *D*, Result 2 months postoperatively. Note residual erythema and pigmentary change. *E*, Result 17 months postoperatively. Note erythema and pigmentary change has resolved. The graft is cosmetically acceptable, and the donor site is imperceptible. This is an excellent result.

priate antibiotics. Routine antibiotic prophylaxis is not required nor are postoperative narcotic analgesics. Regular or extra-strength acetaminophen is usually sufficient. Bleeding may occur as with any surgical procedure but with adequate hemostasis is usually minimal. Epidermal slough is not uncommon, and occasionally superficial dermal necrosis may develop. One to 2 weeks postoperatively, the graft may look red and boggy or even purple. This does not necessarily mean that the graft has failed but does mean that wound care with topical antibiotic ointments should be

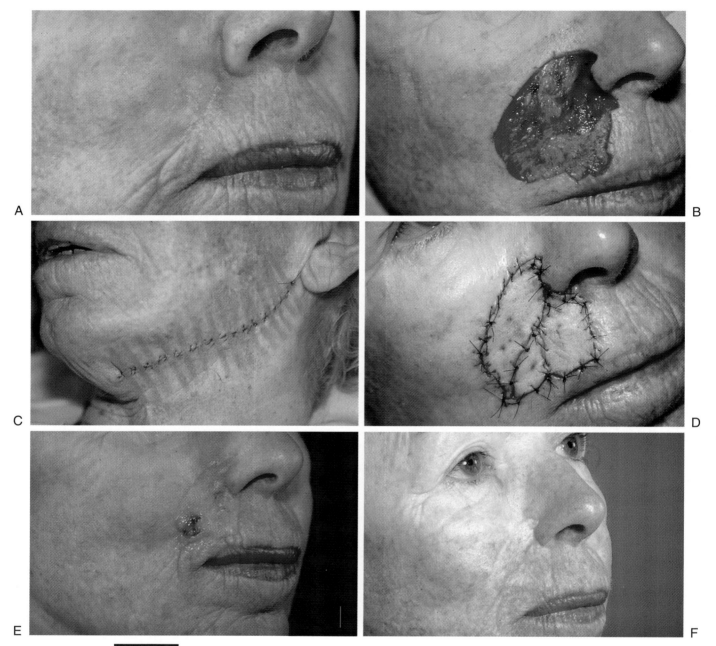

CASE 2

FIGURE 14–4. *A*, Recurrent morphea-type basal cell carcinoma on the right cheek and upper lip crossing the nasolabial fold in a patient with chronic radiation dermatitis. *B*, Defect resulting after Mohs' micrographic surgery. *C*, Donor site for the full-thickness skin graft in the left submandibular area. Note that the excision is long and narrow. *D*, Donor skin is cut into three smaller grafts that are pieced together partially along skin tension lines like a jigsaw puzzle. *E*, Result 6 weeks postoperatively. Note that the graft partially dehisced and that it is still thick, as expected during the contraction stage of wound healing. *F*, Result 8 months postoperatively is excellent.

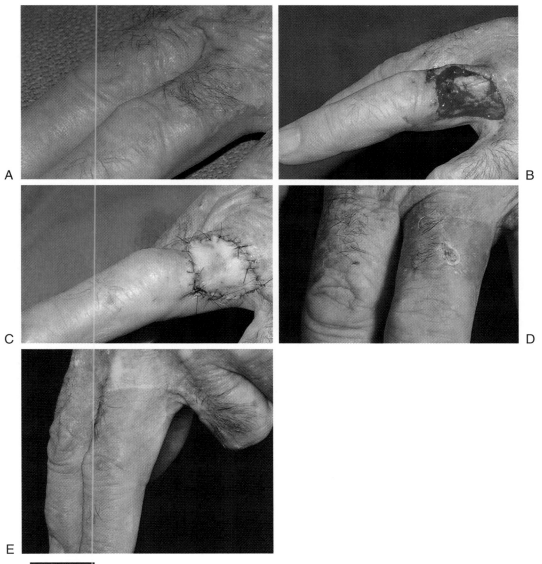

CASE 3

FIGURE 14–5. *A,* Squamous cell carcinoma on the dorsal aspect of the left third finger in the proximal intraphalangeal area. *B,* Defect after Mohs' micrographic surgery. Note the thin synovium that overlies the extensor tendon. Fat still remains at the periphery of the defect. *C,* Result postoperatively after placement of a full-thickness skin graft. The donor site for these grafts is typically the antecubital fossa or the anterior axillary area. *D,* Result 7 weeks postoperatively. Note that the majority of the graft has taken. However, over the central portion of the graft there was some dehiscence where it had been tacked to the synovium and extensor tendon. This was treated with standard topical wound care only. *E,* Result 17 months postoperatively shows good function and cosmetic result.

continued until all crusting or erosion has healed. This may take several days in the case of epidermal slough or 2 to 4 weeks for dermal necrosis (Table 14–5).

Hypertrophic scar formation is uncommon. Corticosteroids intralesionally or topically may be used during the contraction stage of wound healing (2 to 4 months postoperatively) to decrease thickness, but this will resolve spontaneously regardless of therapeutic intervention. The patient may massage the graft once or twice daily for 20 minutes, but medical intervention is not routinely necessary as the graft matures. With proper planning and technique, these grafts are usually very cosmetically acceptable once healed. Modification with dermabrasion remains an option for cases in which a less than satisfactory outcome results.

TABLE 14-4. Full-Thickness Skin Grafts: Postoperative Care

Pain Management
Acetaminophen, regular or extra-strength

Dressings
Keep bolster dressing clean and dry.
Cleanse donor site with dilute hydrogen peroxide twice daily followed by antibiotic ointment.
Cover with gauze and tape at bed time and if risk of soiling.

Complications
Pain
Infection
Bleeding
Epidermal slough
Superficial dermal necrosis
Complete dehiscence with scarring

TABLE 14-5. Full-Thickness Skin Grafts: Causes of Graft Failure

Technical errors
  Improper thickness
  Hematoma
  Poor immobilization
Poor graft bed
  Bone, cartilage, fat, tendon
  Necrotic debris
Improper patient care
  Trauma
  Dependent position
Infection

References

1. Wheeland RG. Skin grafts. In: Roenigk RK, Roenigk HH Jr, eds. Dermatologic Surgery: Principles and Practice. New York: Marcel Dekker, 1989;323–345.
2. Johnson TM, Ratner D, Nelson BR. Soft tissue reconstruction with skin grafting. J Am Acad Dermatol 1992;27:151–165.
3. Hill TG. Reconstruction of nasal defects using full thickness skin grafts: A personal reappraisal. J Dermatol Surg Oncol 1983;9:995–1001.
4. Booth SA, Zalla MJ, Roenigk RK, Phillips PK. The nasolabial fold donor site for full-thickness skin grafts of nasal tip defects. J Dermatol Surg Oncol 1993;19:553–559.
5. Beare BLB, Bennett JP. The nasolabial full thickness graft. Br J Plast Surg 1972;25:315–317.
6. Johnson TG. Contouring of donor skin in full-thickness skin grafting. J Dermatol Surg Oncol 1987;13:883–888.
7. Wright JK, Brawer MK. Survival of full-thickness skin grafts over avascular defects. Plast Reconstr Surg 1980;66:428–431.

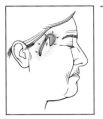

chapter 15

Composite Graft

ANN F. HAAS and RICHARD G. GLOGAU

Composite grafts contain two or more tissue layers. The type of composite graft that comes immediately to mind is the skin–cartilage graft usually used to replace alar rim defects; however, the harvested donor plug used in hair transplantation is also technically a composite graft (Table 15–1). Composite grafts are selected for areas where the various layers provide appropriate contour, thinness (or thickness, depending on recipient area and type of composite graft chosen), and structural support. Because of the high risk of failure secondary to the high metabolic demand, surgical technique and hemostasis are extremely important to protect the tenuous vascular supply. In addition, like other types of grafts, composite grafts are harvested from a donor site usually remote from the recipient site, so there is a second (and sometimes quite painful, in the case of auricular donor sites) surgical incision. Because of the need for proximity of the graft to vascular tissue, the composite graft should probably be no larger than 1.5 to 2 cm (see Table 15–1). A complete patient preoperative discussion is listed in Table 15–2.

TABLE 15-1. Composite Graft: Indications, Contraindication, Limitations

Indications
Alar defects
Auricular defects
Eyebrow repair
Scalp hair loss
Contraindication
Defect size greater than 1.5–2.0 cm
Limitations
Reduced size of ear
High risk of failure due to metabolic demands

TABLE 15-2. Composite Graft: Patient Preoperative Discussion

1. Healing will be in phases. Initially (first week) the graft can vary in color from dark to pink. The stitches will be removed usually at the end of the first week.
2. Then the graft may become puffy and gradually flatten over 2 to 3 months.
3. During the week after surgery, you may have packing in your nose. This packing can be changed daily for the first 48 hours and then can be discontinued. A minimal bandage will cover the surface of your nose.
4. During the week after surgery, you should sleep with your head flat, if possible, and limit exercise to walking (for a nasal tip graft).
5. Cessation of smoking before the surgery is of significant importance in successful outcome after the surgery.

REPAIR OF NASAL DEFECTS

Alar rim defects can be very difficult to reconstruct, because not only must the thickness and contour of the alar rim be taken into consideration but also the structural support requirements need to be considered so that the alar rim will not collapse on inhalation. The most common donor sites for composite grafts to reconstruct the alar rim come from the ear. The most commonly used sites include the helical crus, the helical rim, the anthelix, the tragus, and the earlobe, but any area can be used depending on defect size and necessary contour (Fig. 15–1). Note that the rim of the helix has an anterior roll that can be problematic (and may make the straighter helical crus a better contour choice for grafting). In addition, taking a significant amount of skin from the helical rim shortens the ear, which may present a cosmetic problem.

The initial step in composite grafting involves either making a careful measurement of the recipient defect or making a template of the donor site on the nonadherent

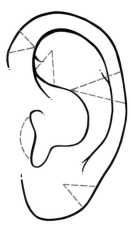

FIGURE 15-1. Donor sites commonly used on the external ear for harvesting composite skin–cartilage–skin grafts. The earlobe yields a composite graft of skin–fat–skin without the structural support of cartilage. Other sites having a rich vascular supply may be used as donor sites (e.g., eyelid and nose). Because of the high visibility of the eyelid and nose, these donor sites are used less frequently than the ear.

(Telfa) or gauze pad, which is then transferred to the donor site. The graft is then harvested from the donor site and placed into cold sterile saline until transferred to the recipient site. The donor site is then closed. The recipient site on the alar rim must be de-epithelialized and scar tissue removed to facilitate the amount of surface area that is exposed to the graft. Depending on the extent of the defect, it may be necessary to manipulate the recipient defect to make available more tissue to increase the surface area that is to come in contact with the graft. Skouge[1] discussed the "tongue in groove" placement of the graft edge into the recipient site as well as use of a turndown, hinged flap to provide vascular lining for large nasal defects. The composite graft is sutured in layers, starting with the mucosal layer, using an absorbable suture (we like 6-0 fast absorbing gut). The needle should pass through the mucosa, then through the graft edge, so that the knots are tied external to the graft (Fig. 15–2).[2] For small grafts (<1 cm in diameter), the cartilage does not need to be sutured to the recipient cartilage. For larger grafts, placement of small Dexon sutures through the cartilage may add mechanical stability to the graft–wound interface. The skin edges of the wound are sutured to the anterior skin edges of the graft with small, nonabsorbable sutures (6-0 Prolene) that are removed at 1 week. There should be minimal handling of the graft, and sutures should be placed so that small amounts of tissue are incorporated with each suture, so as not to strangle the tissue.

The postoperative appearance is characterized by blanching at placement, followed by development of a pink color at about 6 hours. By 24 hours they are cyanotic, and at 3 to 7 days a pink color develops in grafts that will survive. In those that fail, an eschar develops on the epidermis and either the entire graft or the cartilage necroses and sloughs (Table 15–3).

We have used an alternate form of composite grafting

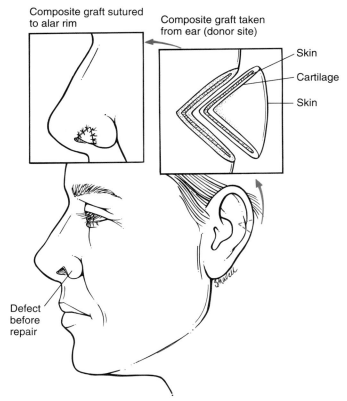

FIGURE 15-2. The composite graft from the helical rim donor site is a skin–cartilage–skin "sandwich." It is sutured into the alar rim defect in layers, starting with the mucosal layer. Smaller grafts may not require suturing of cartilage as is shown. Lastly the skin edges of the wound are sutured to the anterior skin edges of the graft.

quite successfully in alar rim repair. Our variation involves taking a skin–fat composite graft that is harvested as a rectangular full-thickness skin graft from the donor area.[3] Donor areas we prefer include the inner upper arm, the supraclavicular area, and the earlobe (Fig. 15–3). We find that the rectangular shape of the graft facilitates better approximation into the frequently encountered wedge-shaped defect. Modifications of the rectangular shape can be easily made to better accommodate variations in the wedge-shaped recipient site. The graft is minimally defat-

TABLE 15-3. Composite Graft: Postoperative Care

Pain Management
Acetaminophen with codeine for pain in the ear (donor site)
Dressing
Ointment-coated nasal packing changed daily
External nonadherent (Telfa) dressing and ointment without compression
Complications
Graft blackens; allow eschar to form and slough.
High risk of infection warrants perioperative antibiotics.

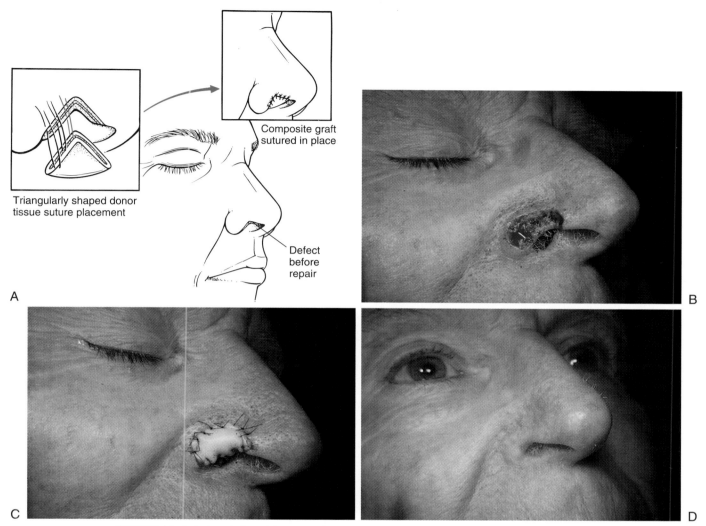

Triangularly shaped donor
tissue suture placement

Composite graft
sutured in place

Defect
before
repair

A

B

C

D

FIGURE 15–3. *A,* A variation of the composite graft uses a "skin–fat–skin" sandwich obtained from the upper inner arm. This donor site is harvested as a rectangle and folded onto itself to form a triangle. The composite graft is sutured into the alar rim defect in two steps: (1) mucosa to skin and (2) skin edges of wound to skin edges of the graft. The first suture placed is designated in red. *B,* Loss of alar rim after resection of a basal cell carcinoma. The defect is a full-thickness loss approximately 1.8 cm in length. *C,* After placement of a skin–fat composite graft from a supraclavicular donor site, the graft is blanched white. The alar rim contour has been restored by the bulk of the skin–fat "sandwich." *D,* The final result shows restoration of the contour of the alar rim without significant retraction of the alar rim.

ted if necessary to approximate the contour of the alar rim.

The initial step in suturing the graft to the edge of the defect is to suture one tip of the graft, epidermis down (forming the "new" nasal mucosa), to the edge of the nasal mucosa. Again, the needle should pass through the mucosa first, then through the edge of the graft, allowing the knot to be tied external to the graft; in this manner the knot will not be buried between the graft and the recipient bed (see Fig. 15–3A). We prefer again to use 6-0 fast-absorbing gut for this suture. The next step is to fold the graft over onto itself, fat against fat, creating a sort of "fat sandwich." This allows the "fold" of the graft to reap-

proximate the missing alar rim. The anterior part of the graft can be trimmed to size. It is wise to leave a little extra bulk and not trim the graft precisely to size, since the graft does contract slightly with healing. A simple suture of 6-0 Prolene can be used to tack the graft into position. A running suture of 6-0 fast-absorbing gut completes the closure. The same type of dressing as previously discussed is applied to this graft, and again the Prolene sutures are removed at 1 week.

There are several advantages of this skin–fat variation of composite graft for alar rim repair. The thickness of the donor tissue provides both mechanical stability and an acceptable alar contour without the extent of metabolic demand or the painful donor defect created by the usual cartilaginous composite graft. In addition, the donor tissue is easily harvested and can be selected from a site of the body yielding the thickness desired for alar rim reconstruction. The donor site scar can be hidden (unless the earlobe is selected as the donor site) and will not result in the cosmetic liability of mismatched earlobes.

The earlobe, as we have mentioned, can be used as a skin–fat composite graft to repair alar rim defects. Wedge-shaped donor grafts from the lateral earlobe can be ''filleted'' to produce a lenticular-shaped graft of sufficient bulk to restore the contour of the nasal tip.[4] Earlobe composite grafts have also been used to reconstruct the columella and unilateral earlobe defects by using a composite graft from the opposite earlobe.

AURICULAR DEFECTS

For reconstruction of partial auricular defects, composite grafting from the opposite ear can be performed (or a cartilage graft combined with a banner flap can be done). For reconstruction of significant auricular defects, however, generally another donor source of cartilage, such as costal cartilage, must be used.

COMPOSITE GRAFTS TO EYEBROW

Several techniques using skin–fat composite grafts have been used to reconstruct the eyebrow. What may be more important than the techniques selected is the presence of scar at the recipient site. In a severely scarred area, a graft restricted to 5 mm in width has been suggested because of the decrease in vascularity versus a graft of 1 cm in width that could survive in an area with no scarring. The presence of a contralateral eyebrow assists in both graft texture and planning the shape and height of graft placement.

Strip grafting, performed with local anesthesia, uses a donor site chosen from the scalp. The appropriate donor area is selected based on hair quality and is planned so that the long axis of the graft runs in the cephalocaudad direction, with the medial part of the graft most cephalad (Fig. 15–4). This graft will be oriented with lateral growth; and even though the normal eyebrow has a somewhat multidirectional growth, most of it is lateral so the graft will be cosmetically acceptable. The proposed brow is measured at the recipient site and then marked on the patient's scalp with a template. The hair of the donor area is trimmed to permit visualization of the hair shaft angle, in a similar fashion to the hair transplantation procedure. The incision is made parallel to the hair shafts and carried down to periosteum. The graft is removed, trimmed so that there is a small amount of fat below the hair follicles, and placed into cold sterile saline. The donor site is closed in a layered fashion. The premeasured strip of skin at the recipient site is excised, and after hemostasis the trimmed

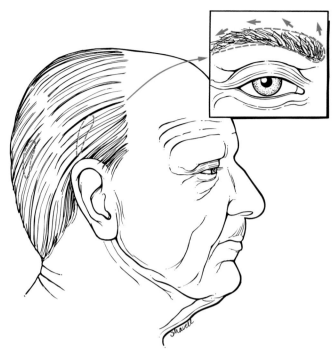

FIGURE 15–4. Strip grafting using a composite graft from scalp donor sites can be used to reconstruct the eyebrow. The donor area is selected based on hair quality and orientation of the hair. The medial part of the graft is the most cephalad.

graft is placed into the recipient defect. The graft is secured in place using nonabsorbable sutures and then dressed with antibiotic ointment and a light compression dressing. Sutures are removed at 1 week.

A full-thickness eyebrow graft from the opposite eyebrow can also be used as a type of composite graft to correct a partially resected eyebrow, particularly if the defect is circular or oval (such as the defect after completion of Mohs' micrographic surgery).[5] If possible, the donor site is taken from the location corresponding to the resected area of the contralateral brow. The donor graft is excised at a level below the hair follicles. It is then placed into the recipient defect and rotated until the orientation of the hair alignment is the same as that of the recipient site. The graft is then sutured in place after undermining of the recipient site. The donor site is closed primarily.

References

1. Skouge JW. Skin Grafting. New York: Churchill Livingstone, 1991.
2. Tromovich TA, Stegman SJ, Glogau RG. Flaps and Grafts in Dermatologic Surgery. Chicago: Year Book Medical Publishers, 1989.
3. Haas AF, Glogau RG. A variation of composite grafting for reconstruction of full-thickness nasal alar defects. Presented at the American College of Mohs Micrographic Surgery and Cutaneous Oncology annual meeting, Charleston, South Carolina, 1993.
4. Lipman SH, Roth RJ. Composite grafts from earlobes for reconstruction of defects in noses. J Dermatol Surg Oncol 1982;8:135–137.
5. English FP, Forester TDC. The eyebrow graft. Ophthalmic Surg 1979;10(7):39–41.

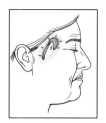

chapter 16

Cultured Epidermal Grafts

KATIA C. ONGENAE and TANIA J. PHILLIPS

All dermatologists and surgeons concerned with wound healing have a major objective—rapid healing of acute and chronic skin defects.[1] Cultured epidermal autografts, grown from a small biopsy sample of the patient's own skin, were first used successfully to cover burn wounds[2] and later also skin ulcers.[3] A further development in this area was the use of allografts, cultured in vitro from allogeneic donor skin to cover skin defects of varying etiologies (Fig. 16–1; Tables 16–1 through 16–3).[1,3,4–15]

Autografts can be grown from a skin sample as small as 1 cm² harvested under local anesthesia.[16] The skin sample is then transported in culture medium to the laboratory

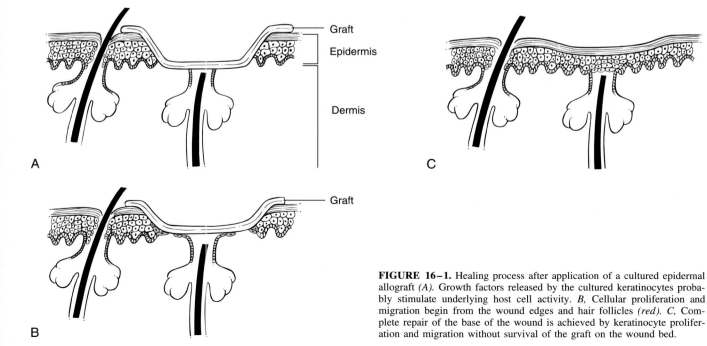

FIGURE 16–1. Healing process after application of a cultured epidermal allograft *(A).* Growth factors released by the cultured keratinocytes probably stimulate underlying host cell activity. *B,* Cellular proliferation and migration begin from the wound edges and hair follicles *(red). C,* Complete repair of the base of the wound is achieved by keratinocyte proliferation and migration without survival of the graft on the wound bed.

**TABLE 16-1. Cultured Epidermal Grafts:
Indications, Contraindications, Limitations**

Indications

Autografts (commercially available)

Burn wounds—properly prepared wound bed excised at an
early stage

Refractory skin ulcers[3]

Junctional-type epidermolysis bullosa[6]

Large excisional wounds (e.g., giant congenital nevi)[7]

Allografts (not yet FDA approved)

Burn wounds[8]

Recalcitrant skin ulcers of various origin[1,4]:

    Venous, arterial, mixed ulcers[9]

    Amputation stump ulcers

    Decubitus ulcers

    Ulcers due to systemic conditions: rheumatoid arthritis, scle-
roderma

Traumatic skin defects[4]

Tattoo CO_2 laser removal sites[4]

Split-thickness skin graft donor sites[10]

Epidermolysis bullosa (recessive dystrophic type)[11,12]

Contraindications

Evidence of infection in the wound bed

Cellulitis[1,19]

Excessive swelling of the extremity[9]

Acute dermatitis of surrounding skin

Absence of clean wound bed and healthy granulation tissue

Limitations

Labor-intensive and time-consuming laboratory techniques

Costs

Culture technique used influences graft quality[13]

Delay in transplantation negatively affects the outcome[13]

Cultured epidermal grafts are not considered as a first-line
treatment

Limited experience with this emerging technique

Autografts

Biopsy is needed

Three- to 4-week interval for culture in vitro

In burn wounds, nonexcised, chronic granulating and fibrotic
beds give poor results[13]

Grafts are vulnerable and susceptible to shear forces and
pressure[14]

Poor growth of elderly keratinocytes in vitro[15]

Graft loss mainly due to infection[13]

Allografts

Ulcer depth (down to fascia and tendon), wound size (>40
cm^2), chronicity (>10 years) negatively affect prognosis[1]

Theoretical possibility of disease transmission[16]

(Fig. 16-2).[5] Full-term neonates of healthy mothers without known risk for transmissible disease are the foreskin
donors for the allografts.[13]

Based on the findings of Rheinwald and Green,[17] it is
possible to grow in vitro large epidermal sheets suitable for
grafting from a small skin sample.[18] After removal of subcutaneous tissue and as much dermis as possible, the skin
is minced and trypsinized[2] to yield disaggregated epidermal
cells.[16] These are seeded on 3T3 cells, which are lethally

**TABLE 16-2. Cultured Epidermal Grafts:
Patient Preoperative Discussion**

The grafts act as a kind of biologic wound dressing that
stimulates healing.

For autografts, a small skin sample is taken (from your thigh
or inner arm) under local anesthesia and is sent to the laboratory. It then takes 3 to 4 weeks to grow sufficient skin for the
graft.

The grafting procedure is painless and does not usually require any anesthesia or sutures. There is no guarantee that this
procedure will result in healing of the wound.

After graft placement, healing can take up to 8 weeks.[1]
Depending on the wound size and depth, the ulcer may not
heal completely with one graft. Repeat graft sessions can be
considered if the first one appears to help wound healing.

1. After the graft procedure patients with lower leg grafts
need to avoid any walking. They will leave the area of the
procedure in a wheel chair and will be accompanied by
a person who can drive them home.

2. Patients must rest in bed for 48 hours, with leg elevation if
the graft site is on the leg. After that, walking is allowed but
physical activity should be limited until the first dressing
change 5 to 7 days later.

3. Dressing changes during this time are unnecessary unless a
lot of exudate occurs.

4. A first follow-up visit is scheduled for 5 to 7 days later. At this
time, the dressings are removed.

---

irradiated mouse fibroblasts known to support rapid growth
of keratinocytes (see Fig. 16-2). Cultures are then fed
with required mitogens, and the medium is changed at
given intervals.[1] In a few weeks, a 1-cm^2 skin sample can
provide enough epithelium to cover the whole body surface

**TABLE 16-3. Cultured Epidermal Grafts:
Operative Issues**

Preoperative Evaluation

Ulcer history

    Etiology

    Duration

    Localization

    Size

    Depth

Previous treatment, grafts

The patient is usually treated with saline dressing for at least 1
week before grafting.

Preoperative Equipment Needs

Lidocaine 2% gel

Sterile scissors and forceps or No. 6 curette

Sterile saline solution and 4 × 4-inch gauze pads

Sterile scissors and forceps to cut the graft if needed

Nonadherent gauze (Adaptic)

Sterile gauze squares

Sterile gauze conforming bandages

Unna boot or elastic bandage

Intraoperative Needs

Two pairs of sterile forceps to manipulate the graft

Sterile field

Pair of sterile gloves

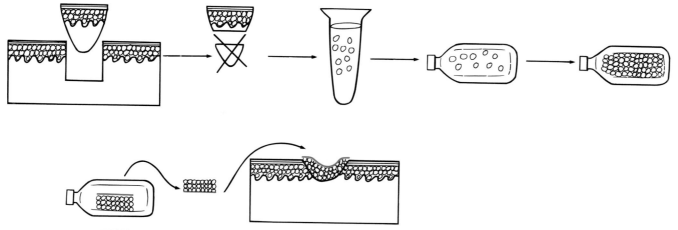

FIGURE 16-2. Cultured epidermal grafting procedure in vitro. Subcutaneous tissue is removed from a small donor skin sample, the epidermis is disaggregated, and single cells are seeded onto irradiated 3T3 mouse fibroblasts in a flask. The epidermal sheets are detached from the flask when confluence is reached and backed with a nonadherent gauze *(red)* before grafting.

area.[16] Cultures are screened for human immunodeficiency virus and other viruses as well as bacteria.[4]

When the cultures reach confluence, the epidermal sheets are detached intact from the tissue culture dish by treatment with the enzyme Dispase (Fig. 16–3A and B).[1,16] The grafts, consisting of four to five stratified layers of keratinocytes, are then placed, basal side up, on a nonadherent gauze pad cut to size (Fig. 16–3C).[1,16] Surgical clips are used to attach the edge of the epidermal sheet to the gauze (Fig. 16–3D and E).[5] The grafts are placed in dishes with just enough serum-free medium to cover the basal layer. A jar that contains several dishes is sealed by flushing the gas phase with 10% carbon dioxide and used for transportation (Fig. 16–3F).[2]

After application of 2% lidocaine gel under occlusion for 10 to 15 minutes, gentle debridement of the wound is performed with a No. 6 curette or forceps and scissors until healthy granulation tissue appears. The wound is subsequently thoroughly cleaned with normal saline.

Grafting is performed using sterile technique, frequently in the outpatient setting. To facilitate handling, two pairs of forceps are used to place the graft with the basal cell surface next to the wound bed (Fig. 16–3G). Although some surgeons like to suture the graft in place, we use no sutures for small leg ulcer wounds. The grafts are held in place by a nonadherent gauze pad covered with an overlay of dry 4 × 4-inch gauze and wrapped with a conforming gauze bandage (Fig. 16–3H and I). A flexible/rigid paste bandage (Unna boot) is correctly applied, followed by a Coban wrap (Fig. 16–3J). An elastic Ace wrap can be used if an Unna boot is not indicated for the patient (Fig. 16–3K).

Dressings are cautiously removed first at 5 to 7 days (Table 16–4).[4,13,19] If there is excessive exudate, the outer dressing can be changed more frequently, but the cultured graft should be left undisturbed. If the dressings are adherent, they should be soaked in normal saline to facilitate removal. The technique can be repeated as necessary (Case 1, Fig. 16–4A through D).

TABLE 16-4. Cultured Epidermal Grafts: Postoperative Care

Pain Management

The grafting procedure is painless and usually results in considerable pain relief immediately after grafting.[4]

Dressings

Change at day 5 to 7, then weekly for leg ulcers. If there is a lot of exudate, dressings can be changed more frequently.

Removal of adherent dressings is easier when soaked with saline.

At the first dressing change, carefully remove the backing material, making sure that the graft is left in place.

Wound is cleaned weekly by carefully dripping normal saline over the wound surface.

Dressings:
   Nonadherent (Adaptic) gauze
   4 × 4-inch dry gauze pads
   Conform wrap
   Unna boot (stopped at week 3) and Coban wrap or Ace wrap

Complications

Infection with increasing pain after grafting is the main cause of graft failure,[19] especially in autografts.[3]

A wound culture is taken and appropriate antimicrobial therapy is started.

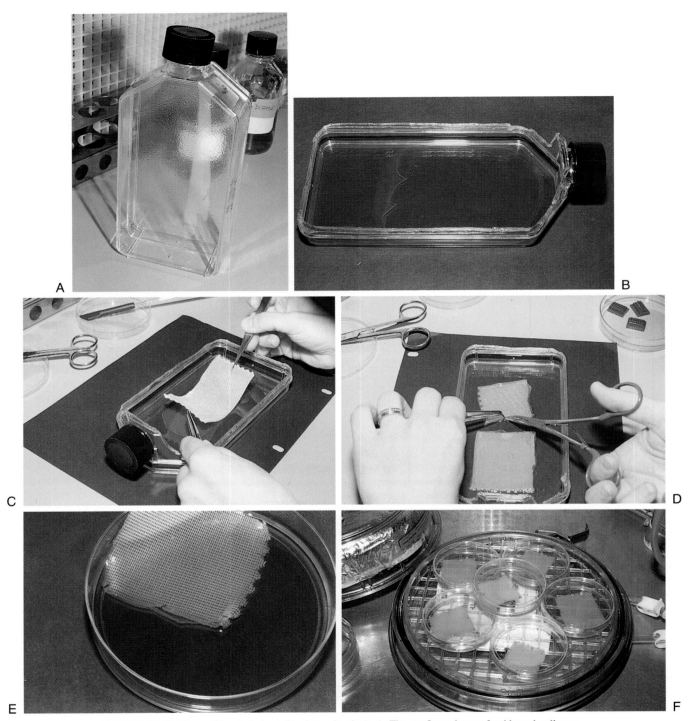

FIGURE 16–3. The grafting technique (in vitro—in vivo). *A,* The confluent layer of epidermal cells can be seen as an opaque sheet on the wall of the culture flask. *B,* Treatment with Dispase enzyme detaches the epidermal sheet from the flask. *C,* A nonadherent dressing is cut to size and placed on the epidermal side of the graft. *D,* Surgical clips are used to attach the edge of the graft to the gauze. *E,* The graft appears as a translucent sheet clipped to a nonadherent gauze basal side up. *F,* The dishes containing the grafts are transported in a sealed container flushed with CO_2.

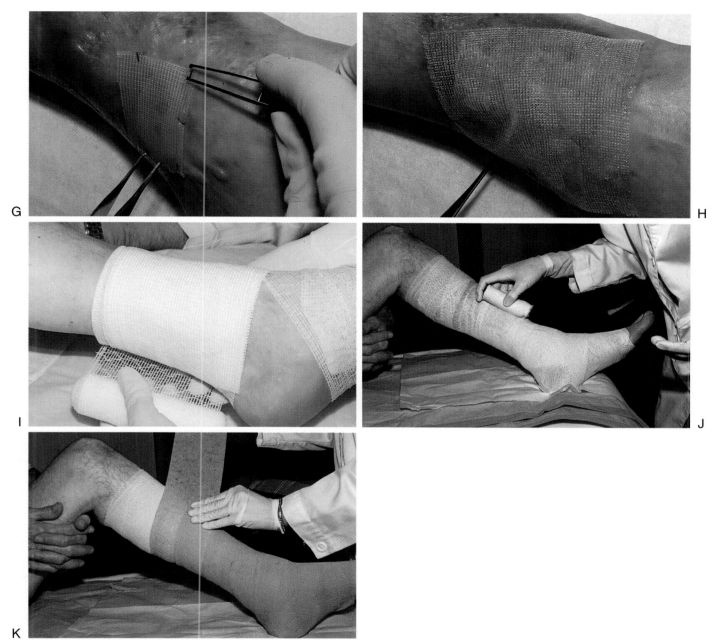

FIGURE 16–3 *Continued G,* Using sterile technique, the graft is placed basal side down on the wound bed. *H,* The graft is covered with an Adaptic nonadherent dressing. *I,* Sterile gauze pads and a sterile gauze conforming bandage hold the graft in place. *J,* An Unna boot is applied starting from the toes and ascending proximally, wrapping the bandage upward with an optimal amount of tension. Irregularities are smoothed by cutting or folding the wrap continuously. *K,* An elasticized wrap, such as Coban, covers the boot, to provide added compression.

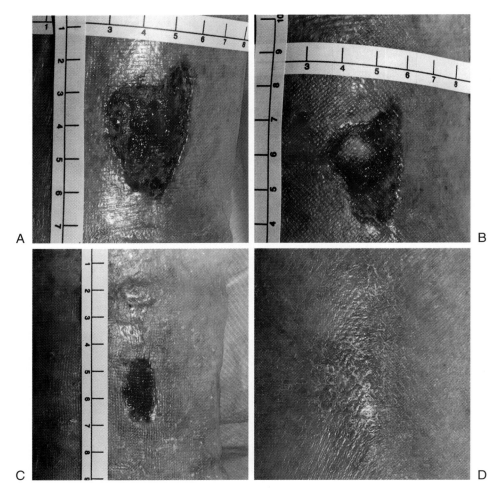

CASE 1

FIGURE 16-4. Recalcitrant venous ulcer present for 8 months in a 74-year-old woman. Two allografts were applied at 9-week intervals. *A,* Appearance of ulcer before first graft. *B,* At 4 weeks after the first allograft the ulcer size decreased and a central island of epithelium has formed. *C,* At 4 weeks after the second allograft the island joined the ulcer edge. Further gradual decrease in size resulted in healing 10 weeks later. *D,* Follow-up 2.5 months after closure shows that the ulcer remains healed.

References

1. Phillips TJ, Gilchrest BA. Cultured allogenic keratinocyte grafts in the management of wound healing: Prognostic factors. J. Dermatol Surg Oncol 1989;15:1169–1176.
2. O'Connor NE, Mulliken JB, Banks-Schlegel S, et al. Grafting of burns with cultured epithelium prepared from autologous epidermal cells. Lancet 1981;1:75–78.
3. Hefton JM, Caldwell D, Biozes DG, et al. Grafting of skin ulcers with cultured autologous epidermal cells. J Am Acad Dermatol 1986;14:399–405.
4. Phillips TJ, Kehinde O, Green H, et al. Treatment of skin ulcers with cultured epidermal allografts. J Am Acad Dermatol 1989;21:191–199.
5. Gallico GG, O'Connor NE, Compton CC, et al. Permanent coverage of large burn wounds with autologous cultured human epithelium. N Engl J Med 1984;311:448–451.
6. Carter DM, Lin AN, Varghese MC, et al. Treatment of junctional epidermolysis bullosa with epidermal autografts. J Am Acad Dermatol 1987;17:246–250.
7. Gallico GG, O'Connor NE, Compton CC, et al. Cultured epithelial autografts for giant congenital nevi. Plast Reconstr Surg 1990;84:1–9.
8. Hefton JM, Madden MR, Finkelstein JL, et al. Grafting of burn patients with allografts of cultured epidermal cells. Lancet 1983;2:428–430.
9. Marcusson JA, Lindgren C, Berghard A, et al. Allogeneic cultured keratinocytes in the treatment of leg ulcers. Acta Derm Venereol 1992;72:61–64.
10. Phillips TJ, Provan A, Colbert D, et al. A randomized single-blind controlled study of cultured epidermal allografts in the treatment of split-thickness skin graft donor sites. Arch Dermatol 1993;129:879–882.
11. McGuire J, Birchall N, Cuono C, et al. Successful engrafting of allogeneic keratinocytes in recessive dystrophic epidermolysis bullosa. Clin Res 1987;35:702A.
12. McGrath JA, Schofield OMV, Ishida-Yamamoto A, et al. Cultured keratinocyte allografts and wound healing in severe recessive dystrophic epidermolysis bullosa. J Am Acad Dermatol 1993;29:407–419.
13. Teepe RGC, Kreis RW, Koebrugge EJ, et al. The use of cultured autologous epidermis in the treatment of extensive burn wounds. J Trauma 1990;30:269–275.
14. Phillips TJ. Cultured skin grafts: Past, present, future. Arch Dermatol 1988;124:1035–1038.
15. Leigh IM, Purkis PE, Cultured grafted leg ulcers. Clin Exp Dermatol 1986;1:650–652.
16. Phillips TJ, Gilchrest BA. Cultured epidermal grafts in the treatment of leg ulcers. Adv Dermatol 1990;5:33–50.
17. Rheinwald JG, Green H. Serial cultivation of strains of human epidermal keratinocytes: The formation of keratinizing colonies from single cells. Cell 1975;6:331–334.
18. Green H, Kehinde O, Thomas J. Growth of human epidermal cells into multiple epithelia suitable for grafting. Proc Natl Acad Sci USA 1979;76:5665–5668.
19. Duhra P, Blight A, Mountford E, et al. A randomized controlled trial of cultured keratinocyte grafts for chronic venous ulcers. J Dermatol Treat 1992;3:189–191.

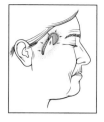

chapter 17

Surgical Techniques for Repigmentation

RAFAEL FALABELLA

SUCTION BLISTER GRAFTS

Epidermal grafts obtained by suction are suitable for surgical treatment of stable forms of vitiligo and other types of leukoderma. The aim of this procedure is to replace the achromic epithelium by normal epidermis bearing melanocytes obtained by 2 to 3 hours of suction at 200 to 300 mm Hg. A standard suction pump or vacuum, usually available in operating rooms, provides enough negative pressure for this purpose.[1-4] When the temperature is raised to around 40°C to 41°C, blistering time is shortened to approximately 1 hour.[5] The suction device allows harvesting multiple grafts simultaneously (Figs. 17–1 through 17–3; Tables 17–1 through 17–3).

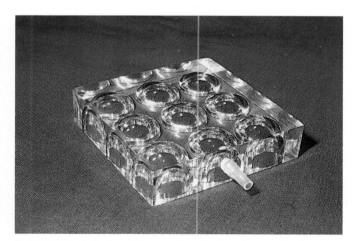

FIGURE 17–1. Suction blister grafting. Suction device with nine interconnected cups of 20-mm diameter each. Standard model without heating appliances is shown.

In removing the achromic epidermis, liquid nitrogen freezing, by either a cryosurgical instrument or a cotton swab, should be done. Two days before grafting, freezing is performed to the entire achromic area or to small 0.5 to 1.0-cm islands, separated at a similar distance from each other.[6] Freezing causes blistering of the epidermis. After the inflammatory changes induced by freezing subside, grafting is performed by removing the top of the blister with iris scissors (Figs. 17–4 and 17–5).

On the grafting day, surgical procedures are performed at both the donor and recipient sites. When the blisters of the donor skin of the medial aspect of the thigh or gluteal region are ready, the bullae of the recipient site are unroofed. The epidermis of the recipient site is discarded. Next, each one of the epidermal grafts bearing melanocytes is freed from the donor area with iris scissors, transferred and extended onto a microscope glass slide that is used as a carrying instrument (Fig. 17–6), and placed on the denuded achromic skin with fine-tipped forceps (Fig. 17–7). Large epidermal sheets can be cut in smaller fragments with a No. 23 surgical blade, when needed (Fig. 17–8). After the procedure is completed (Table 17–4), nonadherent (Telfa) dressings are placed at both recipient and donor sites and are secured in place with elastic bandages. Dressings are removed 5 to 7 days later when healing is accomplished. Since the dermis is not wounded during this procedure, scarring does not occur, at either donor or recipient sites. Repigmentation is observed shortly after grafting. Color matching with only surrounding skin occurs throughout the following months and remains indefinitely[7-9] (Case 1, Fig. 17–9; Case 2, Fig. 17–10). Suction blister grafting should be avoided in active vitiligo because there is failure to restore the normal skin color and koebnerization of donor sites may develop.[10]

175

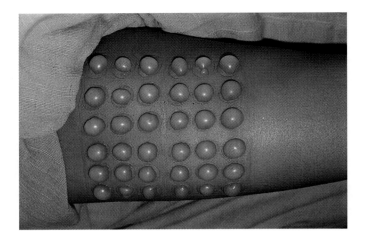

FIGURE 17-2. Suction blister grafting. Thiry-six blisters obtained 3 hours after using four suction devices as shown in Figure 17-1.

TABLE 17-1. Suction Blister Grafts: Indications, Contraindications, Limitations

Indications

Vitiligo[6,7]
  Segmental
  Focal
  Bilateral (old, quiescent, very stable forms)
Leukoderma
  Post burn[2]
  Post dermabrasion[8]
Piebaldism[9]

Contraindications

Active vitiligo[10]
Tendency to develop excessive hyperpigmentation

Limitations

Extensive areas of vitiligo or leukoderma (multiple sessions are possible)
Best results are obtained in monochromic defects. Multiple skin tones within area of leukoderma may lead to a polychromic appearance when repigmented.
More difficult to perform in children younger than age 14.
Regrafting may be necessary between some grafts. (Minigrafting may be useful for additional grafts in small spots.)

TABLE 17-2. Suction Blister Grafts: Patient Preoperative Discussion

1. Healing should take 1 week. During this time bandages will be in place.
2. The surgical area must be kept dry until bandages are removed.
3. If the treated area is on the lower leg, leg elevation when at rest and a reduction in physical activities is recommended. When grafts are placed on joint areas, immobilization may be necessary.
4. When bandages are removed, thin dry sheets of epidermis may fall off the grafts. This material corresponds to dead superficial skin layers, but the grafts remain alive.
5. Initially, the treated area is light colored. Gradually, after a few minutes of daily sunlight exposure, the grafts will darken. Natural skin color, spreading from the edges, will cover the entire defect within a few weeks.

TABLE 17-3. Suction Blister Grafts: Operative Issues

Preoperative Evaluation

History
  Hepatitis, human immunodeficiency virus infection
  Activity of disease (must be stable)
  Previous failure with medical therapy
  Psychological stability
  Reasonable patient expectations from procedure
  Negative history of persistent postinflammatory hyperpigmentation
A preoperative minigrafting test with 3 to 4, 1.2-mm punch grafts, with evaluation 3 to 4 months later, is recommended, to determine the possibility of repigmentation

Preoperative Equipment Needs

Suction pump or vacuum available
Suction device with or without intrinsic heating
Cryosurgical unit (if cotton swab not used)
Iris scissors, curved, thin blades
Fine-tipped forceps
Microscopy glass slides, sterile
Magnifying loupes
Local anesthesia (optional)

Intraoperative Needs

Mild sedation may be necessary.
Lidocaine may be topically applied after unroofing the blisters.
If pain is not controlled, lidocaine may be infiltrated.

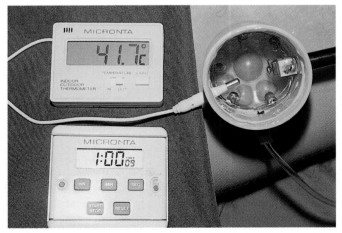

FIGURE 17-3. Suction blister grafting. Suction device with five, small 12-V bulbs inside for heat generation. Timer and thermometer display 1-hour suction time at 41.7°C, respectively. Blisters are ready for grafting, as visualized through the acrylic top of the suction instrument.

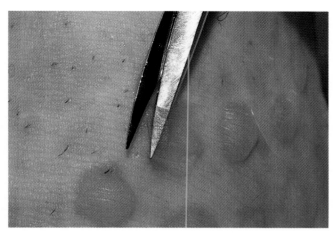

FIGURE 17–4. Suction blister grafting: recipient site. Two days after freezing the leukodermic areas with liquid nitrogen the achromic epidermis is removed with iris scissors just before grafting.

MINIGRAFTS

Minigrafting is a simple, office procedure for repigmenting stable forms of vitiligo and other types of leukoderma (Tables 17–5 through 17–7). This technique resembles the physiologic mechanism of perifollicular repigmentation often seen in vitiligo or after epithelialization following thermal burns, by artificially creating a new source of melanocytes with very small implants of split-thickness skin, harvested with a 1.0- or 1.2-mm punch.[11] No hair follicles are required in these grafts, since epidermal melanocytes migrate and colonize a surrounding area of about 2 mm beyond the graft edges; thus, a repigmented area around 5 mm in diameter will form (Fig. 17–11). When set at a distance of 4 to 5 mm from each other, coalescence of minigrafts, acting as melanocyte and pigment spreading islands, may restore the normal pigmentation of leukodermic defects.[11–15] By using small punches, not larger than 1.2 mm, the "cobblestone" effect of grafts becomes minimal and the resulting appearance is more aesthetically accepted.

Very simple instruments are required: iris scissors, fine-tipped forceps (Carmalt type), and 1.0- or 1.2-mm dermal punches. The grafting site is prepared by infiltration of 1% lidocaine without epinephrine, followed by perforation of recipient holes of 1.0 to 1.5 mm in depth and 4 to 5 mm apart from each other. After this, normal saline compresses are placed, to keep the surgical area clean and free from clots or dried blood. Minigrafts are harvested from the gluteal region (hidden area), with a punch of a similar size to that of the recipient site, very close to each other, transferred to a nonadherent gauze (Telfa) pad moistened with normal saline (Case 3, Fig. 17–12A), and placed within the recipient holes. Monsel's solution is then applied to the entire treated surface to seal serum leakage around the grafts; and after the surgical area is dried, sterile Micropore adhesive tape is used as the only dressing without gauze to immobilize the grafts (Fig. 17–12B; Table 17–8). Dressings are removed 15 days later (Fig. 17–12C), and gradual sunlight exposure is initiated to stimulate melanogenesis and pigment spread (Case 3, Figs.

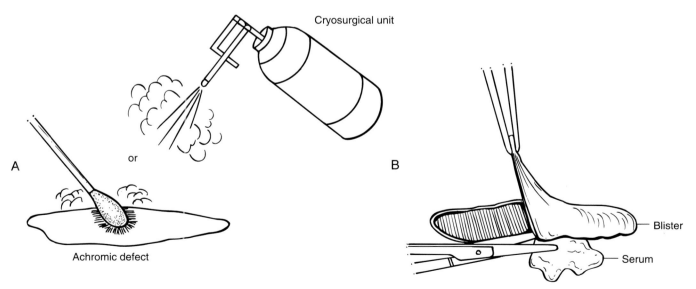

FIGURE 17–5. Recipient site. *A,* Freezing is performed with cotton swab or cryosurgery unit for about 5 seconds at the recipient site. *B,* After a few days, blistering occurs in leukodermic area. The blister is unroofed with iris scissors 2 to 3 days later, just before grafting. Freezing should not be used to raise a blister at the graft donor site since depigmentation can result from freezing.

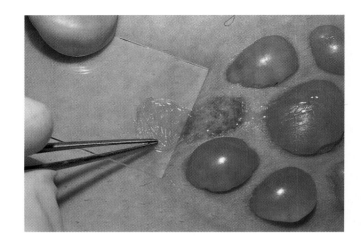

FIGURE 17–6. Suction blister grafting: donor site. Harvesting the suction epidermal grafts is accomplished by cutting the blister edge with iris scissors, followed by spreading the free epidermis onto a microscope glass slide used as a carrying instrument.

A

B

C

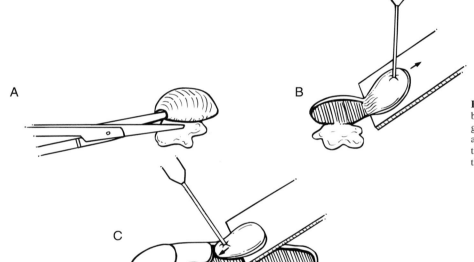

FIGURE 17–7. Grafting procedure. *A,* Suction blister is cut around its periphery. *B,* Next, the graft is extended onto a microscope slide used as a carrying instrument. *C,* The graft is placed on the recipient site, with dermal side down, and the glass slide is slowly moved away.

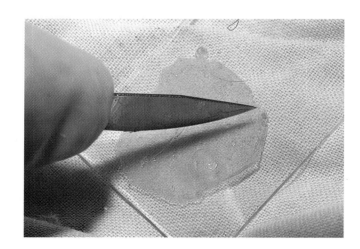

FIGURE 17–8. Suction blister grafting. Large epidermal grafts can be cut with a No. 23 surgical blade to provide a smaller graft when needed to fit recipient sites.

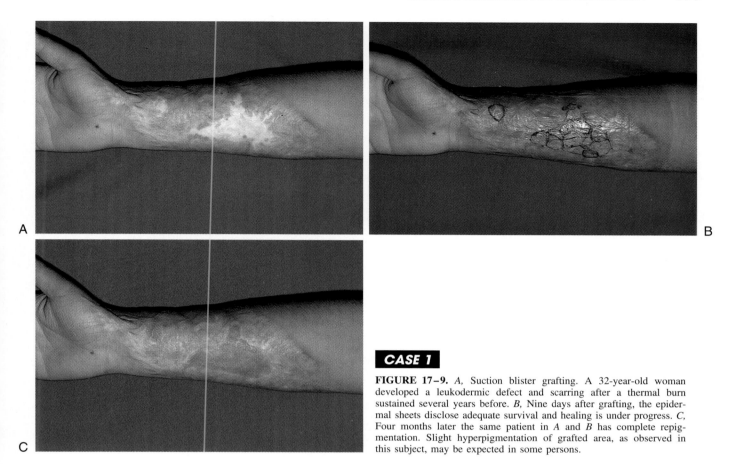

A

B

C

CASE 1

FIGURE 17–9. *A,* Suction blister grafting. A 32-year-old woman developed a leukodermic defect and scarring after a thermal burn sustained several years before. *B,* Nine days after grafting, the epidermal sheets disclose adequate survival and healing is under progress. *C,* Four months later the same patient in *A* and *B* has complete repigmentation. Slight hyperpigmentation of grafted area, as observed in this subject, may be expected in some persons.

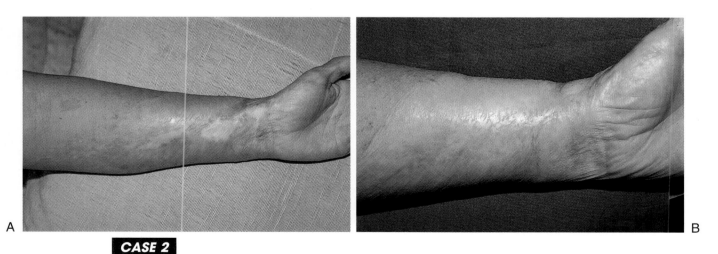

A

B

CASE 2

FIGURE 17–10. *A,* Suction blister grafting. This 40-year-old woman developed an area of leukoderma on her forearm after a gasoline burn sustained 10 years earlier. *B,* At 14 years after grafting, complete repigmentation is evident.

**TABLE 17-4. Suction Blister Grafts:
Postoperative Care**

Pain Management
Acetaminophen (not needed very often)
Dressings
Donor area: nonadherent (Telfa) or impermeable dressings
   (Opsite). Discontinue when healed, in 7 to 10 days.
Recipient area: nonadherent dressings until healing in 5 to 7
   days.
Complications
Koebnerization of donor site in active vitiligo[10]; treat with mid-
   potency topical steroids.
Excessive hyperpigmentation in prone individuals (slight dark-
   ening may be expected). Treat with long-term topical 1%
   hydrocortisone. Avoid excessive sunlight exposure.
Infections are infrequent but may occur. Treat with appropri-
   ate antibiotics when needed.

**TABLE 17-5. Minigrafts: Indications,
Contraindications, Limitations**

Indications
Vitiligo[12,13]
   Segmental
   Focal
   Bilateral (old, quiescent, very stable forms)
Leukoderma
   Post burn[11,14,16]
   Post cryosurgery
   Healed discoid lupus erythematosus[11]
   Post hydroquinone monobenzyl ester toxicity[11,14]
   Post dermabrasion[8]
   Piebaldism[9]
Contraindications
Active vitiligo[10]
Tendency to develop excessive hyperpigmentation
Tendency to develop keloids
Limitations
Extensive areas of vitiligo or leukoderma (multiple sessions are
   possible).
Best results are obtained in monochromic defects. Multiple
   skin tones within area of leukoderma may lead to a po-
   lychromic appearance when repigmented.
More difficult to perform in children younger than age 14.
Regrafting may be necessary between some grafts.

**TABLE 17-6. Minigrafts: Patient Preoperative
Discussion**

1. Healing should take 2 weeks.
2. Dressings (Micropore) must be carefully held in place during these 2 weeks.
3. If dressings (Micropore) are not kept in place as indicated,
   minigrafts may detach with adhesive tape removal. Dressing removal must be done by a physician.
4. The surgical area must be kept dry until the bandage is removed.
5. If the treated zone is in the lower leg, moderate rest is recommended with leg elevation. When grafts are placed on
   joint areas, immobilization may be necessary.
6. When removing the Micropore dressings, very small scabs
   on the surface of the surgical tape may be seen. This is
   due to dried blood or detachment of dead superficial
   layers of skin.
7. Repigmentation around minigrafts is clearly visible 1 to 2
   months postoperatively. Coalescence of pigmentation from
   each graft will be complete in 4 or 6 months. Minigrafts
   usually become darker than desired a few weeks after
   grafting, but this effect will gradually fade over the ensuing
   few months.

TABLE 17-7. Minigrafts: Operative Issues

Preoperative Evaluation
Coagulation disorders.
Negative history of keloid formation
Hepatitis, human immunodeficiency virus infection
Activity of disease (must be stable)
Previous failure with medical therapy
Psychologic stability
Reasonable patient expectations from procedure
Negative history of persistent postinflammatory hyperpigmen-
   tation
A preoperative minigrafting test with three to four 1.2-mm
   punch grafts, with evaluation 3 to 4 months later is recom-
   mended, to detect possibility of repigmentation
Preoperative Equipment Needs
Iris scissors
Fine-tipped forceps (Carmalt type)
1.0 to 1.2-mm dermal punches
Lidocaine without epinephrine
Magnifying loupes
Nonadherent (Telfa) dressings for transfer of grafts from donor
   area to recipient site
Micropore adhesive tape for use as surgical dressings
Intraoperative Needs
Mild sedation (seldom needed)
Avoid epinephrine with local anesthesia in (post-burn) leuko-
   derma or in presence of scarring. It may induce skin necro-
   sis in large areas.

17-12D and E; Case 4, Fig. 17-13; Case 5, Fig. 17-14).
As in other types of grafts, some degree of hyperpigmentation may be expected.[16] A few complications arise when
indications or adequate selection of punches are overlooked
(Case 6, Fig. 17-15; Case 7, Fig. 17-16; Case 8, Fig.
17-17).

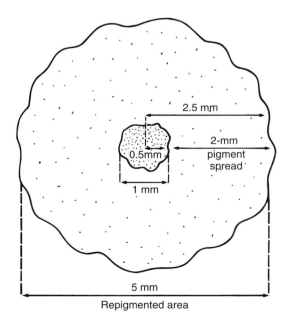

Repigmented area

FIGURE 17-11. Minigrafting. Repigmentation ratio: size of repigmented
area is divided by size of original graft area. A 1-mm diameter graft
repigments an area of approximately 5 mm diameter of depigmented skin.
The repigmented area is 25 times larger than the original graft, as determined with the formula for the area of a circle ($A = \pi r^2$).

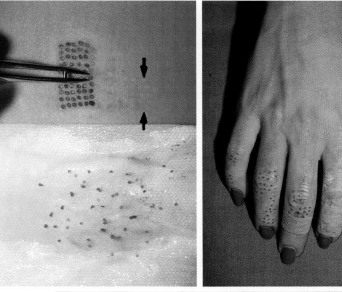

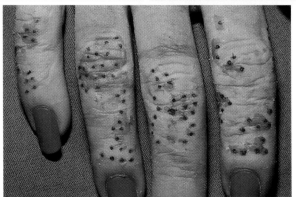

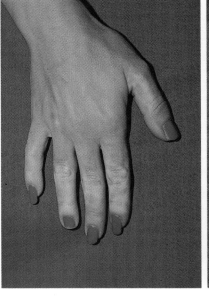

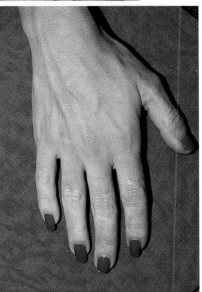

CASE 3

FIGURE 17–12. Minigrafting. *A,* donor site. Multiple 1.2-mm minigrafts are harvested from the gluteal region in a pattern very close to each other. After grafts are cut free with iris scissors, minigrafts are placed on a Telfa gauze pad moistened with normal saline solution and later transferred to the recipient site. Area between arrows was used as a donor site 3 months earlier. *B,* Recipient site. Leukoderma after burn, immediately after grafting. Monsel's solution was applied to seal the surgical space between the graft and the surrounding skin of recipient site; this prevents transudates that might interfere with Micropore dressings. Three fingers have already been covered with tape dressings. *C,* Fifteen days later, Micropore dressings are removed gently and tangentially to avoid detachment of grafts. Small crusts should be left in place until spontaneous elimination occurs. *D,* Preoperative appearance of this 25-year-old woman shows leukoderma on the dorsal aspect of several fingers. The burn was sustained 7 years earlier. *E,* Repigmentation is observed 10 months after grafting. (*A* from Falabella RF. Mini-injertos: Una solucion simple para el problema de las leucodermias estables. Rev Soc Colombiana Dermatol 1992;1:110–116.)

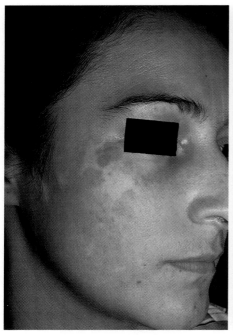
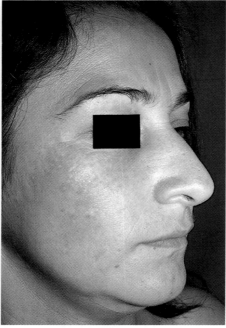

A   B

FIGURE 17–13. Minigrafting. *A,* A 34-year-old woman developed segmental vitiligo on the malar area 4 years before consultation. *B,* Two years later, and after one grafting session, repigmentation of entire area was attained. (*A* and *B* from Falabella RF. Mini-injertos: Una solucion simple para el problema de las leucodermias estables. Rev Soc Colombiana Dermatol 1992;1:110–116.)

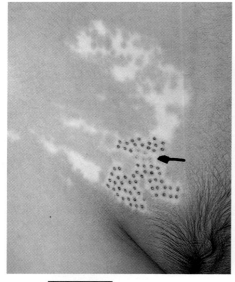
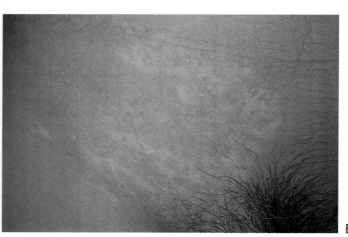

A   B

FIGURE 17–14. Minigrafting. *A,* A 12-year-old girl developed segmental vitiligo on the right lower abdomen that became stable after 8 months of progressive depigmentation. Sixty-two minigrafts were implanted on the lower portion of the achromic lesion. Arrow shows repigmentation of a test area with five minigrafts placed 4 months earlier. *B,* Achromic lesion became completely repigmented, as seen 2 years later after three grafting sessions.

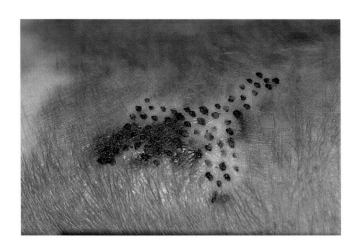

CASE 6

FIGURE 17–15. Complication of minigrafting: recipient site. Necrosis occurred 5 days after using epinephrine with local anesthesia in a leukodermic lesion with mild fibrosis after a thermal burn. (From Falabella RF. Mini-injertos: Una solucion simple para el problema de las leucodermias estables. Rev Soc Colombiana Dermatol 1992;1:110–116.)

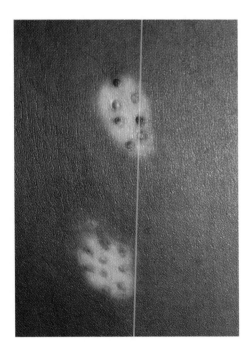

CASE 7

FIGURE 17–16. Complication of minigrafting: recipient site. Several 4-mm punch grafts, implanted within active lesions of a patient with symmetrical vitiligo, resulted in a noticeable ''cobblestone'' effect and repigmentation failure. The smaller size punch grafts may prevent cobblestoning.

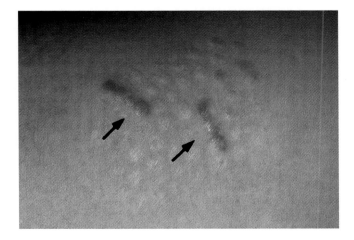

CASE 8

FIGURE 17–17. Complication of minigrafting: donor site. After a 4-mm punch was used to harvest grafts, this patient had unsightly hypertrophic *(arrows)* and atrophic scars.

TABLE 17-8. Minigrafts: Postoperative Care

Pain Management

Acetaminophen (seldom needed)

Dressings

Donor area: nonadherent (Telfa) or impermeable dressings (Opsite). Discontinue when healed, in 7 to 10 days.

Recipient area: Micropore directly on minigrafts and skin. Remove slowly and tangentially after 15 days to avoid graft detachment. No further dressings are needed.

Complications

Koebnerization of donor site when dealing with active vitiligo. Treat with 1% hydrocortisone.

``Cobblestone'' appearance of grafted surface when using large grafts (3–4 mm). Treat by ``shaving off'' top of grafts. Try a test area to evaluate results.

Necrosis of recipient site when using anesthetic with epinephrine. Treat with debridement and compresses.

Excessive hyperpigmentation in prone individuals. (Slight darkening may be expected.) Treat with long-term topical 1% hydrocortisone.

Infections are seldom seen. Treat with appropriate antibiotics when necessary.

References

1. Kiistala U. Suction blister device for separation of viable epidermis from dermis. J Invest Dermatol 1968;50:129–137.
2. Falabella R. Epidermal grafting: An original technique and its application in achromic and granulating areas. Arch Dermatol 1971; 104:592–600.
3. Falabella R. Repigmentation of leukoderma by autologous epidermal grafting. J Dermatol Surg Oncol 1984;10:136–144.
4. Falabella R. Grafting and transplantation of melanocytes for repigmenting vitiligo and other types of leukoderma. Int J Dermatol 1989;28:363–369.
5. Skouge JW, Morison WL, Diwan RV, Rotter S. Autografting and PUVA: A combination therapy for vitiligo. J Dermatol Surg Oncol 1992;18:357–360.
6. Suvanprakorn P, Dee-Ananlap S, Pongsomboon CH, et al. Melanocyte autologous grafting for treatment of leukoderma. J Am Acad Dermatol 1985;13:968–974.
7. Koga M. Epidermal grafting using the tops of suction blisters in the treatment of vitiligo. Arch Dermatol 1988;124:1656–1658.
8. Falabella R. Postdermabrasion leukoderma. J Dermatol Surg Oncol 1987;13:44–48.
9. Selmanowitz VJ, Rabinowitz AD, Orentreich N, et al. Pigmentary correction of piebaldism by autografts: Procedures and clinical findings. J Dermatol Surg Oncol 1977;3:615–622.
10. Hatchome N, Kato T, Tagami H. Therapeutic success of epidermal grafting in generalized vitiligo is limited by the Koebner phenomenon. J Am Acad Dermatol 1990;22:87–91.
11. Falabella R. Repigmentation of stable leukoderma by autologous minigrafting. J Dermatol Surg Oncol 1986;12:172–179.
12. Falabella R. Repigmentation of segmental vitiligo by autologous minigrafting. J Am Acad Dermatol 1983;9:514–521.
13. Falabella R. Treatment of localized vitiligo by autologous minigrafting. Arch Dermatol 1988;124:1649–1655.
14. Falabella R. Repigmentation of leukoderma by minigrafts of normally pigmented, autologous skin. J Dermatol Surg Oncol 1978;4:916–919.
15. Orentreich N, Selmanowitz VJ. Autograft repigmentation of leukoderma. Arch Dermatol 1972;105:736–784.
16. Mir Y, Mir L. The problem of pigmentation in the cutaneous graft. Br J Plast Surg 1961;14:303–307.

section three

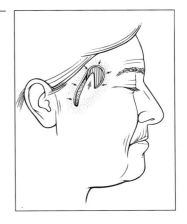

Specialized Anatomic Units and Specialized Techniques

JUNE K. ROBINSON

SPECIALIZED ANATOMIC UNITS

Certain regions of the body surface have complex anatomic arrangements. The nail and ear are two areas with skin closely juxtaposed to deep relatively avascular structures. With aging and with medical conditions, such as diabetes, the blood supply to these areas becomes even more tenuous. In the ear, the dermis rests on the perichondrium and the terminology used to describe the external anatomy refers to the curls of the underlying cartilage (Fig. III–1). Similarly, the dermis of the nail unit rests on the

periosteum of the distal tuft of the terminal phalanx (Fig. III–2A) and the insertion of the central slip of the extensor tendon lies just proximal to the proximal edge of the matrix, only a few millimeters beneath the cutaneous surface (see Fig. III–2B). These sites require careful attention to atraumatic tissue handling to preserve the vascular supply, prevent nerve injury, and prevent injury to perichondrium and periosteum.

Surgery of the ear requires special care because injury to the ear cartilage can lead to perichondritis and chondritis.[1] *Pseudomonas aeruginosa* is a natural colonizing organism

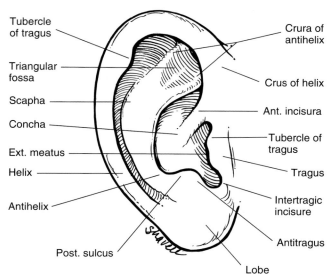

FIGURE III–1. The anatomy of the external ear.

of the external auditory canal.[2] *Pseudomonas* can easily infect the surgical site and cause chondritis.[3,4] *Pseudomonas* infections of the external ear (i.e., malignant otitis externa) can spread to the base of the skull and pose a risk of death if treatment is delayed or inadequate.[5]

Chondritis is more likely to occur in elderly or diabetic patients. The patient presents with a warm exquisitely tender ear, complains that the temporal scalp is sensitive to pain, and cannot stand to comb his or her hair. The area of erythema of the external ear spares the lobe (Fig. III–3).

Treatment of true malignant otitis externa consists of debridement of the necrotic ear cartilage, which may liquefy. Disfigurement or loss of the external ear results from this disease.[3,4] Oral ciprofloxacin[6] may be used to prevent or treat bacterial chondritis, including *Pseudomonas,* before it evolves into full-fledged malignant otitis externa. This may be combined with appropriate topical antibacterial agents (polymyxin B, gentamicin, or 1% acetic acid solution wet to dry dressings).

The hand and digit are not routinely colonized as is the ear canal; thus, the risk of infection for surgical procedures about the nail unit is not increased.[7] Although there is no need for preoperative antibiotics in performing nail surgery, some patients merit consideration of antibiotic administration because the result of a hand infection is disastrous. Patients at increased risk of infection are those with diabetes mellitus, immunosuppression, steroid therapy, and diseases causing vascular compromise. Because of the particular anatomy of the region, a tenosynovitis or acute tendon sheath infection may rarely occur in the postoperative period.[8] There is severe pain and throbbing with massive edema and slight flexion of the digit.[9] Any local pressure or movement of the digit causes severe pain, similar to that of the pain of external otitis. Infection spreads rapidly along the tendons and is usually caused by *Staphylococcus aureus* or *Streptococcus pyogenes.*[10] If treatment is delayed or inadequate, extensive damage may occur. Appropriate antibiotics should be started immediately after culture and sensitivity of the drainage is done. A

hand surgeon should be consulted for possible synovial sheath exposure and irrigation.

SPECIALIZED TECHNIQUES

Some procedures require resources for equipment purchase (e.g., lasers) or support personnel and special equipment (e.g., histopathology technologist and cryostat for Mohs' micrographic surgery). Additional training may be required. For these reasons, specialized procedures may not be readily practiced by all dermatologists. Similarly, in the next section, in which cosmetic cutaneous surgery is presented, there are special equipment needs and training requirements that may place some procedures outside the realm of many dermatologists. Nonetheless, the procedures are part of the spectrum of cutaneous surgery.

The expense of the equipment and devotion of personnel to each of these specialized procedures makes it very hard for one person to deliver a high standard in the full range of cutaneous surgical procedures. This is best exemplified by the array of surgical lasers. Thirteen lasers at 15 wave-

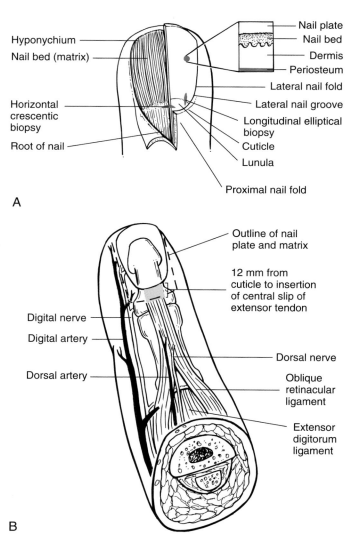

FIGURE III–2. *A,* The nail unit. *B,* The anatomy of the digit.

lengths are used in dermatology today (Table III–1). The clinical applications range from the treatment of vascular malformations in infants and the removal of some pigmented lesions without scarring to precise vaporization of tissue. The clinical applications of laser surgery will continue to evolve, and the question of whether laser surgery is more efficacious than conventional surgery will be asked for each indication.

The key clinical difference in the way lasers destroy tissue relates to which pigments are targeted in the skin, the pulse characteristics, and the wavelength of the light. The target in the tissue is water when vaporizing skin surface lesions with the carbon dioxide laser, hemoglobins when coagulating vascular lesions with the pulsed dye laser, or melanin when treating pigmented lesions and tattoo inks with the short-pulsed laser. Some lasers do not merely duplicate the range of others (see Table III–1) because they may vary in the duration of the pulse or the amount of energy. Shorter pulses are more target specific and are therefore less tissue destructive.

The laser most commonly used in practice is the carbon dioxide laser. Carbon dioxide laser vaporization is similar in many ways to electrosurgery, which is another way of destroying tissue with thermal energy. The precision possible with the carbon dioxide laser is greater than with electrosurgery; however, such precision may be necessary for only few clinical applications. Vaporization of rhinophyma, actinic cheilitis, and Bowen's disease may be controlled with CO_2 laser ablation to prevent excessive depth of destruction. Scarring is infrequent.

Lasers specialized for selective photothermolysis are designed around a single use and are expensive. They are the therapy of choice for specific conditions (e.g., flash lamp pumped pulsed dye laser for port-wine hemangiomas and

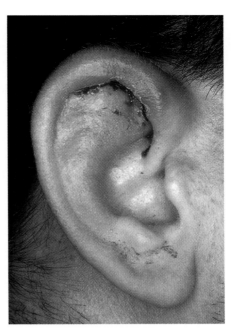

FIGURE III–3. Acute chondritis of the external ear following electrosurgical removal of a cyst of the helix. The cartilage was injured with the curette and left exposed. The *Pseudomonas* infection responded to oral ciprofloxacin. No debridement was necessary.

the Q-switched ruby, neodymium:yttrium-aluminum-garnet [Nd:YAG], or alexandrite laser for some benign pigmented lesions, especially dermal pigmented lesions such as tattoos and the nevus of Ota). No single laser treats all the colors in a professional tattoo.

TABLE III-1. Lasers Used in Cutaneous Surgery

Laser	Wavelength (nm)	Indications
Carbon dioxide (continuous wave)	10,600	Coagulation, vaporization, cutting of tissue for benign and malignant lesions
Nd:YAG (continuous wave)	1064	Deep tissue coagulation
Q-switched Nd:YAG (pulsed)	1064	Blue and black tattoos (usually amateur) Some dermal pigmented lesions*
Q-switched alexandrite (pulsed)	755	Epidermal and dermal pigmented lesions* Blue, black, green tattoos
Q-switched ruby (pulsed)	694	Epidermal and dermal pigmented lesions* Blue, black, green tattoos
Argon-pumped tunable dye (continuous)	577–690	Telangiectases, port-wine stains with irregular or elevated surface Photodynamic therapy
Flashlamp-pumped pulsed dye (long-pulsed)	585	Flat port-wine stains, port-wine stains in children, telangiectases
Copper vapor (pseudocontinuous)	578	Telangiectases, port-wine stains in adults
Krypton (continuous)	568	Telangiectases, port-wine stains in adults
KTP (pseudocontinuous)	532	Telangiectases, port-wine stains in adults Epidermal pigmented lesions
Frequency-doubled Q-switched Nd:YAG (pulsed)	532	Epidermal pigmented lesions Red tattoos
Krypton (continuous)	521,531	Epidermal pigmented lesions
Copper vapor (pseudocontinuous)	511	Epidermal pigmented lesions
Flashlamp-pumped dye (short-pulsed)	510	Epidermal pigmented lesions Red tattoos
Argon (continuous)	488,514	Telangiectases, thick port-wine stains in adults Epidermal pigmented lesions

* Dermal pigmented lesions such as melasma and postinflammatory hyperpigmentation do not routinely respond. Nevus of Ota does respond.

An emerging area of the clinical application of laser surgery is photodynamic therapy. In this treatment, long-wavelength photosensitizing drugs plus light causes local tissue necrosis. The major emphasis in this experimental treatment has been on developing usable photosensitizing drugs. Initially Photofrin, a hematoporphyrin derivative, was used. Now, a number of other drugs (e.g., phthalocyanines, chlorins, purpurins, porphyrin derivatives, and aminolevulinic acid) are undergoing phase I and II trials for treatment of cancer and viral, vascular, and inflammatory hyperproliferative disorders.

In their own special niche, each specialized procedure consistently delivers high-quality results. Now the question is, Can we afford to deliver this care? How can we as a society afford not to deliver that which we are capable of providing?

References

1. Stenuria BH, Marcus MD, Lucenta FE. Disease of The External Ear, 2nd ed. New York: Grune & Stratton, 1980:59–60,96.

2. Weinberg AN, Swartz MN. Gram negative coccal and bacillary infections. In: Fitzpatrick TB, et al., eds. Dermatology in General Medicine, 3rd ed. New York: McGraw-Hill, 1987:2126.

3. Dowling JA, Foley FD, Moncrief JA. Chondritis of the burned ear. Plast Reconstr Surg 1968;42:115–122.

4. Salasche SJ. Acute surgical complications: Cause, prevention, and treatment. J Am Acad Dermatol 1986;15:1163–1185.

5. Zaky DA, et al. Malignant external otitis, a severe form of otitis in diabetic patients. Am J Med 1976;61:298–302.

6. Noel SB, Scanllan P, Meadors MC, et al. Treatment of *Pseudomonas aeruginosa* auricular perichondritis with oral ciprofloxacin. J Dermatol Surg Oncol 1989;15:633–637.

7. Ratz JL, Yetman RJ. The hand. In: Roenigk RK, Roenigk HM, eds. Dermatologic Surgery: Principles and Practice. New York: Marcel Dekker, 1989;26:257–547.

8. Pollen AG. Acute infections of the tendon sheaths. In: Tubiana R, ed. Complications in Hand Surgery. Philadelphia: WB Saunders Co., 1981:6–21.

9. Kanavel AB. Infections of the Hand: A Guide to the Surgical Treatment of Acute and Chronic Suppurative Processes in the Fingers, Hand, and Forearm, 7th ed. Philadelphia: Lea & Febiger, 1983.

10. Hooper G, Pollen AG. Infections of the hand. In: Lamb DW, Hooper G, Kuczynski K, eds. The Practice of Hand Surgery. Oxford: Blackwell Scientific, 1989;37:599–613.

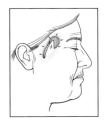

chapter 18

Nail Unit Surgery

STUART J. SALASCHE

NAIL AVULSION AND MATRIX EXPLORATION

Nail avulsion refers to the partial or complete surgical removal of the nail plate to expose the underlying nail bed and whatever portion of the distal nail matrix extends beyond the proximal nail fold (Tables 18–1 through 18–4). Complete visualization and exploration of the matrix requires retraction of the proximal nail fold. This is accomplished by making bilateral, full-thickness incisions at the junction of the proximal and lateral nail folds (Case 1, Fig. 18–1A). These incisions should extend from the free distal edge of the proximal nail fold to the proximal end of the proximal nail groove. The matrix can then be fully exposed for proper examination and biopsy by flipping back the fold with retraction stitches, forceps, or skin

hooks (Fig. 18–1B). At the end of the procedure, the incisions are sutured or secured in place with Steri-Strips (Fig. 18–1C). Matrix exploration is usually accomplished after avulsion of the nail plate. However, the surgeon may wish to inspect the matrix and the proximal nail groove with the plate intact. It is then possible to biopsy a suspicious area through the plate (Case 2, Fig. 18–2).

Complete nail avulsion may be achieved by either the distal or the proximal approach. With either technique, the key is to remove the nail plate as atraumatically as possible, not only to keep bleeding to a minimum but also to not damage the underlying bed and matrix. The longitudinal tongue and groove bonds between the nail bed and the overlying plate constitute the strongest attachment points. Lesser connections exist between the plate and the proximal and lateral nail folds. There is hardly any adherence between the newly formed nail plate and the matrix.

The nail unit is anesthetized, prepared in a sterile manner, and isolated with a sterile barrier. With the distal technique, an instrument, ideally a Freer septum elevator, is inserted beneath the free edge of the nail plate and

TABLE 18–1. Nail Avulsion: Indications, Contraindications, Limitations

Indications

To visualize the nail bed, matrix, and proximal and lateral nail folds

As a prelude to a biopsy or matricectomy

To relieve symptoms of a dystrophic or hypertrophied nail plate

For onychomycosis as an adjunct to systemic antifungal agents

Contraindications

No absolute contraindications

Limitations

Fingernails will take up to 6 months to regrow. Function (e.g., ability to pick up small objects) will be decreased.

Toenails will take up to a year to regrow. Volar soft tissue tends to ''round up,'' making walking uncomfortable.

Nail plate may regrow and display same pathology.

If matrix biopsy is performed, permanent dystrophy may ensue.

TABLE 18–2. Nail Avulsion: Patient Preoperative Discussion

1. Discuss indications and outline procedure.
2. Discontinue anticoagulants and other drugs affecting coagulation before surgery.
3. Dressing will be bulky. If fingernail is involved hand functions may be limited. Dressings on toe will require open shoe or slipper, which should be brought with you.
4. Daily dressing changes will be required. There will be some discomfort and blood-tinged oozing.
5. Physical activities will have limitations, especially if toenails are removed.
6. Nail bed will thicken and harden before real nail begins to grow. This pseudo-nail often confuses patient (see Fig. 18–4F).

TABLE 18-3. Nail Avulsion: Operative Issues

Preoperative Evaluation

History
    Bleeding diathesis
    Hepatitis, human immunodeficiency virus infection
    Prosthesis, artificial valves
    Allergies
    Peripheral vascular disease
    Peripheral neuropathy
Physical examination
Assessment of nail plate to determine best technique

Preoperative Equipment Needs

Local anesthesia
Antibacterial scrub preparation
Barrier protection

Intraoperative Needs

Freer septum elevator, dental spatula, or blunt hemostat
Iris scissors
Skin hooks or fine-toothed forceps
Scalpel blade and handle
Electrocautery unit
Needle holder and suture material

TABLE 18-4. Nail Avulsion: Postoperative Care

Pain Management

Plain or extra-strength acetaminophen for pain
Acetaminophen with codeine if pain is particularly strong

Dressings

Thin film of antibiotic ointment (Polysporin, Bacitracin)
Nonadherent pad (Release, Telfa)
Layer of folded gauze to add bulk
Layers of expansile tube dressing (Surgitube, X-Span)
Changed daily

Complications

Persistent bleeding
Persistent or excessive pain
Permanently dystrophic nail
No nail growth

---

advanced back toward the matrix in the cleavage plane between the plate and bed (Case 3, Fig. 18–3). Since this requires some force, the digit is best stabilized with the surgeon's other hand. Caution must be exercised as the matrix area is approached. The pushing force should be lessened because of the very loose attachment in this area.

It is possible to jam the instrument back into the cul-de-sac of the proximal nail groove and damage tissue. On reaching the end of the proximal nail groove, the elevator is removed and reinserted under the adjacent free edge. It is again advanced as above and repeated as often as necessary until the entire contact surface of nail and plate is freed up. Too much ripping and damage is caused if only a single insertion is made with forcible movement of the elevator from side to side. Next, the elevator is inserted under the proximal nail fold to the back of the cul-de-sac (see Fig. 18–3C). Here, the instrument may be swept from

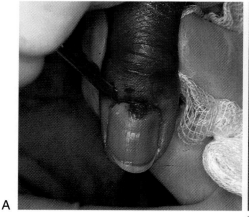

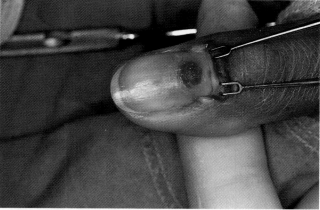

A

B

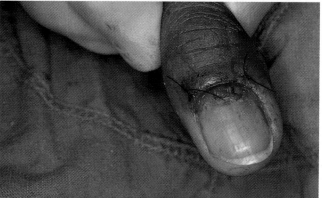

C

CASE 1

FIGURE 18-1. *A*, Matrix exploration: incision of proximal nail fold. *B*, Pyogenic granuloma of matrix exposed as fold is reflected with skin hooks. It is treated. *C*, Proximal fold replaced and sutured.

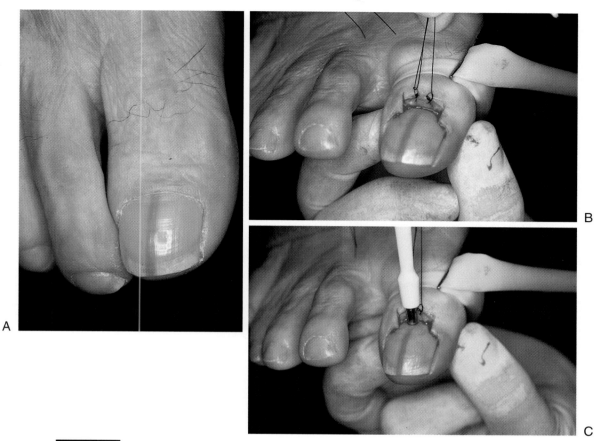

CASE 2

FIGURE 18–2. *A*, Pigmented streak of nail plate of the great toe. *B*, Proximal nail fold reflected with retraction sutures. *C*, Punch biopsy of proximal matrix through nail plate.

side to side without injury to the soft tissue. Thus freed, the nail plate is grasped with a hemostat and retracted distally and removed (see Fig. 18–3*D* and *E*). If any soft tissue connections remain, they can be snipped with an iris scissors.

The proximal approach is somewhat more difficult and is most useful when there is no distal free margin, as occurs with severely dystrophic nails, nails with fungal infection, or previously avulsed nails (Case 4, Fig. 18–4*A*). In this approach the elevator is inserted under the proximal nail fold (see Fig. 18–4*B* and *D*), advanced proximally to the end of the proximal nail groove, and flipped under the proximal edge of the new nail plate (see Fig. 18–4*C*). This is done by feel. The elevator tip is now in the breach between the loosely adherent plate and the underlying matrix. It is advanced distally until it emerges from under the distal edge of the nail (see Fig. 18–4*E*). Caution must be exercised not to push the elevator into the substance of the nail bed. This is best accomplished by pushing upward against the undersurface of the plate as it is moved distally.

In a partial avulsion, the nail plate is split lengthwise and a complete longitudinal segment is removed. This technique can be used as a prelude to biopsy, but it is most

useful for treating ingrown toenails and is discussed in more detail in that section.

NAIL UNIT BIOPSY

There are three types of biopsy of the nail unit that are sufficiently different from routine skin biopsies to warrant detailed discussion. These are (1) biopsy of the nail matrix; (2) biopsy of the nail bed; and (3) combined biopsy of the lateral nail fold, lateral nail matrix, and proximal nail fold. The latter procedure is really a complicated excision. Its use is usually restricted to eradication of Bowen's disease or squamous cell carcinoma of the lateral fold area or to help histologically define a nail unit condition such as Darier's disease or Reiter's syndrome.

Biopsy of the nail matrix is not to be taken lightly because of the real possibility a permanently altered nail plate may ensue. Although indications should be clear and the patient fully cognizant of the potential consequences, biopsy should not be delayed or withheld when the results would influence appropriate management (Tables 18–5 through 18–8). In general, permanent dystrophy will be minimized if the biopsy is limited to 3 mm or less, ori-

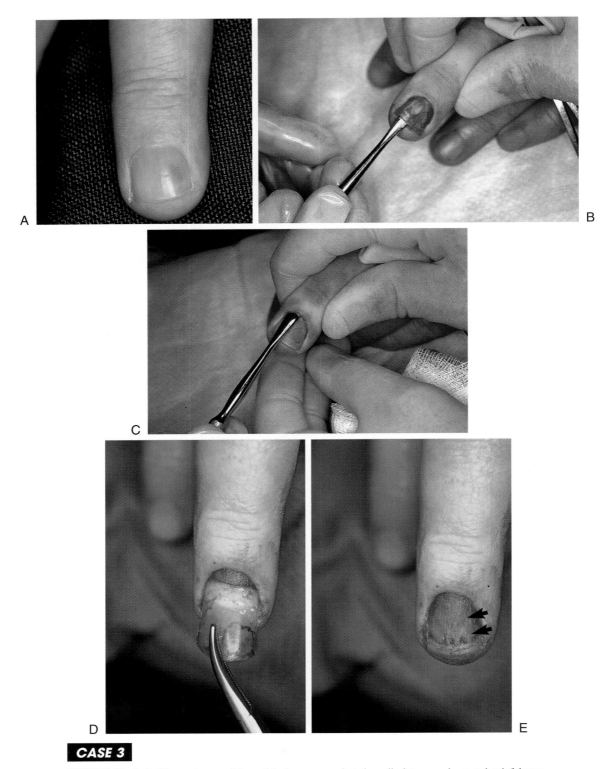

CASE 3

FIGURE 18–3. *A,* Glomus tumor of the nail bed presses against the nail plate as a cherry-red painful area. *B,* Septum elevator advanced back under free edge of nail plate. *C,* Instrument advanced under proximal nail fold. *D,* Nail plate removed with hemostat. *E,* Atraumatic nail avulsion; glomus tumor of the nail bed is exposed *(between arrows).*

ented transversely, situated distally near the far edge of the lunula, and arched to reiterate the distal convexity of the matrix. However, if these ideal conditions are not possible, suturing the defect minimizes the chances of a dystrophic nail.

The most compelling indication for a matrix biopsy is to rule out malignant melanoma when there is a longitudinal pigmented streak of the nail plate. Tumors arising in the matrix area and unexplained full-length nail plate deformities constitute the other reasons to biopsy the matrix.

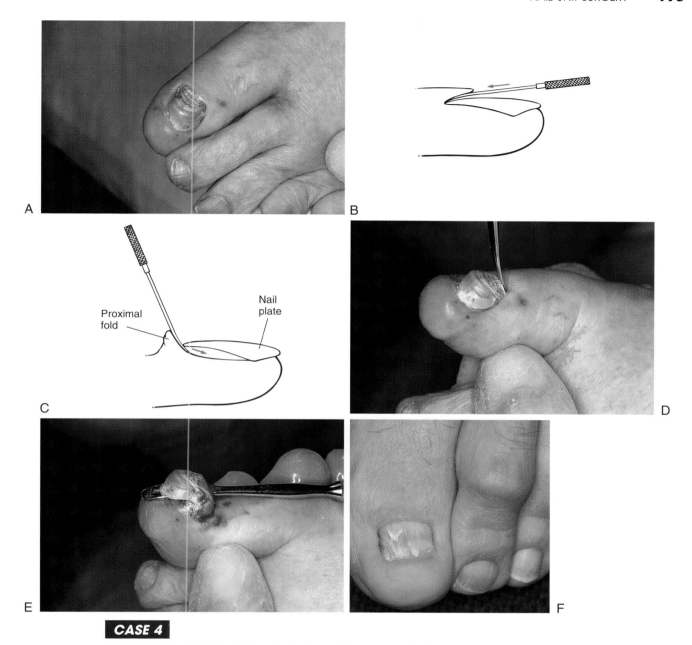

CASE 4

FIGURE 18-4. *A*, Painful, thickened nail plate of the great toenail without clear-cut distal free edge. *B*, The elevator is atraumatically inserted under the proximal fold. *C*, The elevator pushes the loosened fold back, feels the edge of the nail plate, and flips under it. Motion of instrument is indicated by red arrows. *D*, Septum elevator inserted into proximal nail groove. *E*, After the instrument is rotated under nail plate, it is advanced distally. *F*, Many months later, pseudonail forms after avulsion of onychogryphotic nail plate with removal of the matrix.

Biopsy of the matrix can be done with the proximal nail fold retracted and the plate still in place (see Figs. 18–2*C* and III–2*A*). This requires a punch or excision through the newly formed nail plate. The punch should extend down to the periosteum of the terminal phalanx. Although relatively easy to perform, if the biopsy is in the proximal matrix, the nail plate will grow out with a defect that may become permanent since suturing is impossible. In most instances, the plate will be avulsed first and the proximal fold retracted for complete visualization (Case 5, Fig. 18–5). Alternately, if the lesion is asymmetrically disposed, a partial avulsion and retraction of the proximal fold on the

ipsilateral side will allow good surgical access. The exact dimensions of the biopsy can be planned; and after removal of the specimen, undermining in the plane above the periosteum can be done and the defect sutured. Care should be taken to use delicate-toothed forceps when removing the specimen because the tissue is crushed easily. Maintaining orientation of the specimen is also critical for proper histologic interpretation. A simple solution is to tattoo the epithelial surface with an appropriate sterile surgical dye (gentian violet) before the biopsy specimen is removed.

Biopsy of the nail bed involves less risk. The usual

TABLE 18–5. Nail Biopsy: Indications, Contraindications, Limitations

Indications
Pigmented streaks of the nail plate
Space-occupying lesions; benign and malignant tumors
Unexplained nail unit conditions; to establish diagnosis

Contraindications
Same as for avulsions, depends on urgency and importance

Limitations
Same as it is for avulsion if included as part of biopsy procedure
Possible permanent nail split or other longitudinal dystrophy with matrix biopsy

TABLE 18–7. Nail Biopsy: Safety Issues

Preoperative Evaluation
Same as for avulsion of nail plate
Preoperative Equipment Needs
Same as for avulsion of nail plate
Intraoperative Needs
Same as for avulsion of nail plate
Punches of various sizes: 2 mm, 3 mm, and 4 mm
Scalpel blade and handle: Beaver handle with No. 67 blade
Fine-toothed forceps: Graeffe, Bishop-Harmon
Suture material
Suture scissors
Surgical marking dye (sterile)
3/8-inch sterile Penrose drain for tourniquet

indications are a tumor of some sort, but on occasion biopsy is required to identify a disease process. Biopsies should be oriented longitudinally and if possible specimens should be 3 mm or less in width (Fig. 18–6). Suturing is easily performed after the tissue is mobilized by undermining in the plane above the periosteum.

Bowen's disease frequently arises in the lateral nail fold (Case 6, Fig. 18–7A). Often it is misdiagnosed initially as a fungal infection or a wart. Biopsy is best accomplished by removing the lateral nail plate to expose the fold (see Fig. 18–7B). Depending on the extent of the condition, only the fold and portions of the neighboring bed may require excision. Definitive resection may require a combined lateral excision that involves en bloc removal of the lateral portion of the proximal nail fold, the underlying lateral matrix, the lateral nail fold, and several millimeters of adjacent bed and finger skin (see Fig. 18–7C). The incisions are in the vertical dimension through the nail bed and transverse through the lateral skin (see Fig. 18–7D). They should extend down to periosteum and meet at a point to ensure removal of the entire specimen as a single piece (see Fig. 18–7E). The defect may be sutured or allowed to heal by second intention (Fig. 18–7F and G).

CHEMICAL MATRICECTOMY

Destruction of the nail matrix will prevent regrowth of the nail plate. As a planned procedure, this may involve either the entire matrix or only a portion of it. These are referred to as total or partial matricectomies, respectively (Table 18–9). In the latter situation, only the corresponding portion of the nail plate will fail to re-form. Matrix

ablation is accomplished by several modalities. These include surgical excision, CO_2 laser excision utilizing the focused mode or ablation with the defocused mode, electrosurgery, or chemical chemocautery. Chemocautery utilizes fully saturated (88%) liquefied phenol applied directly to the exposed nail matrix. Overall, it is the simplist, least traumatic, and most successful procedure for the majority of practitioners and is the modality discussed here in detail.

The partial chemical matricectomy is most frequently used for recalcitrant ingrown toenails but also finds application in the treatment of pincer or incurvated nails. On occasion, it is useful to obliterate one portion of the nail plate in cases of permanently split nails of various etiologies. This condition is particularly disturbing since the split nail catches and snags on most everything (Fig. 18–8A).

The procedure is done in an outpatient setting under local anesthesia and utilizing proper sterile preparation, surgical site isolation, and universal precautions (Tables 18–10 through 18–12). To gain access to the nail matrix, a partial nail avulsion is done. This is best accomplished with an English nail splitter (see Figs. 18–7B and 18–8B). This instrument, which looks like heavy-duty scissors, is unique in that the lower blade has an anvil-like platform instead of cutting surface. It slides under the free edge of the nail plate and is advanced proximally in the cleavage plane between the plate and the nail bed (Case 8, Fig. 18–9C). When the proximal nail fold is reached, the instrument is clamped shut and the plate is split to this point (see Fig. 18–9C). The blades are then advanced under the cuticle to the end of the proximal nail groove and again

TABLE 18–6. Nail Biopsy: Patient Preoperative Discussion

1. Discuss indications for biopsy and sequelae of not doing biopsy.
2. Outline procedure.
3. Inform of possible long-term dystropy as result of biopsy, especially if matrix is involved.
4. May require sutures and return visit for suture removal.
5. Physical limitations same as for avulsion if part of procedure.

TABLE 18–8. Nail Biopsy: Postoperative Care

Pain Management
Plain or extra-strength acetaminophen
Acetaminophen with codeine if pain is excessive
Dressings
Same as for nail avulsion
Complications
Bleeding and pain
Infection
Persistent nail plate deformity resulting from biopsy

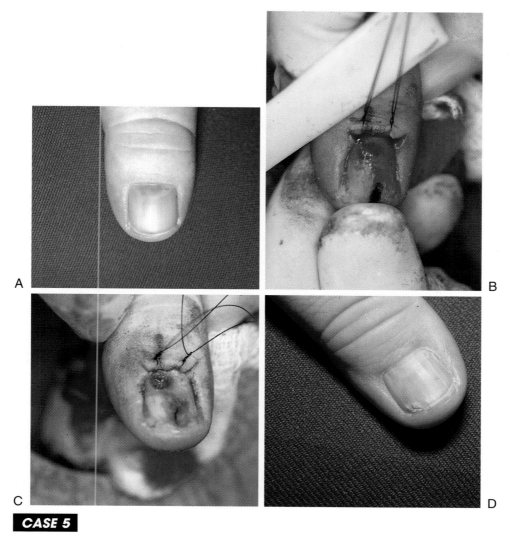

CASE 5

FIGURE 18–5. *A*, Painful glomus tumor of the nail matrix. Thumb is exerting pressure to better delineate the tumor. *B*, Tumor exposed after avulsion and matrix exposure. *C*, Punch biopsy removal of distal matrix glomus tumor. Surgical defect allowed to heal by second intention. *D*, New nail growth at 6 months.

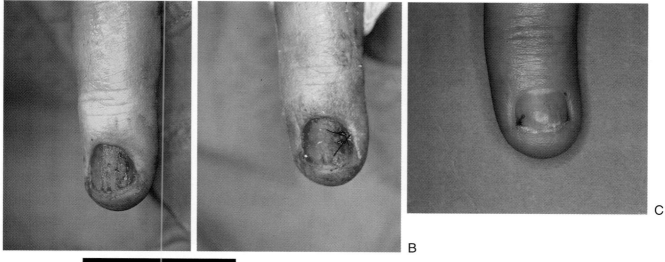

CASE 3 (Continued)

FIGURE 18–6. *A*, Proposed excision of glomus tumor of nail bed (same patient as Fig. 18–3). The longitudinally oriented excision is carried down to the periosteum. The total width of the excision does not exceed 3 mm. *B*, Defect sutured with interrupted sutures. *C*, Healing at 1 year: no recurrence.

195

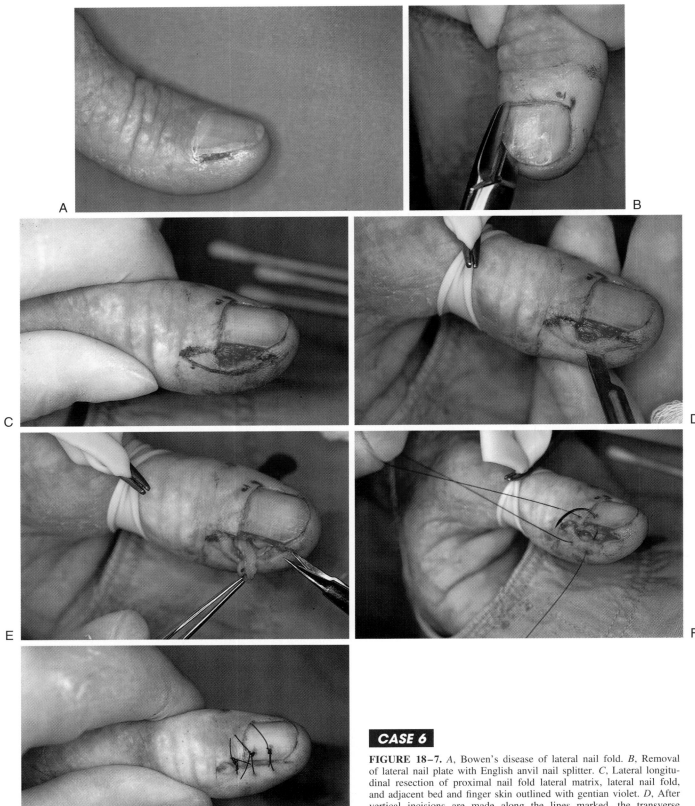

CASE 6

FIGURE 18–7. *A*, Bowen's disease of lateral nail fold. *B*, Removal of lateral nail plate with English anvil nail splitter. *C*, Lateral longitudinal resection of proximal nail fold lateral matrix, lateral nail fold, and adjacent bed and finger skin outlined with gentian violet. *D*, After vertical incisions are made along the lines marked, the transverse incision across the bottom of the lesion is made. *E*, Removal of the en bloc specimen is performed with scissors, and the tip of the specimen is elevated with a forceps. *F*, Placement of sutures. *G*, Suturing completed.

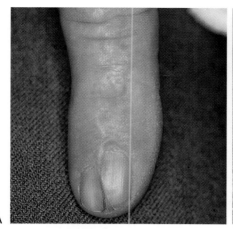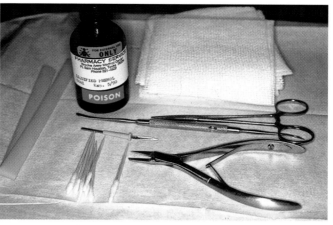

CASE 7

FIGURE 18–8. *A*, Pterygium and split nail secondary to trauma. *B*, Nail matricectomy tray: English nail splitter, Freer septum elevator, cotton-tipped toothpicks, tourniquet, hemostat.

clamped shut to complete the longitudinal splitting of the nail. The appropriate portion of nail is then peeled off with a hemostat (see Fig. 18–9*D*).

With the lateral nail plate removed, the surgeon has easy access to the matrix. As phenol acts to denature the protein component of the matrix epithelium, a dry bloodless surface facilitates good contact with the chemocauterant. This can be accomplished by firm, bilateral digital pressure. Alternately, one can use a tourniquet fashioned from a 3/8-inch Penrose drain. The drain is tightened around the proximal digit and secured with a straight hemostat. It is best to apply the tourniquet just before the application of the phenol so it is in place for only a short time (no more than 10 minutes) and only when needed. The phenol is

applied to the matrix by inserting the phenol-soaked cotton-tipped toothpick into the channel under the proximal nail fold and pressing it directly and firmly against the matrix for about 30 seconds (Fig. 18–9*E*). After neutralizing with alcohol and drying, the procedure is repeated. The phenol frosts the matrix epithelium a white color. It can damage any other portion of the nail unit it contacts, so special care should be taken to avoid application to the surrounding nail bed or folds.

The indications for a total matricectomy are often dictated by the patient's frustration with a functionally or cosmetically disabling altered nail plate (Case 9, Fig. 18–10). To perform a total matricectomy the entire nail plate must first be avulsed (see Fig. 18–10*B*). In this procedure the matrix is divided into halves or thirds and each segment is treated in the same manner as described earlier (see Fig. 18–10*C* and *D*). Healing follows a set pattern. The first week to 10 days the wound is similar to a second-degree burn with denudation of the epidermis. Over the next several weeks epithelialization occurs (see Fig. 18–10*E*). Often and especially on the toenails, there is formation of a thickened, hyperkeratotic nail bed–matrix area. This protective response is called a pseudonail (see Fig. 18–4*F*).

After either partial or total phenol matricectomies patients experience considerable pain and often develop a

TABLE 18-9. Chemical Matricectomy: Indications, Contraindications, Limitations

Indications
Partial matricectomy
   Ingrown toenails (onychocryptosis)
   Pincer or incurvated nails (bilateral partial matricectomies)
   Persistent split nails (usually smaller segment destroyed)
Total matricectomy
   Severely dystrophic nails—functional and cosmetic problems:
      Onychogryphosis: Ram's horn nail
      Onychauxis: thickened or hypertrophic nails
      Onychomycosis, psoriasis, some congenital nails
Contraindications
Severe peripheral vascular disease
Limitations
Permanent absence of the nail plate
   Fingernails
      Cosmetic deficiency
      Functional problems with delicate tasks
   Toenails
      Volar pulp of terminal digit may roll up and cause discomfort (see Fig. 18–11).

TABLE 18-10. Chemical Matricectomy: Patient Preoperative Discussion

1. Discuss indications and outline nature of procedure.
2. Explain finality of outcome: nail will not regrow.
3. Explain cosmetic and functional consequence of permanent loss of nail plate.
4. Open shoe or slippers required after surgery for toenails.
5. Discuss pain probabilities and medications to be used.
6. Discuss need to limit activities.
7. Preliminary discussion of dressing changes.

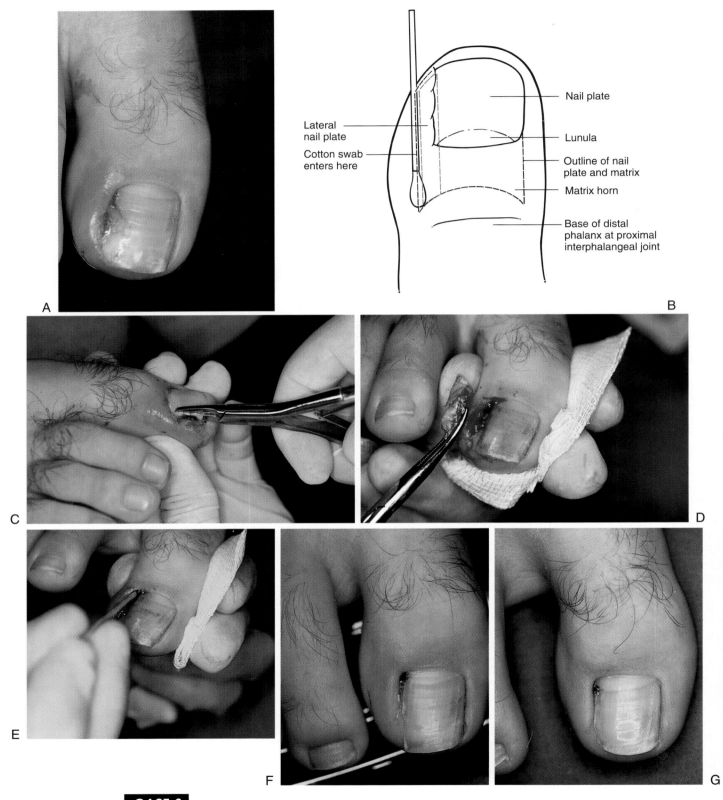

Nail plate

Lateral
nail plate

Cotton swab
enters here

Lunula

Outline of nail
plate and matrix

Matrix horn

Base of distal
phalanx at proximal
interphalangeal joint

CASE 8

FIGURE 18–9. *A*, Ingrown toenail in teenage boy. *B*, Exuberant tissue of the lateral nail fold is curetted away in the area outlined by the red broken line. After the nail plate is removed, the phenol is applied by a cotton swab to the matrix for 30 seconds. The swab follows a channel under the proximal nail fold to reach the matrix horn. *C*, Lateral nail plate split longitudinally. *D*, Lateral nail plate removed with hemostat. *E*, Phenol-soaked applicator destroys matrix. *F*, Appearance several days postoperatively. *G*, Appearance of nail 6 months later.

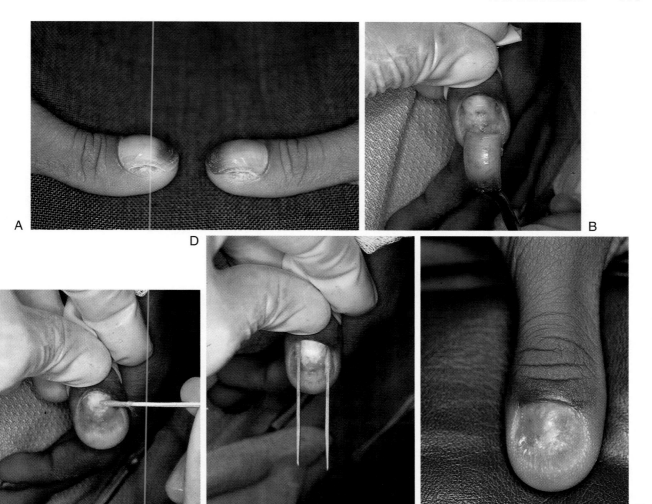

CASE 9

FIGURE 18–10. *A*, Congenitally dystrophic nails with hidrotic ectodermal defect. *B*, Avulsion of nail plate: note hypertrophic matrix. *C*, Phenol applied to central matrix. *D*, Phenol applied to both lateral matrix zones. *E*, Long-term healing.

TABLE 18-11. Chemical Matricectomy: Operative Issues

Preoperative Evaluation

History: Same as nail avulsion
Physical examination: Evidence of vascular insufficiency or peripheral neuropathy

Preoperative Equipment Needs

Local anesthesia
Antibacterial scrub preparation
Barrier protection

Intraoperative Needs

English nail splitter
Liquefied phenol, 88%—fresh, in darkly tinted bottle
Sharp-tipped toothpicks
Loose cotton balls (sterile)
Straight hemostat
Sterile 3/8-inch Penrose drain
Electrocautery unit
Cotton-tipped applicators
Alcohol swabs
Syringe containing 0.6 mL of 0.5% bupivacaine and 0.4 ml of dexamethasone with 30-gauge needle

TABLE 18-12. Chemical Matricectomy: Postoperative Care

Pain Management

Elevate foot or hand
Bulky dressing
Acetaminophen with codeine often required

Dressings

Apply film of antibiotic ointment
Pack proximal nail groove with moistened 1/4-inch Nu Gauze strips, Xeroform gauze, or absorbable collagen pads (Instat)
Cover nail unit with a nonadherent pad (Release, Telfa)
Layer of folded 2×2-inch gauze to add bulk
Several layers of tube dressing (Surgitube, X-Span)
Daily dressing changes: gauze pads usually not replaced after first dressing change

Complications

Pain or bleeding
Lymphangitis
Failure to prevent regrowth of nail plate
Regrowth of small nail plate spicules (see Fig. 18–12)

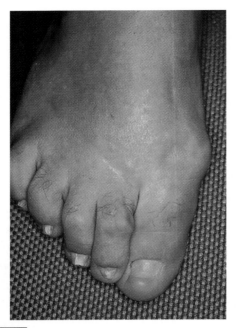

CASE 10

FIGURE 18–11. Distal pulp may ''roll up'' after permanent matricectomy.

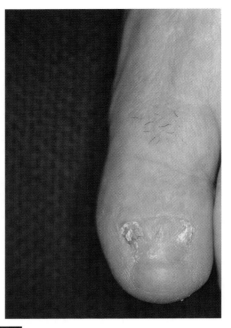

CASE 11

FIGURE 18–12. Spicules of nail plate from inadequate lateral solehorn ablation.

chemical lymphangitis on the dorsum of the digit arising from the proximal nail fold. These symptoms can be prevented by injection of a combination of long-acting local anesthetic and corticosteroid into the proximal nail fold at the completion of the phenol matricectomy. This mixture is made from 0.6 mL of 0.5% bupivacaine and 0.4 mL of dexamethasone. Only about 0.5 mL needs to be injected.

Suggested Readings

1. Daniel CR III. Basic nail plate avulsion. J Dermatol Oncol Surg 1992;18:685–688.
2. Salasche SJ. Surgery of the nail. In: Scher RK, Daniel CR III, eds. Nails: Therapy, Diagnosis, Surgery. Philadelphia: WB Saunders Co., 1990:258–280.
3. Baran R. Surgery of the nail. Dermatol Clin 1984;2:271–284.
4. Siegle RJ, Swanson NA. Nail surgery: A review. J Dermatol Surg Oncol 1982;8:659–666.
5. Albom MJ. Avulsion of the nail plate. J Dermatol Surg Oncol 1977;3:34–35.
6. Baran R. More on avulsion of the nail plate. J Dermatol Surg Oncol 1981;7:854.
7. Scher RK. Surgical avulsion of nail plates by a proximal to distal approach. J Dermatol Surg Oncol 1981;7:296–297.
8. Rich P. Nail biopsy: Indications and methods. J Dermatol Surg Oncol 1992;18:673–682.
9. Baran R, Sayag J. Nail biopsy: Why, when, where, how? J Dermatol Surg Oncol 1976;2:322–324.
10. Scher RK. Biopsy of the matrix of the nail. J Dermatol Surg Oncol 1980;6:19–21.
11. Bennett RG. Technique of biopsy of the nails. J Dermatol Surg Oncol 1976;2:325–326.
12. Scher RK. Longitudinal resection of the nails for purposes of biopsy and treatment. J Dermatol Surg Oncol 1980;6:805–807.
13. Siegle RJ, Harkness JJ, Swanson NA. The phenol alcohol technique for permanent matricectomy. Arch Dermatol 1984;120:348–350.
14. Ceilley RI, Collison DW. Matricectomy. J Dermatol Surg Oncol 1992;18:728–734.

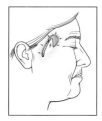

chapter 19

Common Problems of the Ear

Surgical Treatment of Chondrodermatitis Nodularis

Clifford M. Lawrence

The patient presents with a small painful lump on the ear. Chondrodermatitis nodularis lesions are discrete and oval with a raised, rolled edge and central ulcer or depression that usually contains a crust or scale[1,2]; with a few exceptions,[3-5] most are unilateral and occur on the side that the patient sleeps on.[4] Any site may be affected, although the helix in men and the anthelix in women are most common.[4]

Chondrodermatitis nodularis is a benign condition, and treatment is only required if pain interferes with sleep (Table 19-1). Initially topical and intralesional steroids should be tried.[4] Blindly destructive therapies such as electrosurgery, radiation therapy, and curettage result in relapse rates of 38%,[6] 80%,[6] and 31%,[5] respectively. Elliptical excision results in an 18% to 50% recurrence rate[6-8]; curetting off necrotic cartilage after elliptical skin excision may be more effective.[9] Wedge excision[2,10] is deforming and unnecessary. These relatively ineffective surgical therapies should be abandoned in favor of cartilage excision alone.[4,11,12] The aim of such surgical therapy is to expose the affected cartilage without excising any skin, to remove the cartilage around the nodule leaving a smooth cut edge, and then to suture the skin edges. The advantage of the technique is the good cosmetic result and high cure rate.

INSTRUCTIONS FOR PATIENTS

The procedure takes 30 to 45 minutes, with lesions on the anthelix taking longer. Sutures are required, and these will be removed at around 5 days. A small local dressing will be applied and removed with the sutures. Postopera-

TABLE 19-1. Surgical Treatment of Chondrodermatitis Nodularis: Indications, Contraindications, Limitations

Indications
Painful nodule causing sleep disturbance
Failed medical therapy
Recurrence after previous surgery
Contraindications
None
Limitations
Recurrence rate of 5% on the helix
Recurrence rate of 30% on the anthelix
Recurrence more likely on anthelix sites in women
Recurrences more likely after previous surgery
Lesions may improve but not disappear completely

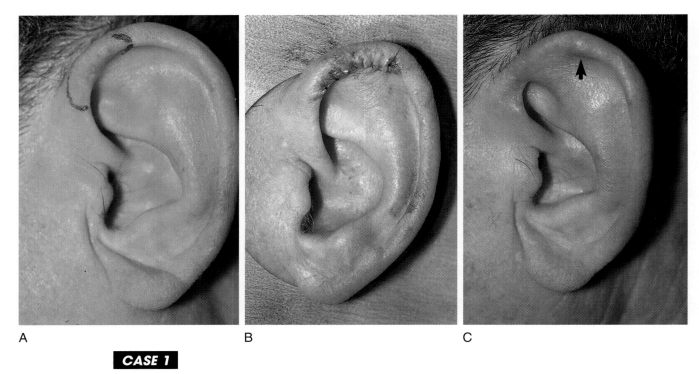

A   B   C

CASE 1

FIGURE 19–1. Recurrence of helix chondrodermatitis. This lesion had recurred after earlier elliptical excision *(A)*. It was excised *(B)* but recurred at the tip of the cartilage excision 3 months later *(arrow in C)*.

tive pain is not usually a problem; if necessary, acetaminophen can be taken. After the successful treatment of lesions on the helix, pain relief is almost immediate; pain usually persists with anthelix lesions for several weeks. Patients should avoid sleeping on the affected side until the sutures have been removed; thereafter, the wound can be washed with warm water and soap as required. Second lesions sometimes occur on the same or opposite ear (Case 1, Fig 19–1). It may be helpful if the patient can vary his or her sleeping position so that different ears and sites are rested on; a soft pillow may also be helpful. Although recurrences may occur, this is less likely on the helix, where cure rates of 93% are reported. Lesions on the anthelix are more difficult to treat, and the risk of recurrence is higher at approximately 30%. In some patients pain is reduced postoperatively so that sleep is no longer disrupted, but the ear may still be painful when squeezed. In this circumstance no further treatment is required. If necessary, further surgery can be done at the site of a recurrence.

SAFETY ISSUES

Local anesthetic with epinephrine should be used to help limit bleeding and ensure adequate visualization (Table 19–2). The blood supply to the ear is such that ischemic complications are not a problem, with the possible exception of diabetic patients with small vessel disease. No patient sedation is required. As with all skin surgical procedures one must be aware of the hazards of human immunodeficiency virus infection or hepatitis and operating on patients with a bleeding diathesis or infected skin. If a large dressing is required after surgery of anthelix lesions, the dressing must go behind as well as in front of the ear to cushion the pinna.

SURGICAL TECHNIQUE (Table 19–3)

Helix

An incision up to 20 mm either side of the nodule is made along the rim of the helix. If a biopsy sample is taken that includes cartilage, a thicker sliver of helix carti-

---

TABLE 19–2. Surgical Treatment of Chondrodermatitis Nodularis: Equipment Required

Local anesthetic: epinephrine
No. 15 blade and scalpel handle
Fine-toothed forceps or skin hooks
Damp gauze to hold the slippery ear steady
Bipolar hemostasis
Blunt, curved scissors
Needle holder
5-0 monofilament nylon suture material
Optional extra: serrated edge scissors for cutting cartilage

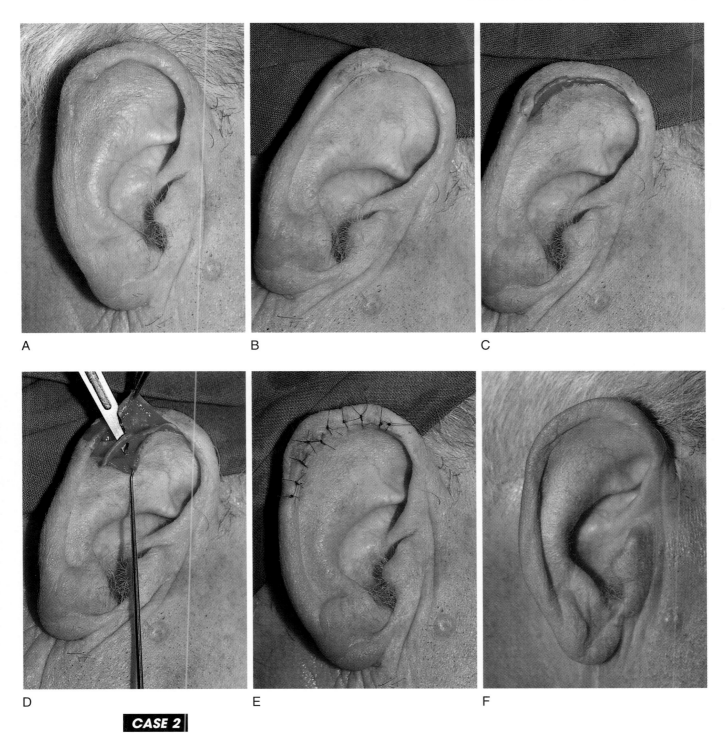

A
B
C

D
E
F

CASE 2

FIGURE 19--2. Surgical treatment of chondrodermatitis on the helix. *A,* Preoperative appearance. When taking a punch biopsy try not to go too deep into the cartilage because the cartilage excision will have to go beneath the punch hole to ensure that the cut edge is smooth. *B,* An incision is made along the helix rim. *C,* The skin is dissected back over the perichondrium to expose the cartilage. This is the most time-consuming part of the procedure; the skin on the lateral surface of the ear is very fragile and if there has been previous surgery will be tightly bound down. It is best to hold the ear steady with the forefinger behind the ear and the thumb everting the helical rim. Bluntly dissect on the lateral surface first and then find the plane between the perichondrium and the dermis on the rim of the helix and gently work along the length of the helix dissecting onto the medial surface of the ear to expose the cartilage. *D,* The blade is held horizontally, and a slice of cartilage is removed and the cartilage edges checked for smoothness. If necessary, the cartilage can be cut using very sharp serrated-edged scissors rather than a blade. *E,* The skin edges are sutured; a running cuticular suture can often be used. If necessary, the skin incision can be extended to enable sufficient excision of cartilage to get a smooth edge of the cartilage. *F,* Appearance at 5 months.

TABLE 19–3. Surgical Treatment of Chondrodermatitis Nodularis: Specific Considerations of Technique

1. Use local anesthetic with epinephrine.
2. Inject the anesthetic between the perichondrium and dermis. This hydrodissects the skin off the cartilage and makes blunt dissection easier.
3. Get good hemostasis. Do not be lulled into a false sense of security by the short-lived effect of the epinephrine.
4. Anesthetize an adequate area preoperatively—at least 20 mm on either side of the nodule—so the incision can be extended if required.
5. Cut the cartilage holding the blade horizontally to help produce flat cartilage edges.
6. Check the cut cartilage edges with a fingertip to ensure smoothness.
7. Recurrences occur where the cartilage is irregular or the cut edge is not gently tapered enough. On the helix leave smooth, gently tapering edges at the tips of the cartilage excision.
8. Remove enough cartilage. On the helix a 20-mm sliver of cartilage is probably the minimum.

lage will have to be excised to get below the punch biopsy margins to ensure a smooth contour. The skin is dissected off to reveal the helix cartilage. A sliver of cartilage approximately 3 mm thick at the ulcer and shelving steadily to the normal cartilage is removed (Case 2, Fig. 19–2). It is essential that the cut cartilage edge and particularly the tips of the cartilage excision are left smooth and gently tapering; rough or protuberant edges will result in recurrence (Case 1, Fig. 19–1). Nonprotuberant, smooth cartilage edges are achieved by holding the blade horizontal where possible, cutting the cartilage with a carving rather than a slicing motion, and checking with the fingertip that the cut edge feels smooth. If the edge is rough, further cartilage shaves must be taken. In this way a sliver of cartilage with gradually tapering ends, up to 40 mm long, will be excised. Hemostasis should be obtained with dia-

thermy and the skin edges sutured. With the use of this technique cosmesis is excellent and the cure rate is over 90%.[4]

Anthelix

Anesthetic must be injected into the lateral and medial surfaces of the ear because tissue on both ear surfaces will be handled and must be numb. To expose cartilage on the anthelix a flap approximately 25 mm wide and 15 mm long has to be raised, with its attached margin directed toward the helix (Case 3, Fig. 19–3) and the ulcerated area at its center. Basing the flap on the anthelix does not give such good exposure but the flap vascularization is the same. The perichondrium-covered cartilage is thus exposed, and an area of cartilage can be excised, revealing the dermis and fat on the medial side of the ear. The size of the piece of cartilage excised will be determined by the amount of cartilage that has to be removed to produce a smooth ear contour without protuberant cartilage edges. The operator must attempt to produce smooth, nonprotruding cartilage edges by using the scalpel blade as close to the horizontal as possible and checking the smoothness of cartilage edges with the fingertip. After obtaining hemostasis, the flap is re-sited and sutured. Ulcerated areas of skin do not need to be excised and can be left to heal by second intention or sutured. Lesions on the anthelix are more difficult to treat than those on the helix. This procedure results in a 70% cure rate.[4] The cosmetic result is good with a retained ear shape (Case 4, Fig. 19–4).

Recurrences

Postoperatively painful areas always occur away from the original lesion site and at the edge of the cartilage excision.[6,13] It is thus essential that all efforts are made to ensure that these are not palpable before wound closure. Recurrences can be treated using the same principle of cartilage excision or intralesional steroids.[4]

CASE 3 ▶

FIGURE 19–3. Surgical treatment of chondrodermatitis on the anthelix. *A,* The flap with the biopsied nodule at its center was designed and dissected off the perichondrium to expose the cartilage. *B,* Note the ulcerated cartilage. Avoid making the mistake of designing the flap too small. The bigger it is, the better it is to expose the affected cartilage. There is little risk of skin necrosis since the flap is very broad based and will receive additional blood supply from the dermal blood vessels on the posterior surface of the ear when cartilage is excised. *C,* A piece of cartilage *(red broken line)* is excised by holding the blade horizontally and using a slicing motion to remove the cartilage. The red arrow shows the forward motion of the blade. *D,* The dermis and fat on the posterior surface of the ear are exposed. It was also necessary to extend the skin incision so that more cartilage could be removed to get smooth cut edges and a nonprotruding cartilage contour. *E,* The skin edges and ulcer were sutured with a central tacking suture. *F,* A simple local dressing was applied. *G,* Appearance at 1 month.

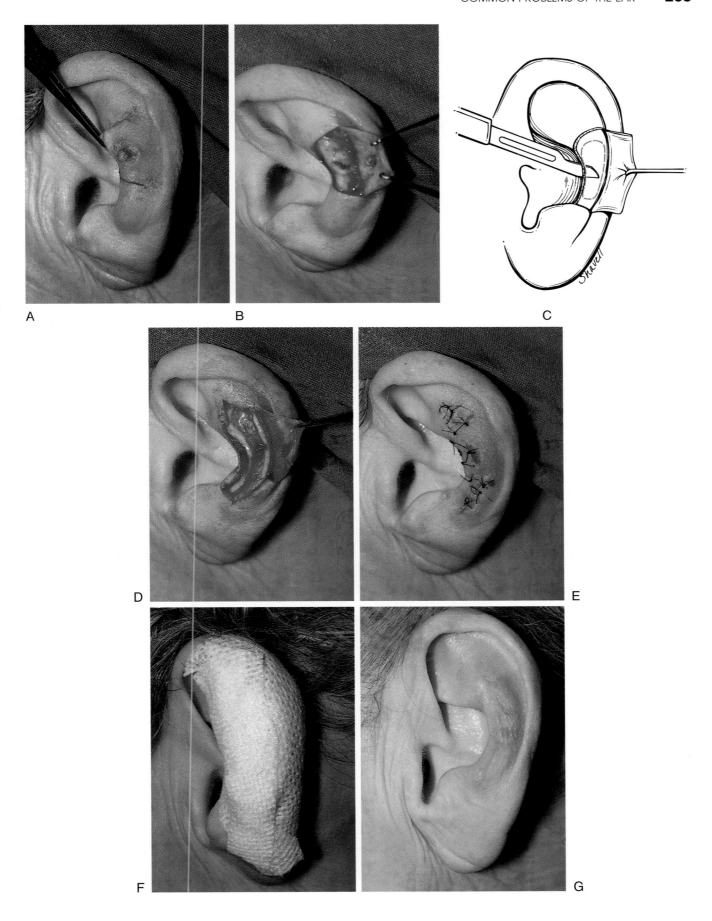

A

B

C

D

E

F

G

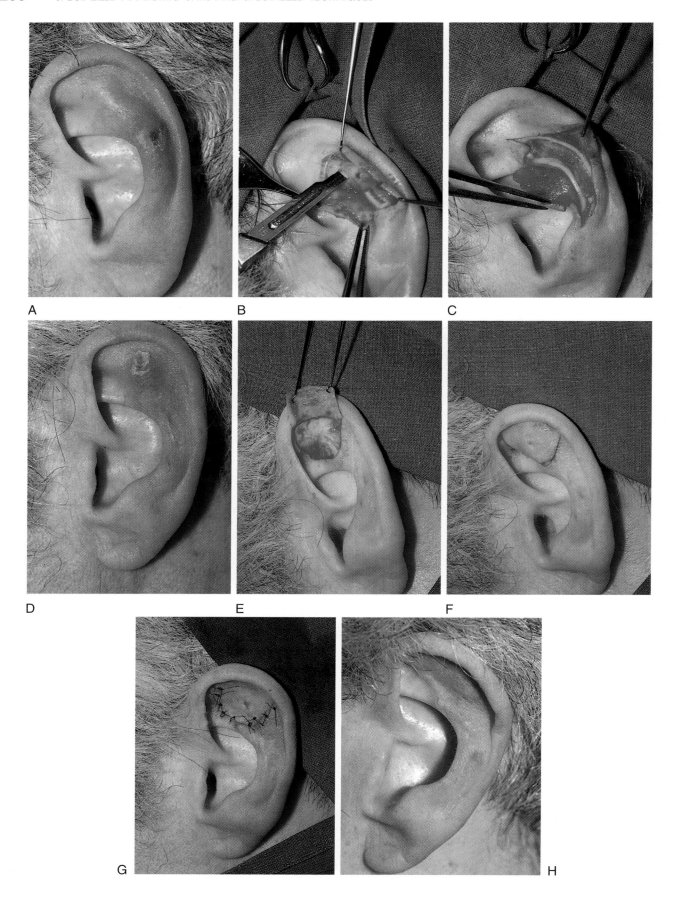

A

B

C

D

E

F

G

H

◀ **CASE 4**

FIGURE 19–4. Surgical treatment of recurrent chondrodermatitis on the anthelix. Chondrodermatitis of the anthelix *(A)* being excised for the first time *(B)*. *C,* Note that the flap had to be extended to allow adequate cartilage exposure. *D,* Seven months later there was a recurrence at the upper pole at the edge of the cut cartilage. *E,* At a second operation a flap was designed to allow access to the affected portion of cartilage. *F,* The flap was dissected off the cartilage and the cartilage was excised leaving no protuberant edges. *G,* The skin flap was re-sited. *H,* Appearance 15 months later.

Split Earlobe Repair

June K. Robinson

Pierced ears are fashionable for men as well as women. Earlobes as well as other portions of the pinna are pierced. In time, the weight of the earring may elongate the pierced hole into a slit or a downward traumatic event transects the lobe resulting in a split earlobe.

The repair of elongated splits involves excision of the epidermis of the slit and suture of the wound side to side. No subcutaneous buried sutures are necessary. The ear is pierced in 4 to 6 weeks. The patient can wear clip-on earrings during this interval.

At the time of ear piercing, the patient brings an earring with a stainless steel post that is cleansed with alcohol. The site of the new piercing is selected in consultation with the patient but is usually medial to the repair. A local anesthetic is injected. A 14- or 16-gauge needle is inserted from back to front. The thin post of the earring is inserted into the barrel of the needle and pulled through. The patient leaves these earrings in place for 10 days. Newly created epithelial tracts are formed during this time. The earring is turned daily by 180 degrees to prevent adhesions.

If the split earlobe is repaired by excising the epithelium and sutured side to side, a slight dimple in the rim of the ear may result as the incision line undergoes scar contraction. This dimple is not frequently remarked about by the patient. To prevent this contraction the repair can be planned with incorporating a Z-plasty on the rim (Fig. 19–5) or by using the technique of interlocking "Ls" to break up the force of contraction on the rim (Case 5, Fig. 19–6).

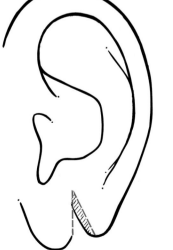
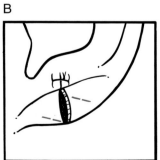
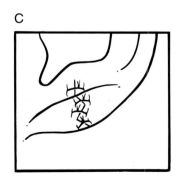

FIGURE 19–5. Z-plasty incorporated into repair to prevent dimpling of the rim. *A,* The epithelial tract is excised and closed on the anterior and posterior surfaces of the ear with interrupted sutures. Incision lines are shown as broken red lines. *B,* Small triangles are planned at the inferior portion of the incision as it joins the rim of the ear. Incision lines *(broken red lines)* form the two transposition flaps. *C,* Triangles are transposed and inset with tip stitches.

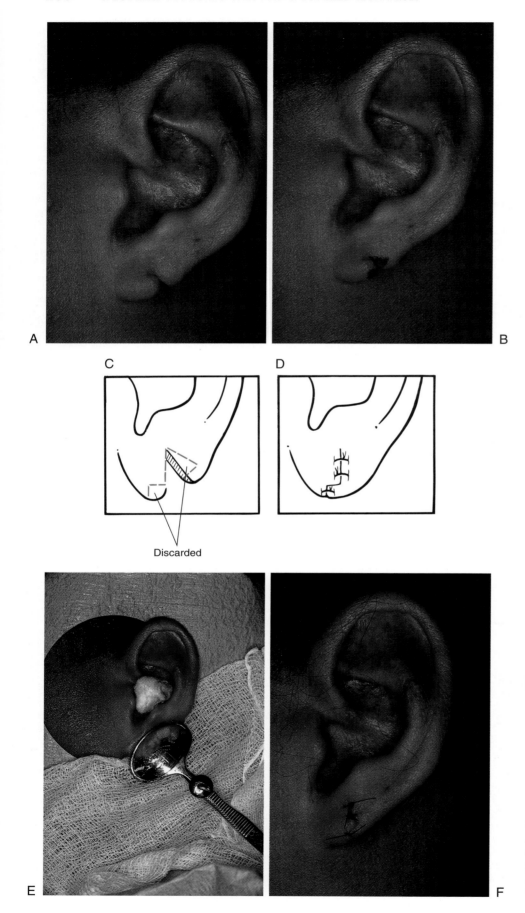

Discarded

FIGURE 19–6. Interlocking ''L'' technique to prevent dimpling of the rim. *A,* Split earlobe in an African-American woman with systemic lupus erythematosus and very small earlobes. *B,* Excision with interlocking ''Ls'' marked in gentian violet. *C,* Planning the incisions and portion to be discarded. *D,* Because the incision is not a straight line but rather is ''stepped,'' the future contraction of the scar will not produce dimpling along the rim of the lobe. *E,* A chalazion clamp is used to stabilize the earlobe as the incisions are made. The clamp also provides hemostasis. *F,* Because the tips of the flaps are extremely small it was not possible to inset them with tip stitches.

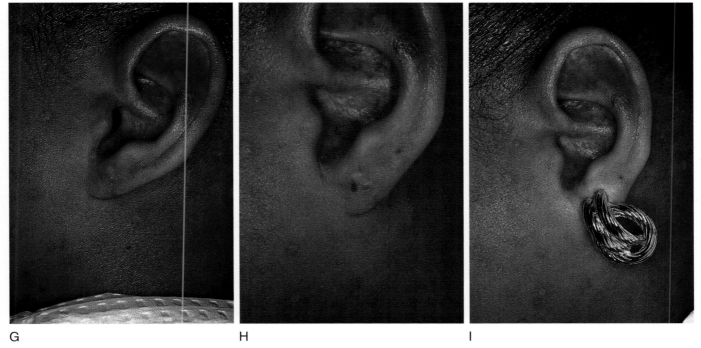

G   H   I

FIGURE 19–6 *Continued*
G, Six weeks after the repair was performed there is no evidence of keloid formation. The incision line is well healed with minimal retraction or "dimpling" of the rim. *H,* At the 6-week visit, the patient and physician select the site of piercing, which is not in the incision line. The site is marked with gentian violet. *I,* With the use of local anesthesia the ear is pierced and the earring is placed.

References

1. Lawrence CM. Chondrodermatitis nodularis. In: Arndt KA, LeBoit PE, Robinson JK, Wintoub BU, eds. Cutaneous Medicine and Surgery. Philadelphia: WB Saunders Co., 1996.
2. Metzger SA, Goodman ML. Chondrodermatitis helicis: A clinical re-evaluation and pathological review. Laryngoscope 1976;86:1402–1412.
3. Bard JW. Chondrodermatitis nodularis chronica helicis. Dermatologica 1981;163:376–384.
4. Lawrence CM. The treatment of chondrodermatitis nodularis with cartilage removal alone. Arch Dermatol 1991;127:530–535.
5. Kromann N, Hoyer H, Reymann F. Chondrodermatitis nodularis chronica helicis treated with curettage and electrocauterization: Follow-up of a 15-year material. Acta Derm Venereol 1983;63:85–87.
6. Newcomer VD, Steffen CG, Sternberg TH, et al. Chondrodermatitis nodularis chronica helicis. Arch Dermatol Syph 1953;68:241–255.
7. Shuman R, Helwig EB. Chondrodermatitis helicis. Am J Clin Pathol 1954;24:126–144.
8. Strack MF, Bourke JF, Graham-Brown RAC. Treatment of chondrodermatitis nodularis helicis. Br J Dermatol 1993;129(Suppl 42):39.
9. Coldiron BM. The surgical management of chondrodermatitis nodularis chronica helicis. J Dermatol Surg Oncol 1991;17:902–904.
10. Kitchens GG. Auricular wedge resection and reconstruction. Ear Nose Throat J 1989;68:673–674, 677–679, 683.
11. Zimmerman MC. Chondrodermatitis nodularis chronica helicis, a nondeforming surgical cure for painful nodule of the ear. Arch Dermatol 1958;78:41–46.
12. Ceilley RI, Lillis PJ. Surgical treatment of chondrodermatitis nodularis chronica helicis. J Dermatol Surg Oncol 1979;5:384–386.
13. Barker LP, Young AW, Sachs W: Chondrodermatitis of the ears: A differential study of nodules of the helix and antihelix. Arch Dermatol 1960;81:53–63.

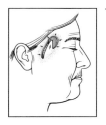

chapter 20

Mohs' Micrographic Surgery

ROY C. GREKIN

Mohs' micrographic surgery is a meticulous technique for surgically removing selected cutaneous malignant lesions (Tables 20–1 through 20–6). The procedure requires combining the skills of surgeon and pathologist in one physician who has had extensive training in the technique.

TABLE 20–1. Mohs' Micrographic Surgery: Indications, Contraindications, Limitations

Indications
Epithelial tumors
  Basal cell carcinoma (See Table 20–2)
  Squamous cell carcinoma
  Keratoacanthoma
  Bowen's disease
Adnexal carcinomas
  Microcystic adnexal carcinoma
  Adenocarcinoma
  Extramammary Paget's disease
  Eccrine carcinoma
Dermal tumors
  Dermatofibrosarcoma protuberans
  Malignant fibrous histiocytoma

Contraindications
Tumors not assessable by frozen section examination
Tumors with discontiguous growth patterns
Patient intolerant to local anesthesia
Large or deeply invasive tumors into bone or other body cavity
Poor patient health

Limitations
Mapping errors
Technician sectioning error
Microscopic interpretation error

TABLE 20–2. Indications for Mohs' Micrographic Surgery of Basal Cell Carcinoma

Tumors at Higher Risk for Recurrence with Other Therapies
Recurrent basal cell carcinoma
Histologic variants
  Sclerosing (morpheaform), infiltrative, micronodular
Location
  H-zone of face: periorbital, nasal tip/alae, lips, ears, periauricular, melolabial folds
Perineural spread
Size greater than 2.0 cm
Tumors in Areas Where Tissue Conservation Is Important
Eyelids, ears, nose, lips
Fingers
Genitalia

This training is often a 1- or 2-year fellowship after completion of residency.

Mohs' micrographic surgery involves several precise steps. The tumor is first excised and carefully mapped as to location (Fig. 20–1). The excisional specimen is cut into pieces small enough to fit on a microscope slide, and its edges are stained to allow proper orientation. A technician within the surgical unit then performs frozen horizontal (as opposed to standard vertical) sectioning of the entire undersurface and edges of the tissue specimens (Fig. 20–2). This provides for examination of 100% of the surgical margin of the resected tissue, as compared with 0.2% to 0.5% of margins with vertical sectioning. Microscopic examination of hematoxylin and eosin (or toluidine blue)–stained sections allows for precise localization of residual

TABLE 20-3. Mohs' Micrographic Surgery Patient Preoperative Discussion

Physician Concerns
1. Delineation and documentation of indications
   a. Histologic proof of diagnosis (biopsy)
   b. Precise localization of tumor and size
2. Prior procedures in areas
3. Patient health history (see Table 20-4)
4. Patient desires

Patient Concerns
1. Explanation of indications for Mohs' micrographic surgery and alternative procedures
2. Explanation of techniques and indications
   a. Anesthesia
   b. Stage I, II, III, etc.; time for each
   c. Repair options after tumor extirpation
   d. Dressings
3. Postoperative course
   a. Wound care, activity limitations
   b. Pain management
   c. Suture removal
   d. Touch-up repair procedures
   e. Complications (see Table 20-6)

tumor at any margins. This is noted on the surgical map, and further tissue is excised only in those areas with residual tumor. The stepwise process is repeated until all margins are clear (see Table 20-5). Each stage may require from 1 to 2 hours, depending on tumor size. Excision of

TABLE 20-4. Mohs' Micrographic Surgery: Operative Issues

Preoperative Evaluation
Medical history
  Hepatitis, human immunodeficiency virus infection
  Medications
  Allergies
  Immunosuppression
  Prosthetics
  Cardiac valve disease
  Bleeding problems
  Smoking history
  Other significant medical illnesses
  Aspirin avoidance

Intraoperative Needs

Well-equipped Surgical Suite
Surgical light
Adjustable table
Suction
Electrosurgical device
Appropriate high-quality instruments
Mapping, tissue staining materials
Anesthesia, adjunctive medications
Emergency equipment
Dressing materials

Tissue Preparation Laboratory
Histology technician
Cryostat
Staining equipment manual or automated
Microscope
Slide storage

TABLE 20-5. Mohs' Micrographic Surgery: Procedural Steps

1. Delineate tumor with a marking pen.
2. Administer anesthesia, 1% lidocaine with epinephrine.
3. Clean and drape the area.
4. Debulk the tumor with curette or scalpel (see Fig. 20-1A).
5. Remove a 1- to 3-mm layer of tissue around the curetted area.
   a. Perform a 30-degree beveled cut under the tumor.
   b. Obtain 1- to 3-mm margins depending on size and infiltrative histology (see Fig. 20-1B).
   c. Obtain hemostasis with electrodesiccation.
   d. Place a dressing.
   e. Draw surgical map (see Fig. 20-1C).
   f. Cut excised tissue into specimens appropriate for processing (see Fig. 20-1D).
   g. Stain nonepidermal edges with dyes (red color used in Fig. 20-1D to indicate a dye).
6. Give tissue to histology technician.
   a. Place specimens deep side up on cryostat (see Fig. 20-2A).
   b. Freeze specimens.
   c. Perform horizontal sectioning across entire tissue undersurface and through epidermal margin (see Fig. 20-2B).
   d. Stain the slides (see Fig. 20-2C).
7. Interpret the slides.
8. Note areas of remaining tumor on surgical map (see Fig. 20-2D).
9. Repeat steps 5 through 8 in areas of residual tumor as indicated.
10. Discuss repair options with patient.

TABLE 20-6. Mohs' Micrographic Surgery: Postoperative Care

Dressings
Antibiotic ointment
Steri-Strips
Telfa
Gauze, cotton balls
Tapes
Occlusive dressings

Pain Management
Acetaminophen
Acetaminophen with codeine
Hydroxycodone (Vicodin)
Oxycodone (Percocet)
Meperidine (Demerol)

Complications

Early
Pain
Bleeding
Hematoma
Nerve damage

Intermediate
Infection
Necrosis
Dehiscence

Late
Hypertrophic scar
Contracture
Ectropion

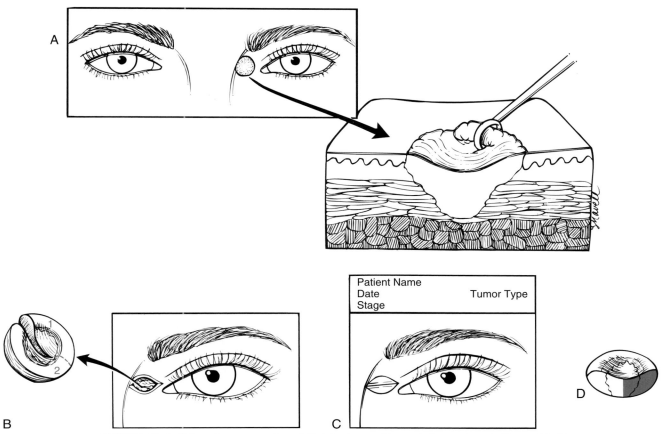

FIGURE 20–1. Schematic representation of Mohs' micrographic surgical procedure. *A,* Tumor debulking with a curette removes all clinically visible tumor. *B,* From the wound thus created, a thin layer of tissue is excised. This saucer- or bowl-shaped layer carefully encompasses the entire wound surface created by the curette. *C,* A map of the tumor location and its size is created. As colored dyes are applied to the cut nonepidermal surfaces of the specimen, the location of the dye is marked on the map *(red)* to maintain orientation. *D,* The layer is cut into specimens of a size that can be processed in a cryostat.

larger tumors (greater than 2–3 cm) may exceed 2 hours per stage. Multiple stages, done with the use of local anesthesia, can be performed in 1 day (Case 1, Fig. 20–3).

Advantages of this type of surgery are related to the 100% marginal examinations and precise mapping of tumor location. These provide for the highest possible cure rates (95%–99%) and maximal tissue conservation since no standard safety margins need to be included. Disadvantages include increased operating expenses due to equipment (cryostat, microscope, advanced operating room equipment), longer operating periods, and additional personnel (see Table 20–4).

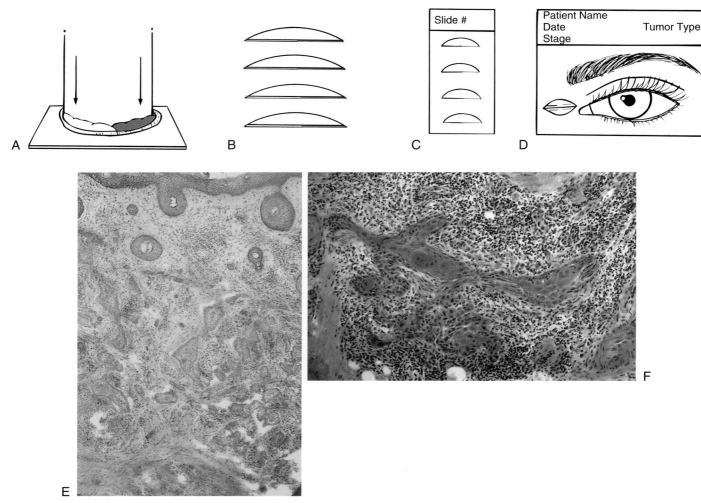

FIGURE 20–2. Schematic representation of frozen section preparation of the tissue. *A*, The specimen is inverted, flattened, and chilled in the cryostat. *B*, Multiple frozen sections are cut from the block. *C*, The frozen sections are placed onto a glass slide and stained with either hematoxylin and eosin or toluidine blue. *D*, The prepared frozen sections are interpreted by the surgeon, and the location of residual tumor is marked onto the map. Additional surgery or stages are then continued at the precise location of the residual cancer. Subsequently removed tissue is processed and examined as described in *A* through *D*. *E*, Frozen section of sclerosing (morpheaform) basal cell carcinoma stained with toluidine blue demonstrates metachromasia of the stroma around the tumor chords and nests in the dermis. The epidermal edge (superior) assists in orienting the specimen. Black and red dyes used to stain the borders of the specimen are not shown in this view. *F*, Hematoxylin and eosin preparation of a frozen section of a well-differentiated squamous cell carcinoma shows tumor nests present at the deep margin stained with black dye.

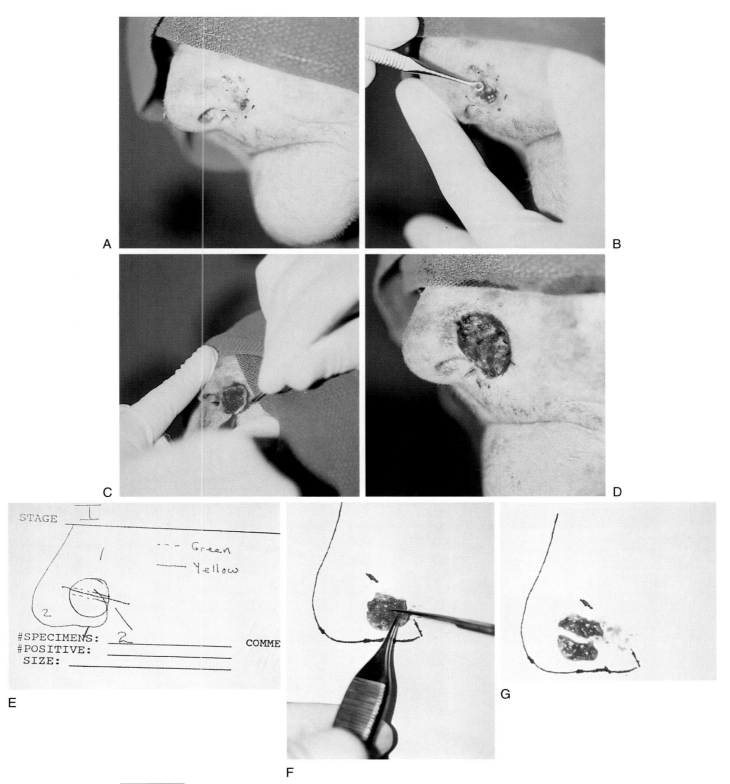

STAGE I

---- Green
——— Yellow

#SPECIMENS: 2
#POSITIVE:
SIZE:

COMME

CASE 1

FIGURE 20–3. *A*, Preoperative photograph of left nasal alar basal cell carcinoma. *B*, Debulking of basal cell carcinoma with curette. *C*, Stage I excision. Note 30- to 45-degree angle of knife blade and 2-mm margin of normal-appearing skin around debulked area. *D*, Stage I excision completed. Note scoring of epidermis at medial and lateral margins corresponding to division of specimen into sections appropriate for processing. *E*, Map orienting tissue specimen and denoting dye-marking of nonepidermal margins. *F*, Division of specimen. *G*, Divided specimen showing orientation. Compare with map in *E*.

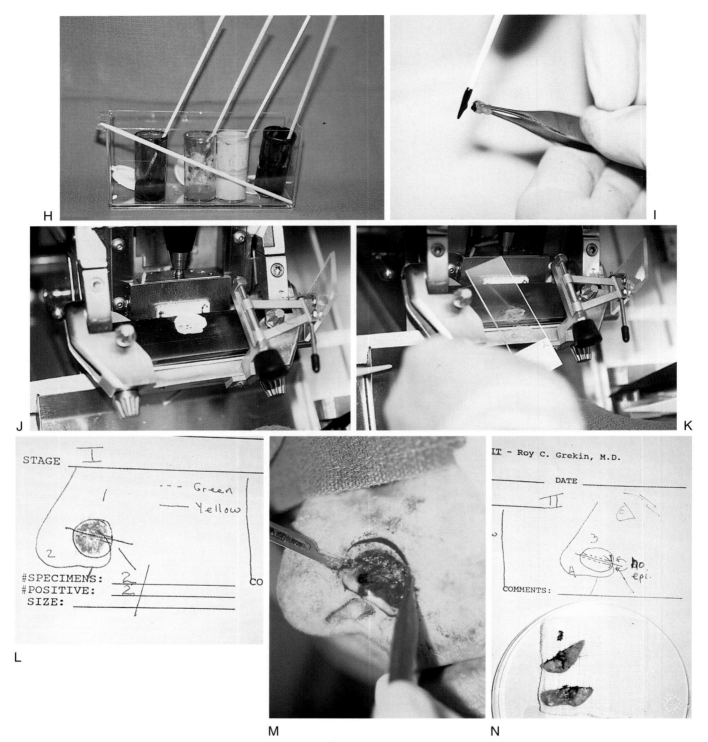

FIGURE 20–3. *Continued H*, Tissue dyes. *I*, Dye-marking of nonepidermal margins with black ink. *J*, Sectioning of frozen specimens. *K*, Frozen sections adhering to glass slide. *L*, Residual tumor in specimen margins noted by coloring the area red on map in *E*. *M*, Stage II excision. Right lateral epidermis spared under the suction device, which is a glass eyedropper filled with blood in the photograph. *N*, Stage II specimens and map.

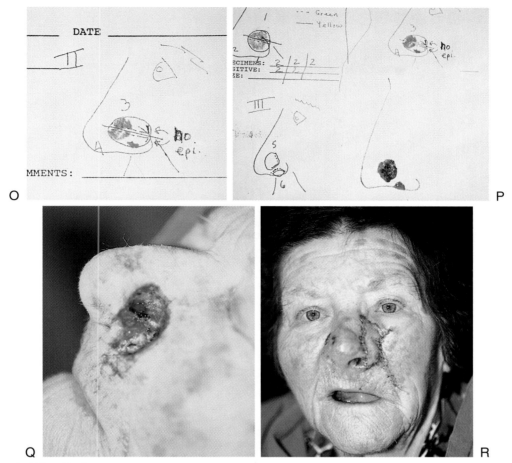

FIGURE 20–3. *Continued O*, Residual tumor after stage II noted on map after prepared specimens are interpreted by the surgeon. *P*, Stage III excisional specimens and map. *Q*, Postoperative defect after stage III. *R*, Repair of defect by nasolabial fold transposition flap.

Suggested Readings

1. Albom MJ. Squamous cell carcinoma of the finger and nail bed: A review of the literature and treatment by the Mohs surgical technique. J Dermatol Surg Oncol 1986;12:972–974.
2. Brown MD, Zachary CB, Grekin RC, Swanson NA. Genital tumors: Their management by micrographic surgery. J Am Acad Dermatol 1988;18:115–122.
3. Cottel WI, Bailin PL, et al. Essentials of Mohs micrographic surgery. J Dermatol Surg Oncol 1988;14:11–13.
4. Hanke CW, Wolfe RL, Hochman SA, et al. Perineural spread of basal cell carcinoma. J Dermatol Surg Oncol 1983;9:742–747.
5. Lang PG, Osguthorpe JD. Mohs micrographic surgery of the head and neck. Dermatol Clin 1989;7(4).
6. Lang PG, Maize JC. Histologic evolution of recurrent basal cell carcinoma and treatment implications. J Am Acad Dermatol 1986;14:186–196.
7. Levine JL, Bailin PL. Basal cell carcinoma of the head and neck: Identification of the high-risk patient. Laryngoscope 1980;90:955–961.
8. Levine HL, Ratz JL, Bailin P. Squamous cell carcinoma of the head and neck: Selective management according to site and stage—skin. Otolaryngol Clin North Am 1985;18:499.
9. Maloney ME. The dermatologic surgical suite, design and materials. In: Grekin RC, ed. Practical Manuals in Dermatologic Surgery. New York: Churchill Livingstone, 1991.
10. Mikhail GR. Mohs Micrographic Surgery. Philadelphia: WB Saunders Co., 1991.
11. Mohs FE. Chemosurgery: Microscopically Controlled Surgery for Skin Cancer. Springfield, IL: Charles C Thomas, 1978.
12. Mohs FE, Snow SN. Microscopically controlled surgical treatment for squamous cell carcinoma of the lower lip. Surg Gynecol Obstet 1985;160:37–41.
13. Niparko JK, Swanson NA, Baker SR, et al. Local control of auricular, periauricular, and external canal cutaneous malignancies with Mohs surgery. Laryngoscope 1990;100:1047–1051.
14. Robins P, Rodriguez-Stains R, Rabinovitz H, Rigel D. Mohs surgery for periocular basal cell carcinomas. J Dermatol Surg Oncol 1985;11:1203–1207.
15. Roenigk RK. Mohs micrographic surgery. Mayo Clin Proc 1988;63:175–183.
16. Roenigk R, Roenigk H. Current surgical management of skin cancer in dermatology. J Dermatol Surg Oncol 1990;16:136–151.
17. Rowe DE, Carroll RJ, Day CL Jr. Mohs surgery is the treatment of choice for recurrent (previously treated) basal cell carcinoma. J Dermatol Surg Oncol 1989;15:424–431.
18. Salasche SJ, Amonette RA. Morpheaform basal-cell epitheliomas: A study of subclinical extensions in a series of 51 cases. J Dermatol Surg Oncol 1981;7:387–394.
19. Swanson N. Mohs surgery technique, indications, applications, and the future. Arch Dermatol 1983;119:761–773.
20. Swanson NA, Grekin RC, Baker SR. Mohs surgery: Techniques, indications and implications in head and neck surgery. Head Neck Surg 1983;6:683.
21. Swanson NA, Tromovitch TA, Stegman SJ, Glogau RG. A novel method of re-excising incompletely excised basal carcinomas. J Dermatol Surg Oncol 1980;6:438–439.

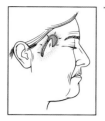

chapter 21

Laser Treatment of Vascular Lesions

ROY G. GERONEMUS

PULSED-DYE LASER TREATMENT

Treatment of Port-Wine Stains

Flashlamp-pumped pulsed-dye laser therapy is considered the treatment of choice for many different types of port-wine stains (Table 21–1). The low risk of scarring and of permanent pigmentary alteration from the use of this laser has made it possible to treat these congenital malformations in young infants, children, and adults. The incidence of scarring is believed to be far less than 1%, while pigmentary alteration (hypopigmentation and hyperpigmentation) occurs in less than 2% of patients. The pulsed-dye laser is effective in lightening most port-wine stains; however, complete clearing cannot always be obtained (Case 1, Fig. 21–1). The therapeutic response often depends on the anatomic location of the port-wine stain, with the central portion of the face and distal extremities responding more slowly, in terms of the degree of lightening, compared with other anatomic areas. Multiple treatment sessions are usually required to obtain the maximum benefit. Approximately 75% lightening is seen in most patients after two to three treatment sessions. Maximum lightening or clearing, however, may take many additional treatment sessions. Some patients require repetitive treatments (sometimes between 10 and 20) to obtain the maximum therapeutic response.

Treatment with the pulsed-dye laser is characterized by post-treatment darkening that resembles purpura. This darkening of the skin can last for 5 to 14 days, depending on the diameter of the laser beam utilized during the treatment. Smaller-diameter spot sizes (3 mm) respond with more rapid clearing than larger-diameter spot sizes (5–7 mm). When the appropriate energy fluences are used, the skin does not slough or crust and no postoperative wound care is required. Makeup can be worn after a pulsed-dye laser procedure if crusting has not occurred. Cosmetic camouflage may be difficult during the immediate postoperative time period when the darkening is at its peak; however, opaque cosmetic foundations may be of some value to those patients concerned with their postoperative appearance.

Postinflammatory hyperpigmentation may be seen over the malar areas of the cheeks and extremities in some patients. Hypopigmentation can occur temporarily, more commonly being evident on the neck and extremities.

Treatment of Hemangiomas

The pulsed-dye laser has been effective in the treatment of superficial hemangiomas during their proliferative and involutional phases (see Table 21–1). In view of its limited depth of vascular injury (1.2 mm), the pulsed-dye laser does not penetrate deeply enough to affect the deeper component of most hemangiomas. Its greatest use has been for those hemangiomas that have a superficial component or those with combined superficial and deep components. The use of this laser during the proliferative phase of growth may be helpful in limiting the superficial proliferation of the hemangioma, but proliferation of the deeper component may continue despite treatments.

Pulsed-dye laser treatment of infants and children with hemangiomas can take place in most instances without local or topical anesthesia. Larger hemangiomas may require topical, local, or general anesthesia to aid in the immobilization of the patient (Table 21–2). Repetitive treatments are required to obtain the maximum benefit. During the proliferative phase of growth, treatments at 2- to 3-week intervals are beneficial in limiting the proliferation. During the involutional phase, treatment intervals can be scheduled more widely apart (1–2 months). The postoperative appearance is limited by the dark color, which may persist for 1 to 2 weeks after treatment.

TABLE 21–1. Pulsed-Dye Laser Treatment:
Indications, Contraindications, Limitations

Indications	Contraindications	Limitations
Port-wine stains	Thrombocytopenia Type VI phototype skin	Postoperative darkening Complete clearing may not be obtained Hypertrophic port-wine stains may not respond.

Hemangiomas
  Superficial (proliferative and involutional
    phases)
  Superficial and deep (proliferative and
    involutional phases)
	Thrombocytopenia	Complete resolution may not be obtained.
		Deep or cavernous hemangiomas do not respond.
		Depigmentation may be found at the treated site.

Telangiectases
  Spider telangiectases
  Linear telangiectases
  Poikiloderma of Civatte
  Red noses
	Thrombocytopenia
	Anticoagulation
		Larger-diameter vessels (more than 100 μm) do not
		  generally respond to this treatment.
		Telangiectases and superficial varicosities of the
		  lower extremities usually do not respond, with
		  the exception of telangiectatic mats and very
		  small diameter vessels, seen on the thighs and
		  ankles.

Postoperative wound care is not usually required. If crusting occurs, topical antibacterial ointment can be used (Table 21–3).

Treatment of Telangiectases

The pulsed-dye laser may be safely and effectively used for treatment of small- and medium-diameter vessels (up to 100 μm in diameter) (see Table 21–1). It is ideally suited for spider telangiectases in children and adults and for diffuse small-diameter vessels that are commonly found on the cheeks and nose (Case 2, Fig. 21–2; Case 3, Fig. 21–3). This treatment results in post-treatment discoloration similar to purpura, which may be unsettling to some patients. Treatment responses are usually seen within one to two sessions. The degree of darkening depends on the size of the laser beam spot used during the procedure. Smaller-diameter spot sizes of 2 to 3 mm allow for a 5- to 7-day period of postoperative discoloration, while the larger-diameter spot sizes of 5 to 7 mm will leave discoloration present for a longer period of time (7–14 days). Makeup may be worn after these procedures, but cosmetic camouflage can be difficult for the first few postoperative days.

The advantages of this laser treatment are the absence of scarring and pigmentary alteration. Postinflammatory hyperpigmentation may be seen over the malar areas and distal extremities, while hypopigmentation may be seen more commonly over the neck and extremities.

CONTINUOUS-WAVE LASER THERAPY

Treatment of Port-Wine Stains

Continuous-wave lasers can be used in the treatment of port-wine stains, particularly when the vessels involved are hypertrophic or of large diameter (Table 21–4). Continuous-wave lasers include the argon, continuous-wave dye, copper vapor, krypton, KTP, and neodymium : yttrium-

TABLE 21–2. Pulsed-Dye Laser Treatment:
Operative Issues

Preoperative Evaluation
History of bleeding diatheses
Use of anticoagulation

Preoperative Equipment Needs
Calibrated and maintained pulsed-dye laser
Local or topical anesthesia

Intraoperative Needs
Protective eyewear
Metal ocular shields should be used when the eyelids are
  being treated
Wavelength-specific eye protection for patients and staff

TABLE 21–3. Pulsed-Dye Laser Treatment:
Postoperative Care

Pain Management
Topical application of hydrogel dressings (Spenco Second Skin
  or Vigilon)
Ice may be used for topical alleviation of discomfort.
Acetaminophen or acetaminophen with codeine may be re-
  quired for treatment of larger areas.

Dressings
Dressings are generally not required
Vigilon will provide symptomatic relief.
If crusting occurs, antibacterial ointment will be beneficial

Complications
Atrophic scarring is rare but most commonly found in young
  infants and children.
Crusting is treated with the use of topical antibacterial ointments.
Hyperpigmentation or hypopigmentation usually resolves
  spontaneously.

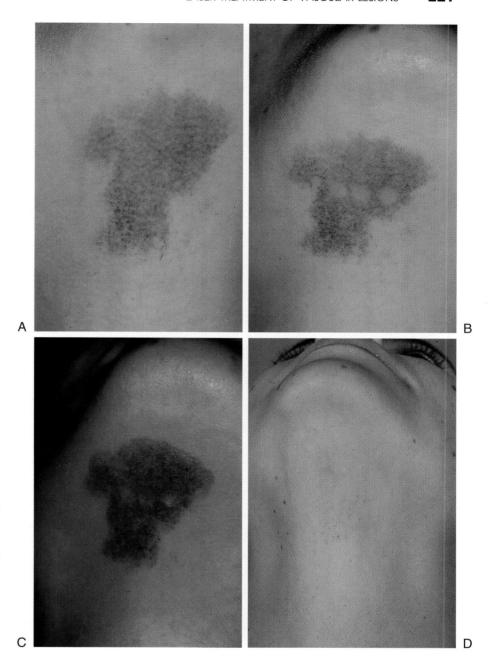

CASE 1

FIGURE 21–1. *A*, Port-wine stain on the neck of a 25-year-old woman. *B*, Clearing and absence of textural change noted at all three test sites 1 month after test treatment. The energies utilized were as follows: 6.75 J/cm^2—left; 7.0 J/cm^2—middle; 7.25 J/cm^2—right. *C*, Pulsed-dye laser treatment of entire area at 7 J/cm^2. Note purpuric darkening of entire treated area with surrounding erythema. *D*, Clearing after six treatment sessions. (From Dover JS, Arndt KA, Geronemus RG, et al. Illustrated Cutaneous Laser Surgery: A Practitioner's Guide. Norwalk, CT: Appleton & Lange, 1990:111, 112.)

aluminum-garnet (Nd:YAG) lasers. These lasers emit light continuously and can be shuttered to minimize the exposure time to the skin surface. Light emitted from these continuous-wave light sources can also be delivered through a robotized scanning device, which further minimizes the thermal damage to the vascular tissue.

The freehand technique of the use of the continuous-wave light sources allows for the tracing of individual vessels through magnification or standard use. Immediate blanching of the vessel is seen, and slight crusting can occur. This crusting should last 5 to 7 days. A gradual lightening of the treated area will take place for 3 to 4 months after the treatment session. The risks of this procedure include hypertrophic or atrophic scarring, permanent depigmentation, and transient hyperpigmentation.

Treatment of Hemangiomas

Continuous-wave lasers have also been used in the treatment of superficial and deep hemangiomas. Although good results have been noted on occasion, the risk of scarring and permanent pigmentary alteration does exist. All of the continuous-wave lasers, except the Nd:YAG, are limited to the treatment of superficial hemangiomas. With its greater depth of nonspecific tissue injury, the Nd:YAG

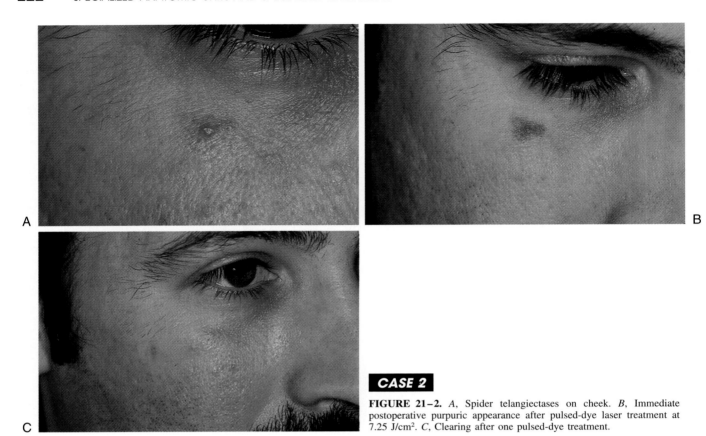

CASE 2

FIGURE 21–2. *A*, Spider telangiectases on cheek. *B*, Immediate postoperative purpuric appearance after pulsed-dye laser treatment at 7.25 J/cm². *C*, Clearing after one pulsed-dye treatment.

TABLE 21–4. Continuous-Wave Laser Treatment:
Indications, Contraindications, Limitations

Indications	Contraindications	Limitations
Port-wine stains 　Hypertrophic port-wine stains 　Port-wine stains of the face in adults with the exception of the upper lip and mandible 　Port-wine stains in children and flatter port-wine stains when robotized scanning devices are used in conjunction with the continuous-wave light sources	Children (except when robotized scanning devices are used) Impaired wound healing Type VI skin phototype	Complete clearing may not be obtained. Hypertrophic, atrophic scarring, and depigmentation may be seen. Telangiectases and superficial varicosities of lower extremities usually do not respond, with the exception of telangiectatic mats and very small diameter vessels, seen on the thighs and ankles.
Hemangiomas 　Superficial hemangiomas (lasers with and without robotized scanning devices) 　Deep hemangiomas (Nd:YAG laser)	Anatomic areas prone toward hypertrophic scarring	Scarring and pigmentary loss may be seen. Most continuous-wave light sources will not treat the deeper or more cavernous components of a hemangioma.
Telangiectases 　Large-diameter vessels of the head and neck 　Spider telangiectases 　Smaller-diameter vessels and spider telangiectases in children when robotized scanning devices are used	History of impaired wound healing Type VI skin phototype	Hypertrophic and atrophic scarring may occur, as well as permanent depigmentation. Smaller-diameter vessels cannot be treated unless the robotized scanning devices are utilized. Telangiectases and superficial varicosities of the lower extremities usually do not respond, with the exception of telangiectatic mats and very small diameter vessels, seen on the thighs and ankles.

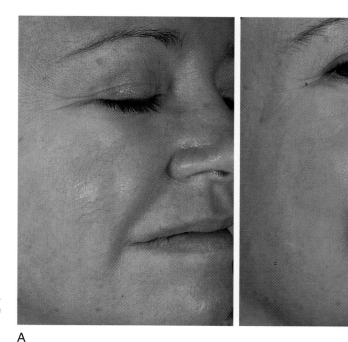

CASE 3

FIGURE 21–3. *A*, Facial telangiectasia. *B*, Clearing after treatment with the continuous-wave dye laser (577 nm) at 0.1 mm spot, 0.8 watt.

A

B

laser has been used to treat deeper vascular lesions, but scarring can occur.

The procedure requires local anesthesia (Table 21–5). Postoperative crusting occurs, and healing takes place within 1 to 2 weeks. Additional treatment sessions may be necessary to obtain the maximum benefit.

Treatment of Telangiectases

Continuous-wave lasers have been used in the treatment of a variety of telangiectases. They are most efficacious in large-diameter telangiectases by individual tracing of the vessel. The use of robotized scanning devices with the continuous-wave lasers minimizes the risk of scarring in the treatment of spider telangiectases in children as well as smaller-diameter telangiectases in adults. After treatment, immediate blanching or whitening of the vessel occurs, followed by a slight degree of crusting for 5 to 7 days. Postoperative antibacterial ointment is required to facilitate healing (Table 21–6).

Patients may prefer this form of continuous-wave laser treatment over the pulsed-dye laser treatment of telangiectasia because there is no postoperative purpura. Since the

TABLE 21–5. Continuous-Wave Laser Treatment: Operative Issues

Preoperative Evaluation
History: Bleeding diathesis
Preoperative Equipment Needs
Calibrated and maintained laser
Topical antibacterial ointment
Local anesthesia, topical anesthesia
Intraoperative Needs
Appropriate eye protection for patients and staff, including the use of ocular shields when treating the eyelids

area treated is usually smaller than the area treated for a hemangioma, the risk of atrophy or permanent depigmentation is easily tolerated because there is less immediate postoperative change in the appearance. A comparison of safety and efficacy of facial telangiectases with laser treatment versus electrocautery has not yet been done, but it is my impression that the appropriate use of laser treatment offers an improved therapeutic outcome with fewer potential side effects.

TABLE 21–6. Continuous-Wave Laser Treatment: Postoperative Care

Pain Management	Dressings	Complications
Topical hydrogel dressings Ice Acetaminophen with codeine for discomfort	Topical antibacterial ointment until healing has occurred. Larger areas should be covered with semiocclusive dressing.	Hypertrophic and atrophic scarring may be seen, as well as permanent depigmentation; transient hyperpigmentation may also be noted.

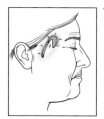

chapter 22

Continuous-Wave Lasers

SUZANNE OLBRICHT

THE CO$_2$ LASER USED FOR ABLATION

The continuous-wave CO$_2$ laser can be used for ablation of common cutaneous tumors that are above the surrounding surface of the skin. The laser energy produces vaporization of tissue by heating intracellular and extracellular water quickly to above the boiling point of water, releasing a plume of tissue fragments and steam (Case 1, Fig. 22–1). The wound is shallow because the energy is absorbed very superficially. The base of the wound contains coagulated tissue. The CO$_2$ laser produces hemostasis as it ablates. The volume of tissue vaporized varies directly with power density at the tissue level. The width of the zone of thermal damage of adjacent tissue, however, varies directly in relationship to duration of exposure. Short laser exposures with a high-power density vaporize the same volume of tissue as longer exposures at a lower-power density but with much less adjacent thermal damage. By moving quickly and increasing the power density and completing a number of passes over the tissue, the surgeon can create a defect of any size and depth, thus making the CO$_2$ laser a very sensitive tool. Modifications, such as the use of the Superpulse or Ultrapulse CO$_2$ lasers, further limit lateral tissue damage (Tables 22–1 through 22–5).

CO$_2$ LASER USED FOR EXCISION

The continuous-wave CO$_2$ laser can also be used for excision, in a manner similar to a cold steel knife. The handpiece contains a mirror that focuses the beam. If the beam is used at its focal point on the skin surface, the spot size at the skin surface is very small (generally 0.2 mm in diameter) and the power density is very great, creating a narrow incision as the beam is drawn along the skin surface (Fig. 22–2). The lateral damage is minimal, such that the specimen is adequate for histologic review, but great enough to allow hemostasis in the wound as cutting proceeds. Vessels smaller than 0.5 mm in diameter are sealed during the incision, and larger vessels can be grasped with a forceps and easily welded shut. If this fails to control bleeding, then suture ligation may be used (see Table 22–3 and Tables 22–6 through 22–9).

ARGON LASER

The argon laser emits a continuous-wave beam of light at six different wavelengths from 457.9 to 514.5 mn in the blue-green portion of the visible spectrum. In most argon laser systems for clinical use, two options are available: either all six wavelengths are delivered as blue-green light or a filter can be introduced that permits only green (514 nm) light to be delivered. The argon light is delivered to the tissue through a fiberoptic cable that is connected to a variety of terminal handpieces. The beam is a continuous wave, but it may be mechanically shuttered to produce brief "pulses" of energy.

Argon laser energy is absorbed by two chromophores in the skin: melanin and hemoglobin. In a lightly pigmented individual, the light may penetrate up to 1 mm into the tissues (Case 2, Fig. 22–3). In darkly pigmented skin, the energy may be absorbed almost completely in the pigment. Absorption produces heat that damages the target structure. Because the duration of exposure in this system cannot be as short as the pulsed or Q-switched lasers, this heat also spreads beyond the target structure to the adjacent tissue (Tables 22–10 through 22–14).

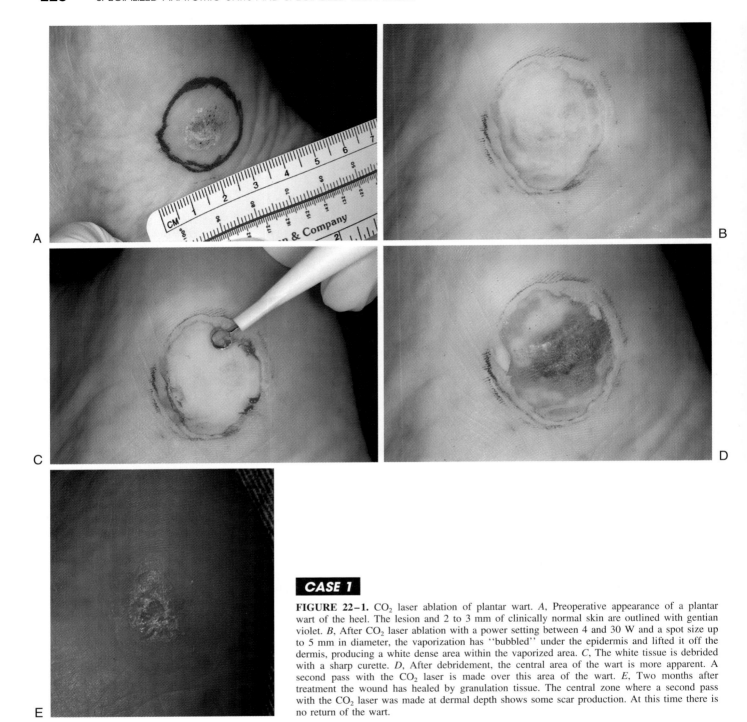

CASE 1

FIGURE 22–1. CO_2 laser ablation of plantar wart. *A,* Preoperative appearance of a plantar wart of the heel. The lesion and 2 to 3 mm of clinically normal skin are outlined with gentian violet. *B,* After CO_2 laser ablation with a power setting between 4 and 30 W and a spot size up to 5 mm in diameter, the vaporization has "bubbled" under the epidermis and lifted it off the dermis, producing a white dense area within the vaporized area. *C,* The white tissue is debrided with a sharp curette. *D,* After debridement, the central area of the wart is more apparent. A second pass with the CO_2 laser is made over this area of the wart. *E,* Two months after treatment the wound has healed by granulation tissue. The central zone where a second pass with the CO_2 laser was made at dermal depth shows some scar production. At this time there is no return of the wart.

CONTINUOUS-WAVE DYE LASER

Continuous-wave dye lasers in clinical practice for dermatology most often emit energy in the 573 to 640 nm range and are usually tuned to wavelengths of 577 or 585 nm for the treatment of vascular lesions. These wavelengths are produced by the organic fluorescent compounds dissolved in solvents such as alcohol or water. Narrow spectra are created by prisms and filters. Continuous-wave dye energy is delivered to the tissue through a fiberoptic cable. The beam is a continuous wave, but it can be mechanically shuttered to produce brief impulses of energy. Scanning devices have been attached as terminal delivery systems that deliver these impulses in a computerized random pattern to simulate the pulsed-dye laser; however, these shuttered impulses do not have a high peak energy and are delivered for longer durations and thus do not have the same tissue or therapeutic effect.

TABLE 22-1. CO_2 Laser Used for Ablation: Indications, Contraindications, Limitations

Indications

Epidermal or Mucosal Disorders

Actinic cheilitis
Erythroplasia of Queyrat
Oral florid papillomatosis
Sublingual keratosis
Bowenoid papulosis
Balanitis xerotica obliterans
Bowen's disease or squamous cell carcinoma in situ
Superficial basal cell carcinoma
Epidermal nevus
Nail ablation
Lichen sclerosus et atrophicus
Zoon's balanitis
Hailey-Hailey disease
Darier's disease
Porokeratosis

Warts

Verruca vulgaris
Verruca plantaris
Periungual warts
Widespread condylomata acuminata
Recalcitrant warts

Dermal Processes

Syringomas
Granuloma faciale
Trichoepitheliomas
Neurofibromas
Xanthelasma
Adenoma sebaceum
Myxoid cysts
Apocrine hidrocystoma
Angiolymphoid hyperplasia
Pearly penile papules
Cowden's disease
Chrondrodermatitis nodularis helicis
Debridement of granulation tissue
Cutaneous infections (e.g., botryomycosis, leishmaniasis)

Vascular Lesions

Lymphangioma circumscriptum
Pyogenic granulomas
Angiokeratomas

Miscellaneous

Red tattoo reactions
Cutaneous resurfacing
De-epithelialization before reconstructive surgical procedure
Aging hands
Sterilization of infected wounds

Contraindications

Keloid formation
Sites where second intention healing is not appropriate
Process for which there is no definitive clinical or pathologic diagnosis

Limitations

Large tumor size may preclude use of this modality because of poor wound healing and scarring
Ablation does not yield a specimen for pathologic examination

TABLE 22-2. CO_2 Laser Used for Ablation: Patient Preoperative Discussion

1. Procedure requires local or regional anesthesia.
2. Postoperative pain is usually minimal but may require use of oral medication.
3. The wound may require 2 to 6 weeks to heal depending on its size and site.
4. Daily wound care is required until complete healing has ensued.
5. If the wound is on the lower extremity, the leg should be elevated while resting.
6. Depending on the site, scarring may be minimal, atrophic, or sometimes hypertrophic. If the site is around the nail, a distorted nail may result.
7. Treated process may recur.

TABLE 22-3. CO_2 Laser for Ablation and Excision: Operative Issues

Preoperative Evaluation

History:
    Hepatitis, human immunodeficiency virus infection, immuno-suppression
Examine other scars for healing

Preoperative Equipment Needs

CO_2 laser with power output of 15 to 30 W for ablation; 25-40 W for excision
Smoke evacuation system
Barrier protection
Laser safety masks
Clear or plastic goggles
Gloves
Local anesthesia
Wound care materials

Intraoperative Needs

Sterile water or saline in a basin
Gauze sponges
Sterile instruments—tissue scissors, curette for ablation
For excisional use of CO_2 laser—a standard surgical tray of sterile instruments and closure materials

TABLE 22-4. CO_2 Laser Used for Ablation: Technique

1. Surgical plan: determine desired endpoint.
2. Preparation of site: lesion and necessary margins may be outlined with surgical marking pen and cleaned with normal saline.
3. Anesthesia: local, regional, or general.
4. Draping: wet sponges for prevention of inadvertent burns.
5. Power output setting: 4 to 30 W depending on lesion and site.
6. Waveform: continuous-wave, shuttered beam, or super-pulsed beam.
7. Spot size at the tissue surface: 0.5- to 5-mm diameter defocused beam, depending on distance of handpiece from tissue surface.
8. Vaporization with beam defocused:
    a. Continuous-wave beam or pulsed beam used with air brush–like movements.
    b. Shuttered beam directed to single site.
9. Debridement: wipe with wet sponge (saline, sterile water, hydrogen peroxide) to clean off tissue fragments, char, or coagulum.
10. Repeat treatment: vaporization and debridement repeated as necessary to achieve desired depth of tissue removal.
11. Surgical dressing: appropriate for size and site of wound.
12. Postoperative instructions for wound care: appropriate for size and site of wound.

Energy at 577 and 585 nm penetrates into the dermis in fair-skinned individuals and is absorbed by oxyhemoglobin. As with the argon laser, the energy may be absorbed almost completely in pigmented skin. Absorption produces heat that damages the target structure. Also similar to the argon laser, the duration of exposure in this system cannot

TABLE 22-5. CO$_2$ Laser Used for Ablation: Postoperative Care

Pain Management

Acetaminophen (Tylenol)
Elevation of extremity
Narcotics are not generally required.

Wound Care

Daily cleansing with mild soap and water or diluted hydrogen peroxide
Apply bacitracin or Neosporin ointment and cover with Telfa pad secured by tape or Band-Aid or use semipermeable occlusive dressing.
Continue wound care until tissue has completely reepithelialized.

Complications

Hypertrophic scarring or keloid formation
Prolonged wound healing
Bleeding
Infection
Excessive growth of granulation tissue
Recurrence

TABLE 22-6. CO$_2$ Laser Used for Excision: Indications, Contraindications, Limitations

Indications

Patients:
With bleeding disorders or taking anticoagulants in whom epinephrine is contraindicated
With pacemakers or other electronic monitoring devices that limit the use of electrosurgery
For whom blood loss may be life threatening
Sites:
Vascular lesions
Vascular tissues
Infected sites

Contraindications

Similar to standard cold steel surgery

Limitations

Wound healing begins somewhat slower in laser wounds than scalpel cut wounds, so that sutures may need to be left in place longer.
Use of articulated arm system and hand piece feels awkward at first.
Undermining may be more easily accomplished with a mirror attachment that angles the beam.
Low-power output lasers may not allow use of a power density great enough to move quickly and make an incision with minimal lateral damage.

TABLE 22-7. CO$_2$ Laser Used for Excision: Patient Preoperative Discussion

1. Procedure requires local, regional, or general anesthesia.
2. Postoperative pain is usually minimal.
3. The wound may require somewhat longer to heal than a scalpel cut wound.
4. If second intention healing is intended, daily wound care is required until complete healing has ensued.
5. If the wound is on the lower extremity, the leg should be elevated while resting.
6. Scarring will be similar to a scalpel cut wound. Depending on the site, scarring may be minimal, atrophic, or sometimes hypertrophic.

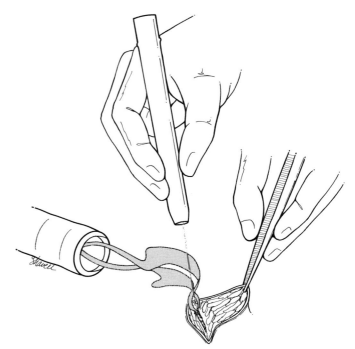

FIGURE 22-2. When the CO$_2$ laser is used as an excisional tool, the beam (red) is focused with a power setting between 25 and 40 W and a spot size of 0.2 mm. This power density creates a narrow incision as the beam moves along the skin. Hemostasis of vessels smaller than 0.5 mm is achieved as the laser beam creates the incision. The surface skin is lifted back with a forceps to allow the base of the wound to be seen and the laser beam to access deeper tissues. The smoke evacuator (tube) is placed very close to the path of the beam for maximum removal of vaporized particles and smoke. The wound will be sutured closed after excision of the specimen with the CO$_2$ laser.

TABLE 22-8. CO$_2$ Laser Used for Excision: Technique

1. Surgical plan: determine extent of desired incision/excision.
2. Preparation of site: clean site with an antibacterial preparation and dry it. Margins may be marked with a surgical marking pen.
3. Anesthesia: local, regional, or general.
4. Draping: sterile cloths and wet sponges close to the wound edges.
5. Power output setting: 25 to 40 W.
6. Waveform: continuous-wave or Superpulsed or Ultrapulsed beam.
7. Spot size at the tissue surface: use the beam at the focal point, generally yielding a spot size of 0.2 mm in diameter. Most handpieces have focal length guides to mark the distance from the handpiece to the skin surface at the focal point.
8. Incision: draw the beam across the skin surface to cut, moving quickly to produce little lateral tissue damage. No char should be appreciable.
9. Debridement: wipe with wet sponge to clean off tissue fragments or coagulum. Dry with gauze sponge.
10. Repeat treatment: apply a little traction and repeat as needed to complete incision.
11. Excision: the base of a wedge excision is separated similarly. Undermining can also be accomplished.
12. Repair: use standard techniques if wound is to be closed primarily.
13. Surgical dressing: layered dressing consisting of bacitracin, Telfa, and protective padding of gauze, secured by tape or rolled gauze.

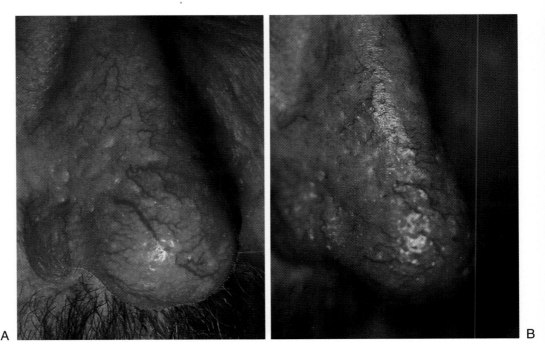

CASE 2

FIGURE 22–3. Argon laser surgery for telangiectasia. *A,* Preoperative appearance of telangiectasia of the nasal tip. The size of these vessels, which are greater than 0.5 mm in diameter, makes the argon laser particularly useful. *B,* Six weeks after treatment with the argon laser some vessels are cleared but others are only partially cleared. Another treatment with the argon laser will be performed. There is no scarring from the prior treatment.

be as short as the pulsed or Q-switched lasers so that heat spreads beyond the target structure to the adjacent tissue.

Treatment indications, technique, and results are equivalent to the use of the argon laser. Of great importance is the use of safety goggles designed especially for these wavelengths. They are not the same as the ones used for the argon laser.

COPPER VAPOR LASER

The copper vapor laser was first introduced in industry but is useful as a medical laser because it emits light at 578.2 nm (yellow light) and 511 nm (green light). Light is produced by the interaction of electrons from a gas dis-

charge with atoms of copper vaporized by a high-voltage pulsed electronic circuit. Both wavelengths are produced at one time and may be transmitted through a fiberoptic cable together or singly with the use of a filter. The copper vapor laser is a pulsed laser that emits a train of very short

TABLE 22–9. CO₂ Laser Used for Excision: Postoperative Care

Pain Management
Tylenol
Elevation
Narcotics are not generally required.

Wound Care
Standard surgical dressing applied to closed wounds for stability and protection
For secondary intention wounds, daily cleansing with mild soap and water or diluted hydrogen peroxide, followed by application of bacitracin ointment or Polysporin and a Band-Aid or Telfa dressing

Complications
Hypertrophic scarring or keloid formation
Prolonged wound healing
Bleeding
Infection

TABLE 22–10. Argon Laser Surgery: Indications, Contraindications, Limitations

Indications
Port-wine stains of the face:
  Thick
  Dark red to purple
  Mature
Telangiectasia of the face, particularly lesions that are greater than 0.5 mm in diameter
Spider angiomas
Telangiectatic mats
Cherry angiomas
Venous lakes
Red adenoma sebaceum

Contraindications
Patients younger than 17 years old
Lesions of the upper lip and neck

Limitations
Argon laser treatment generally lightens dark red and purple port-wine stains and reduces abnormally thickened areas but does not produce completely normal skin.
Multiple treatment sessions may be required.
Telangiectases may require more than one treatment due to either partial clearing or recurrence.
Faint red or flat vascular lesions, vascular lesions with telangiectasias 0.1 to 0.5 mm in diameter are currently best treated with pulsed vascular lasers.
Treatment of pigmented lesions with this laser may produce excessive heat and unnecessary tissue damage. Better laser systems also exist for their treatment.

TABLE 22–11. Argon Laser: Patient Preoperative Discussion

1. Treatment of small areas causes a burning sensation that is usually tolerable without anesthesia. Larger areas may require pretreatment with EMLA cream or injection of local anesthesia.
2. Non–sun-tanned skin improves with treatment better than sun-tanned skin. Treated sites may not suntan well after treatment.
3. A test site is done first and then evaluated 4 months later.
4. The treated site will be dusky in color and edematous for several days. A thin crust will then form that sloughs in 7 to 10 days.
5. Improvement may not be appreciated for several months but may continue for up to 1 year.
6. Repeat treatment with this laser or other laser systems may be required for optimal improvement.
7. Scarring can result.
8. The test area is sometimes not representative of what occurs with treatment of the rest of the lesion.

pulses with a duration of 20 ns, an interval between pulses of 67 to 125 μs, and 10,000 to 15,000 pulses per second. A single pulse does not have enough energy to coagulate a blood vessel, and the train of pulses produces tissue effects equivalent to the argon and continuous-wave dye lasers. The spot diameter of the beam varies from 100 to 800 μm.

Energy at 578 nm coincides with a peak in the absorption spectrum of oxyhemoglobin and is relatively well absorbed by hemoglobin and poorly absorbed by melanin. The energy of 511 nm is better absorbed by pigment. However, in neither case is there selective photothermolysis such as that which occurs with the flash lamp pulsed-dye laser or Q-switched lasers.

Treatment indications, technique, and results are equivalent to the use of the argon laser. Energies less than 15 J/cm^2 are used to limit adjacent thermal destruction. Again, the safety goggles used must be designed especially for these wavelengths and are not the same as the ones used for the argon laser.

TABLE 22–12. Argon Laser: Operative Issues

Preoperative Evaluation

History of recent sun tan or prolonged sun exposure may require delaying the procedure.

Preoperative Equipment Needs

Argon laser with dermatologic handpieces
Orange colored, argon-light absorbing, polycarbonate safety goggles
Anesthesia
Plastic eyeshield and ophthalmic topical anesthetics and ointments if treating eyelids

Intraoperative Needs

Sterile water or saline in a basin
Gauze sponges
Wound care materials

TABLE 22–13. Argon Laser: Technique

Test Area for Treatment of Port-Wine Stains

1. Choose an inconspicuous area that is representative of the entire lesion, and draw a circle 1 to 2 cm in diameter with a blue or green felt-tipped pen. Consider treating two test areas, one with full spectrum of argon energy and one with green light only.
2. Administer anesthesia.
3. Set the laser beam spot size to 1 mm in diameter and use 0.8-W power output.
4. Hold the handpiece perpendicular to the skin's surface at the distance that produces a 1-mm spot. For most handpieces, this is about 2 cm from the skin surface.
5. Move the laser beam across the test area either with continuous back-and-forth horizontal or vertical passes or with enlarging concentric rings. The handpiece should be moved just slowly enough to produce a slight opalescent color.
6. Avoid overlapping treatments.
7. Apply bacitracin or Polysporin ointment.
8. Evaluate results at 4 months.

Treatment of Large Areas of Port-Wine Stains

1. Evaluate treated test site for improvement and textural changes. Discuss if further treatment is warranted. If more than one test area has been treated, use the parameters that yielded the best early result for continued therapy.
2. Decide the extent of the treatment to be done at this session. Areas as large as 5×5 cm can be treated at one time. It is advisable to treat different cosmetic units at different sessions.
3. Administer anesthesia.
4. Use same laser parameters as used in test area: generally a 1-mm spot size and 0.8-W power output.
5. Move the handpiece just slowly enough to produce the opalescent discoloration. It may be moved in a continuous back-and-forth horizontal or vertical motion or in concentric circles. Do not overlap treatment sites. The beam can be shuttered into ``pulses,'' but this technique requires more time, is tedious, and does not improve the results.
6. Nodules may be treated with somewhat higher power outputs, such as 1.0 to 1.2 W.
7. Apply an ice pack or cool wet cloth if patient complains of burning.
8. Apply bacitracin or Polysporin ointment.
9. Reevaluate for further treatment of other sites in 6 weeks when healing is complete, but re-treatment of the same site should be deferred for 1 year.

Treatment of Telangiectasias

1. Determine which vessels are to be treated. Vessels greater than 0.5 mm in diameter may respond better to this technique than to other laser systems (see Fig. 22–3).
2. Anesthesia is not usually required.
3. Choose a laser spot size equal to or slightly larger than the diameter of the vessel. Telescoping handpieces are generally available for most laser models.
4. Set the power output from 0.4 to 0.8 W.
5. Hold the handpiece perpendicular to the surface of the skin and trace the vessel. If the vessel does not seal and shrink, increase the power as needed.
6. Reactive erythema may occur, obscuring vessels to be treated in adjacent locations.
7. Apply an ice pack or cool wet cloth if patient complains of burning.
8. Apply bacitracin or Polysporin ointment.
9. Reevaluate for further treatment in 6 weeks.

TABLE 22-14. Argon Laser: Postoperative Care

Pain Management

Acetaminophen (Tylenol)
Narcotics are not generally required.

Wound Care

Wash treated area twice a day with mild soap and water, avoiding friction.
Apply bacitracin or Polysporin ointment immediately after cleansing.
Bandaids or Telfa dressing may be used depending on the site and size of the area treated. Semipermeable dressings that do not contain an adhesive may also be used.
Continue wound care until reepithelialization is complete.

Complications

Pigmentary changes
Atrophic scarring
Hypertrophic scarring or keloid formation, incidence increased in patients younger than 17 and in those with lesions of the upper lip and neck
Bleeding
Infection
Pyogenic granulomas

Selected Readings

1. Arndt KA. Argon laser therapy of small cutaneous vascular lesions. Arch Dermatol 1982;118:220–224.
2. Dinehart SM, Waner M, Flock S. The copper vapor laser for treatment of cutaneous vascular and pigmented lesions. J Dermatol Surg Oncol 1993;19:370–375.
3. Dover JS, Arndt KA, Geronemus RG, et al. Illustrated Cutaneous Laser Surgery, a Practitioner's Guide. Norwalk, CT: Appleton & Lange, 1990.
4. Ferenczy A, Bergeron C, Richart RM. Carbon dioxide laser energy disperses human papillomavirus deoxyribonucleic acid onto treatment fields. Am J Obstet Gynecol 1990;163:1271–1274.
5. Fitzpatrick RE, Goldman MP. CO_2 laser surgery. In: Goldman MP, Fitzpatrick RE. Cutaneous Laser Surgery: The Art and Science of Selective Photothermolysis. St. Louis: CV Mosby, 1994:198–258.
6. Lanigan SW, Carwright P, Cotterill JA. Continuous wave dye laser therapy of port-wine stains. Br J Dermatol 1989;121:343–352.
7. McBurney EI. Clinical usefulness of the argon laser for the 1990s. J Dermatol Surg Oncol 1993;19:358–362.
8. McDaniel DH. Clinical usefulness of the Hexascan: Treatment of cutaneous vascular and melanocytic disorders. J Dermatol Surg Oncol 1993;19:312–319.
9. Noe JM, Barsky SH, Geer DE. Port-wine stains and the response to argon laser therapy: Successful treatment and the predictive role of color, age and biopsy. Plast Reconstr Surg 1980;65:130.
10. Olbricht SM, Stern RS, Tang SV, et al. Complications of cutaneous laser surgery: A survey. Arch Dermatol 1987;123:345–349.
11. Reid R. Physical and surgical principles governing carbon dioxide laser surgery on the skin. Dermatol Clin 1991;9:297–304.
12. Ross M, Watcher MA, Goodman MM. Comparison of the flashlamp pulsed-dye laser with the argon tunable dye laser with robotized handpiece for facial telangiectasia. Lasers Surg Med 1993;13:374–397.
13. Waner M, Dinehart SM. A comparison of the copper vapor and flashlamp pulsed-dye lasers in the treatment of facial telangiectasia. J Dermatol Surg Oncol 1993;19:992–998.
14. Wheeland RG. Treatment of port-wine stains for the 1990s. J Dermatol Surg Oncol 1993;19:348–356.

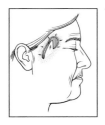

chapter 23

Laser Surgery for Pigmented Lesions

GEORGE J. HRUZA

Laser treatment of benign skin lesions can be accomplished with several different lasers. Although pigmented lesions have been treated with the argon laser for 20 years,[1] the theory of selective photothermolysis and technologic advances have led to a great increase in the number of lasers that can be used to treat pigmented lesions with minimal risk of adverse sequelae. Selective photothermolysis states that if a chromophore such as a melanosome is irradiated with a very brief laser light pulse of an appropriate wavelength, the target can be destroyed without causing collateral damage.[2] For melanosomes, the laser light pulse should be less than 1 μs long. Because melanin absorbs light from the ultraviolet through the visible and into the near infrared portions of the electromagnetic spectrum, lasers with various wavelengths can be used for the treatment of pigmented lesions.[3,4] Clinically used lasers that achieve selective photothermolysis of melanosomes include pulsed-dye (510 nm), frequency doubled Q-switched neodymium:yttrium-aluminum-garnet (Nd:YAG) (532 nm), Q-switched ruby (694 nm), Q-switched alexandrite (755 nm), and Q-switched Nd:YAG (1064 nm) lasers (Table 23–1).[5–8]

Benign epidermal pigmented lesions can be treated with almost all lasers used in dermatology. For best results, the short pulse lasers are preferred because they confine their damage to the pigmented cells while sparing the underlying dermis.[9–12] Laser irradiation results in epidermal necrosis with an intact basement membrane followed by reepithelialization from adnexal structures and the periphery.[7] Continuous wave lasers including the argon (488 and 514 nm),[1] tunable dye (500+ nm),[13] and krypton (521 and 531 nm) lasers as well as quasi–continuous wave lasers such as the copper vapor bromide (511 nm)[14] and KTP (532 nm) lasers can also be used to remove epidermal pigmented lesions. These lasers work by achieving relatively nonspecific epidermal necrosis with variable amounts of damage to the underlying dermis. Therefore, the margin of safety is somewhat narrower, requiring more exacting attention to laser parameters than with the short pulse lasers. A modification of the continuous and quasi–continuous wave lasers has been the addition of computerized scanning devices (Dermascan, Hexascan) that move the beam around a hexagonal irradiation field to achieve shorter dwell times and more even irradiation than when these lasers are used freehand.[13]

TABLE 23–1. Lasers and Laser Parameters Used for Benign Pigmented Lesion Treatment

Laser	Wavelength	Mode	Pulse Duration	Pulse Rate	Energy Fluence
Pulsed tunable dye	510 nm	Pulsed	400 ns	1 Hz	2–4 J/cm²
Frequency doubled Q-switched Nd:YAG	532 nm	Pulsed	5–10 ns	10 Hz	2–4 J/cm²
Q-switched ruby	694 nm	Pulsed	20–40 ns	1 Hz	4–10 J/cm²
Q-switched alexandrite	755 nm	Pulsed	100 ns	1–8 Hz	4–10 J/cm²
Q-switched Nd:YAG	1064 nm	Pulsed	5–10 ns	10 Hz	4–10 J/cm²
Argon	488/514 nm	Continuous	30–50 ms	Hexascan	10–14 J/cm²
Tunable dye	500+ nm	Continuous	30–50 ms	Hexascan	10–14 J/cm²
Copper vapor	511 nm	Quasi-continuous	20 ns	15,000 Hz	Not reported
			30–50 ms	Hexascan	10–14 J/cm²
KTP	532 nm	Quasi-continuous	30–50 ms	Hexascan	10–14 J/cm²
Krypton	521/531 nm	Continuous	0.2 second continuous	Continuous	Not reported

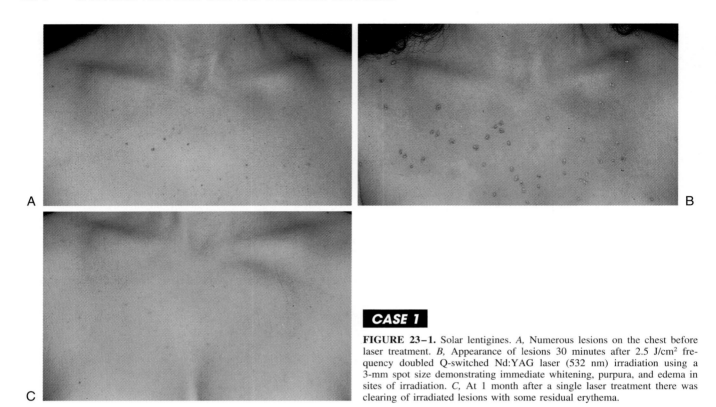

CASE 1

FIGURE 23–1. Solar lentigines. *A,* Numerous lesions on the chest before laser treatment. *B,* Appearance of lesions 30 minutes after 2.5 J/cm² frequency doubled Q-switched Nd:YAG laser (532 nm) irradiation using a 3-mm spot size demonstrating immediate whitening, purpura, and edema in sites of irradiation. *C,* At 1 month after a single laser treatment there was clearing of irradiated lesions with some residual erythema.

TABLE 23–2. Benign Pigmented Lesions Responsive to Laser Treatment

Indications	Laser(s)	Contraindications	Limitations
Epidermal Lesions	***Pulsed Lasers***	Tendency for postinflammatory hyperpigmentation	Occasional incomplete fading of lesion with need for additional treatments
Lentigines (see Cases 1 and 2, Figs. 23–1 and 23–2)	Pulsed tunable dye	History of keloid formation if chest lesions are to be treated	Recurrence of ephelides and lentigines with new ultraviolet light exposure
Ephelides	Frequency doubled Q-switched Nd:YAG		
Café-au-lait macule (see Case 3, Fig. 23–3)	Q-switched ruby		
Becker's nevus	Q-switched alexandrite		Frequent repigmentation of café-au-lait macules and Becker's nevi
Nevus spilus (lentiginous component only)	***Continuous Wave Lasers***		
	Argon		
	Tunable dye		Nevus spilus variable response
Postinflammatory hyperpigmentation (epidermal only)	Krypton		
	Quasi-continuous Wave Lasers		
	Copper vapor		
	KTP		
Dermal Lesions	***Pulsed Lasers***	Skin type V and VI epidermal hyperpigmentation may interfere with laser light penetration into dermis reducing laser effectiveness	Usual need for multiple treatments
Nevus of Ota (see Case 4, Fig. 23–4)	Q-switched ruby		Fading may take 4 to 12 months after treatment to become evident
Nevus of Ito	Q-switched alexandrite		
Mongolian spot	Q-switched Nd:YAG	Dark tan	
		Tendency for postinflammatory hyperpigmentation	

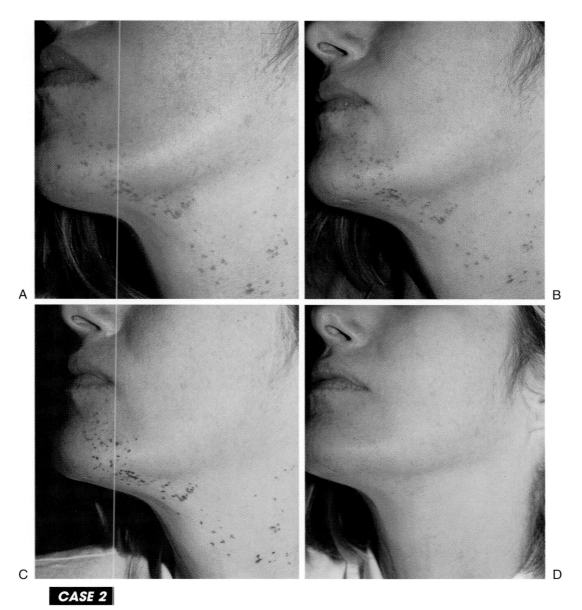

CASE 2

FIGURE 23-2. *A,* Left neck unilateral segmental lentiginosis before laser treatment. *B,* Appearance of lesions immediately after freehand 511-nm copper vapor laser irradiation shows the desired lasing endpoint of slight darkening of the lentigines. Irradiation parameters consisted of 200 mW average power, a 150-μm spot size, and 200-ms pulse duration. *C,* Four days after laser treatment fine crusts have formed in the treated sites that will separate within 10 to 14 days. *D,* Several weeks after two laser treatments there is almost total clearing of the treated lesions. (*A* to *D* courtesy of Milton Waner, M.D.)

Ephelides, lentigines (Case 1, Fig. 23-1), and unilateral segmental lentiginosis lesions (Case 2, Fig. 23-2)[14] fade with one to two laser treatments. Café-au-lait macules (Case 3, Fig. 23-3) and Becker's nevi fade with laser treatment, but there is a variable rate of reappearance of the lesions.[9] The lentiginous component of nevus spilus responds to laser treatment.[10] The response of postinflam-matory hyperpigmentation and melasma has been variable, ranging from good fading to no effect or even worsening of the hyperpigmentation observed.[9,10] The best results have been achieved in the treatment of epidermal postin-flammatory hyperpigmentation (Table 23-2).[15]

Dermal pigmented lesions such as nevus of Ota (Case 4, Fig. 23-4), nevus of Ito, and Mongolian spot can be

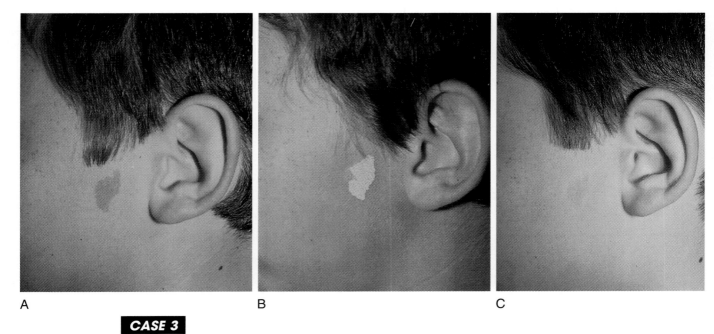

A   B   C

CASE 3

FIGURE 23–3. *A*, Café-au-lait macule of the left preauricular cheek before laser treatment. *B*, Appearance of lesion immediately after 3.5 J/cm² frequency doubled Q-switched Nd:YAG laser (532 nm) irradiation using a 2-mm spot size shows the desired immediate temporary whitening that serves as a useful endpoint of treatment. *C*, At 3 months after a single laser treatment there was significant fading of the lesion. Repigmentation in the future is a strong possibility. (*A* to *C* courtesy of Milton Waner, M.D.)

TABLE 23–3. Laser Surgery for Pigmented Lesions: Patient Preoperative Discussion

1. The laser treatment will feel like multiple pinpricks or like a rubber band snapping against the skin. For rapidly pulsing lasers (Q-switched Nd:YAG at 1064 or 532 nm, continuous wave and quasi–continuous wave lasers), the sensation may be more of heat of varying intensity.
2. A topical anesthetic cream placed under an occlusive dressing may be applied 1 to 2 hours before treatment to reduce the discomfort of laser treatment.
3. Immediately after treatment, the skin will temporarily turn white (see Fig. 23–3*B*) after treatment with the short pulse lasers or slightly gray (Fig. 23–1*B*) after treatment with the continuous wave of quasi–continuous wave lasers. This is followed a few minutes later by redness and slight swelling in the area. Stinging akin to a sunburn may be experienced for several hours after treatment. Additionally after treatment with the frequency doubled Q-switched Nd:YAG or pulsed tunable dye laser, prominent bruising in the area of treatment will develop (see Fig. 23–1*B*). To minimize this bruising, no aspirin or aspirin-containing products should be taken for at least 2 weeks before treatment. Other anti-inflammatory drugs such as ibuprofen should not be taken for at least 24 hours before treatment. Acetaminophen is an acceptable alternative if pain medication is needed.
4. Although the laser leaves the skin surface mostly intact, a fine scab usually forms. Care should be taken to prevent trauma to the treated area for the first week after treatment. Manipulation of the area should be minimized until the fine scab has separated, which usually occurs after 1 to 2 weeks. Make-up should be applied and removed very gently. The area may get wet, but drying should be very gentle so as not to disrupt the healing. There are no physical activity restrictions.
5. No dressings are usually needed. However, if the treated area significantly scabs up, a light coat of Polysporin ointment may be gently applied daily until the area has healed.
6. Sun exposure should be minimized for at least 2 weeks after treatment. If sun exposure cannot be avoided, protective clothing (e.g., hat) and high sun protective factor sunscreens should be worn. A sun tan will increase the risk of laser treatment area darkening.
7. If areas around the eye(s) have been treated, an ice pack should be placed on the laser treated site for 10 minutes each hour for 6 hours after treatment to decrease the amount of swelling.
8. After the scab has fallen off, the area may be pink for several weeks. This gradually fades back to normal skin color. Occasionally the area may develop a tan color that may take several months to completely fade (Case 5, Fig. 23–6).
9. Scarring and permanent loss of pigment in the treated area develops very rarely.
10. If the treated area becomes increasingly tender, red, swollen, or purulent, contact the surgeon's office immediately since this may represent an infection that may require treatment.
11. After 6 to 8 weeks for epidermal lesions and after 4 to 6 months for dermal lesions, the treated site should be evaluated for additional laser treatment as needed. Not all lesions will respond to the laser, and some lesions may repigment after initial fading.

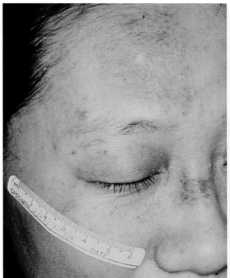 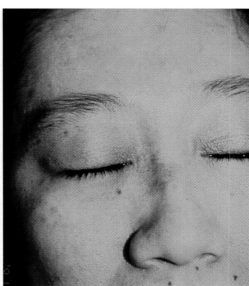

FIGURE 23–4. *A,* Nevus of Ota in the right forehead and periorbital region before laser treatment. *B,* One year after a 7.5 J/cm² Q-switched ruby laser (694 nm) treatment using a 5-mm spot size there is more than 80% fading in the irradiated areas. The nose and eyelid areas were not treated. (*A* and *B* courtesy of R. Rox Anderson, M.D.)

A   B

effectively faded with short pulse lasers through selective photothermolysis. The melanosomes within nevus cells are shattered with death of the nevus cell. The melanosome fragments are picked up by macrophages and gradually transported away through lymphatic drainage. One to several treatments are required for maximal fading, which may take as long as 12 months after the last treatment to become evident. Dermal pigmented lesions respond to treatment with the Q-switched ruby (694 nm), Q-switched Nd:YAG (1064 nm), and Q-switched alexandrite (755 nm) lasers; these wavelengths have selectivity for melanin and penetrate to a depth of 1 to 2 mm into the dermis.[16] Lasers with wavelengths shorter than 600 nm would be expected to be less effective due to the reduced depth of penetration.[2] Continuous and quasi–continuous wave lasers are not effective for the treatment of dermal pigmented lesions since thermal diffusion from the irradiated melansomes causes dermal necrosis with resultant scar formation (Tables 23–3 through 23–5).

The treatment of compound, junctional, and congenital nevi with lasers is controversial. Clearly any lesion of uncertain biologic potential must not be treated with laser without a biopsy that establishes the benign nature of the lesion. Long-term effects of laser light on potentially premalignant lesions such as congenital or dysplastic nevi are unknown. If such lesions are treated, careful long-term follow-up is advisable.

The actual treatment technique depends on the type of laser used. For pulsed lasers, the handpiece is held perpendicular to the skin surface with the spacer bar resting against the skin surface (Fig. 23–5). The lesion is irradiated with individual, slightly overlapping laser pulses. The clinical endpoint is intense whitening at the impact site, which may represent gas formation (see Fig. 23–3B). This whitening reaction resolves within 10 to 45 minutes. It protects the lesion from overtreatment since additional irradiation will be diffusely reflected from the skin surface with minimal penetration.[9,10,16]

TABLE 23–4. Laser Surgery for Pigmented Lesions: Operative Issues

Preoperative Evaluation

Allergies
Medications
Immunosuppression
Human immunodeficiency virus infection
Hepatitis infection
Coagulopathy
Syncopal history
Herpes infection in area of proposed treatment
Keloid formation
Impaired wound healing
Skin type I–VI
Postinflammatory hyperpigmentation
Previous treatments and outcomes

Preoperative Needs

Appropriate laser turned on and warmed up in standby mode
Appropriate clean laser handpiece
Laser warning signs
Extra laser safety glasses should be placed on the outside of laser room door.
Laser is tested and/or calibrated as per laser operator manual.
Make-up is removed from proposed treatment area.
Standby local anesthetic
If working on eyelids, stainless steel eyeshields are placed between conjunctiva and eyelid under topical anesthesia.
Number of persons in laser room is kept to a minimum.

Intraoperative Needs

Wavelength specific laser safety glasses or goggles are worn by the patient and all personnel in laser room.
Door is closed and laser warning signs are prominently displayed outside the door.
Foot is removed from foot pedal whenever lasing is stopped to avoid inadvertent laser pulses outside designated treatment area.
At the conclusion of treatment, laser is turned off or returned to standby mode before laser safety glasses are removed.
For dermal lesions treated with high-energy fluences, irradiation is carried out through a clear barrier dressing such as Vigilon to capture ejected debris, or, alternatively, a plastic cone attached to the laser handpiece can capture the debris.

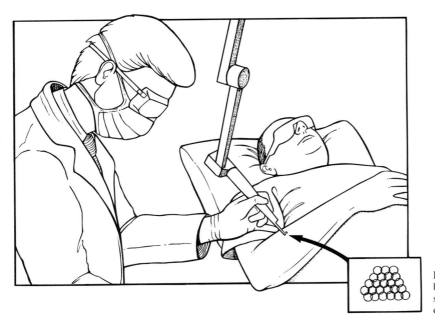

FIGURE 23–5. A short-pulse pigmented lesion laser being used with the handpiece perpendicular to the skin surface and the pulses placed to achieve complete filling of the treatment field by 10% to 20% overlap.

The continuous wave and quasi–continuous wave lasers can be used either with a freehand technique often under loupe magnification or with the aid of an automated scanning device. Freehand the lesion is traced or "painted" with the handpiece generally using an individual pulse mode (e.g., 0.2 second on and 0.2 second off). The freehand technique requires extensive experience to achieve reproducible results with minimal adverse effects. The use of an automated scanning device (e.g., Hexascan) has improved the risk–benefit ratio. The automated scanning device scans the laser beam across a hexagonal area while it is resting against the skin surface. Once a hexagon has been completed, the handpiece is moved to an adjacent area that is irradiated. This process is repeated until the entire lesion has been treated. The endpoint with both techniques is a barely perceptible darkening, graying, or opalescence of the lesion's surface (see Fig. 23–1B).[13,14,17]

Anesthesia is usually not needed but can be easily achieved with the application of EMLA cream or 40% lidocaine in acid mantle cream to the proposed treatment area under occlusion for 1 to 2 hours before treatment. Young children may have to be treated under deep sedation or even general anesthesia. As these treatments are usually done for cosmetic reasons, waiting until the child is old enough to have treatment done under local anesthesia may be preferable.

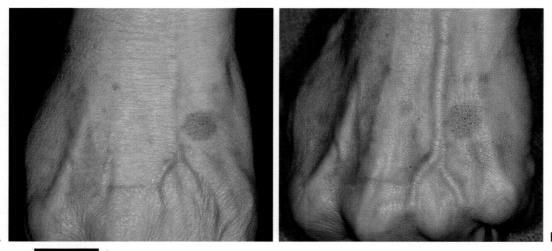

CASE 5

FIGURE 23–6. Complication. *A*, Several solar lentigines of the left dorsal hand before laser treatment. *B*, Three months after 3.6 J/cm² frequency doubled Q-switched Nd:YAG laser (532 nm) treatment using a 2-mm spot size there is significant postinflammatory hyperpigmentation aggravated by sun exposure after laser therapy. The congenital nevus was not treated.

TABLE 23-5. Laser Surgery for Pigmented Lesions: Postoperative Care

Pain Management

Acetaminophen as needed for discomfort in area of treatment

For periorbital area treatment, ice packs for 6 hours after laser irradiation

Dressings

None needed

Optional: Polysporin ointment applied daily for 1 week

Complications

Occasional postinflammatory hyperpigmentation, which is usually self-limited. It is managed with avoidance of sun exposure and, if persistent, with hydroquinones, isotretinoin, and topical corticosteroids (see Fig. 23-6).

Permanent hypopigmentation is very rare with pulsed lasers but more frequent with continuous wave and quasi-continuous wave lasers. No effective treatment is available. Prevention is by using pulsed lasers and low energy fluences for treatment.

Occasional scarring after continuous wave and quasi-continuous wave laser treatment can develop. Prevention is by using pulse lasers that have not been associated with scarring (for this indication). Also, low-energy fluences should be used for treatment. Flat atrophic scars need no management. Hypertrophic scars usually respond to daily massage of the treated area. If the scar is persistent, intralesional 10-40 mg/mL triamcinolone acetonide injections may flatten the scar.

References

1. Apfelberg DB, Maser MR, Lash H, Rivers J. The argon laser for cutaneous lesions. JAMA 1981;245:2073-2075.
2. Anderson RR, Parrish RR. Selective photothermolysis: Precise microsurgery by selective absorption of pulsed radiation. Science 1983;220:524-527.
3. Parrish JA, Anderson RR, Harrist T, et al. Selective thermal effects with pulsed irradiation from lasers: From organ to organelle. J Invest Dermatol 1983;80(Suppl):75-80.
4. Sherwood KA, Murray S, Kurban AK, Tan OT. Effect of wavelength on cutaneous pigment using pulsed irradiation. J Invest Dermatol 1989;92:717-720.
5. Margolis RJ, Dover JS, Polla LL, et al. Visible action spectrum for melanin-specific selective photothermolysis. Lasers Surg Med 1989;9:389-397.
6. Anderson RR, Margolis RJ, Watanabe S, et al. Selective photothermolysis of cutaneous pigmentation by Q-switched Nd:YAG laser pulses at 1064, 532, and 355 nm. J Invest Dermatol 1989;93:28-32.
7. Hruza GJ, Dover JS, Flotte TJ, et al. Q-switched ruby laser irradiation of normal human skin: Histologic and ultrastructural findings. Arch Dermatol 1991;127:1799-1805.
8. Kurban AK, Morrison PR, Trainor SW, Tan OT. Pulse duration effects on cutaneous pigment. Lasers Surg Med 1992;12:282-287.
9. Goldberg D. Benign pigmented lesions of the skin: Treatment with the Q-switched ruby laser. J Dermatol Surg Oncol 1993;19:376-379.
10. Grekin RC, Shelton RM, Geisse JK, Frieden I. 510-nm pigmented lesion dye laser: Its characteristics and clinical uses. J Dermatol Surg Oncol 1993;19:380-387.
11. Goldberg D. Treatment of pigmented and vascular lesions of the skin with the Q-switched Nd:YAG laser. Lasers Surg Med 1993;13(Suppl 5):55.
12. Brauner GJ, Schliftman AB. Treatment of pigmented lesions of the skin with alexandrite laser. Lasers Surg Med 1992;12(Suppl 4):72.
13. McDaniel D. Clinical usefulness of the Hexascan. J Dermatol Surg Oncol 1993;19:312-319.
14. Dinehart SM, Waner M, Flock S. The copper vapor laser for treatment of cutaneous vascular and pigmented lesions. J Dermatol Surg Oncol 1993;19:370-375.
15. Fitzpatrick R, Goldman M. Laser treatment of benign pigmented lesions using a 300 nanosecond pulse and 510 nm wavelength. J Dermatol Surg Oncol 1993;19:341-346.
16. Kasai KI, Notodihardjo HW. Analysis of 200 nevus of Ota patients who underwent Q-switched Nd:YAG laser treatment. Lasers Surg Med 1994;14(Suppl 6):50.
17. McDaniel DH, Mordon S. Hexascan: A new robotized scanning laser handpiece. Cutis 1990;45:300-305.

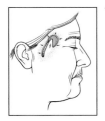

chapter 24

Keloid Surgery

A. PAUL KELLY

The first rule of keloid therapy is prevention by use of appropriate planning and technique.[1] Nonessential cosmetic surgery should not be performed in patients with a history of keloid formation; however, persons with only earlobe keloids should not be considered prone to development of keloids elsewhere.

Prevention of keloids lies in planning surgical procedures to minimize wound tension. Orienting incision lines to reduce tension by following skin creases will reduce the risk of keloid formation. Additionally, incisions should not cross joint spaces such as the knee, ankle, or shoulder and the presternal high tension area. Using meticulous surgical technique to reduce excessive tissue necrosis will also minimize the risk of keloid formation.

Physicians are often reluctant to perform keloid surgery because of the fear that the keloid may recur and grow to a size larger than the excised lesion (see Case 3, Fig. 24-3). If tissue sparing is not essential, a standard elliptical excision technique will suffice. However, when tissue sparing is preferred or when earlobe lesions have a base wider than 1 cm, excision with closure using the skin overlying the keloid as a split-thickness graft is preferred.[2,3] Since the keloid acts as a tissue expander to the overlying skin, this autograft technique is suitable for most excisions regardless of lesion configuration. Effective keloid management often combines medical, surgical, and radiologic methods (Table 24-1).[4-8]

Simple surgical excision is often combined with intralesional corticosteroids, external pressure, or silicone gel dressings. An emerging therapy is intralesional interferon gamma, 0.01 to 0.1 mg, given three times a week for 3 consecutive weeks.[9]

Silicone gel sheeting (Epi-Derm and Silastic) and silicone occlusive sheeting (SIL-K and Morelle SOS) may be used either as a nonsurgical method of treating keloids primarily or as a postoperative adjunct to prevent keloid regrowth after surgical removal. The silicone gel or occlusive sheeting seems to work best on new keloids (i.e., those less than 6 months old). It is placed over the keloid and held in place by tape. Pressure is not necessary. The silicone sheeting is left on the skin for 12 to 20 hours at a time, cleansed daily with suds from a glycerin-based soap, dried while the keloid is washed, and reapplied. Hairy areas should be avoided because the silicone occlusion often leads to folliculitis. Even if there is no reduction in keloid size, the silicone gel or sheeting usually relieves most of the symptomatology. A new piece of gel must be used every 1 to 2 weeks, whereas one piece of sheeting can be used for the duration (6-12 months) of therapy.[10-12]

External compression with elastic garments, stretchable dressings, or pressure earrings can help prevent the growth of keloids after surgical resection. Pressure is maintained for 4 to 6 months after surgery and is often combined with intralesional corticosteroid injections.[13]

Cryotherapy may also serve as a primary mode of therapy or an adjunct. When used primarily the lesion is anesthetized with topical anesthesia (EMLA) and then local 1% lidocaine. The keloid is frozen long enough for a thaw time of 30 to 45 seconds. Sometimes a second freeze-thaw cycle in 4 to 6 weeks is necessary for a better resolution of the keloid. Due to the necrotic slough, it usually takes 2 to 3 weeks for the postoperative site to heal. Following cryosurgery, injecting the base of the keloid with triamcinolone, 40 mg/mL, helps prevent keloid recurrence. The injections should be given after the slough and every 2 weeks for a series of three injections. Before treating any dark-skinned patients with liquid nitrogen, the

TABLE 24-1. Keloid Surgery: Indications, Contraindications, Limitations

Indications
Pain
Tenderness
Cosmetic concern
Cancer phobia
Contraindications
Impaired wound healing
Hemophilia
Infection of keloid, overlying or surrounding tissue
Other medical problem when surgery is contraindicated
Limitations
May recur
Postoperative intralesional corticosteroid injections and pressure or silicone sheeting is imperative

TABLE 24-3. Keloid Surgery: Operative Issues

Preoperative Evaluation
History
　Bleeding diathesis
　Human immunodeficiency virus infection, hepatitis
　Immunosuppression
　Pacemaker
　Artificial valve
　Hypertension
　Diabetes
　Allergies
Preoperative Equipment Needs
30-gauge needle
Local anesthesia
Barrier protection
Electrocautery with tip
Scissors
Surrounding area injected with triamcinolone, 10 mg/mL
Intraoperative Needs
Labeled specimen bottle
Sterile surgical tray, including sutures, needle holder, No. 15 or 15C scalpel, scalpel handle, curved Gradle scissors, and Adson forceps (1 × 2 teeth)

patient should be informed that freezing more than 25 seconds will usually result in hypopigmentation that may last 18 months or longer. Prolonged freezing destroys the melanocytes (Table 24-2).[14,15]

Cryotherapy may also be an adjunct to intralesional steroid therapy. Freezing for 10 to 15 seconds will produce edema of the tissue 5 to 10 minutes later, and this edema seems to create an epidermodermal plane, which in turn, makes intralesional injections much easier. To be most effective, the triamcinolone is injected directly into the papillary dermis of a very firm keloid. This may cause hypopigmentation, which may last 6 months or longer.

Ionizing radiation may be used in conjunction with surgical resection to reduce the risk of regrowth. Delivery is by superficial x-ray, electron beam, or interstitial implantation.[16,17] Although there are risks to using ionizing radiation for a benign process, substantial improvement may result.

SURGICAL THERAPY FOR EARLOBE KELOIDS

Surgical resection of keloids of the earlobe is unique because the contour of the lobe must be preserved.[18] If the

TABLE 24-2. Keloid Surgery: Patient Preoperative Discussion

1. Postoperative care (cleanse with alcohol three times a day followed by application of a topical antibiotic) is necessary to prevent infection.
2. Healing should take 2 weeks.
3. No dressing is necessary on earlobe lesions after 24 hours.
4. Contact sports and swimming should be avoided until 1 week after suture removal.
5. Other physical activity is unlimited unless the anatomic area of the excision will be compromised.
6. You must come for your postoperative injections every 2 or 3 weeks to help prevent keloid regrowth.
7. The lesion may recur, especially on presternal and shoulder areas.

keloid is small enough (generally having a base of less than 1 cm and not located near to the helical or lobule rim), it can be excised and heal by second intention. When the contour of the lobe would be distorted by second intention healing, then excision with closure is performed (Case 1, Fig. 24-1).

In other instances, preservation of contour is best achieved by using the skin overlying the keloid as an autograft (Case 2, Fig. 24-2).

When preparing to do earlobe keloid surgery (Cases 1 and 2; Figs. 24-1 and 24-2; Table 24-3) triamcinolone, 40 mg/mL, is injected into the base of the keloid every 2 to 3 weeks for at least two times before performing surgery. This helps prevent recurrence. At the time of surgery the keloid and surrounding area is anesthetized with a mixture of equal parts of 2% lidocaine and triamcinolone, 10 mg/mL. Cotton is placed in the external auditory canal to prevent blood from clogging the canal and sometimes causing temporary hearing loss. The operative site is then prepared and draped in a sterile fashion. When performing autografting, a half-moon or tongue-like incision of the approximate size of the base of the lesion to be excised is made from the border of the flattest and smoothest part of the keloid (see Fig. 24-2C). This lip of skin overlying the keloid tissue is carefully dissected from the underlying, white, glistening fibrous tissue with a No. 15 or 15C scalpel, No. 65 Beaver blade, or sharp iris or Gradle scissors to a distance slightly past the border of the keloid (see Fig. 24-2D). The keloid is then excised at the border between the keloid and clinically normal skin. For keloids on the earlobe, care must be taken not to excise all of the dermal tissue on the opposite side of the lobe for the autograft to have an adequate tissue and vascular base. Also, a

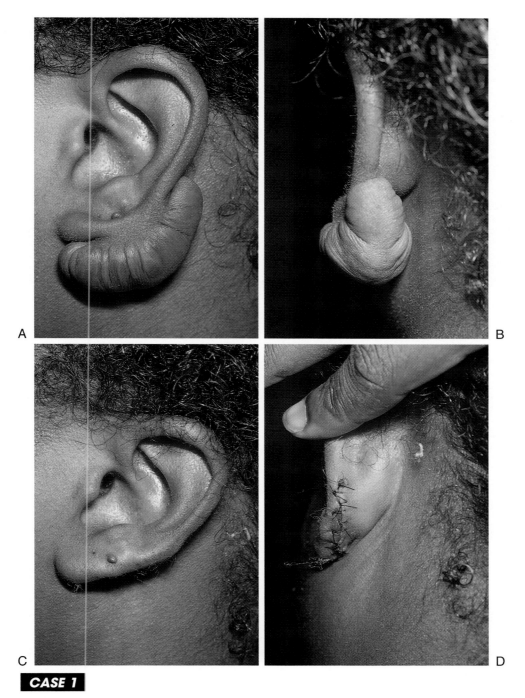

A

B

C

D

CASE 1

FIGURE 24–1. *A,* Large pendulous keloid of the left lobe distorts the contour of the lobe. *B,* Posterior view. *C,* Keloid resection by excision and closure restores the rim and contour of the lobe. Careful attention during the resection prevents excision of dermal tissue from the anterior surface of the lobe. *D,* Appearance 1 week after surgery. There is no edema.

through-and-through wide excision would be hard to heal and would heal with marked deformity of the ear. The saved overlying skin is then approximated to the border of the excision with interrupted nylon, polypropylene, or polybutester interrupted sutures (see Fig. 24–2E). Sometimes the same suture material is used to tack down the central part of the autograft to the underlying dermis to ensure

adhesion of these two surfaces in the event of postoperative bleeding or serous fluid accumulation. The sutures are left in place for 12 to 14 days because earlier removal may be fraught with wound dehiscence (Table 24–4).

One to 2 weeks after suture removal, the postoperative site is injected with triamcinolone, 40 mg/mL, and repeated every 2 to 3 weeks. Four postoperative injections

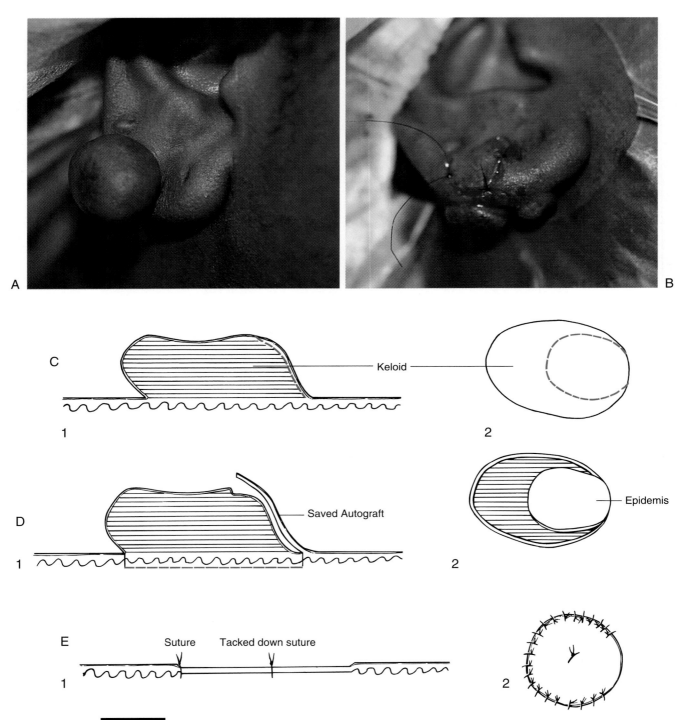

CASE 2

FIGURE 24–2. *A,* Keloid of the anterior surface of the right earlobe resulted from ear piercing. *B,* Immediately after keloid excision with the use of the overlying skin as an autograph the keloids of the posterior surface of the ear and rim of the lobe are more visible. These will be removed after the anterior surgical site is well healed. The cotton ball was removed from the ear canal before taking this photograph. *C,* A half-moon or tongue-like incision of the approximate size of the base of the lesion to be excised is made from the flattest and smoothest border of the keloid. *1,* Side view (cross-section). *2,* Top view. *D, 1* and *2,* The overlying lip of skin is carefully reflected from the keloid. The keloid is excised across its base. *E, 1* and *2,* The wound is closed with the lip of the autograph skin that is tacked down with a central suture.

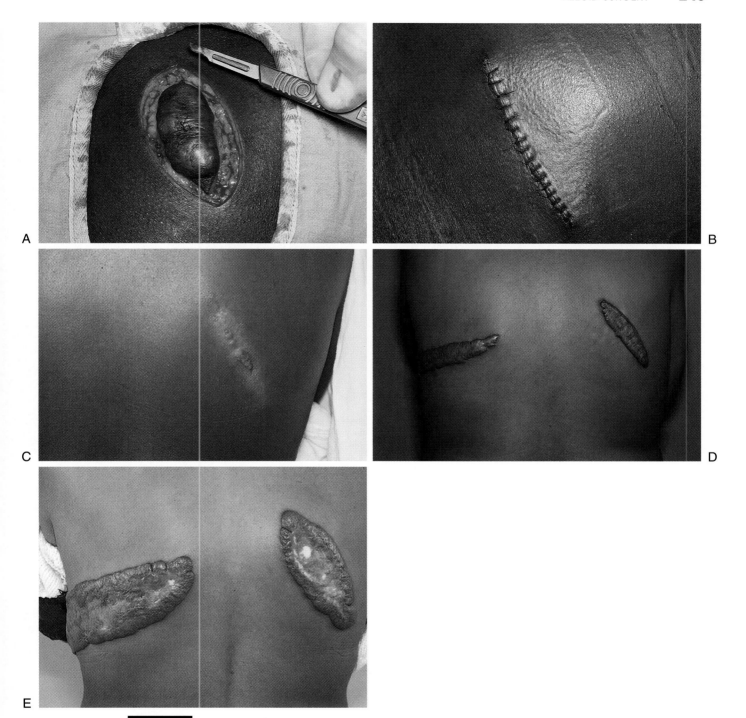

CASE 3

FIGURE 24–3. Complication. *A*, Keloid of the right upper back is excised with an elliptical excision. *B*, Appearance immediately after undermining and closing the wound with 4-0 interrupted nylon sutures. There is no excess tension on the wound edges of the excision of the keloid. *C*, Four months after surgery, hypopigmentation was caused by three triamcinolone injections. There is slight recurrence of the keloid. The patient refused more injections and did not use external compression garments as advised. Silicone gel was not available at this time. *D*, Five years after surgery there is regrowth of the right back lesion and a left flank keloid. This left flank keloid was excised concomitantly with the one shown in *A*. Both lesions are tender and painful. *E*, Ten years after surgery, the lesions stopped enlarging but are still tender and painful. The patient is now starting silicone gel therapy but refuses surgery.

TABLE 24-4. Keloid Surgery: Postoperative Care

Pain Management

Acetaminophen

Nonsteroidal anti-inflammatory agent

Avoid aspirin because of possible bleeding complications.

Dressings

Postoperative antibacterial ointment and gauze dressing

After 24 hours earlobe dressing not needed

Dressing after 24 hours in other locations only to prevent clothing or physical activity irritation

Complications

Regrowth of keloid

Ecchymosis

Wound dehiscence if sutures removed too soon or if trauma

Possible wound infection if not properly following postoperative care instructions; treat with appropriate antibiotic.

---

seem to be sufficient to prevent most recurrences. Another adjunct for preventing keloid recurrence is the use of pressure earrings for earlobe postoperative sites or pressure-gradient elastic garments on other anatomic areas for at least 8 hours but preferably 16 hours a day for 4 to 6 months. Silicone gel or silicone sheeting applied to the postoperative site 12 hours a day for 4 to 6 months is another successful preventive measure. Although advised not to, some patients insist on repiercing their earlobe. In this situation, the piercing site is injected with a combination of equal parts of 2% lidocaine and triamcinolone, 10 mg/mL, and the ear is pierced by the physician. Once the piercing site has healed the patient should have injections of triamcinolone, 10 mg/mL, into the piercing site every 3 weeks for three injections.

References

1. Murray JC, Pollack SV, Pinnell SR. Keloids: A review. J Am Acad Dermatol 1981;14:461–470.
2. Apfelberg DB, Maser MR, Lash H. The use of epidermis over a keloid as an autograft after resection of the keloid. J Dermatol Surg Oncol 1976;2:409–411.
3. Kelly AP. Surgical treatment of keloids secondary to ear piercing. J Natl Med Assoc 1978;70:349.
4. Cosman B, Wolf M. Correlation of keloid recurrence with completeness of local excision. Plast Reconstr Surg 1972;50:163–165.
5. Kelly AP. Keloids. Dermatol Clin 1988;6:413–424.
6. Stucker FJ, Shaw GY. An approach to management of keloids. Arch Otolaryngol Head Neck Surg 1992;118:63–67.
7. Pollack S. Management of keloids. In: Wheeland R, ed. Cutaneous Surgery. Philadelphia: WB Saunders Co., 1993:688–697.
8. Nemeth AJ. Keloids and hypertrophic scars. J Dermatol Surg Oncol 1993;19:738–746.
9. Granstein RD, Rook A, Flotte TJ, et al. A controlled trial of intralesional recombinant interferon gamma in the treatment of keloidal scarring: Clinical and histologic findings. Arch Dermatol 1990;126:1295–1302.
10. Ahn ST, Monato WN, Mustoe TA. Topical silicone gel: A new treatment for hypertrophic scars. Surgery 1989;106:781–787.
11. Hirshowitz B, Ullmann Y, Har Shai Y, et al. Silicone occlusive sheeting (SOS) in the management of hypertrophic and keloid scarring, including possible mode of action of silicone, by static electricity. Eur J Plast Surg 1993;16:5–9.
12. Mercer NSG. Silicone gel in the treatment of keloid scars. Br J Plast Surg 1989;42:83–87.
13. Kischer CW, Shetlar MR, Shetlar CL. Alteration of hypertrophic scars by mechanical pressure. Arch Dermatol 1975;111:60–64.
14. Rusciani L, Rossi G, Bono R, et al. Use of cryotherapy in the treatment of keloids. J Dermatol Surg Oncol 1993;19:529–534.
15. Zouboulis CC, Blume U, Buttner P, et al. Outcomes of cryosurgery in keloids and hypertrophic scars. Arch Dermatol 1993;129:1146–1151.
16. Nicolai JP, Bos MT, Bronkhorst FB, Smale CE. A protocol for the treatment of hypertrophic scars and keloids. Aesthetic Plast Surg 1987;11:29–32.
17. Malaker K, Ellis F, Paine CH: Keloid scars: A new method of treatment combining surgery with interstitial radiotherapy. Clin Radiol 1976;27:179–183.
18. Salasche ST, Grabski WJ. Keloids of the earlobes: A surgical technique. J Dermatol Surg Oncol 1983;9:552–556.

section four

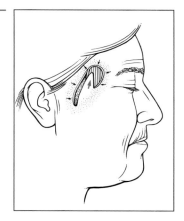

Cosmetic Cutaneous Surgery

JUNE K. ROBINSON

Cosmetic surgery is part of the realm of dermatologic surgery. The procedures discussed in this section require varying skill levels and have different risks associated with performing them. Some, such as dermabrasion and hair replacement surgery, have been developed and practiced for decades by dermatologists. Others are new techniques that dermatologists have quickly mastered and subsequently made their own contributions (e.g., liposuction surgery). All cosmetic procedures require similar considerations by the patient and the surgeon. The principles required to form the appropriate expectations are outlined in the following discussion.

In approaching the patient seeking improvement in his or her appearance caused by aging or diseases such as acne, the physician has differing concerns than in treating malignancies and a changing role in providing information and counseling the patient. The physician must ascertain if the patient's desires are the result of serious, mature consideration with an understanding of what can be achieved or simply a passing fancy or trend. The patient's motives in seeking the surgery may often be uncovered by asking the following:

- Who originally suggested that the cosmetic surgery be performed?
- What do you expect the surgery to do for you?
- In what way will the surgery help you?
- How long have you liked or disliked this? Have you changed your mind about it, or have you constantly liked or disliked it?

If patients tend to be constantly experimenting with new glasses or hair color, it is likely that they will not remain satisfied with the permanent results brought about by cosmetic surgery. The patient should be the one voicing the desire for surgery and not feel that the procedure will change his or her image, popularity, relationships, or potential for success in their occupation.

There is no standard questionnaire to use in the evaluative interview. Every surgeon must interview the patient according to his or her own style and personality. One useful principle to remember while conducting the consultation is to have empathy and give the patient permission to fully state the desired outcome as well as any anxieties and concerns. By using the consultation visit to listen to the patient and uncover the reasons the patient desires cosmetic surgery, the surgeon gains insight into the patient's needs and concerns. This cosmetic consultation must do more than exchange information about the procedure being considered. Ideally, the patient should talk more than the surgeon. Candid, open-ended questions of the who, what, when, and why type can prompt responses from patients that will allow the surgeon to decide if the anticipated surgical result can meet the patient's expectations or fantasies.

In bringing the consultation interview to closure, the surgeon discusses the limitations of and alternatives to surgery as well as general discussion of complications. At the end of the session, the surgeon may pause and then ask the patient, ''Is there anything else I should know about you?'' This final sincere question, asked after the doctor–patient relationship has been established, may produce new and relevant information.

Since cosmetic surgery is elective, it may be delayed until both the doctor and the patient are comfortable with one another and with the anticipated result. If the patient has other stressful situations in his or her life, then surgery can be delayed until these situations have been resolved. Establishing a mutual bond of trust may take more than one consultation visit. The actual length of the visit may vary from 30 to 60 minutes: some persons need time to elapse to be able to frame their concerns. For these persons, two separate visits are helpful.

The initial interview establishes the framework for the surgery and postoperative care. The surgeon makes the patient responsible for his or her decisions, expectations, and behavior during the procedure and during the healing period. If the surgeon is intuitively uncomfortable with a patient or in performing the procedure that offers the best solution to the problem, the surgeon can either give the patient a future appointment or refer the patient to another physician. If the second appointment is not satisfactory or is still uncomfortable for the surgeon, it may be best not to operate on the patient. The optimal way to do this is not to reject the patient but to merely postpone the decision, which generates less hostility and ill will.

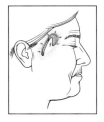

chapter 25

Tattoo Removal

RONALD G. WHEELAND

GENERAL DESCRIPTION

The introduction of foreign pigments and other materials into the dermis as tattoos has long been performed as a sign of tribal marking, as body ornamentation, or as an expression of personal rebellion.[1,2] Numerous archeologic finds have scientifically established that tattooing has existed since prehistoric times.[3] At present, it is estimated that 10 million persons in the United States have at least one decorative tattoo, and that number is rising rapidly.[4,5] In addition, tattooing is also performed today as a cosmetic procedure to enhance the lip lines and to simulate mascara on the eyelids or rouge on the cheeks.[6] Medical tattooing may be used for areolar reconstruction after mastectomy and to accurately identify radiation ports for performing radiation therapy for deep malignancies. Traumatic tattoos can also occur when asphalt is introduced into the skin in motor vehicle accidents or when carbon particles are forcibly introduced into the skin from firecrackers, accidental

backfiring of black powder firearms, or with other types of explosions.[7,8] Regardless as to the mechanism by which it has been acquired, at some point many individuals become interested in seeking the effective removal of their tattoo. As a result, a large and varied number of techniques have been employed over the years for removing tattoos, including ablative techniques (Table 25–1), nonablative techniques (Table 25–2), traditional excisional surgical removal (Table 25–3), and laser surgical procedures (Table 25–4).

PATIENT CONSULTATION

When treating a person with a decorative tattoo, a number of different factors must be considered to help the patient decide what is the most ideal technique to use for removing his or her particular tattoo (Table 25–5). As with all surgical procedures, to ensure that informed con-

TABLE 25–1. Ablative Techniques for Tattoo Removal

Technique	Advantages	Disadvantages
Chemical destruction	Simple, safe, effective for all colors	Incomplete pigment removal; scarring; alopecia
Salabrasion	Low cost, simple, effective for all colors, no anesthesia required	Incomplete pigment removal; requires multiple treatments; scarring, alopecia
Dermabrasion	Simple technique, low cost, uses equipment already available	Incomplete pigment removal, scarring, alopecia; must be repeated; larger area must be treated due to large size of fraizes
Chemabrasion	Simple technique, low cost, reduces number of re-treatments	Multiple treatments; scarring, dyschromia usually follows
Curettage	Simple, low cost	Anesthesia required; incomplete pigment removal; must be repeated; results in scarring
Cryosurgery	Simple, low cost	Painful; incomplete pigment removal; must be repeated, hypopigmentation follows; scarring
Electrosurgery	Simple, low cost	Incomplete removal; hypopigmentation and scarring may result
Infrared coagulator	Relatively low cost, simple technique	Anesthesia required, long healing time, incomplete pigment removal, re-treatment often necessary, alopecia may result, special equipment required
Chemical peeling	Low cost	Unpredictable results, re-treatment is likely

TABLE 25-2. Nonablative Techniques for Tattoo Removal

Technique	Advantages	Disadvantages
Overtattooing	Camouflaging of name or design possible for some colors	Trades one tattoo for another; may reduce effectiveness of subsequent removal techniques
Tattoo supplementation	Camouflaging of name or design possible for some colors	Increases quantity of pigment; may reduce effectiveness of subsequent removal techniques
Scarification	Simple, low cost	Results are unpredictable; retreatment is likely

TABLE 25-3. Excisional Surgery Techniques for Tattoo Removal

Technique	Advantages	Disadvantages
Simple excision with primary closure	Simple, low cost, predictable result, little morbidity	Limited to small tattoos; produces linear scars
Staged excision with primary closure	Larger tattoos can be treated; linear scar is predictable	Entire removal process is greatly lengthened; increases overall morbidity and cost
Tissue expansion with primary closure	Larger tattoos can be effectively treated	Multiple visits required for inflation of expander; geometric scar results; increased cost
Excision with random pattern flap closure	Small and medium-sized tattoos can be treated in one procedure	Geometric scar results; increased cost
Excision with skin graft repair	Large tattoos can be treated	Two scars will result; long healing time; increased cost; pain
Tangential excision	Quick, simple, even large tattoos can be treated	Geometric scar results; long healing time required; limited to flat anatomic sites; not good for small tattoos

TABLE 25-4. Laser Surgical Techniques for Tattoo Removal

Laser System	Wavelength	Output	Advantages	Disadvantages
Argon	488–514 nm	Continuous wave or "long" pulses	None	Incomplete removal; permanent hypopigmentation; scars; long healing time; multiple treatments required
Carbon dioxide	10,600 nm	Continuous wave or short pulses	One treatment; low cost; complete removal; good for allergic granulomas	Safety hazards to eyes and plume risks; scars; long healing time (18 months); dyspigmentation; local anesthesia required
Ruby	694 nm	Q-switched	No scars; no anesthesia; good for green colors and traumatic tattoos; minimal postoperative care	Temporary hypopigmentation; multiple treatments; not good for red colors or allergic granulomas; splatter hazard; cosmetic tattoos may darken
Nd:YAG	1064 nm and 532 nm	Q-switched	No scars; no anesthesia; good for red colors and traumatic tattoos; minimal postoperative care	Temporary hyperpigmentation; multiple treatments; not good for green colors or allergic granulomas; splatter hazard; cosmetic tattoos may darken
Alexandrite	755 nm	Q-switched	Same as for ruby laser system	Same as for ruby laser system

TABLE 25-5. Factors Influencing Choice of Tattoo Removal Techniques

Size and anatomic location
Desired postoperative appearance and patient deadlines
Nature of the tattoo
    Type of tattoo: amateur, professional, traumatic, or
      cosmetic
    Pigment density
    Pigment depth
    Multiplicity of colors
Duration of tattoo
Past history of adverse scarring
Skin type
Anticipated cost
Presence of allergic granulomas

sent has been given, each patient with a tattoo must be told in great detail about the nature of the problem; the treatment options that are available, including the option of doing nothing since in most cases tattoo removal is purely an elective procedure; the risk of each of the different forms of treatment that are available; the benefits of the various treatments; the known complications of each type of treatment; and the potential for scarring. Only by carefully evaluating each individual patient and his or her particular tattoo can the most ideal treatment plan be formulated so as to have the greatest opportunity to achieve complete patient satisfaction.

VARIABLES AFFECTING TREATMENT MODALITIES FOR TATTOO REMOVAL

Size and Anatomic Location

Two of the most important considerations in selecting the proper form of treatment for a tattoo are its size and anatomic location.

Small Tattoos

In many cases, the best treatment for removing a small tattoo is simple elliptical excision followed by primary closure.[9] Not only is this a simple, safe, quick, and inexpensive procedure to perform, but it is also generally associated with little surgical risk in a healthy person and results in minimal postoperative pain while requiring only a limited amount of wound care during the short time period required for healing. Simple surgical excision has the additional benefit of being able to completely remove all of the tattoo pigment in a small tattoo (Case 1, Fig. 25–1) in only one treatment session while simultaneously leaving a generally acceptable, short, linear scar.[10]

Large Tattoos

Unfortunately, simple surgical excision is not typically an effective form of treatment for larger tattoos or tattoos found on anatomic locations where there is great tension or

where the skin is thick and tight. In these situations, complete removal in a single excisional surgery procedure is unlikely since primary wound closure is usually not possible and if the wound is closed under tension a poor cosmetic result can generally be anticipated. However, surgical excision can still be an effective form of treatment for larger tattoos if it is performed as a series of staged procedures spread out over a relatively long period of time (Case 2, Fig. 25–2) or when it is combined with tissue expansion[11] to permit primary wound closure once sufficient excess tissue has been generated. Unfortunately, when these two modifications of the simple surgical excision procedure are employed for the removal of large tattoos, the required repetitious nature of the procedure is associated with a concomitant increase in both the expense of the procedure and the time required to perform it. The individual must also show remarkable patience since multiple return office visits for the secondary procedures or inflation of the expander are required. Even then, when

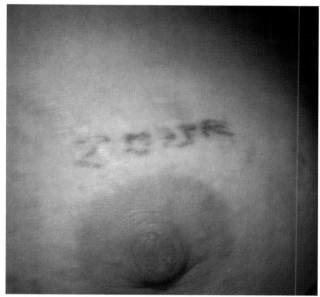

A

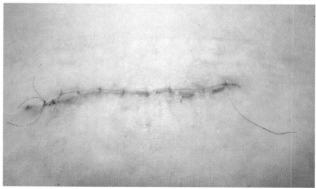

B

CASE 1

FIGURE 25–1. *A,* Preoperative appearance of a small, roughly linear amateur tattoo on the breast. *B,* Immediate appearance of wound after simple side-to-side closure of an elliptical excision.

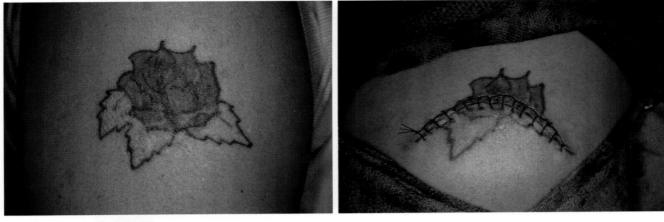

A   B

CASE 2

FIGURE 25–2. *A*, Preoperative appearance of a medium-sized multicolored professional tattoo on the arm.
B, Immediate appearance of sutured wound after closure of the first phase of a staged surgical excision.

either of these treatment modifications is utilized to remove larger tattoos, the patient is still ultimately left with a large and visible scar, which may be a source of discontent.[12]

The use of random pattern flaps or skin grafts to treat larger tattoos can minimize the need to perform multistaged procedures. Although this technique allows immediate closure of these larger wounds, the patient is left with highly visible geometric scars at the operative site or scars at the skin graft donor site. For these reasons, when dealing with large tattoos or difficult anatomic locations, the use of ablative techniques such as cryosurgery,[13,14] chemical destruction,[15–17] chemical peels,[18] carbon dioxide (CO_2) laser vaporization,[19,20] or combinations of chemical and laser treatments[21,22]; salabrasion[23–25]; dermabrasion alone[26,27] or combined with curettage[28]; infrared coagulation[29,30]; tangential (dermatome) excision[31]; or Q-switched laser surgery[4–6,32–36] becomes the preferred form of treatment.

Desired Cosmetic Appearance and Patient Deadlines

The patient's desired outcome as to the final appearance of the treated site is a major consideration when deciding on the type of treatment for any tattoo. Although the tattooed patient will generally desire complete removal of a tattoo, in some cases, a patient may wish to have only a small, particularly offensive portion of a larger tattoo removed to eliminate a name, symbol, or a color to which the patient has developed an allergic reaction. Regardless into which category the patient falls, the most important decision is whether the patient wishes to have the tattoo removed with or without the creation of a permanent scar. This fundamental question has only recently become relevant because of the ability of the new Q-switched laser surgical techniques that permit fading or complete tattoo removal without a significant risk of scarring. Unfortunately, the biggest disadvantage of these new Q-switched laser surgical techniques is that an unpredictable number of

re-treatments, performed at 6- to 8-week intervals, will generally be required to fade or remove the tattoo entirely.

For this same reason, if the patient has a particular time frame or special deadline to meet for having the tattoo removed, then the newer Q-switched laser surgical procedures should be avoided since there is, at present, no accurate way to predict either the ultimate response or how many treatments may be required to achieve the goal of complete removal. When a deadline has been established by the patient as to when he or she would like the tattoo to be completely removed, and the ultimate cosmetic appearance is only of secondary importance, use of one of the ablative procedures that ensures complete and total pigment removal in a single procedure, such as elliptical or tangential excision (Case 3, Fig. 25–3) or CO_2 laser vaporization, should be considered.

Nature of the Tattoo

Types of Tattoos

There are four major categories of tattoos: amateur, professional, traumatic, and cosmetic. Each type is associated with a slightly different set of potential risks, benefits, and complications that must be considered before actually deciding on any given form of treatment (Table 25–6). *Amateur tattoos* are typically black since they are often applied with some form of penetrating wound using India ink or some other form of carbonized material. Their small size commonly makes simple surgical excision possible in many cases. Because the pigment is variably deposited at different levels within the dermis, superficial ablative procedures such as salabrasion, dermabrasion, chemical peels, and even tangential excision are commonly ineffective since deep residual pigment will often be retained focally within the dermis. However, CO_2 laser vaporization can be an extremely effective form of treatment for these types of tattoos since focal deeper deposits of pigment can be removed without damaging the surrounding normal tissue (Case 4, Fig. 25–4). Because relatively large carbon parti-

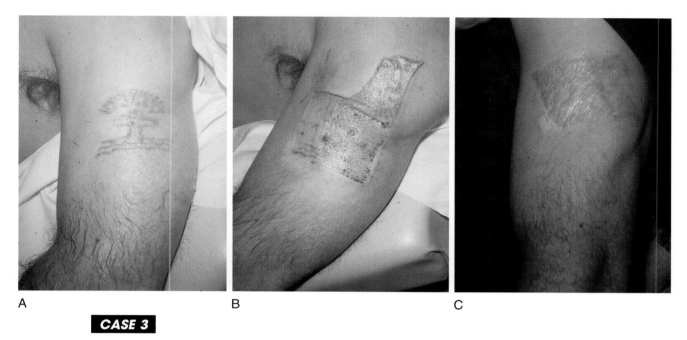

CASE 3

FIGURE 25–3. *A,* Clinical appearance of a large professional tattoo on the upper arm before tangential excision. *B,* Intraoperative appearance showing complete pigment removal after one split thickness of skin has been tangentially excised using a dermatome. *C,* Clinical appearance 3 months postoperatively showing a soft, flat, geometric scar with no residual tattoo pigment.

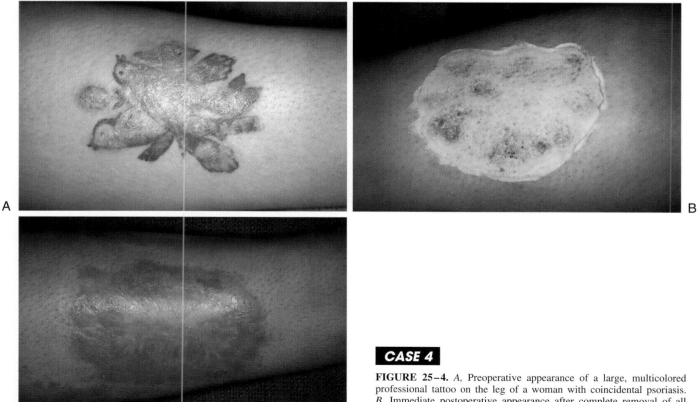

CASE 4

FIGURE 25–4. *A,* Preoperative appearance of a large, multicolored professional tattoo on the leg of a woman with coincidental psoriasis. *B,* Immediate postoperative appearance after complete removal of all pigment with carbon dioxide laser vaporization. *C,* Soft flat scar is seen 4 months later without residual tattoo pigment or psoriasis.

TABLE 25-6. Anticipated Results of Tattoo Treatment by Type

Type of Tattoo	Treatment	Anticipated Response
Amateur	Excision	Excellent: one treatment for small tattoos, linear scar results
	Q-switched laser	Good/excellent: three to four re-treatments; no scarring; minimal postoperative care
	Dermabrasion	Fair/good: re-treatment likely
	CO_2 laser	Fair/good: one treatment; scar may duplicate the original tattoo
	Salabrasion	Fair: re-treatment necessary
Professional	Q-switched laser	Good/excellent: six to eight re-treatments; no scarring; minimal postoperative care; incomplete pigment removal possible, especially red, green, yellow, and white; should not be used in allergic granulomas; cost cannot be accurately determined in advance
	Dermabrasion	Fair/good: incomplete pigment removal and re-treatment likely; geometric scars
	CO_2 laser	Fair/good: one treatment; scar may duplicate the original tattoo 18 months before final cosmetic result is obtained
	Tangential excision	Fair/good: quick; low cost; may leave residual pigment; geometric scars; long healing time
	Excision	Poor except for small tattoos; large tattoos treated only with staged excision or tissue expansion
	Salabrasion	Poor: re-treatment necessary; incomplete pigment removal likely; scars and hypopigmentation will develop
Traumatic	Dermabrasion	Good/excellent: if performed early after injury
	Q-switched laser	Good/excellent: one to two treatments; no scarring; minimal postoperative care
	Excision	Good: only for linear areas; punch technique can be used for focal pigment deposits
	CO_2 laser	Fair/poor: may leave depressed scar; difficult to treat large areas
	Salabrasion	Poor: difficult to control uniformity; hard to treat small areas
Cosmetic	Q-switched laser	Good/excellent: re-treatments are necessary; no scarring; minimal postoperative care; incomplete removal and pigment darkening are possible
	Dermabrasion	Fair/good: incomplete pigment removal and re-treatment likely; technically difficult to perform on some anatomic areas
	CO_2 laser	Fair/good: may be useful in certain anatomic sites, may produce scars
	Excision	Poor: except for small tattoos

cles are responsible for producing the black color found in most amateur tattoos, impacts from the various Q-switched lasers (Case 5, Fig. 25–5) can easily break them into smaller fragments and produce substantial lightening after only a small number of treatments.[37]

The issues that surround successful treatment of *professional decorative tattoos* relate to the greater total quantity of tattoo pigment that is typically present, the density and depth of the pigment, and the common use of multiple pigments to produce different colors. Professional tattoo pigments are generally applied over a narrower range of depths within the dermis than which is seen with amateur tattoos. The depth of pigment deposition is based on the different reflective properties of the various pigment colors being used and the individual experience of the tattoo artist.[25] However, because there is greater uniformity in the deposition of pigment particles in professional tattoos, the

ablative treatments, such as salabrasion (Case 6, Fig. 25–6), dermabrasion, and tangential excision, often provide excellent results.

The presence of multiple colors or high pigment density found in professional tattoos does not impact on the potential effectiveness of the traditional ablative procedures used in their removal. However, both of these factors can have a significant negative impact on the success of the new Q-switched laser techniques. This is a result of how the short pulses from these high-powered lasers interact with tattoo pigment. Although the mechanism of action for these newer lasers is still somewhat unclear, it appears that certain colors found in professional tattoos (notably green, red, yellow, and white) are resistant to the impacts of these lasers and are not fragmented into smaller pieces as readily as are the carbon particles found in amateur tattoos. This not only makes the need for multiple re-treatments more

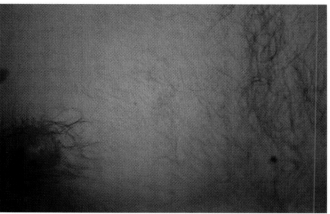

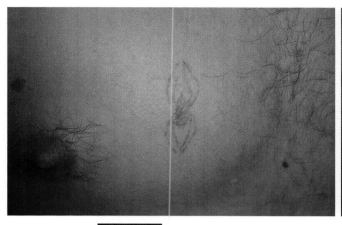

A   B

CASE 5

FIGURE 25–5. *A,* Preoperative appearance of a black amateur tattoo on the chest. *B,* Complete tattoo pigment removal without scarring or changes in texture has been achieved after two treatments with the Q-switched Nd:YAG laser.

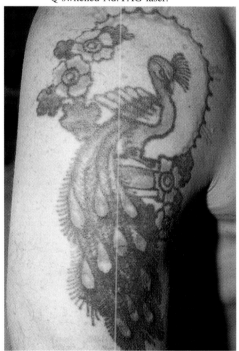

CASE 6

FIGURE 25–6. *A,* Preoperative appearance of a large multicolored professional tattoo on the arm. *B,* Thick eschar containing much of the tattoo pigment has separated from the site 3 weeks after salabrasion. *C,* Faint tattoo pigmentation can still be seen through a slightly scaling surface 4 weeks after the second salabrasion.

A

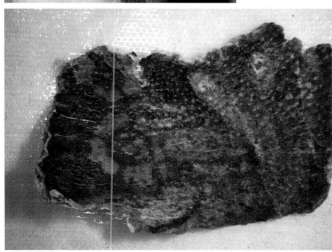

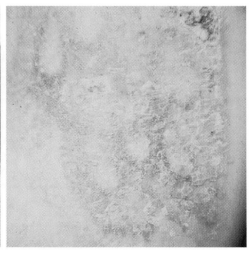

B   C

common for certain pigments, it may also be the reason that some colors can never be completely removed. Furthermore, differences in wavelength may make one of these Q-switched laser systems more effective in the treatment of one tattoo pigment color, but the same system may be ineffective in treating a different color. Despite the successful application of these newer devices in the treatment of many tattoos, at present there is no single laser system that can treat all tattoo pigments with equal success.

Traumatic tattoos are characterized by the presence of multiple, small speckles or lines of blue or black pigment commonly on the exposed portions of the face and hands that generally represent carbon particles that have become embedded in the dermis after some form of trauma, explosion, or penetrating wound.[7] Most often, in the context of immediate emergency care provided in a hospital setting, these wounds are typically cleansed with the use of anesthesia with vigorous scrubbing using antiseptic cleansers to remove as much of the gross pigmentation as possible. As the wounds heal, additional pigment will typically be lost within the resolving surface crust. The residual pigment that is identifiable once wound healing is complete can be managed by dermabrasion, chemical peels, punch excision,[38] or one of the Q-switched lasers.[39]

A technique has developed in which various mixtures of materials containing iron oxide are injected into different anatomic sites using tattoo needles to produce red, tan, brown, black, and flesh-colored pigments for the purpose of cosmetic enhancement. These *cosmetic tattoos* are used on the eyelids to simulate mascara in patients allergic to certain cosmetics, on the eyebrows to re-create a normal hairline, on the lips for better definition of the margin (Case 7, Fig. 25–7), for areolar reconstruction after mastectomy, and to hide a variety of other scars and blemishes. Unfortunately, because of changes in fashion, poor surgical technique resulting in unsatisfactory pigment placement, or general disenchantment with the cosmetic appearance that has been obtained, some persons will ultimately seek removal of their cosmetic tattoos. The only two forms of treatment that have been able to provide satisfactory results in these conditions are excisional and laser surgery. The biggest advantage of the newer Q-switched laser surgical techniques is their potential ability to remove this pigment without producing a visible scar. However, the way the laser light interacts with these types of tattoo pigments may result in a change in the chemical composition of the iron oxide in the tattoo. This may convert it from the red ferric oxide to the black ferrous oxide.[6] Furthermore, the black ferrous oxide that forms may be very resistant to subsequent removal with further treatment using the Q-switched lasers.

Duration of the Tattoo

All tattoos fade over time as a result of the natural phagocytosis process of the foreign particles that remove them by way of the lymphatics.[40] This process of phagocytosis and removal from the tissue is probably enhanced by the use of certain ablative tattoo treatment techniques such as salabrasion, dermabrasion, and the new Q-switched

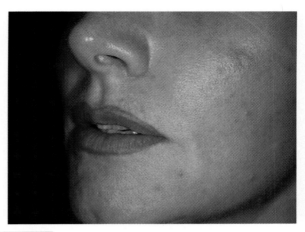

CASE 7

FIGURE 25–7. The lip line has been augmented through the injection of iron oxide pigment as a cosmetic tattoo. The lighter area of the left upper lip between the vermilion and the outline of the tattoo is the patient's cutaneous lip with partial coloration by the tattoo pigment.

lasers.[4,5,37,39] Knowing the duration of the tattoo may help to more accurately predict the likely response to treatment.

Older tattoos of 10 or 20 years' duration may be more difficult to remove with traditional ablative procedures since the pigment may extend deeper or wider in the dermis than is initially apparent. This is especially important in excisional surgery since it may be difficult to define precisely the true extent of the surgical margins and a more aggressive procedure may be required to effect complete eradication of the tattoo. Conversely, the older tattoos can be expected to respond better and faster to the Q-switched lasers, which seem to stimulate phagocytosis by breaking the tattoo particles into smaller fragments (Cases 8 and 9, Figs. 25–8 and 25–9). However, newly applied tattoos of less than 1 year's duration may be more resistant to this treatment because appreciable phagocytosis may have not yet had the opportunity to occur. The newer tattoos may also be somewhat refractory to treatment with the newer Q-switched lasers because of the use of more brilliant and vibrant colors that may be composed of a host of different pigments derived from organic dyes, uncommon metals, or other materials that do not uniformly respond to the laser impacts.

Past History of Adverse Scarring

The most common and greatest concern expressed by patients who are seeking removal of their tattoo is the element of scarring. Despite the development of the Q-switched lasers, which can effectively fade or remove most tattoos without a significant risk of permanent scarring, many of the older techniques are still commonly used today because of the advantages that they offer as to cost, limited number of re-treatments, and simplicity of performance. For this reason, it remains of great importance to determine each patient's past medical history in regard to adverse scarring so that some preoperative determination of

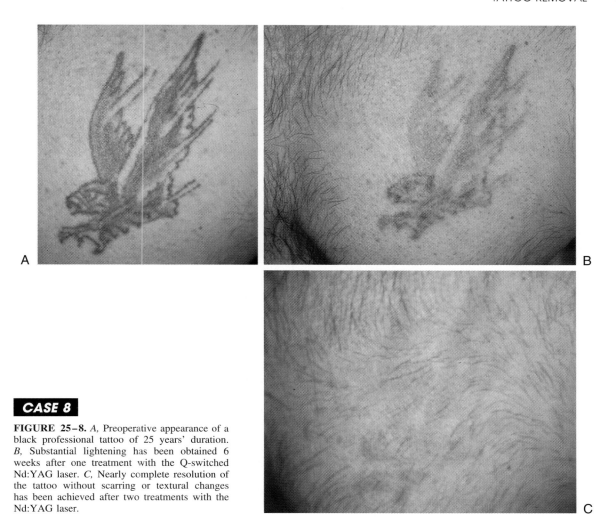

CASE 8

FIGURE 25–8. *A,* Preoperative appearance of a black professional tattoo of 25 years' duration. *B,* Substantial lightening has been obtained 6 weeks after one treatment with the Q-switched Nd:YAG laser. *C,* Nearly complete resolution of the tattoo without scarring or textural changes has been achieved after two treatments with the Nd:YAG laser.

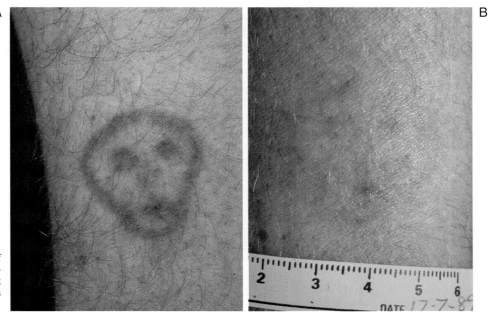

CASE 9

FIGURE 25–9. *A,* Preoperative appearance of an amateur tattoo on the arm. *B,* Nearly complete resolution has been obtained without scarring or alopecia following two treatments with the Q-switched ruby laser.

that risk can be given. For purposes of greatest safety, the ablative procedures that are commonly employed for removing tattoos should probably not be used to treat patients who give a positive past history of hypertrophic scarring or keloid formation following trauma or surgery. However, this finding does not appear to preclude the safe use of the Q-switched lasers in these same patients. Despite the apparent low risk of adverse scarring following tattoo treatment with the Q-switched lasers, no guarantees as to the potential outcome should ever be given to patients in this regard.

Skin Type

The patient's skin type is probably only of indirect importance when discussing possible techniques for tattoo removal because of the known greater predilection for patients of darker skin types to develop keloids or hypertrophic scars following trauma or any other type of surgical procedure. However, the skin type does play an important role in determining the potential effectiveness of the Q-switched lasers in removing tattoos. This is a result of absorptive interference caused by large quantities of melanin within the epidermis of persons with dark skin types. In these persons, certain wavelengths of light, especially those produced by the ruby, alexandrite, and frequency-doubled yttrium-aluminum-garnet (YAG) lasers, may be blocked by the melanin in the epidermis from penetrating into the dermis. This results in inadvertent damage to the epidermis, which is manifested initially by crusting and later by temporary hypopigmentation. It also decreases the quality of the response seen in the tattoo with less lightening than would otherwise be expected. Obviously, since pigment irregularities can be seen in all skin types with any of the different forms of treatment, this concern should always be stressed to each patient during the consultative visit.

Anticipated Cost

Most patients who seek information about having their tattoo removed will want to be given some estimate of the anticipated cost of the procedure, since in almost all cases this elective procedure will not be covered by medical insurance. This can be a relatively straightforward determination when simple elliptical excision is the method chosen for treatment. Similarly, for the destructive techniques that completely eliminate virtually all tattoo pigment in a single procedure, such as tangential excision, excision and grafting, or CO_2 laser vaporization, the anticipated cost can accurately be determined by the size of the tattoo and the amount of operative time required to perform the procedure. However, for those techniques that frequently have to be repeated several times or more, such as salabrasion, dermabrasion, chemical peeling, cryosurgery, infrared coagulation, and Q-switched laser surgery, the determination of the anticipated cost represents a much more difficult task. It is standard policy in some practices to quote the patient a fixed fee that covers the cost of the entire procedure required for complete tattoo removal. There are obvious advantages to this approach. However, the unpredict-

ability of the response to some forms of tattoo treatment, especially with the Q-switched lasers, which makes multiple re-treatments a necessity in virtually all cases, suggests the benefit of charging a fee for each treatment. In this way, the patient knows in advance that there is no accurate way to predict the response to treatment and that he or she will ultimately determine when the desired maximal degree of improvement has been achieved. It is often advisable, as it is for every elective surgical procedure, to require payment for the procedure at least 1 week in advance. This will reduce the number of cancelled appointments or patients who fail to keep their appointments.

Presence of Allergic Granulomas

Certain tattoo pigments can result in localized allergic reactions at the tattooed site (Case 10, Fig. 25–10), which can cause pruritus and chronic eczematous changes as well as systemic symptoms and lymphadenopathy.[41] Although these reactions have been reported in association with many different tattoo pigments, the most common reactions occur with mercury used to make the red pigment,[42–44] manganese used to make the purple pigment,[45,46] chromium used to make the green pigment, cobalt used to make the blue pigment, and cadmium used to make the yellow pigment. Previously, patients with localized allergic reactions to any of the tattoo pigments were typically treated with topical or intralesional corticosteroids. However, if the reaction persisted despite these maneuvers, the offending portions of the tattoo could be removed using curettage, local excision, or CO_2 laser vaporization.[43,47]

The mechanism of action for the treatment of tattoos with the Q-switched lasers consists of fragmentation of the intracellular tattoo pigments by selective photothermolysis[48] and cavitation, which results in extracellular deposition of the smaller tattoo particles.[37] These particles are dispersed throughout the dermis where they are engulfed by macrophages and subsequently removed from the skin. However, the net result of these actions may stimulate the immune system and serve to worsen a preexisting allergic reaction to a particular tattoo pigment. For that reason, it has now been recommended that allergic granulomas not be treated with the new Q-switched lasers but rather be removed with some form of ablative treatment to ensure complete removal of the offending pigment.

POSTOPERATIVE WOUND CARE AND PAIN MANAGEMENT

As could be expected, the type and amount of postoperative wound care following tattoo removal vary tremendously with the technique that is chosen for the procedure. For most of the ablative techniques (see Table 25–1), daily cleansing with 3% hydrogen peroxide followed by an application of an antibiotic ointment and a simple absorbent dressing is all that is required until the wound heals completely in 1 to 2 weeks. When salabrasion or infrared coagulation is used, the same wound care is continued on a daily basis until the thick eschar separates spontaneously in 2 to 4 weeks. Postoperative pain following most of the

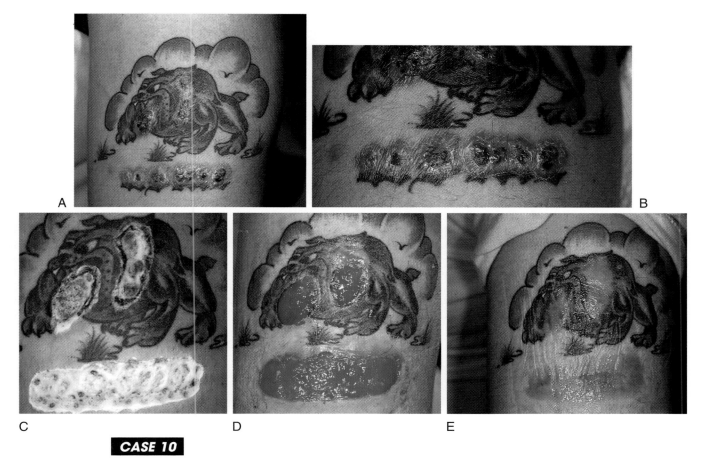

A

B

C

D

E

CASE 10

FIGURE 25–10. *A,* Preoperative appearance of a multicolored professional tattoo with a granulomatous reaction limited to the areas of red pigment deposition. *B,* Close-up view of the largest granulomas. *C,* Complete ablation of the granulomas has been achieved using the carbon dioxide laser in the vaporizational mode. *D,* After 2 weeks the treated sites show excellent granulation tissue and early reepithelialization beginning at the margins of the wounds. *E,* Complete reepithelialization has occurred by 2 months without any recurrence of the allergic granulomas.

ablative procedures is generally insignificant, but on occasion, acetaminophen with codeine may be required for the first 24 to 48 hours postoperatively. Few restrictions are placed on the patient's physical activities, and most patients can resume normal functions in 1 week.

For the nonablative techniques, which are used only on a limited basis, minimal wound care is typically required. In these cases, pigment removal is largely dependent on the ensuing inflammatory reaction and not the actual destruction of the soft tissue that contains the tattoo. For this reason, wound care consists only of soap and water cleansing once a day and no limitations in the patient's physical activities are generally required.

For the surgical excision procedures, traditional wound care and postoperative limitations on physical activities are employed. However, after treatment of larger tattoos, in which more complicated random pattern flaps, long incisions with geometric closures, or tissue expansion have been utilized, limited physical activity for 1 to 2 weeks is generally an important requirement. This is especially important in patients treated with the tissue expansion technique since rupture or extrusion of the device has been reported after trauma. In addition, prophylactic antibiotics

are sometimes recommended during tissue expansion, but the absolute need for this precaution has not been firmly established.

Since full-thickness wounds are produced with both the argon and CO_2 laser surgical techniques, routine twice-daily cleansing and sterile dressing applications are necessary. Long-term wound care is required when the CO_2 laser is used, since complete reepithelialization may not occur for 4 to 6 weeks after treatment of some larger tattoos. Typically there is little postoperative pain for the first 3 to 4 days after CO_2 laser treatment. However, significant pain and pruritus may develop after 1 week that may require use of acetaminophen and codeine for several days to provide the patient with maximum comfort.

The Q-switched lasers share the common feature of little or no postoperative pain in most cases and rapid healing without a need for traditional surgical dressings. Since tissue splatter occurs as the high-powered laser pulses impact on the skin surface during treatment, immediate postoperative bleeding is generally seen. However, this ceases almost immediately and by 24 to 48 hours a fine crust or scale has developed that generally resolves in 7 to 10 days using only soap and water. In some cases, a sterile hydrogel dressing is employed during the Q-switched laser treatment to contain the splatter. This dressing may be left in place at the completion of the procedure and serve as the initial dressing for the first 24 hours.

COMPLICATIONS

Patient dissatisfaction with the various procedures used to treat tattoos generally has to do with incomplete pigment removal or adverse scarring. As with most surgical procedures, this dissatifation can usually be prevented by performing a thorough preoperative consultation and evaluation and providing the patient with as much information as possible about the procedure. For every elective procedure, including tattoo removal, it is absolutely imperative that patients do not have unrealistic expectations and that they have given true informed consent based on a complete understanding of the various treatment options and procedures available to them.

Most of the complications associated with common procedures such as dermabrasion, simple excision, staged ex-

cision, excision and grafting, and excision with tissue expansion can also be seen when these same techniques are also used to treat tattoos. Fortunately, these complications, such as hypertrophic scarring (Case 11, Fig. 25–11), are managed in an identical fashion as with other procedures and no special precautions must be taken. However, as previously mentioned, one of the unique complications seen specifically with tattoo removal using the Q-switched lasers is pigment darkening. This occurs most commonly with the cosmetic tattoos[6] but can also be seen with red, green, white, and yellow tattoos as well. In these situations, prevention should be the number one goal since once the tattoo pigment has darkened it may be extremely refractory to subsequent treatment. For this reason, when dealing with cosmetic tattoos that are made from the injection of iron oxide, a small test site in an inconspicuous location should be treated first. Generally, the pigment darkening occurs either immediately or within approximately 30 minutes. Thus, if after that interval no darkening has occurred, the treatment can be continued. For maximal safety, however, it may be advisable to postpone the first treatment for a short interval to ensure that this complication has not oc-

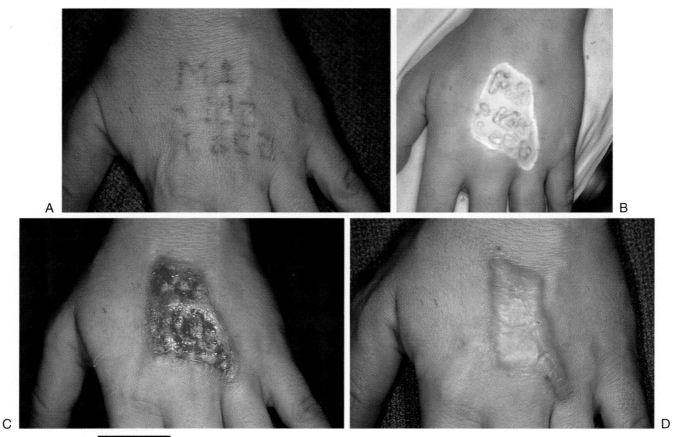

CASE 11

FIGURE 25–11. *A,* Preoperative appearance of an amateur tattoo on the hand. *B,* Complete tattoo pigment removal has been accomplished with carbon dioxide laser vaporization. The shape of the treatment site has been altered so the resultant scar will not duplicate the letters and words of the original tattoo. *C,* The wound has contracted and partially reepithelialized by 4 weeks. *D,* After 4 months, the wound has contracted farther and developed slight hypertrophic scarring, which was treated with intralesional steroid injections, external pressure, and massage.

curred. Finally, whenever lasers are employed for any purpose, there is always a risk of inadvertent injury to the eyes. This potential complication can be eliminated through the use of appropriate eyewear that provides protection against the wavelengths of light being used.[49]

References

1. Goldstein N. Psychological implications of tattoos. J Dermatol Surg Oncol 1979;5:883–888.
2. Levy J, Sewell M, Goldstein N. A short history of tattooing. J Dermatol Surg Oncol 1979;5:851–856.
3. Roberts D. The ice man: Lone voyager from the copper age. Natl Geogr 1993;183:36–67.
4. Kilmer SL, Lee MS, Grevelink JM, et al. The Q-switched Nd:YAG laser effectively treats tattoos: A controlled, dose–response study. Arch Dermatol 1993;129:971–978.
5. Kilmer SL, Anderson RR. Clinical use of the Q-switched ruby and the Q-switched Nd:YAG (1064 nm and 532 nm) lasers for treatment of tattoos. J Dermatol Surg Oncol 1993;19:330–338.
6. Anderson RR, Geronemus R, Kilmer SL, et al. Cosmetic tattoo ink darkening: A complication of Q-switched and pulsed-laser treatment. Arch Dermatol 1993;129:1010–1014.
7. Agris J. Traumatic tattooing. J Trauma 1976;16:798–802.
8. Hanke CW, Conner AC, Probst EL Jr, Fondak AA. Blast tattoos resulting from black powder firearms. J Am Acad Dermatol 1987;17:819–825.
9. Bailey BN. Treatment of tattoos. Plast Reconstr Surg 1967;40:361–371.
10. Harrison PV. The surgical removal of amateur tattoos. Clin Exp Dermatol 1985;10:540–544.
11. Roenigk RK, Wheeland RG. Tissue expansion in cicatricial alopecia. Arch Dermatol 1987;123:641–646.
12. Zimmerman MC. Suits for malpractice based on alleged unsightly scars resulting from removal of tattoos. J Dermatol Surg Oncol 1979;5:911–912.
13. Dvir E, Hirshowitz B. Tattoo removal by cryosurgery. Plast Reconstr Surg 1980;66:373–378.
14. Colver GB, Dawber RP. Tattoo removal using a liquid nitrogen cryospray. Clin Exp Dermatol 1984;9:364–366.
15. Scutt RWB. The chemical removal of tattoos. Br J Plast Surg 1972;25:189–194.
16. Penoff JH. The office treatment of tattoos: A simple and effective method. Plast Reconstr Surg 1987;79:186–191.
17. Fogh H, Wulf HC, Poulsen T, Larsen P. Tattoo removal by overtattooing with tannic acid. J Dermatol Surg Oncol 1989;15:1089–1090.
18. Stegman SJ, Tromovitch TA. Cosmetic dermatologic surgery. Arch Dermatol 1982;118:1013–1016.
19. Bailin PL, Ratz JL, Levine HL. Removal of tattoos by CO_2 laser. J Dermatol Surg Oncol 1980;6:997–1001.
20. Apfelberg DB, Maser MR, Lash H, et al. Comparison of argon and carbon dioxide laser treatment of decorative tattoos: A preliminary report. Ann Plast Surg 1985;14:6–15.
21. Dismukes DE. The "chemo-laser" technique for the treatment of decorative tattoos: A more complete dye-removal procedure. Lasers Surg Med 1986;6:59–61.
22. Ruiz-Esparza J, Goldman MP, Fitzpatrick RE. Tattoo removal with minimal scarring: The chemo-laser technique. J Dermatol Surg Oncol 1988;14:1372–1376.
23. Crittenden FM. Salabrasion: Removal of tattoos by superficial abrasion with table salt. Cutis 1971;7:295–300.
24. Manchester GH. Removal of commercial tattoos by abrasion with table salt. Plast Reconstr Surg 1974;53:517–521.
25. Koerber WA Jr, Price NM. Salabrasion of tattoos: A correlation of the clinical and histological results. Arch Dermatol 1978;114:884–888.
26. Chai KB. The decorative tattoo: Its removal by dermabrasion. Plast Reconstr Surg 1963;32:559–563.
27. Clabaugh W. Removal of tattoos by superficial dermabrasion. Arch Dermatol 1968;98:515–521.
28. Ceilley RI. Curettage after dermabrasion: Techniques of removal of tattoos. J Dermatol Surg Oncol 1979;5:905.
29. Colver GB, Cherry GW, Dawber RPR, Ryan TJ. Tattoo removal using infrared coagulation. Br J Dermatol 1985;112:481.
30. Groot DW, Arlette JP, Johnston PA. Comparison of the infrared coagulator and the carbon dioxide laser in the removal of decorative tattoos. J Am Acad Dermatol 1986;15:518–522.
31. Wheeland RG, Norwood OT, Roundtree JM. Tattoo removal using serial tangential excision and polyurethane membrane dressing. J Dermatol Surg Oncol 1983;9:822–826.
32. Goldman L, Wilson RG, Hornby P, et al. Radiation from a Q-switched ruby laser: Effect of repeated impacts of power output of 10 megawatts on a tattoo of man. J Invest Dermatol 1965;44:69–71.
33. Reid WH, McLeod PJ, Ritchie A, et al. Q-switched ruby laser treatment of black tattoos. Br J Plast Surg 1983;36:455–459.
34. Taylor CR, Gange RW, Dover JS, et al. Treatment of tattoos by Q-switched ruby laser: A dose–response study. Arch Dermatol 1990;126:893–899.
35. Scheibner A, Kenny G, White W, Wheeland RG. A superior method of tattoo removal using the Q-switched ruby laser. J Dermatol Surg Oncol 1990;16:1091–1098.
36. Fitzpatrick RE, Ruiz-Esparza J, Goldman MP. The alexandrite laser for tattoos: A preliminary report. Lasers Surg Med 1992;12s:72.
37. Taylor CR, Anderson RR, Gange RW, et al. Light and electron microscopic analysis of tattoos treated by Q-switched ruby laser. J Invest Dermatol 1991;97:131–136.
38. Kaufmann R. The mini-punch technic: A method for late removal of traumatic facial tattooing. Hautarzt 1990;41:149–150.
39. Quan MB, Wheeland RG. Treatment of traumatic tattoos using the Q-switched Nd:YAG laser. J Dermatol Surg Oncol, in press.
40. Altemus DA. Unusual tattoo reaction may be a first. Cosmet Dermatol 1993;6:38–40.
41. Goldstein N. Complications from tattoos. J Dermatol Surg Oncol 1979;5:869–878.
42. Biro L, Klein WP. Unusual complications of mercurial (cinnabar) tattoo. Arch Dermatol 1967;96:2.
43. Kyanko NE, Pontasch MJ, Brodell RT. Red tattoo reactions: Treatment with the carbon dioxide laser. J Dermatol Surg Oncol 1989;15:652–656.
44. Brodell RT. Retattooing after the treatment of a red tattoo reaction with the CO_2 laser. J Dermatol Surg Oncol 1990;16:771.
45. Ravits HG. Allergic tattoo granuloma. Arch Dermatol 1962;86:287–289.
46. Schwartz RA, Mathias EG, Miller CH, et al. Granulomatous reaction to purple tattoo pigment. Contact Dermatol 1987;16:199–202.
47. Koranda FC, Norris CW, Diestelmeier MF. Carbon dioxide laser treatment of granulomatous reactions in tattoos. Otolaryngol Head Neck Surg 1986;94:384–387.
48. Anderson RR, Parrish JA. Selective photothermolysis: Precise microsurgery by selective absorption of pulsed irradiation. Science 1983;220:524–527.
49. Wheeland RG, Bailin PL, Ratz JL, Schreffler DE. Use of scleral eye shields for periorbital laser surgery. J Dermatol Surg Oncol 1987;13:156–158.

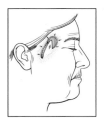

chapter 26

Sclerotherapy

ROBERT A. WEISS

Sclerotherapy, a procedure most commonly employed for treatment of superficial telangiectases and venulectases, is performed by direct injection of a small quantity of an irritating solution into an abnormally enlarged or stretched vein with immediate application of compression to keep the solution in contact with the endothelium and the sclerosant within the injection site. The solution disrupts the endothelium and penetrates further into the vessel wall, causing vessel wall destruction and edema within minutes.[1-3] An intravascular coagulum is subsequently formed by red blood cells in the vessel lumen. Weeks to months may pass before disappearance of the treated vessel by histiocyte digestion. Progress may be monitored by a combination of physical examination and Doppler ultrasonography. Sclerotherapy may also be used to treat larger varicosities as long as certain guidelines are followed[4,5] (Tables 26–1 and 26–2).

The materials and instruments required to treat telangiectases, venulectases, and varicosities by sclerotherapy include 3-mL syringes, transparent-hub 27- and 30-gauge needles, cotton balls for immediate compression, and tape to affix the cotton balls to the injection site. Tapes most commonly used include hypoallergenic paper tape and Transpore tape. After the application of cotton balls, graduated compression is applied to the entire leg.[4] This may

TABLE 26-1. Principles of Varicose Vein Sclerotherapy

Larger veins treated before smaller veins
Proceed from most proximal veins distally
Reflux points determined initially and treated specifically
Vein must be emptied of blood by various maneuvers before injection
Direct finger pressure in a spreading and compressing motion after injection
Entire varicosity is treated at one session
Immediate and adequate compression

TABLE 26-2. Sclerotherapy: Indications, Contraindications, Limitations

Indications
Varicose veins: source of reflux must be monitored
Reticular veins
Telangiectasia: causative source of reflux must be eliminated simultaneously

Contraindications
Bedridden patient
Severe arterial obstruction
Diabetes (severity dependent)
History of deep venous obstruction
Allergy to sclerosing agent or urticaria after previous treatment
Hypercoagulable states may predispose to thrombosis extending into the deep system
Pregnancy (compression is treatment of choice)
Poor tolerance of support hose

Limitations
Reflux at saphenofemoral junction
Reflux at saphenopopliteal junction
High rate of blood flow such as arterial spider angiomas
Recurrence or new varicosity formation likely over time
Exogenous estrogen or progesterone may decrease procedure effectiveness

be accomplished by expert wrapping with a short stretch compression bandage such as Comprilan. Graduated compression is accomplished by the application of an increased number of layers at the ankle with decreasing layers as the wrap is applied up to the thigh.

More commonly employed are support hose that are manufactured to provide graduated compression to precisely defined pressures at the ankles. Manufacturers of support hose are listed in Table 26–3. Guidelines for selection of degrees of compression for various sites and sizes of vessels are listed in Table 26–4.

PRINCIPLES AND GUIDELINES FOR DOPPLER ULTRASONOGRAPHY

Continuous-wave Doppler ultrasonography emits a continuous beam of ultrasound waves that detect red blood cells moving within the targeted vein or artery. Optimal frequencies for examining superficial vessels are 8 to 10 MHz while deeper vessels require a lower frequency of 4 to 5 MHz.[6,7] A probe angle of 30 to 45 degrees relative to blood flow yields the most consistent waveform height since flow velocity waveform relates to the probe angle.[6]

The venous system is a series of wide channels experiencing slow flow, unlike the high-pressure contractile pipes of the arterial system. Venous flow is generated by muscle contractions occurring at irregular intervals. At rest, spontaneous flow signals are difficult to hear by Doppler ultrasonography. Exceptions are large veins in the groin communicating with abdominal veins that are influenced by excursions of the diaphragm (S or spontaneous sounds). To generate or augment an audible signal of flow, a maneuver such as manual compression of the calf to simulate muscle contraction must be performed by the examiner (A or augmented sounds). When compression is released, gravitational hydrostatic pressure causes reverse flow to cease within 0.5 to 1.5 seconds when valves are competent, but a long flow sound is audible when valves are incompetent (Fig. 26–1).

TABLE 26–3. Support Hose Manufacturers

Jobst
Jobst (A Beiersdorf Company)
P.O. Box 471048, 5825 Carnegie Blvd.
Charlotte, NC 28247-1048
704-554-9933

Sigvaris
Sigvaris
P.O. Box 570, 32 Park Drive East
Branford, CT 06405
800-322-7744

JUZO
Julius Zorn, Inc.
P.O. Box 1088
Cuyahoga Falls, OH 44223
800-222-4999

Medi
Medi USA, L.P.
76 W. Seegers Rd.
Arlington Heights, IL 60005
800-633-6334

Venosan
Venosan North America, Inc.
1617 North Fayetteville Street
PO Box 4068
Asheboro, NC 27204-4068

SEQUENCE OF DOPPLER ULTRASONOGRAPHY

Groin and Thigh

With the patient standing or sitting up and using the 4 to 5-MHz transducer in a warm room, examination begins in the medial groin at the inguinal ligament by locating the femoral arterial signal. Moving the transducer slightly medially over the common femoral vein, one may hear normal respiratory excursions of venous flow. Distal manual thigh compression with the hand not holding the transducer briefly enhances the signal. The patient is then requested to perform a Valsalva maneuver. A long reflux sound is indicative of femoral venous reflux, which can be confirmed with a duplex ultrasound examination.

TABLE 26–4. Sclerotherapy: General Guidelines for Compression

Vessel Type	Compression Type
Telangiectasia (nonprotuberant) not associated with reticular veins	Transpore tape with cotton balls for 24 hours
Telangiectasia (protuberant) associated or not associated with reticular vein	Graduated compression hose of 15 to 18 mm Hg for 1 to 2 weeks with Transpore tape over cotton balls. Cotton balls are removed after 24 hours.
Reticular veins up to 3 mm	Graduated compression hose 15 to 18 mm Hg for 1 to 2 weeks. Cotton balls with tape at injection sites are removed after 24 hours.
Larger reticular veins 4 to 6 mm or minor varicose veins (<6 mm)	Graduated compression hose 20 to 30 mm Hg for 2 weeks. Cotton balls with tape at injection sites are removed after 24 hours.
Varicose veins (>6 mm)	Graduated compression hose 30 to 40 mm Hg for 2 weeks. Foam pads over injection site are held by short stretch bandage for 3 days.

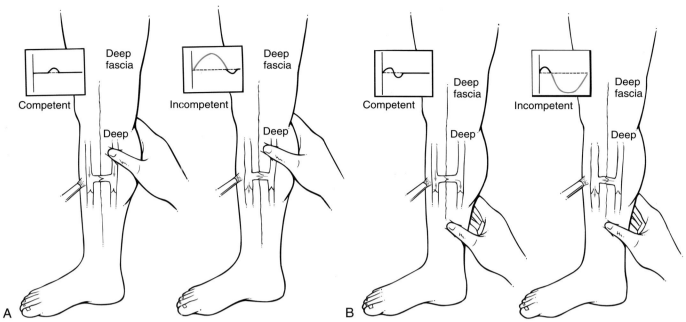

FIGURE 26–1. Principles of venous Doppler examination. *A*, Proximal compression phase. During proximal compression with competent valves, a brief sound is heard (*inset*) that rapidly concludes as blood movement is stopped by competent valves. When incompetent valves are present, a long sound is heard (*inset*) as blood movement (*red arrow*) is detected through a wide-open incompetent valve. The sound continues as long as compression is applied. As compression is released, flow stops. *B*, Distal compression phase. With competent valves, brief normal forward flow is heard. As distal compression is released, blood flows backward under gravity but is rapidly stopped by competent valves. With incompetent valves, a brief normal upward flow is heard; however, as distal compression is released, blood flow continues backward (*red arrow*) with a prolonged sound as incompetent valves are unable to prevent continued flow propelled by hydrostatic pressure (gravity). Schematic insets show bidirectional tracings of sounds produced; flow toward the transducer is shown as positive (*red*) while flow away from the transducer is shown as negative. The hand applying compression palpates for fascial defects in the area of incompetent perforators.

After common femoral vein examination, the transducer is moved distally with light pressure approximately 4 cm to listen below the saphenofemoral junction. While performing a short series of thigh compressions to generate venous flow signals, the transducer is moved side to side to locate the greater saphenous vein. Here a 7- to 8-MHz probe is useful. Gentle external compression and release of the thigh *distal* to the transducer should lead to transient increases in signal frequency (amplitude) followed by rapid cessation of signal as competent valves snap shut. When valvular insufficiency at the saphenofemoral junction is present, initial increase in flow is followed by a prolonged back flow signal.

During a Valsalva maneuver, a continuous and pronounced reflux signal is a reliable sign of valvular insufficiency. However, mild and brief reflux can be found in 15% of normal persons.[8] An equivocal result may require a duplex ultrasound examination for a definitive answer.

When varicosities are seen on the upper thigh but Valsalva maneuver is negative for reflux at the saphenofemoral junction, compression and release maneuvers are repeated to identify sources of reflux. Incompetent communications may exist on the upper thigh, causing varicosities of iliac, pudendal, pelvic, or epigastric veins. Most commonly observed are incompetent hunterian perforating veins causing varicosities in the mid thigh where reflux is usually demonstrated by distal compression and release. For superficial varicosities originating in the lower third of the thigh, Dodd perforating veins are suspected. Common sites of perforating veins are shown in Figure 26–2.

Popliteal Fossa and Knee

The popliteal fossa can be a difficult region to evaluate. Many superficial veins traversing the popliteal space may reveal reflux during distal compression and release. The patient is examined while standing with the leg slightly flexed and weight supported on the opposite leg. The probe is positioned at the upper portion of the popliteal space just lateral to the midline. Constant pulsation of the popliteal artery can be heard. The popliteal vein usually lies deep to the artery. Listening for reflux during distal compression and release will be accomplished by background arterial pulsation. If reflux is heard with the 4- to 5-MHz transducer, then deep flux is probably present. By moving slightly distally, many venous sounds may be heard since gastrocnemius veins, posterior tibial veins, and peroneal veins all converge within a relatively short distance.

At about midportion of the popliteal space, switching to an 8-MHz probe, a similar sequence of external compression and release can be performed for the lesser saphenous vein beginning at its junction with the popliteal vein. Light compression of the calf distal to the Doppler probe is the best method to demonstrate reflux. The Valsalva maneuver is less reliable in this area since proximal valves are often competent. Because the lesser, or short, saphenous vein runs a course down the center of the calf, reflux within it should usually be audible for several centimeters below the saphenopopliteal junction. Only theoretically can this be distinguished from deep reflux. Occasionally, the lesser saphenous vein extends far proximally before terminating into the deep system. The lesser saphenous vein occasionally terminates in the greater saphenous vein on the mid to upper medial thigh through the vein of Giacomini. Distally, the lesser saphenous vein can be followed to its origin just posterior to the lateral malleolus.

On the anteromedial leg, the important site to examine by Doppler is Boyd's perforator group. Located medial to the tibia several centimeters below the knee, this is the *most common site for spontaneous appearance of primary varicose veins*. This region must be investigated for reflux by distal compression and release.

Ankle

The deep veins at the ankle are actually quite close to the surface, often communicate with the posterior arch vein, and can be heard with an 8-MHz probe (legs dependent). Strict adherence to anatomic landmarks should differentiate these from superficial veins. Reflux within the deep system at the ankle is important in evaluation of patients with venous ulceration. The posterior tibial veins lie just posterior to the medial malleolus and surround the posterior tibial artery. Arterial pulsatile sounds are identified, and then distal compression is applied to the foot, or proximal compression to the calf, to identify flow and reflux in these deep veins.

Perforating veins at the ankle of greatest concern are Cockett's perforators and the retromalleolar and inframalleolar perforators. These perforating veins are in communication with the posterior arch vein. Varicosities on the medial ankle can often be traced to reflux in Cockett's perforators. The deep purple "corona phlebectasia" on the dorsal foot can often be traced to reflux in the inframalleolar perforators.

PHOTOPLETHYSMOGRAPHY

The term *plethysmography* describes a number of techniques used to measure volume changes. These are particularly useful to measure the entire venous volume of the leg or selected parts of the venous system. A plethysmograph consists of a mechanism to sense displacement and a modifying unit (transducer), which translates changes from a displacement-sensing device into another form of energy, which is then recorded. Photoplethysmography (PPG) requires a light-emitting diode and a receiving diode to measure changes in blood volume in the subcutaneous venous plexus. These volume changes reflect regional venous volume changes rather than volume changes of the entire leg.[9]

PPG permits quantification of the physiologic significance of Doppler findings, while venous Doppler ultrasonography is used to detect exact sites of valvular incompetence. PPG allows differentiation between superficial and deep venous insufficiency plus has the additional advantage of independence from examiner experience, as is the case with Doppler ultrasound examination.[10,11]

With PPG, a single photoelectric light source illuminates a small area of skin and an adjacent photoelectric sensor measures the reflectance of light.[12] Near infrared (940 nm) is suited for optimal measurement of skin blood content because epidermal absorption at this wavelength is limited to 15% of emitted light. In 1982, Wienert and Blazek[13] introduced an improved device called light reflection rheography (LRR), which decreased variation from surface reflection or external light. LRR included three light diodes rather than one to illuminate the whole venous plexus of a small area of skin with a single sensor measuring the light reflectance and an additional sensor measuring skin temperature.[14] The amount of reflectance was related to the blood volume in the area of the probe. In practice, PPG and LRR yield equivalent results except for a steadier baseline with LRR. Recent advances have led to greater

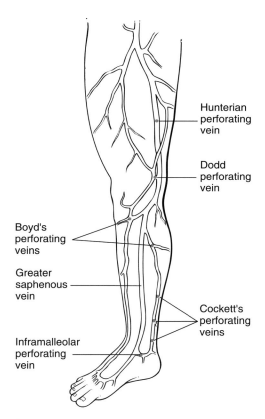

FIGURE 26–2. Common anatomic sites of perforating veins. Inframalleolar perforator incompetence causes the "corona phlebectasia" of multiple purple venulectases on the dorsum of the foot. Cockett's perforators are a group on the medial ankle associated with tributaries of the greater saphenous vein. Boyd's perforator group may be directly associated with the greater saphenous vein or its tributaries. This site is the most common for development of spontaneous primary varicosities in patients genetically susceptible. Hunterian and Dodd perforating vein incompetence must be distinguished from incompetence at the saphenofemoral junction to develop a logical treatment plan.

Labels in figure:
Hunterian perforating vein
Dodd perforating vein
Boyd's perforating veins
Greater saphenous vein
Inframalleolar perforating vein
Cockett's perforating veins

reliability with digital PPG (D-PPG; ELCAT GmbH, Wolfratshausen, Germany) in which a dedicated microprocessor standardizes the signal received by the photoelectric sensor.[15] This arrangement leads to a reproducible, standardized baseline regardless of skin thickness or pigmentation allowing quantitative rather than qualitative venous pump measurements.[15,16] An additional advantage is the ability to follow improvements in venous function after treatment.[16]

For PPG examination, the patient sits relaxed with the knees bent at a 110- to 120-degree angle. By convention, a small probe containing light-emitting and sensing diodes is taped to the medial aspect of the lower leg 8 to 10 cm (4 fingerwidths) above the medial malleolus. After resting the leg for several minutes to establish a constant baseline, the patient then dorsiflexes the foot eight to ten times, activating the calf muscle pump and effecting drainage of the venous system. As the skin venous plexus empties, it causes increased reflectance of light. A tracing is made of the changes in reflected light from the skin under the probe (Fig. 26–3). After the calf muscle pumping ceases, blood refills the skin plexus, which absorbs increasing amounts

of light and venules fill. A direct relationship is assumed between filling of deep leg veins and filling of veins measured in the skin. Excellent correlation of vessel surface filling time (PPG refill time) with direct invasive pressure refill time has been shown.[17] The PPG tracing returns to its initial resting value as the calf venous system refills. A refill time shorter than 25 seconds indicates venous valvular insufficiency. Longer refill times indicate normal venous valve function. Table 26–5 shows suggested standard interpretations of PPG refill times.

When the initial test indicates a refill time less than 25 seconds, the test is repeated at 80 to 100 mm Hg with a tourniquet placed 1 inch above the knee. The refill time should return to normal if the source of reflux is in the superficial system. If the PPG/LRR refill time remains less than 25 seconds with the above-knee tourniquet, the test is repeated with a tourniquet below the knee. Repeating the PPG with a below-knee tourniquet is especially indicated if varicosities are observed near calf or ankle perforating veins. The refill time should normalize if reflux is from the superficial system. A PPG examination that does not nor-

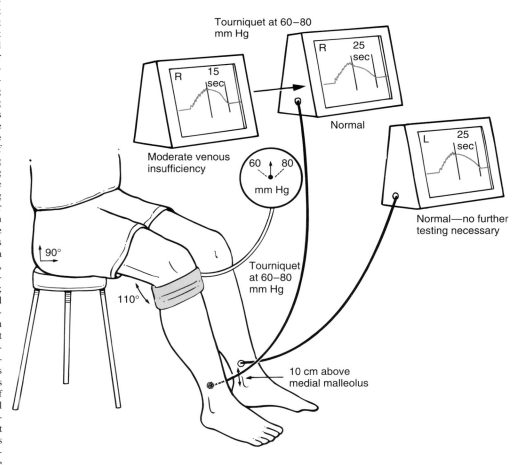

FIGURE 26–3. Photoplethysmography. By convention, the patient sits with the knees bent at a 110- to 120-degree angle. A small probe containing a photoelectric light source is taped to the medial aspect of the lower leg 8 to 10 cm (about four fingerwidths) above the medial malleolus. After resting the leg for several minutes to establish a constant baseline, the patient then dorsiflexes the foot 10 times, activating the calf muscle pump and effecting drainage of the calf deep venous system. A tracing is made of the changes in color intensity of the skin under the probe. After the calf muscle pumping ceases, the tracing slowly returns to its initial resting value as the calf veins refill. Here the left leg is normal, with refilling time longer than 25 seconds after 10 dorsiflexions at the ankle (shown as 10 slowly rising peaks on the tracing). The right leg indicates venous valvular insufficiency with a 15-second refill time. On the right, the test is repeated with a below-knee tourniquet at 60 to 80 mm Hg; the repeat tracing shows a refill time of 25 seconds, which is considered normal. This examination shows the deep valves competent with reflux occurring in the superficial veins on the right. A correctable photoplethysmography predicts that elimination of the varicosities will normalize venous function of the involved leg. T_0 equals the total refill time and has been internationally standardized. V_0, the highest point of the pump curve, equals venous pump power and is a quantitative measurement only for the microprocessor-controlled digital photoplethysmography (see Table 26–5).

malize by application of tourniquets requires further investigation by duplex ultrasonography or other methods before treatment is initiated.

The PPG may give abnormal readings when ankle joint mobility is reduced or when arterial occlusive disease prevents normal inflow to the skin.[8] Present uses of PPG/LRR include (1) forecasting outcome of elimination of varicosities; (2) observing pumping ability of the deep venous system of the calf; and (3) evaluating the success of treatment.

DUPLEX ULTRASONOGRAPHY

The ultimate in noninvasive examination of the venous system is duplex ultrasonography. This allows direct visualization of the veins and identification of flow through venous valves. An image is created by an array of Doppler transducers that are switched on and off sequentially. This is combined with a method to echo-pulse a Doppler signal. The echo-pulse is recorded as a dot that is located on the x and y axes and is brighter in proportion to the intensity of the reflected signal (z axis). This creates a two-dimensional ultrasound image. The Doppler velocity recording allows an image produced by reflection from moving red blood cells to be seen so that blood vessels and flow are shown.[6] Duplex scanning combines echo-pulsing with Doppler velocity recording. Color units have circuitry to indicate flow from the heart in red and toward the heart in blue.

Duplex scanners are found in fully equipped vascular laboratories, but laboratory personnel must be instructed in the examination of the superficial venous system. This must include an assessment of the saphenofemoral junction and the saphenopopliteal junction with the patient standing. A complete duplex ultrasound examination will also map superficial and deep veins with precise identification of sources of venous reflux.[18,19]

Once the evaluation of the patient is complete, the presence and source of significant venous reflux should have been identified. If the patient has significant saphenofemoral reflux, treatment may include surgical control of that reflux before sclerotherapy. Experienced European or Canadian phlebologists may attempt to sclerose the saphenofemoral junction.[20] They have reported a 93% success rate with strong sclerosing solutions not available in the United States.[21-23] However, the most comprehensive comparison of surgery and sclerotherapy caused Hobbs[24] to conclude that saphenous vein insufficiency is best managed by surgery while sclerotherapy is superior for treatment of isolated perforator incompetence. Sclerotherapy, according to Hobbs,[25] is also useful in treatment of residual or recurrent varicose veins after surgery.

TECHNIQUES OF LARGE VEIN SCLEROTHERAPY

The technique presently used most widely is that of Fegan with minor modifications.[4] The patient sits at the end of the examining table with the treated leg dependent. A bulging varicosity is cannulated with a needle, butterfly, or angiocatheter that is held or taped in place. Before

TABLE 26-5. Grades of Venous Insufficiency by Photoplethysmography*

Grade	Refill Time (T_0)	Interpretation
Normal	Greater than 25 seconds	Healthy veins
Grade I	24 to 20 seconds	Slight venous insufficiency
Grade II	19 to 10 seconds	Moderate venous insufficiency
Grade III	Less than 10 seconds	Severe venous insufficiency

* This grading applies only to the "sedentary dorsal extensions" movement routine.

injection, the leg is elevated and supported above cardiac level for 1 to 2 minutes to allow drainage of blood. Then a small amount of blood is drawn back from the syringe to ensure that the needle remains in the varicosity lumen. As the injection of 0.5 to 1.0 mL occurs, finger pressure several centimeters above and below the injection point is applied to confine the action of the sclerosing solution. Finger pressure is maintained for 30 to 60 seconds, followed by the immediate application of compression with a foam pad. The pad is secured by foam-elastic tape or relatively inelastic, wraparound bandage to maintain compression *immediately*. Fegan's method is particularly effective for incompetent perforators. Fascial defects through which perforators course may be palpated and serve as the site of needle entry.

Hobbs[26] believes that multiple puncture sites along the course of a varicosity independent of the perforators lead to varix ablation. When injecting multiple sites along a varicosity, repeat injections are made every 4 to 6 cm until the entire varix has been sclerosed. Cannulation of several sites before injection minimizes inaccessibility of distal segments from postinjection spasm.

Variations of large vessel sclerotherapy include the "air-block technique" in which 0.5 to 1.0 mL of air is injected initially to "clear" the varix of blood[27] or the "foam technique" in which a detergent solution (sodium tetradecyl sulfate [STS]) is shaken for 30 seconds to create a foam.[28] This foam, which develops only in glass syringes, is then injected and allows less volume of sclerosing solution to be used. Theoretically, these techniques enhance contact with the vessel wall, but whether these variations actually improve results remains uncertain.

A widely used variation of Fegan's technique is the marking of varicosities with the patient standing while needle insertion occurs with the patient recumbent (Fig. 26-4, Cases 1 and 2). This minimizes movement of the leg and the inserted needle. To limit possible displacement of the inserted needle but improve likelihood of cannulation, the needle may be inserted with the patient in slight reverse Trendelenburg position on a power table and then moved hydraulically into a venous pressure neutral position. Immediately after injection, the leg can be elevated and compression applied. Direct finger pressure in a spreading and compressing motion outward from both proximal and distal to the injection site is often very useful

FIGURE 26–4. Treatment of varicose veins. *A,* Varicose vein in distribution of Giacomini's vein connecting the greater and the short saphenous veins. Pretreatment Doppler ultrasound examination reveals reflux in this varicose vein segment but absence of reflux at the saphenofemoral or saphenopopliteal junctions. The highest point of reflux correlates with a mid-thigh hunterian perforator. Photoplethysmographic refill time was 20 seconds with normal muscle pump function. A total of 2 mL of 1% sodium tetradecyl sulfate (STS) was injected into several sites along this varicosity. With the patient standing, areas of loud reflux are marked. While the patient is recumbent and the varicosity flattened, the marked areas are specifically cannulated and injected. *B,* Results after two treatments 1 month apart showing good response. Symptoms of focal burning and throbbing subsided within a week after the first injection. Postinjection compression consisted of 2 weeks of 20- to 30-mm Hg graduated compression hose.

FIGURE 26–4. *C,* Varicose vein originating from Dodd's (lower thigh) perforating vein. Pretreatment evaluation with Doppler ultrasonography revealed reflux originating at the highest point seen but absence of reflux at the saphenofemoral or saphenopopliteal junctions. Photoplethysmographic refill time was 35 seconds with normal muscle pump function. Treatment consisted of injection of 1% STS into four sites along this varicosity for a total of 2 mL. After treatment the patient complied with 2 weeks of 30 to 40-mm Hg graduated compression hose. *D,* After two treatments, resolution of this vein is apparent. Long-term follow-up reveals no recurrence after 2 years. Aching after prolonged standing has resolved. The patient continues to wear 15 to 18-mm Hg graduated compression hose daily since she has an occupation that requires a great deal of standing.

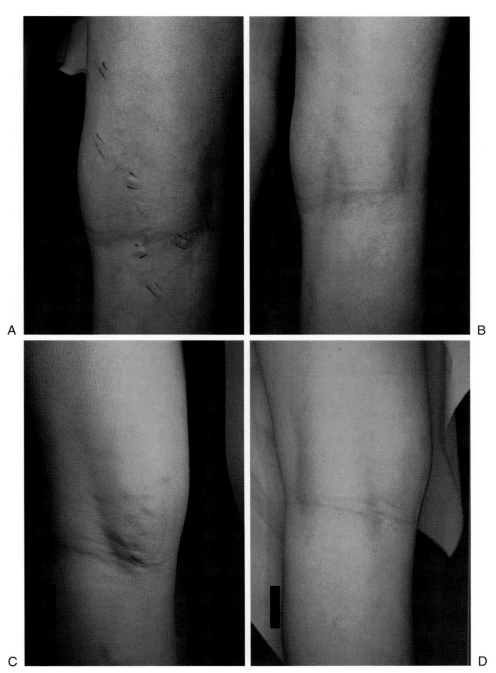

not only to spread the sclerosing solution laterally but also to promote contact with greater endothelial surface area while propelling blood out of the vessel.

A technique frequently used in Europe for sclerosing saphenous junctions is the open-needle Sigg technique.[29,30] A needle not attached to a syringe is inserted into the skin and manipulated until venous blood drips from the hub. Sigg originally advocated further withdrawal of blood by syringe until the vein to be treated was "empty." European phlebologists presently use this open technique to ascertain intravascular placement of the needle and confirmation of venous rather than arterial cannulation.

Rapid, immediate, and adequate compression after injection of sclerosant is very important. For increased compression, bunches of cotton balls may be substituted for foam pads although the use of foam pads (STD-E pads; S.T.D. Pharmaceuticals, Hereford, United Kingdom) probably allows for the strongest, complete, and pressure point free local compression over injection sites. Graduated compression hose, 30 to 40 mm Hg, are usually worn immediately after treatment. These hose are stretched over local compression at the treatment sites. Alternatively, a relatively noncompliant wrap placed to provide graduated compression may be applied. Patients may shower by taping a plastic bag over the compression bandage or stocking.

Although Tournay[31] minimized the importance of compression, several theoretical and practical considerations affirm its necessity. Compression limits flow of blood back into the varicosity, thus decreasing thrombus formation and the tendency for recanalization.[32,33] Additionally, with less thrombus formation, there is less thrombophlebitic reaction and less postsclerosis pigmentation. Compression has been shown to improve the effectiveness with greater resolution per treatment of both small and large varicosities.[34,35] Graduated compression hose also permits the patient complete mobility after treatment and enhances muscle pump function. This rapidly dilutes and removes any sclerosing solution that inadvertently enters the deep system.

The duration of compression is still debated. Fegan[4] recommended 6 weeks, but 3 to 5 days of compression has been suggested as adequate by others.[32,33] A trial comparing compression for 1, 3, and 6 weeks concluded that 3 weeks was optimal,[36] and most phlebologists have patients wear compression hose of 30 to 40 mm Hg for 3 to 6 weeks.

Immediate ambulation after treatment is believed to cause rapid dilution of sclerosing solution, which prevents high concentrations of sclerosing solution from maintaining contact with walls of deep veins. Walking may also lessen risks of deep venous thrombosis by avoiding stagnation of blood flow. In conjunction with graduated compression, ambulation also causes the muscle pump of the calf to reduce venous hypertension in superficial veins by decreasing venous volume. Risks of deep venous thrombosis are also lessened by adhering to the principle of no more than 1.0 mL per injection site, with the usual volume being only 0.5 mL.[37]

TREATMENT OF RETICULAR VARICOSE VEINS

Treatment of reticular veins is very similar to large varicose veins, although the concentration, strength, and volume of sclerosing solution is decreased (Tables 26–6 through 26–8). Subdermic reticular veins are treated only after all sources of reflux have been treated by sclerotherapy and/or surgery. Doppler ultrasonography may also be used as a guide to demonstrate reflux in the reticular veins and to locate those that require treatment.[38] Most reticular veins causing telangiectasia on the lateral thigh and calf are associated with the lateral venous system (Fig. 26–5 and Case 3, Fig. 26–6).[39–41]

With the patient recumbent, the 3-mL syringe with a 27- to 30-gauge needle is inserted into the reticular vein, which is usually superficial and visibly blue; therefore, it usually does not require marking by pen. When the sensation of piercing the vein is felt, the plunger is pulled back gently until blood is seen beginning to back up into the transparent hub. This is possible even with a 30-gauge needle, although a 27-gauge needle is commonly employed. Usually the volume is no more than 0.5 mL per injection site, and it is often considerably less. The sclerosing solution most commonly used is sodium tetradecyl sulfate (STS, Sotradecol) in concentrations of 0.2% to 0.5% (Case 4, Fig. 26–7). Previous reports have suggested that treatment of reticular veins greatly reduces the recurrence rate of telangiectasia associated with them as well as reducing side effects[39] (Case 5, Fig. 26–8; Case 6, Fig. 26–9).

TABLE 26–6. Sclerotherapy: Patient Preoperative Discussion

1. Healing and resolution of the treated area requires a minimum of 4 to 6 weeks but may require months. Your veins may take *multiple* treatments to improve.
2. Appropriate bandaging after the procedure requires total graduated compression of the leg in addition to localized compression with cotton balls or foam rubber pads.
3. Cotton balls are removed within 24 hours, but graduated compression is maintained from 1 to 2 weeks depending on the size of veins treated.
4. Immediate ambulation is requested, but strenuous activity such as high impact aerobics or heavy weight-lifting with your legs is discouraged for 1 week. Hot baths should be avoided for 24 hours.
5. Immediate bruising is expected, which may take several weeks to resolve. Some tenderness of the treated areas may develop but is usually mild, lasts for up to several days, and is easily treated by ibuprofen or similar over-the-counter pain medication. Redness or irritation may develop at the site of tape application. An allergic reaction to the sclerosing solution is possible and results in generalized hives within minutes after injection. A small test dose is administered on the first visit to observe for reactions.
6. Possible complications include failure of the appearance of the veins to improve, development of a pink blush or ''mat'' that can replace the treated vein but will usually spontaneously resolve over months, or development of brown spots at the sites of injection or along the path of a treated vein that may last for months. The brown discoloration may be preceded by accumulations of blood especially in larger veins and is minimized by application of compression. If tender or painful, these bruises may be treated by the doctor by puncture and drainage usually several weeks after the initial treatment. Rarely, this accumulation of blood may form a clot. Although this is trapped in the treated vein but an extremely rare possibility (less than 1%) is the extension of this clot into a deeper vessel. Other possible complications include blistering, secondary infection, ulceration, and scarring, which can occur if the solution leaks out of the treated vein in sufficient quantity. All precautions are taken to minimize this possibility.

TABLE 26-7. Sclerotherapy: Operative Issues

Preoperative Evaluation

History
  Arterial occlusive disease
  Previous trauma to leg
  Family history of large varicose veins
  History of deep venous thrombosis
  Exogenous hormones
  Tolerance of support hose
Physical examination
  Identify varicosities extending into groin
  Identify varicosities extending over long distances
  Examine sites of pain
Diagnostics
  Doppler ultrasonography (determine sites of reflux)
  Photoplethysmography (evaluate deep system and predict results of treatment)

Preoperative Equipment Needs

Isopropyl alcohol to cleanse skin
30- and 27-gauge needles
Sclerosing solutions (see text)
Cotton balls
Tape to secure cotton balls
Support hose or short stretch bandage
Binocular operating loupes (2×–2.5×) with 1.5–2 foot working distance
Doppler ultrasound transducer (8 MHz probe for superficial and 5 MHz for deep)
Photoplethysmography unit (optional but preferred)

Intraoperative Needs

Frequent change of 30-gauge (or 27-gauge) needles
Multiple syringes of sclerosing solutions
Diluent for extravasation (e.g., sterile water for hypertonic saline, 1% lidocaine for Sotradecol), 2%
  nitroglycerin paste (for topical application at suspected extravasation points)

Sclerosing Solutions

Hypertonic Saline. Although approved by the Food and Drug Administration (FDA) only for use as an abortifacient, the most commonly employed solution among dermatologists in the United States is hypertonic saline at a concentration of 23.4%. The advantage of hypertonic saline is its theoretical total lack of allergenicity when unadulter-ated. This agent has been commonly used in various concentrations from 10% to 30%, with the addition of heparin, procaine, or lidocaine. A patented solution, Heparsal, containing 20% hypertonic saline, 100 units/mL of heparin, and 1% procaine was thought to reduce pain and prevent thrombus formation in deep vessels, but a study of 800 patients demonstrated that addition of heparin to hypertonic saline provided no benefit.[42] With claims of pain reduction

TABLE 26-8. Postoperative Care

Pain Management

Compression in treated areas minimizes pain
Ibuprofen or acetaminophen for 3 days to treat localized tenderness

Dressings

Graduated compression bandage or hosiery over cotton balls or foam rubber pads for 1 to 2
  weeks
Cotton balls secured with tape for telangiectasia without associated larger vessels
Cotton balls usually removed within 24–48 hours

Complications

Painful extravasation site treated immediately by infiltration with 1% lidocaine without epinephrine
  and topical application of nitrol paste
Intravascular hematomas or coagula drained by puncture with No. 11 blade or 18-gauge needle
  1 to 3 weeks after treatment
Allergy to sclerosing solution treated by switching to different category of sclerosing solution (e.g.,
  detergent to hypertonic)
Ulceration site treated by daily dressing changes with topical antibiotic and occlusive dressing
  such as polyethylene oxide gel. Occasionally ulcer site is excised and/or grafted
Adhesive tape irritation treated with high-potency topical steroid
Superficial thrombophlebitis treated with graduated compression and nonsteroidal anti-inflamma-
  tory agents for 1 to 2 weeks
Arterial injection must be treated as an emergency with admission for intravenous administration
  of thrombolytic agents

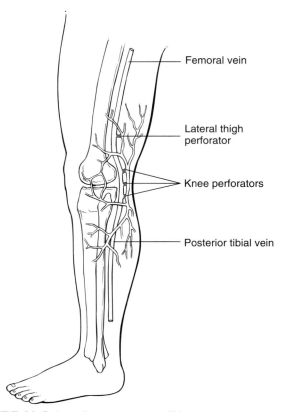

Femoral vein

Lateral thigh
perforator

Knee perforators

Posterior tibial vein

FIGURE 26–5. Lateral venous system. This venous system was first described as separate from the saphenous system responsible for varicosities on the lateral leg by Albanese.[40] A schematic diagram based on Doppler ultrasound findings shows that reflux through incompetent perforating veins (*red*) at the lateral to posterolateral knee transmits increased venous pressure to reticular veins. These expand and transmit pressure to smaller vessels, which become bridges of telangiectatic/venulectatic webs on the thighs and calves. An incompetent small perforating vein (*red*) on the lateral thigh may also contribute to venous hypertension in the subdermic reticular system. These perforators are connected either directly or by means of a network of tributaries to the deep system.[41]

with procaine or lidocaine exaggerated, hypertonic saline is used either unadulterated or diluted to 11.7% with sterile water for smaller telangiectases.[43] A high success rate with hypertonic saline in the treatment of telangiectasia with few complications has been reported in nearly 300 patients[44] (Case 7, Fig. 26–10; Case 8, Fig. 26–11).

Some patients abandon hypertonic saline in spite of the low risk of allergic reactions after experiencing burning pain or muscle cramping immediately after injection. Because hypertonic solutions affect all cells in the path of the osmotic gradient, nerve endings in the vessel adventitia or the underlying muscle may be stimulated, causing a burning pain or a cramping sensation lasting from seconds to minutes and rarely longer than 5 minutes.[44]

With hypertonic solutions, damage of tissue adjacent to injection sites may easily occur. *Large ulcers may be produced by extravasation at the injection site, particularly when injecting the sclerosant very close to the skin surface.* Intradermal injection of 0.1 mL hypertonic saline in rabbit skin produces necrosis.[45] Immediate intense pain on extravasation warns against further injection at the site. Meticulous technique with absolutely minimal extravasation is necessary for the safe use of hypertonic saline.

Hypertonic Dextrose and Hypertonic Saline. Sclerodex (Omega Laboratories, Montreal, Canada) is a mixture of dextrose, 250 mg/mL, sodium chloride, 100 mg/mL, propylene glycol, 100 mg/mL, and phenylethyl alcohol, 8 mg/mL. Sclerodex is a relatively weak sclerosant recommended for local treatment of small vessels, with a total volume of injection not to exceed 10 mL per visit with 0.1 to 1.0 mL per injection site. Sclerodex has been used predominately in Canada and is reported to result in less discomfort than hypertonic saline, although a slightly burning sensation occurs.[46] The lower concentration of saline combined with the nonionic dextrose causes a hypertonic injury without the intense nerve ending stimulation of pure hypertonic saline. Use of Sclerodex has resulted in fewer complications than use of hypertonic saline but in a similar

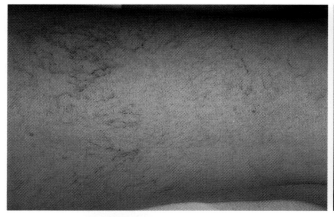
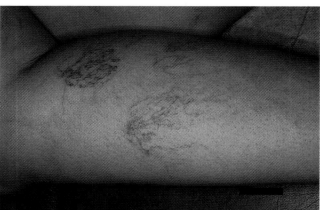

A

B

CASE 3

FIGURE 26–6. *A,* Telangiectatic bridge pattern on the upper lateral thigh. One of the most common patterns, these telangiectases are associated with a subdermic reticular varicosity that demonstrates reflux by Doppler ultrasonography. Reflux can be traced to the lateral knee. *B,* Telangiectatic web pattern on the lateral calf. Treatment must be directed not only toward the telangiectatic web but also toward the associated reticular vein of the lateral subdermic venous system along the lateral calf. Reflux originates at the lateral knee.

incidence of pigmentation as compared with use of polidocanol and STS.[47] The advantage of decreased pain on injection is slightly offset by the potential increased allergenicity of the phenylethyl alcohol component of Sclerodex, with a reported incidence of allergic reactions of 1 in 500.[46] Use in the United States must await FDA approval.

Polidocanol. Although polidocanol (Aethoxysklerol, Chemische Fabrik Kreussler & Co, Wiesbaden-Biebrich, West Germany; Aetoxisclerol, Laboratories Pharmaceutiques Dexo, Nanterre, France; Sclerovein, Resinag AG, Zurich, Switzerland), a urethane compound, was originally developed as an anesthetic, it was found to have the property of sclerosing small-diameter vessels after intradermal injection. Polidocanol contains hydroxypolyethoxydodecane dissolved in distilled water with 5% ethanol as a stabilizer. First used as a sclerosing agent in the late 1960s in Germany, polidocanol is popular worldwide due to a painless injection and the extremely rare incidence of cutaneous necrosis with intradermal injection.[45,48] Polidocanol, however, is *not* approved by the FDA, and its use is presently prohibited in the United States.

In the rabbit ear dorsal vein model, 1% polidocanol is equivalent to 0.5% STS and hypertonic saline.[49] By extrapolating from several clinical studies, when used on human telangiectases 0.5% polidocanol appears to be equivalent to hypertonic saline and 0.1% to 0.2% STS. The higher incidence of hyperpigmentation with 1% polidocanol, compared with hypertonic saline indicates that 1% polidocanol is a stronger sclerosant than hypertonic saline.[50] Lower concentrations of polidocanol have demonstrated a lower incidence of hyperpigmentation than hypertonic saline or STS.

Sodium Tetradecyl Sulfate. STS (Sotradecol, Wyeth-Ayerst Labs, Philadelphia, PA; S.T.D. Injection, S.T.D. Pharmaceuticals, London, England; Thromboject, Omega Laboratories, Montreal, Canada) is a long-chain fatty acid salt with strong detergent properties. It is a very effective sclerosing agent approved by the FDA. Although popular

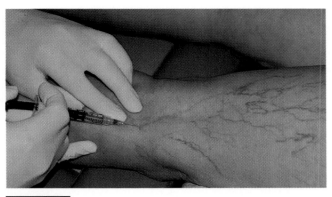

CASE 4

FIGURE 26–7. Proper injection technique. After noninvasive testing demonstrates the absence of reflux at the major junctions of the superficial system and no deep venous disease, the patient may be treated. Reticular varicosity associated with telangiectatic webs demonstrating reflux by Doppler ultrasonography is cannulated with a 30-gauge needle bent approximately 30 degrees. Blood is aspirated into the transparent needle hub to confirm intravascular positioning. The fingers of the nondominant hand stretch and fix the skin. The thumb or forefinger of the nondominant hand can be used as a support for the needle to allow small movements forward and backward (analogous to movement of a cue stick in billiards) for fine adjustments of needle position. After injection of no more than 0.5 mL of sclerosing solution, the telangiectases may be cannulated and injected.

with vascular surgeons since the 1960s[4,24,51] and first described for use in telangiectasia in the 1970s,[52] STS has been unpopular with dermatologists until recently. This is probably because of the relatively high incidence of postsclerosis pigmentation reported at a 1% STS concentration and the possibility of cutaneous necrosis even in the absence of recognized extravasation.[53] Cutaneous necrosis as high as 60% to 70% with 1% STS can be reduced to 3%

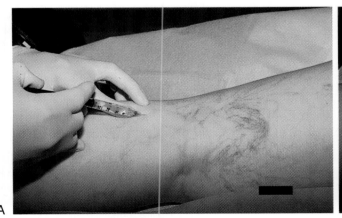

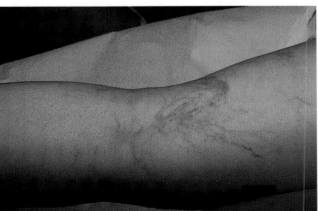

A   B

CASE 5

FIGURE 26–8. Immediate appearance of reticular veins after successful injection. *A,* Injection of reticular network with 0.5% sodium tetradecyl sulfate into three sites separated by 3 to 4 cm with 0.5 mL injected per site. *B,* Reticular veins respond by immediate vasoconstriction. Some sclerosing solution has entered the telangiectatic webs without direct injection. These appear more erythematous.

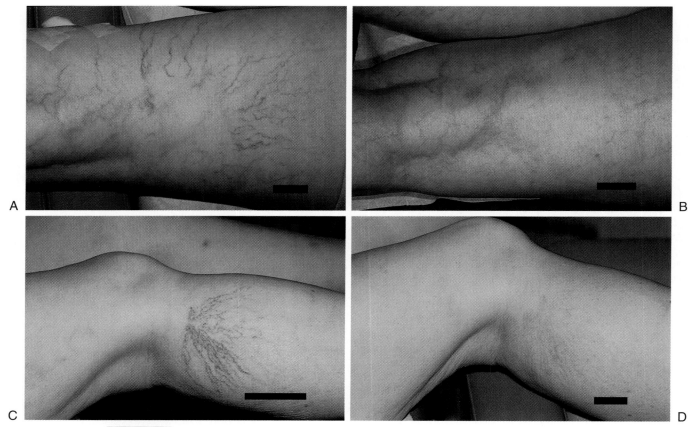

CASE 6

FIGURE 26–9. Short-term results of sclerotherapy of telangiectasia. *A,* Before treatment, typical bridge of telangiectasia with source of reflux through reticular veins on the posterolateral thigh. *B,* Three months after a single treatment with 3 mL of 0.5% sodium tetradecyl sulfate (STS) into the reticular network (no more than 0.5 mL per injection site) and supplemental injection of telangiectases at 6 sites with a total of 0.5 mL of 0.1% STS. Excellent resolution with some residual hyperpigmentation in the largest reticular vein, which required another 6 months to resolve. Compression after treatment consisted of 20- to 30-mm Hg graduated compression hose worn for 2 weeks. *C,* Lateral calf telangiectatic web attributed to lateral subdermic venous system reflux measured by Doppler ultrasonography. *D,* Two months after treatment with 2 mL total of 0.5% STS into reticular veins and supplemental injection of 0.5 mL total of 0.1% STS into base of telangiectatic web directly. Excellent results were obtained, but an additional treatment of 0.1% STS directly into telangiectases was necessary for complete resolution.

by using 0.33% STS.[53] Intradermal injection of 0.5% STS (0.1 mL) into rabbit skin leads to dermal and epidermal necrosis.[45] Although noted to cause allergic reactions such as generalized urticaria, bronchospasm, anaphylactic shock, and even death, the actual incidence of allergic reactions has been estimated at approximately 0.3%.[2,54] Fegan[55] reports 15 cases out of 16,000 in which a stinging pain in the skin with erythema developed 30 to 90 minutes after injection but no anaphylactic reactions. Fegan's positive experience with such large numbers of patients indicates that STS is a relatively safe sclerosing solution.

Interpretation of available data leads to recommendations of use of 0.1% to 0.2% for telangiectases up to 1 mm, 0.2% to 0.5% in reticular veins or small varicosities (1–3 mm diameter), and 0.5% to 3% in larger varicosities related to major sites of valvular reflux. The maximum recommended dosage per treatment session in the package insert is 10 ml of 3% solution.

Sodium Morrhuate. Sodium morrhuate (Scleromate, Palisades Pharmaceuticals, Tenafly, NJ) is a 5% solution of the salts of saturated and unsaturated fatty acids in cod liver oil. Approximately 10% of its fatty acid composition is unknown, and its use by dermatologic surgeons is limited by reports of fatalities secondary to anaphylaxis.[56,57] This agent is used primarily for sclerosis of esophageal varices, but complications including allergic reactions are reported as high as 17% to 48%.[58]

Although sodium morrhuate is approved by the FDA for the sclerosis of varicose veins, use in treatment of telangiectasia is not recommended because of the caustic qualities, with an increased potential for cutaneous necrosis compared with other available solutions.

Chemical Irritants. The chemical irritants polyiodinated iodine (very strong) and chromated glycerine (very weak) are believed to have a direct toxic effect on the endothelium with injury confined primarily around the injection

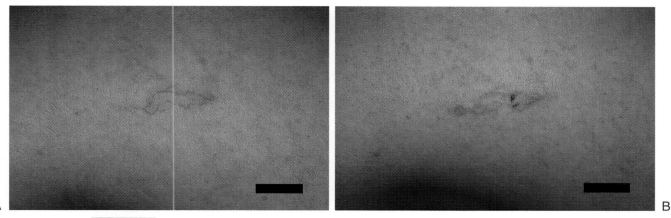

CASE 7

FIGURE 26-10. Immediate appearance of telangiectasia after successful injection. *A,* Before injection. *B,* Five minutes after injection. Urticarial and erythematous appearance after injection with 0.05 mL of hypertonic saline. Urticarial appearance is least apparent with sodium tetradecyl sulfate.

site. After injection of polyiodinated iodine (Varigloban), the endothelium is destroyed within seconds only near the site of injection because of rapid inactivation, exposing the subendothelial layers on which fibrin is rapidly deposited.[58] At the sites of endothelial destruction the chemical can penetrate farther and diffuse into deeper layers of the vessel wall, causing further destruction. A preliminary study indicates that no activation of blood coagulation occurs with sodium iodine, indicating little risk for propagation of a thrombus.[59] The chemical irritants may yet turn out to be the most specific sclerosing agents, targeting injury to the site of injection by quick inactivation by blood proteins accompanied by minimal thrombus formation and deep diffusion into the vessel wall. Use of chemical irritants is presently prohibited in the United States because of lack of FDA approval.

Side Effects

Postsclerotherapy Hyperpigmentation. Postsclerosis pigmentation is defined as the appearance of increased visible pigmentation along the course of a treated vein of any size (see Fig. 26-9). This pigmentation may be the result of sclerotherapy but may also preexist overlying a varicosity to be treated; in this case pretreatment photographs are invaluable. Perivascular hemosiderin deposition and not increased melanin production causes postsclerosis pigmentation.[60] The incidence of pigmentation is variable and has been reported to be dependent on both the dilution and the type of sclerosing agent as well as on the diameter of the treated vessel, with smaller vessels having decreased frequency.[50] The incidence in the treatment of telangiectasia has been reported to be from 11% to 30% using hypertonic

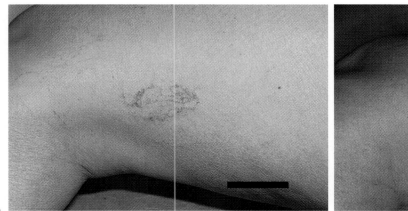
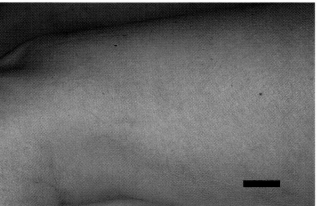

CASE 8

FIGURE 26-11. Long-term results after sclerotherapy. *A,* Appearance before treatment. *B,* Appearance $1\frac{1}{2}$ years after two treatments with hypertonic saline separated by 1 month, 0.1 mL per treatment. The treated area of telangiectases remains resolved. No associated reticular varicosity could be located by Doppler examination or visual inspection.

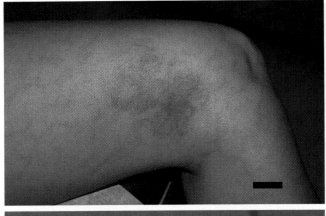

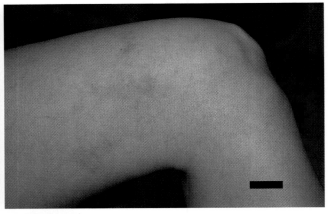

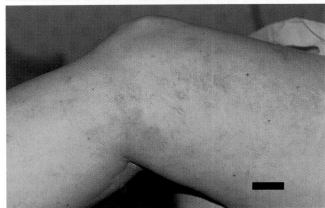

FIGURE 26–12. Telangiectatic matting. *A,* One month after sclerotherapy with 1% polidocanol to a telangiectatic web on the medial thigh, the patient returned with a worsened appearance with many more telangiectases. *B,* Subsequent treatment with 0.2% sodium tetradecyl sulfate into reticular veins identified visually and by Doppler ultrasonography resulted in improvement. Further improvement has occurred over time without additional intervention.

FIGURE 26–12. *C,* Similar matting on the medial thigh in another patient resolved with time and treatment of reticular veins transmitting pressure into the region. The medial thigh appears to be particularly susceptible to telangiectatic matting.

saline,[44,61] 11% to 30% with polidocanol,[62,63] and 30% with STS.[64] Use of 1% STS for treatment of telangiectasia causes a nearly 80% incidence of pigmentation,[52] while with 0.1% STS incidence of pigmentation can be lowered to 11%, comparable to 0.5% polidocanol and hypertonic saline.[50] The incidence of pigmentation may be reduced in varicose veins by expressing the dark, viscous blood thought to be a liquefied coagulum or intravascular hematoma that may accumulate 1 to 4 weeks after sclerotherapy.[30,65]

Pigmentation usually lasts for months but may last for up to 5 years. Follow-up for 1 year in 113 patients in one study demonstrated spontaneous resolution of pigmentation in 70% within 6 months with rare persistence for more than a year.[50] Attempts to hasten resolution of pigmentation have been mostly unsuccessful since the pigment is dermal hemosiderin and not epidermal melanin. Bleaching agents, exfoliants such as trichloroacetic acid or phenol, and cryotherapy have achieved limited success.

Telangiectatic Matting. Telangiectatic matting is defined as the appearance of groups of new, fine (<0.2 mm diameter) telangiectases surrounding a previously treated area in a blush-like manner (Cases 9 and 10, Fig. 26–12). A retrospective analysis of over 2000 patients reports an incidence of 16% in patients treated with hypertonic saline and polidocanol.[66] Resolution usually occurs spontaneously within a 3- to 12-month period, with 70% to 80% spontaneous resolution within the first 6 months.[50,67] Only 10% of patients with matting require repeat treatment of the area.[67]

Matting may also occur as a result of trauma to the leg,

in association with pregnancy or hormonal therapy, or in scars around previous sites of surgical stripping. Sclerotherapy-induced matting has been proposed to be caused by excessive sclerosing solution concentrations, use of overly potent or too much volume of sclerosing solutions, excessive hydrostatic pressure of injection, too much blanching, or improper compression.[50,68] Predisposing factors include predilection for certain areas of the leg, such as the thigh, and a number of epidemiologic factors related to individual susceptibility, including obesity, hormonal therapy with estrogen, family history, and a longer history of telangiectasia.[66] The relative risk factor for development of telangiectatic matting is 3.17 times greater for female patients taking hormonal supplements.[50] Neither estrogen nor progesterone receptors have been found in telangiectases so that another mechanism may be responsible.[69] The only successful treatment of matting has been with the Candela pulsed-dye laser at 585 nm, although temporary hyperpigmentation usually occurs after laser therapy.[70,71] In most cases further treatment is not necessary since matting will resolve spontaneously.

Cutaneous Necrosis and Ulceration. Avoiding the complication of necrosis mostly depends on the skill of the physician; however, cutaneous ulceration (Case 11, Fig. 26–13) may occur with *any* sclerosing solution, even with the most skilled technique. Minimizing extravasation is achieved by stopping further injection at the first sign of a "bleb" or slightest resistance to injection or when a sudden increase in pain is noted by the patient.

Unavoidably, a tiny amount of sclerosing solution may

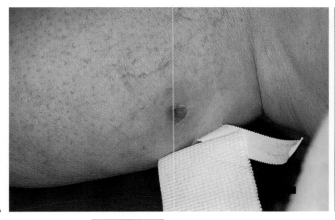
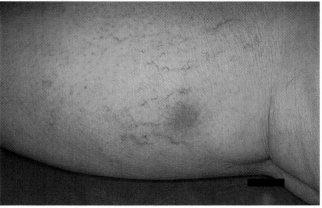

A   B

CASE 11

FIGURE 26–13. Ulceration. *A,* A small area of cutaneous breakdown probably caused by escape of a tiny amount of hypertonic saline intradermally while attempting to cannulate a telangiectasis. Prolonged blanching was seen at the site. Perhaps use of topical nitroglycerin ointment would have minimized the skin breakdown. A safer approach would have been to cannulate the reticular vein associated with the telangiectases. *B,* Within a month after its initial appearance, the ulcer healed with minimal sequelae using conservative wound care of daily dressing changes with a polyethylene oxide gel. Excision of ulcer with grafting would have been considered had healing not occurred within several weeks. Good cosmesis resulted with fading of erythema.

be left along the needle tract as the needle is withdrawn. Sclerosing solution may also leak out into the skin through the small puncture sites of vessel cannulation. Inadvertent puncture through the entire vessel may result in small perforations on the back wall of the treated vein through which more solution may leak. When the treated vein has a particularly fragile, thin wall, a sclerosant may cause rapid full-thickness injury, leading to rupture with perivascular accumulation. Additionally, injection may inadvertently occur into a small arteriole associated with a ''spider'' telangiectasis, with resultant necrosis and ulceration.

When the dermatologic surgeon recognizes that extravasation has occurred, the risk for necrosis can be minimized by injecting normal saline in a ratio of 10:1 into the extravasation site.[67] Extensive massage of small subcutaneous blebs to spread the trapped sclerosing agent as quickly as possible will minimize prolonged blanching of the area. An anecdotal report of topical nitroglycerin paste applied immediately to the extravasation site indicates that necrosis may be reduced or prevented.[72]

Superficial Thrombophlebitis. This complication (Case 12, Fig. 26–14) is most commonly mistaken for the normal nodular fibrosis that occurs with proper sclerotherapy called ''endosclerosis'' by Fegan.[4] After sclerotherapy of larger varicosities (4–8 mm), a *nontender,* nonpigmented, nonerythematous fibrotic cord may be palpable along the course of the vein and may persist for months. Superficial thrombophlebitis, however, is characterized clinically by a very tender, indurated, linear erythematous swelling. Incidence is quite variable, estimated at 1% to 0.01% after sclerotherapy,[73] although one report indicates that the incidence is higher than previously suspected.[5] A liquefied coagulum usually accompanies the presence of superficial thrombophlebitis and should be evacuated. Treatment also consists of leg elevation and/or compression and regular administration of aspirin or other nonsteroidal anti-inflammatory drugs. Extension of superficial thrombophlebitis into the deep system is extremely rare but may occur through the saphenofemoral or saphenopopliteal junctions.

Pulmonary Embolism. Pulmonary emboli probably occur from extension of a superficial thrombus into the deep venous system. Evidence of extension from superficial thrombus to deep thrombophlebitis should be treated promptly by anticoagulation. The incidence of pulmonary embolism has been associated with injection of large quantities of sclerosant at a single site.[74] The incidence is extremely low, with fewer than 1 in 40,000 patients treated.

Exogenous hormonal therapy is well known to increase the risk of deep thrombophlebitis and pulmonary embolism. Oral contraception may increase the risk of emboli for patients undergoing sclerotherapy.[75] Compression followed by immediate ambulation and adherence to the principle of no more than 0.5 to 1 ml of sclerosing solution per injection site is thought to minimize the risks of deep venous thrombosis and subsequent emboli.

Arterial Injection. This dreaded medical emergency is fortunately extremely rare. Warning signs include immediate intense pain far beyond the normal discomfort at the initiation of injection and aspiration of bright red blood into the syringe before injection. Continuous intense burning pain with immediate bone-white cutaneous blanching over a large area is the usual initial sign. Progression to a sharply demarcated cyanosis within minutes confirms arterial injection and must be recognized immediately. Emergency treatment involves immediate application of ice, attempts to flush the inadvertently injected artery with normal saline and/or heparin, injection of 3% procaine to inactivate STS, and emergency consultation with a vascular surgeon for intravenous anticoagulation. Rarely, arterial injection may not be accompanied by the usual signs of

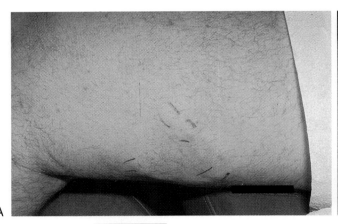
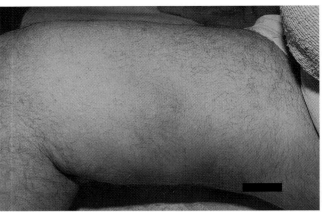

A

B

CASE 12

FIGURE 26–14. Superficial thrombophlebitis. *A,* Incompetent Hunterian perforator causing superficial varicosity beginning in the mid thigh. Doppler ultrasound examination revealed reflux from the mid thigh downward; however, no reflux was detected at the saphenofemoral junction. Photoplethysmographic examination revealed a refill time of 15 seconds, correctable to 30 seconds by application of a thigh tourniquet at 80 mm Hg compressing this varicose vein. *B,* One week after treatment with 2% sodium tetradecyl sulfate, four injections of 0.5 mL each, the patient returns with a tender, erythematous subcutaneous mass at the treatment site. The patient did not comply with use of 30- to 40-mm Hg graduated compression hose for more than 3 days. Treatment consisted of ibuprofen, 400 mg three times a day, reapplication of 30- to 40-mm Hg graduated compression, and visual monitoring for extension every 3 days. Resolution occurred within 10 days. Superficial thrombophlebitis can be distinguished from the normal postsclerotherapy accumulation of an intravascular hematoma or coagulum by the presence of erythema and tenderness. Intravenous anticoagulation with heparin is indicated when a superficial phlebitis extends into the common femoral vein.

immediately intense pain and discoloration.[75] Arterial injection may lead to necrosis of skin, subcutaneous tissue, and muscle.

References

1. Goldman MP. A comparison of sclerosing agents: Clinical and histologic effects of intravascular sodium morrhuate ethanolamine oleate hypertonic saline (11.7%) and Sclerodex in the dorsal rabbit ear vein. J Dermatol Surg Oncol 1991;17:354–362.
2. Goldman MP, Bennett RG. Treatment of telangiectasia: A review. J Am Acad Dermatol 1987;17:167–182.
3. Rotter SM, Weiss RA. Human saphenous vein in vitro model for studying the action of sclerosing solutions. J Dermatol Surg Oncol 1993;19:59–62.
4. Fegan WG. Continuous compression technique of injecting varicose veins. Lancet 1963;2:109–112.
5. Feied CF. Deep vein thrombosis: The risks of sclerotherapy in hypercoagulable states. Semin Dermatol 1993;12:135–149.
6. Partsch H. Primary Varikose der Vena saphena magna und parva. In: Kriessman A, Bollinger A, Keller H, eds. Praxis der Doppler Sonographie. Stuttgart: Thieme, 1982:101–103.
7. Weiss RA. Evaluation of the venous system by Doppler ultrasound and photoplethysmography or light reflection rheography before sclerotherapy. Semin Dermatol 1993;12:78–87.
8. Fronek A. Noninvasive Diagnostics in Vascular Disease. New York: McGraw-Hill, 1989.
9. Rosfors S. Venous photoplethysmography: Relationship between transducer position and regional distribution of venous insufficiency. J Vasc Surg 1990;11:436–440.
10. Weindorf N, Schulz-Ehrenburg U. Der Wert der Photoplethysmographie (Licht Reflexions Rheography) in der Phlebologie. Vasa 1986;15:397–401.
11. McMullin GM, Coleridge Smith PD. An evaluation of Doppler ultrasound and photoplethysmography in the investigation of venous insufficiency. Aust NZ J Med 1992;62:270–275.
12. Hertzman AB. The blood supply of various skin areas as estimated by the photoelectric plethysmograph. Am J Physiol 1938;33:498–499.
13. Wienert V, Blazek V. Eine neue Methode zur unblutigen dynamischen Venedruckmessung. Hautarzt 1982;33:498–499.
14. Neumann HAM, Boersma I. Light reflection rheography: A noninvasive diagnostic tool for screening of venous disease. J Dermatol Surg Oncol 1992;18:425–430.
15. Blazek V, Schmitt HJ, Schultz-Ehrenburg U, Kerner J. Digitale Photoplethysmographie (D-PPG) fur die Beinvenediagnostik: Medizinisch-technische Grundlagen. Phlebol Proktol 1989;18:91–97.
16. Kerner J, Schultz-Ehrenburg U, Lechner W. Quantitative Photoplethysmographie bei gesunden Erwachsenen, Kindern und Schwangeren und bei Varizenpatienten. Phlebol 1992;21:134–139.
17. Abramowitz HB, Queral LA, Flinn WR, et al. The use of photoplethysmography in the assessment of venous insufficiency: A comparison to venous pressure measurements. Surgery 1979;66:434–441.
18. Szendro G, Nicolaides AN, Zukowski AJ, et al. Duplex scanning in the assessment of deep venous incompetence. J Vasc Surg 1986;4:237–242.
19. Nicolaides A. Quantification of venous reflux by means of duplex scanning. J Vasc Surg 1990;10:670–677.
20. de Groot WP. Practical phlebology: Sclerotherapy of large veins. J Dermatol Surg Oncol 1991;17:589–595.
21. Vin F. Echo-sclerotherapy of the external saphenous vein (discussion 90-6). Phlebologie 1991;44:79–84. In French.
22. Raymond-Martimbeau P. Two different techniques for sclerosing the incompetent saphenofemoral junction. A comparative study. J Dermatol Surg Oncol 1990;16:626–631.
23. Schadeck M. Sclerotherapy of great saphenous veins: A 48-month followup (abstract). J Dermatol Surg Oncol 1990;16:87.
24. Hobbs JT. Surgery and sclerotherapy in the treatment of varicose veins: A random trial. Arch Surg 1974;109:793–796.
25. Hobbs JT. A random trial of the treatment of varicose veins by surgery and sclerotherapy. In: Hobbs JT, ed. The Treatment of Venous Thrombosis. Philadelphia: JB Lippincott, 1977.
26. Hobbs JT. Compression sclerotherapy in venous insufficiency. Acta Chir Scand Suppl 1988;544:75–80.
27. Orbach EJ. Sclerotherapy of varicose veins: Utilization of intravenous air block. Am J Surg 1944;66:362–366.
28. Orbach EJ, Petretti AK. Thrombogenic property of foam synthetic anionic detergent (sodium tetradecyl sulfate, N.N.R.). Angiology 1950;1:237–243.

29. Sigg K. Sclerosing treatment of varicose veins. Internist 1967;8:388–398. In German.

30. Sigg K. The treatment of varicosities and accompanying complications. Angiology 1952;3:355–379.

31. Harridge H. The treatment of primary varicose veins. Surg Clin North Am 1960;40:191–202.

32. de Groot WP. Treatment of varicose veins: Modern concepts and methods. J Dermatol Surg Oncol 1989;15:191–198.

33. Fraser IA, Perry EP, Hatton M, Watkin DF. Prolonged bandaging is not required following sclerotherapy of varicose veins. Br J Surg 1985;72:488–490.

34. Shouler PJ, Runchman PC. Varicose veins: Optimum compression after surgery and sclerotherapy (comments). Ann R Coll Surg Engl 1989;71:402–404.

35. Goldman MP, Beaudoing D, Marley W, et al. Compression in the treatment of leg telangiectasia: A preliminary report. J Dermatol Surg Oncol 1990;16:322–325.

36. Reddy P, Terry T, Lamont P, Dormandy JA. What is the correct duration of bandaging following sclerotherapy? In: Negus D, Jantet G, eds. Phlebology '85. London: John Libbey & Co, 1985:141–143.

37. Weiss RA, Weiss MA. Sclerotherapy. In: Wheeland RG, ed. Cutaneous Surgery. Philadelphia: WB Saunders, 1994:951–981.

38. Weiss RA, Weiss MA. Doppler ultrasound findings in reticular veins of the thigh subdermic lateral venous system and implications for sclerotherapy. J Dermatol Surg Oncol 1993;19:947–951.

39. Weiss RA, Weiss MA. Painful telangiectasias: Diagnosis and treatment. In: Bergman JJ, Goldman MP, eds. Varicose Veins and Telangiectasias: Diagnosis and Treatment. St. Louis: Quality Medical Publishing, 1993:389–406.

40. Albanese AR, Albanese AM, Albanese EF. Lateral subdermic varicose vein system of the legs: Its surgical treatment by the chiseling tube method. Vasc Surg 1969;3:81–89.

41. Somjen GM, Ziegenbein R, Johnston AH, Royle JP. Anatomic examination of leg telangiectasias with duplex scanning. J Dermatol Surg Oncol 1993;19:940–945.

42. Sadick NS. Treatment of varicose and telangiectatic leg veins with hypertonic saline: A comparative study of heparin and saline. J Dermatol Surg Oncol 1990;16:24–28.

43. Sadick NS. Sclerotherapy of varicose and telangiectatic leg veins. Minimal sclerosant concentration of hypertonic saline and its relationship to vessel diameter (comments). J Dermatol Surg Oncol 1991;17:65–70.

44. Weiss RA, Weiss MA. Resolution of pain associated with varicose and telangiectatic leg veins after compression sclerotherapy. J Dermatol Surg Oncol 1990;16:333–336.

45. Goldman MP, Kaplan RP, Oki LN, et al. Extravascular effects of sclerosants in rabbit skin: A clinical and histologic examination. J Dermatol Surg Oncol 1986;12:1085–1088.

46. Mantse L. A mild sclerosing agent for telangiectasias (letter). J Dermatol Surg Oncol 1985;11:855.

47. Mantse L. More on spider veins (letter). J Dermatol Surg Oncol 1986;12:1022.

48. Eichenberger H. Results of phlebosclerosation with hydroxypolyethoxydodecane. Zentralbl Phlebol 1969;8:181–183.

49. Goldman MP, Kaplan RP, et al. Sclerosing agents in the treatment of telangiectasia: Comparison of the clinical and histologic effects of intravascular polidocanol, sodium tetradecyl sulfate, and hypertonic saline in the dorsal rabbit ear vein model. Arch Dermatol 1987;123:1196–1201.

50. Weiss RA, Weiss MA. Incidence of side effects in the treatment of telangiectasias by compression sclerotherapy: Hypertonic saline vs. polidocanol. J Dermatol Surg Oncol 1990;16:800–804.

51. Hobbs JT. The treatment of varicose veins: A random trial of injection/compression versus surgery. Br J Surg 1968;55:777–780.

52. Tretbar LL. Spider angiomata: Treatment with sclerosant injections. J Kansas Med Soc 1978;79:198–200.

53. Tretbar LL. Injection sclerotherapy for spider telangiectasias: A 20-year experience with sodium tetradecyl sulfate. J Dermatol Surg Oncol 1989;15:223–225.

54. Passas H. One case of tetradecyl-sodium sulfate allergy with general symptoms. Soc Fr Phlebol 1972;25:19.

55. Fegan WG. Varicose Veins: Compression Sclerotherapy. London: William Heinemann, 1967.

56. Goldman MP. Sclerotherapy: Treatment of Varicose and Telangiectatic Leg Veins. St. Louis: Mosby–Year Book, 1991.

57. Lewis KM. Anaphylaxis due to sodium morrhuate. JAMA 1936; 107:1298–1299.

58. Sarin SK, Kumar A. Sclerosants for variceal sclerotherapy: A critical appraisal. Am J Gastroenterol 1990;85:641–649.

59. Raymond-Martimbeau P, Leclerc JR. Activation of blood coagulation after injection sclerotherapy of the lower extremity: A prospective study (abstract). J Dermatol Surg Oncol 1991;17:91.

60. Goldman MP, Kaplan RP, Duffy DM. Postsclerotherapy hyperpigmentation: A histologic evaluation. J Dermatol Surg Oncol 1987; 13:547–550.

61. Bodian EL. Techniques of sclerotherapy for sunburst venous blemishes. J Dermatol Surg Oncol 1985;11:696–704.

62. Duffy DM. Sclerotherapy: An overview. Clin Dermatol 1992;10: 373–380.

63. Goldman PM. Sclerotherapy for superficial venules and telangiectasias of the lower extremities. Dermatol Clin 1987;5:369–379.

64. Tournay PR. Traitment sclerosant des très fines varicosités intra ou saousdermiques. Soc Fr Phlebol 1966;19:235–241.

65. Goldman PM. Polidocanol (aethoxysklerol) for sclerotherapy of superficial venules and telangiectasias. J Dermatol Surg Oncol 1989;15:204–209.

66. Davis LT, Duffy DM. Determination of incidence and risk factors for postsclerotherapy telangiectatic matting of the lower extremity: A retrospective analysis. J Dermatol Surg Oncol 1990;16:327–330.

67. Duffy DM. Small vessel in sclerotherapy: An overview. In: Callen JP, Dahl MV, Golitz LE et al., eds. Advances in Dermatology. Chicago: Year Book Medical Publishers, 1988:221–242.

68. Ouvry PA, Davy A. The sclerotherapy of telangiectasia. Phlebologie 1982;35:349–359.

69. Sadick NS, Niedt GW. A study of estrogen and progesterone receptors in spider telangiectasias of the lower extremities. J Dermatol Surg Oncol 1990;16:620–623.

70. Goldman MP, Fitzpatrick RE. Pulsed-dye laser treatment of leg telangiectasia: With and without simultaneous sclerotherapy. J Dermatol Surg Oncol 1990;16:338–344.

71. Goldman MP, Martin DE, Fitzpatrick RE, Ruiz-Esparza J. Pulsed dye laser treatment of telangiectases with and without subtherapeutic sclerotherapy: Clinical and histologic examination in the rabbit ear vein model. J Am Acad Dermatol 1990;23:23–30.

72. Goldman MP. Presented before the North American Society of Phlebology, Orlando, FL, 1993.

73. Goldman MP. Sclerotherapy treatment for varicose and telangiectatic leg veins. In: Coleman WP, Hanke CW, Alt TH, Asken S, eds. Cosmetic Surgery of the Skin. Philadelphia: BC Decker, 1991: 197–211.

74. Sigg K. Zur Behandlung der Varicen der Phlebitis und ihrer Komplikationen. Hautarzt 1950;1-2:443–448.

75. Fegan WG. The complications of compression sclerotherapy. Practitioner 1971;207:797–799.

76. Biegeleisen K, Neilsen RD, O'Shaughnessy A. Inadvertent intra-arterial injection complicating ordinary and ultrasound-guided sclerotherapy. J Dermatol Surg Oncol 1993;19:953–958.

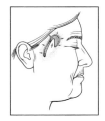

chapter 27

Hair Replacement Surgery

DOMINIC A. BRANDY and KATHRYN L. BRANDY

PUNCH HAIR-GRAFTING

Punch hair transplantation is a technique, based on the theory of donor dominance, that was introduced by Orentreich[1] in 1959. The initial phase of this method involves the harvesting of donor dominant scalp at the proper angle with a motor-driven, cylindrical, carbon-steel trephine (4.0–5.0 mm in diameter that yields 15 to 25 hairs in each graft). In the developmental years, these punch-grafts were removed randomly and allowed to heal by second intention; but the procedure has evolved to the point that the donor dominant grafts are now harvested in a cluster fashion with the remaining defect being closed with a Pierce-type closure (Fig. 27–1A). After excising these donor punch-grafts, including the hair bulb, the fat of the graft is trimmed and stray hairs are removed under magnification. Trimming fat from donor grafts prevents later cobblestoning at the recipient site. The grafts are then placed into slightly smaller holes (0.5–0.75 mm differential) that are created with trephines directed at a 45-degree anterior angle. A circumferential bandage is recommended for compression and the absorption of blood.

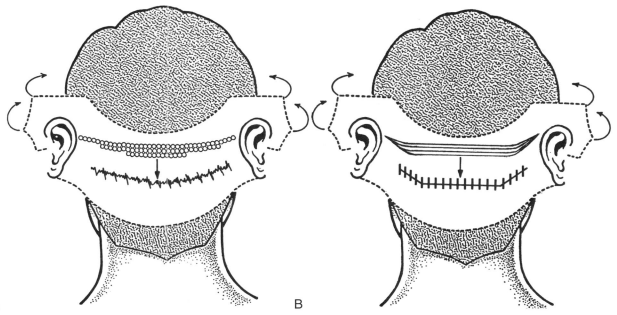

A B

FIGURE 27–1. Punch grafting. *A,* Schematic diagram demonstrating the cluster harvesting technique followed by a Pierce-type closure. *B,* Schematic diagram demonstrating the strip harvesting technique followed by a straight line closure.

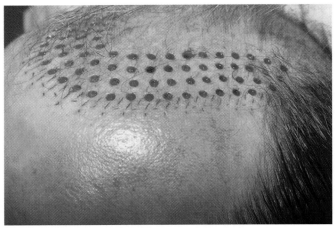

FIGURE 27–2. The first session of punch hair-grafting. The holes are arranged circumferentially, with each hole being separated from the adjacent hole by one hole size. The spaces between rows 1, 3, 5, and 7 are also separated by one hole size. The second session is performed in rows 2, 4, 6, and 8 in the same fashion. The third session is then performed between the first session of growing grafts and the fourth session between the second session. (Reprinted by permission of the publisher from Brandy DA. A three-step punchgrafting approach. J Dermatol Surg Oncol 1992;18:191. Copyright 1992 by Elsevier Science Inc.)

TABLE 27–1. Punch Hair-Grafting: Indications, Contraindications, Limitations

Indications

Male pattern baldness
Cicatricial alopecia[2]
  Burn scars
  Inactive lupus

Contraindications

Dark hair on light skin
Recipient dominant skin disorders
Bleeding diathesis
Anticoagulant treatment
Impaired wound healing

Limitations

Tufted or abrupt hairline common when micrografts are not used anteriorly
Difficult to treat crown effectively
Limited primarily to patients with blond, gray, red, or light brown hair
``Kinkiness'' of hair[3]
``Hyperpigmentation'' of hair[4]

The most common sequencing utilized for the recipient area is a systematic four-step approach that ensures that each alopecic area will be covered with hair on completion of the hair transplantation sessions (Fig. 27–2). Once the graft congeals with the recipient area and revascularizes, the hair in that graft begins growing approximately 3 months from the point of implantation. In regard to timing between transplantation sessions, 4 months is probably ideal, because it allows the scalp to regain full laxity and gives the surgeon the ability to analyze the growth of the previous session. Good results can be achieved when the patient is chosen properly and when strict spatial relationships are maintained throughout the sessions (Case 1, Fig. 27–3) (Tables 27–1 through 27–4).

TABLE 27–2. Punch Hair-Grafting and Mini-Micrografting: Patient Preoperative Discussion

1. Do not use aspirin, fish oils, niacin, or vitamin E or smoke tobacco or marijuana for the 2 weeks before surgery.
2. Do not ingest alcohol or nonapproved drugs 48 hours preoperatively.
3. Start stretching the scalp 30 minutes per day starting 1 month before the surgery.
4. Wash the hair, neck, and face well the night before and the morning before the procedure with povidone-iodine scrub.
5. On the day of the surgery, do not wear a T-shirt or clothing that must be pulled over the head.
6. The initial phase of healing should take approximately 10 days. Hair may be shed from the grafts and will return later.
7. A bandage is worn overnight postoperatively and removed the following day. Start icing the forehead and sides of the head four times per day once the bandage is off.
8. Sleep supine with the head elevated above the heart for 1 week.
9. Avoid sun exposure for 4 weeks after surgery.
10. Do not swim, ingest alcohol or aspirin, exercise vigorously, or smoke for 2 weeks after surgery.
11. Sutures will be removed in 10 days.
12. Take the prescribed antibiotics as directed.
13. Avoid taking hot showers or baths for the first 2 weeks after surgery.
14. Cleanse the grafted area with a 1:1 solution of distilled water and hydrogen peroxide five times per day for 5 days. Clean donor sites in a similar fashion.
15. Hair may be shampooed, using regular tap water on the third postoperative day.
16. Small crusts or scabs may form on top of the grafts. They will fall off in approximately 2 weeks and will contain small amounts of telogen hair.
17. Leave the transplanted area open to the air as much as possible. Avoid hairpieces and hats, during the first week whenever possible.
18. Numbness will occur above the donor incision and behind the area that has been transplanted. Sensation should return in approximately 6 months, though it may take 1 year.
19. The transplanted area may appear pink in the first few weeks. This pinkness will gradually fade.
20. Itching may occur over the transplanted area and along the incision line in the first 2 weeks. A cream can be prescribed for this.
21. Avoid picking the scabs over the grafts.
22. Apply minoxidil (Rogaine) twice daily to the grafted area starting 2 weeks after the surgery. This may shorten the resting phase of the grafted hair.

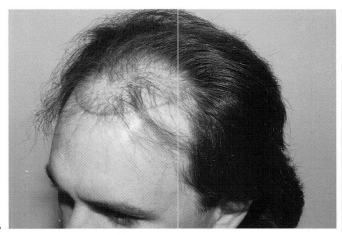
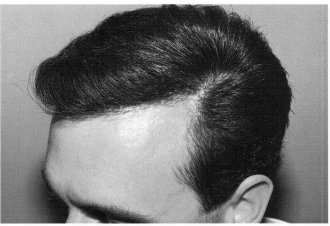

CASE 1

FIGURE 27-3. Punch grafting. *A*, Patient presented with frontal baldness. Planned placement of the anterior hairline is marked on the scalp and shown to the patient. *B*, Appearance after four sessions of organized punch grafting.

TABLE 27-3. Punch Hair-Grafting: Operative Issues

Preoperative Evaluation

History
   Bleeding diathesis
   Poor wound healing
   Hepatitis
   Human immunodeficiency virus infection
   Diabetes
   Mitral valve prolapse
   Prosthetic valve
   Anabolic steroids
   Immunosuppression
   Cardiac arrhythmias

Physical Examination

Examine donor hair-bearing scalp for density, hair quality, and color. Try to project the extent of future baldness by wetting the hair with alcohol. Examine other scars for healing quality.

Preoperative Equipment Needs

Sterile drapes and gowns
Bovie unit
Pron Pillo
Local anesthesia
Sterile instrumentation
   Needle holder
   Suture scissors
   Forceps
   Hemostat
Suture material
Bandaging material
Wall suction
Epinephrine (diluted 1:300,000)
Oral sedation and analgesia
Cardiac monitor
Barrier protection for staff
Carbon steel trephines
   (range, 3.0–5.0 mm)
Hand engine

Intraoperative Needs

Dexamethasone (Decadron), 8 mg (long acting) and 8 mg (short acting) IM for swelling
Cefadroxil (Duricef), 1 g PO
Sterile Petri dishes
Assistant to count number of grafts taken and number of recipient sites bored
Assistant to prepare grafts and place grafts

MINI-MICROGRAFTING

Minigrafts are smaller than punch-grafts (three to eight hairs per graft) and are created by several approaches (Tables 27–5 through 27–7). The approach that Bradshaw[5] described was that of quartering 4.5-mm punch-grafts (Fig. 27–4*A*). This required the surgeon to harvest several 4.5-mm punch-grafts with a motor-driven trephine and then to quadrasect these under magnification with a blade. Other described methods have included bisecting 4.0-mm grafts, trisecting 3.0-mm grafts, and similar dissecting approaches. With all of these techniques, one- to two- haired micrografts are also usually excised from the edge of the conventional grafts and used later to refine the hairline. More recently, the senior author[6] has recommended using a triple- or quadruple-bladed knife to excise two or three 3.0-mm strips (ear to ear) from the donor area (see Fig. 27–1*B*) and subsequently transecting these into 3.0 × 1.5-mm minigrafts and one- to two-haired micrografts (see Fig. 27–4*B*). Each strip will normally yield 80 minigrafts (six to eight hairs per graft) that fit very nicely into No. 15 Bard-Parker incisions, as seen in the anterior hairline of Figure 27–2.

In regard to the organization of the recipient sites for mini-micrografting, the most common approach is to make random incisions or holes and then continue to randomly fill in the spaces during subsequent sessions. We agree that randomness is essential at the hairline, but also feel strongly that order should be the goal posterior to the hairline. To achieve this order, we draw three to four horizontal reference lines on the patient preoperatively. These lines will guide a systematic three-step approach[7] that will allow the surgeon to cover all alopecic areas with hair (Case 2, Fig. 27–5). The initial set of incisions is placed 6.0 mm apart and organized in a fully staggered pattern (Fig. 27–6*A*). Four months after the first session, the second session is performed 2.0 mm to the right of the first session of growing minigrafts (see Fig. 27–6*B*). Four months after the second session, the third session is performed 2.0 mm to the right (and slightly posterior) to the second session of growing minigrafts (see Fig. 27–6*C*). If

TABLE 27-4. Punch Hair-Grafting: Postoperative Care

Pain Management
Hydrocodone (Vicodin) (1 every 3–4 hours) for incisional pain
Extra-strength acetaminophen (1–2 capsules every 6 hours) to augment Vicodin if needed

Dressings
Circumferential head dressing:
    Nonadherent (Telfa) pads over grafted sites
    6 large gynecologic pads
    4 Kling wraps
    1 elastic Kling around the chin to secure the bandage

Complications
Hematoma may occur at donor site.
    Aspirate with 14-gauge needle on a 20-mL syringe; then apply pressure.
    Evacuate if it recurs.
Ingrown hair
    Apply warm compresses twice daily.
Telogen effluvium
    Apply minoxidil (Rogaine) to the areas twice daily.
Infection
    Treat with antibiotic.
Arteriovenous fistula and aneurysm
    Figure-of-eight suture
Permanent hair loss or necrosis
    Revise the area during the subsequent procedure or as a separate procedure.
Hypertrophic scars
    Inject triamcinolone (Kenalog) 10 mg/mL every 2 weeks until scar resolves.
    Mini-micrografting

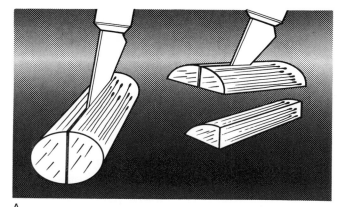

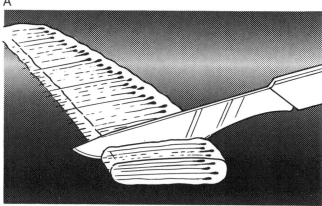

FIGURE 27–4. Mini-micrografting. *A*, Bradshaw's original technique involved quadrasecting 4.5-mm grafts, which created minigrafts containing six to eight hairs. *B*, In the strip technique, each 3.0-mm strip is transected into 3.0 × 1.5-mm rectangular minigrafts, with each containing six to eight hairs. (*A*, reprinted by permission of the publisher from Brandy DA. Conventional grafting combined with minigrafting: A new approach. J Dermatol Surg Oncol 1987;13:61. Copyright 1987 by Elsevier Science Inc.)

a fourth session is desired by the patient, three- to four-haired minigrafts are placed into random 16-gauge NoKor needle incisions. During all of these sessions, 50 to 100 one- to two-haired micrografts are inserted into random 18-gauge NoKor needle incisions anterior to the hairline.

A stencil[8] (Robbins Instruments, Chatham, NJ) is used before the first session and has been found to keep the first session extremely well organized (Case 3, Fig. 27–7). This is extremely important because all secondary procedures will be based on this initial session. During the second session, the surgeon simply makes a small dot over each growing graft from the first session, then makes No. 15 blade incisions 2.0 mm to the right of these marks. During the third session, the surgeon makes larger dots encompassing the first and second sessions of growing grafts, then makes the intraoperative incisions in between these dots and slightly posterior.

SCALP REDUCTION

Scalp reduction involves the treatment of alopecia by excision rather than by hair-grafting (Tables 27–8 through 27–11). After undermining the entire scalp above the nuchal ridge, the surgeon overlaps the undermined scalp to estimate a safe margin for excision. The overlapping bald skin is then excised with a scalpel and is sutured with a two-layered closure. A secure closure at the galea aponeurotica is essential to ensure fine healing at the skin surface. The types of scalp reductions are classified into four basic patterns: (1) the midline sagittal ellipse (Fig. 27–8*A*); (2) the Y-pattern (see Fig. 27–8*B*); (3) the paramedian pattern (see Fig. 27–8*C*); and (4) the circumferential pattern (see Fig. 27–8*D*). All of these procedures, except for

TABLE 27-5. Mini-micrografting: Indications, Contraindications, Limitations

Indications

Male and female pattern baldness (all colors of hair)
Cicatricial alopecia

Contraindications

Same as for punch hair-grafting (see Table 27-1) except that all hair colors can be grafted effectively

Limitations

Is slightly more difficult to achieve the density of punch hair-grafting

TABLE 27-6. Mini-micrografting: Operative Issues

Preoperative Evaluation

Same as punch hair-grafting (see Table 27-3)

Preoperative Equipment Needs

First 12 items from the punch hair-grafting section
No. 15 Bard-Parker blade
NoKor needles (16 and 18 gauge)
McPherson microforceps

Intraoperative Needs

Same as punch hair-grafting (see Table 27-3)

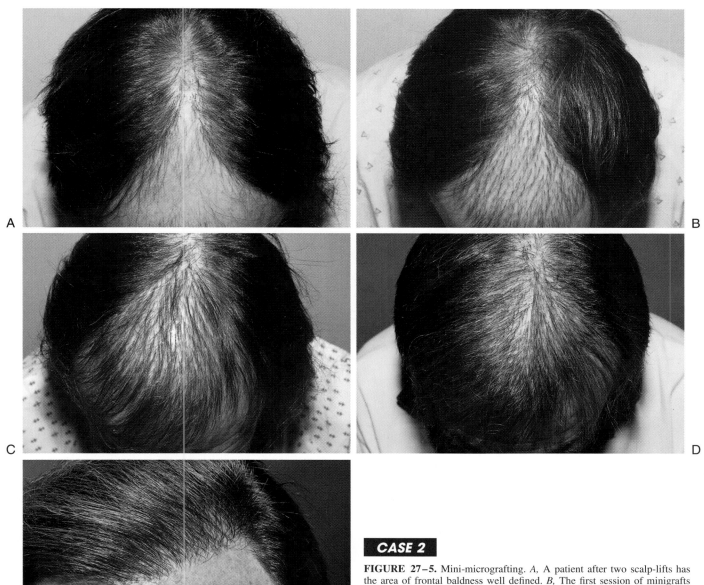

CASE 2

FIGURE 27-5. Mini-micrografting. *A,* A patient after two scalp-lifts has the area of frontal baldness well defined. *B,* The first session of minigrafts is growing. *C,* Two sessions of minigrafts growing. *D,* After three sessions of minigrafts, the anterior hairline and area of frontal baldness are filled in with hair growth. *E,* Same patient as in *D* after three sessions with the hairline exposed. Micrografts are performed anteriorly with each session. (*A* to *E,* reprinted by permission of the publisher from Brandy DA. A new instrument for the expedient production of minigrafts. J Dermatol Surg Oncol 1992;18:491. Copyright 1992 by Elsevier Science Inc.)

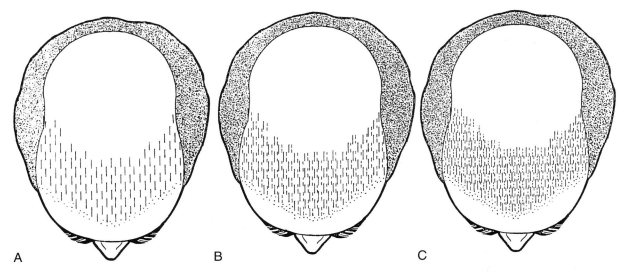

FIGURE 27–6. Mini-micrografting. *A,* The first step of a systematic three-step slit-minigrafting approach involves No. 15 blade slits separated by 6.0 mm and arranged in a fully staggered pattern. Micrografts are placed anteriorly with all sessions. *B,* Four months later the second session is performed 2.0 mm to the right of the first session of growing grafts. *C,* Four months later the third session is performed 2.0 mm to the right and slightly posterior to the second session.

TABLE 27–7. Mini-micrografting: Postoperative Care

Pain Management
Same as punch hair-grafting (see Table 27–4)

Dressings
Same as punch hair-grafting (see Table 27–4)

Complications
Cyst formation
  Excise the cyst.
"Pitted appearance" of graft
  Bore out the pitted graft with a small hand-held trephine and replace the graft.
Ingrown hair
  Apply warm compresses to the area twice daily.

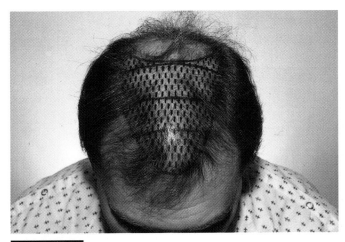

CASE 3

FIGURE 27–7. Mini-micrografting. A stencil is used during the first session to meticulously organize the foundation for the three-step protocol. Notice the important circular configuration posteriorly.

TABLE 27–8. Scalp Reduction: Indications, Contraindications, Limitations

Indications
Pattern baldness
Cicatricial alopecia

Contraindications
Extensive posterior baldness should not be totally treated with midline, paramedian, and Y-pattern scalp reductions.
Impaired wound healing
Bleeding diathesis
Anticoagulant treatment

Limitations
Slot formations[9] with midline, paramedian, and Y-pattern
Stretch-back with midline, paramedian,[10] and Y-pattern
Limitations 1 and 2 make it difficult to treat extensive baldness. Circumferential scalp reduction[11] should be used on most patients with extensive baldness.
If scalp laxity is poor, scalp-lifting or tissue expansion is a better option.
Some elevation of the periauricular hairline

TABLE 27–9. Scalp Reduction: Patient Preoperative Discussion

1. Follow numbers 1 through 13 from Table 27–2 in the punch hair-grafting section.
2. Clean the incision with witch hazel or hydrogen peroxide 4 times per day for 10 days.
3. Apply bacteriostatic K-Y jelly over the incision after incisional cleaning for 10 days.
4. Wash hair daily. This can be done immediately after bandage removal.
5. While healing takes place, the incision will be light red to pink and will gradually fade to a skin tone or lighter shade.
6. Numbness may remain for 6 months to a year and should completely resolve.
7. If scarring is evident, apply Couvre alopecia masking cream until hair-grafting can be performed into the scar.

TABLE 27-10. Scalp Reduction: Operative Issues

Preoperative Evaluation

Same as for punch hair-grafting (see Table 27–3)
Scalp laxity should be good.

Preoperative Equipment Needs

First 12 items from Table 27–3 in punch hair-grafting section
No. 10 scalpel
Facelift scissors
Suction retractor
K-Y Jelly
Hook retractor

Intraoperative Needs

Topical thrombin diluted with 5 mL normal saline (2500 units) under the flaps before closure
Dexamethasone (Decadron), 8 mg (long acting) and 8 mg (short acting) IM
Cefadroxil (Duricef), 1 g PO

TABLE 27-11. Scalp Reduction: Postoperative Care

Pain Management

Same as for punch hair-grafting (see Table 27–4)

Dressings

K-Y Jelly on the incisions
Circumferential head dressing same as for punch hair-grafting (see Table 27–4)

Complications

Same as punch hair-grafting (see Table 27–4)
Necrosis
  Keep clean with diluted hydrogen peroxide until the scab falls off and instruct patient not to pick the scab.
  Later revise.
Hypesthesia
  Inform patient that it may last for up to a year postoperatively.
Slot formation
  Use a Frechet[12] transposition procedure.
Stretch-back
  Use retention sutures[13] or scalp extension techniques[13,14] to prevent.

the circumferential pattern, involve the undermining of bald skin and placing that bald skin under tension.

Midline, Y-pattern, and paramedian scalp reduction procedures are usually recommended for patients desiring elimination of cicatricial alopecia or of mild posterior pattern alopecia or the partial reduction of extensive baldness. All scalp reductions advance hair with its normal uniformity and hair texture; therefore, they should usually be performed posteriorly whenever the circumstances are amenable to the technique. Circumferential scalp reduction, unlike midline, Y-pattern, and paramedian scalp reductions,

can be used for the complete excision of both mild and extensive forms of male pattern baldness (Figs. 27–9 and Case 4, 27–10). The primary reasons for this fact are (1) stretch-back (the stretching back of the alopecic skin) is virtually eliminated because the central bald skin is not undermined, and (2) the posterior donor fringe is elevated approximately 1.5 cm with each procedure (significantly reducing the chances of developing inferior slot formations).

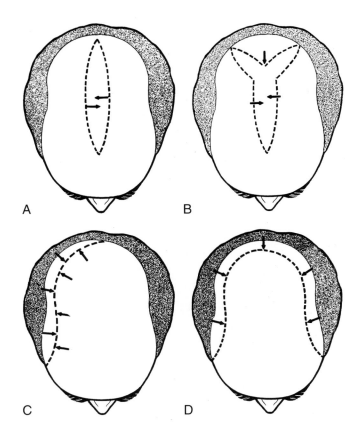

FIGURE 27–8. Scalp reduction. *A,* The midsagittal reduction undermines bald skin and has two primary vectors, indicated by arrows. *B,* The Y-pattern reduction also undermines bald skin but has three primary vectors, indicated by arrows. *C,* The paramedian reduction undermines bald skin on just one side and has two primary vectors, except for the posterior aspect. *D,* The circumferential reduction undermines no bald skin and has multidirectional vectors throughout its entire length.

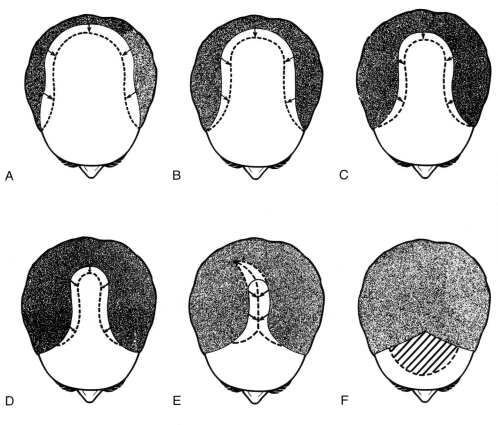

FIGURE 27–9. Serial circumferential scalp reductions (*A* through *D*) followed by a bitemporal scalp reduction (*E*) will accomplish closure on most extensively bald patients with three to five procedures, depending on scalp laxity. Minimicrografting can then be performed frontally (*F*) in the area with the diagonal lines.

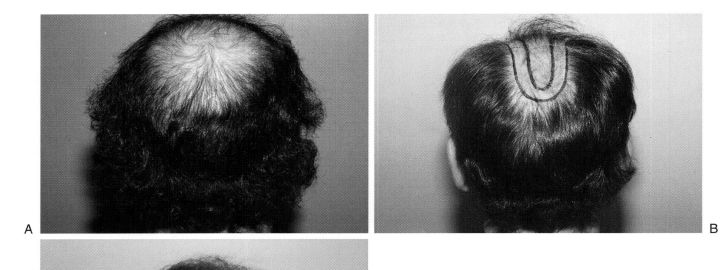

FIGURE 27–10. Scalp reduction. *A*, Patient with extensive baldness posteriorly. *B*, Appearance after two circumferential scalp reductions and immediately before the third procedure. Prior incisions of the two circumferential scalp reduction are indicated by the blue line. *C*, After three circumferential and one bitemporal scalp reduction, the patient has hair coverage. The appearance of hair density is enhanced by a permanent and change to a lighter hair color.

SCALP-LIFTING

Scalp-lifting[15] consists of five basic techniques: (1) the Marzola lateral scalp-lift (Fig. 27–11*A*); (2) the bilateral occipitoparietal scalp-lift (see Fig. 27–11*B*); (3) the bitemporal scalp-lift (see Fig. 27–11*C*); (4) the modified bitemporal scalp-lift; and (5) the frontoparietal advancement scalp-lift (see Fig. 27–11*D*) (Tables 27–12 through 27–15). The primary difference between these procedures and scalp reduction is that the undermining proceeds down to the hairline of the nape. This extra undermining is important because it gives approximately 60% more stretch (Fig. 27–12) primarily because the area below the nuchal ridge is devoid of restrictive galea. The incision and configuration of this procedure is exactly the same as that of the circumferential scalp reduction. It begins at the mid-sideburn anterior to the superficial temporal artery, proceeds around the entire donor dominant fringe, and ends at the mid sideburn on the opposite side. This incision gives the surgeon tremendous visualization and the ability to easily undermine down to the hairline of the nape.

This procedure is primarily indicated for those patients with extensive baldness. Because of the much greater su-

perior and medial advancement (Case 5, Fig. 27–13) with these procedures, most patients with type 5 baldness can have their incisions closed posteriorly with just two procedures (i.e., a bilateral occipitoparietal scalp-lift and a bitemporal scalp-lift). For those with lesser forms of baldness, a modified bitemporal scalp-lift works exceptionally well as a one-step treatment for bitemporal recessions and stable posterior hair. The excision of this procedure is shaped somewhat like a conventional bitemporal lift, but

TABLE 27–12. Scalp-lifting: Indications, Contraindications, Limitations

Indications
Pattern baldness
Cicatricial alopecia

Contraindications
Impaired healing
Bleeding diathesis
Anticoagulant treatment
Poor hair density in the donor fringe
Poor hair quality below the nuchal ridge
High periauricular hairline

Limitations
Scar formation at the sideburns and vertex
Permanent hypesthesia at the vertex that gradually improves
Some elevation of the periauricular hairline
Requires occipital artery ligations performed 2 to 6 weeks before the lift

TABLE 27–13. Scalp-lifting: Patient Preoperative Discussion

1. Follow numbers 1 through 13 from Table 27–2 in the punch hair-grafting section.
2. A large head bandage will be worn overnight and removed the next day in the office. The head is washed, and a second smaller head bandage is applied. This is removed the next day by the patient.
3. Drains are inserted during surgery and will be removed the next day with the bandage removal.
4. A cervical collar is worn for 3 days for 24 hours and then for the next 4 nights.
5. Ice should be applied after the first dressing is removed to the forehead and the back of the neck—never on the top of the head.
6. Clean the incision lines with witch hazel or hydrogen peroxide four times per day for 10 days.
7. Wash the hair in the shower daily starting the second day after the surgery.
8. Apply bacteriostatic K-Y Jelly over the incision.
9. Numbness will be present and can last from 6 months to 2 years. In some cases, there may be some lingering numbness.
10. While healing takes place, the incision line will be pink, fading to a skin tone or lighter shade. This scar can be camouflaged with Couvre cover cream after the sutures are removed and will be grafted at a future date.
11. A small procedure called a bilateral occipital artery ligation will be required 2 to 6 weeks before scalp-lifting surgery. This has been found to greatly decrease the chance of developing permanent hair loss in the hair-bearing scalp.
12. A responsible adult will need to pick the patient up after surgery and stay with him or her that night because of the use of intravenous anesthesia.

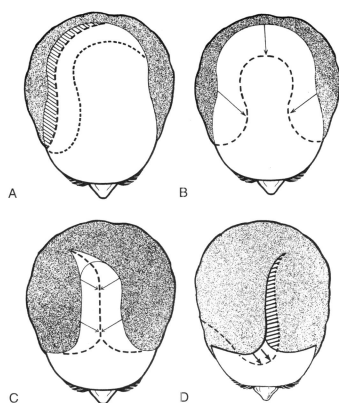

FIGURE 27–11. Scalp-lifting. *A,* The Marzola lateral scalp-lift compared with a paramedian scalp reduction. The significantly improved movement with the Marzola lift is accomplished without undermining bald skin. The paramedian scalp reduction is indicated by the area marked with diagonal lines. *B,* The bilateral occipitoparietal scalp-lift. *C,* The bitemporal scalp-lift. The vectors can be shifted anteriorly to treat bitemporal recessions (modified bitemporal lift). *D,* The frontoparietal advancement scalp-lift must be performed two times for hairline development. The schematic demonstrates the first advancement. The diagonal lines indicate overlap that is excised; the arrows indicate the anterior advancement.

TABLE 27–14. Scalp-lifting: Operative Issues

Preoperative Evaluation
Same as for scalp reduction (see Table 27–10), but pay special attention to the hair quality below the nuchal ridge
Patients with previous hair-grafting should only have Marzola lateral scalp lifts.
Preoperative Equipment Needs
Same as for scalp reduction (see Table 27–10)
Penrose drains
Anesthesia equipment needed for intravenous sedation
Intraoperative Needs
Same as for scalp reduction (see Table 27–10)

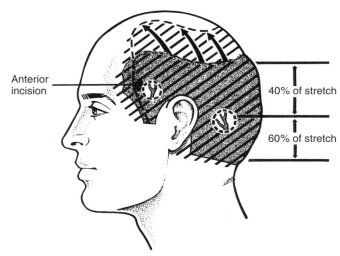

FIGURE 27–12. Scalp-lifting. The extra undermining from the nuchal ridge down to the hairline of the nape contributes approximately 60% of the stretch with scalp-lifting. The hair-bearing scalp is lifted to the anterior incision line, and the redundant non–hair-bearing skin is excised.

the vectors are shifted anteriorly so that more is advanced frontally and less medially. A conventional bitemporal scalp-lift can be used as an excellent treatment for those with type 4 baldness that will not progress in the future. In most cases, however, it is used as a closure procedure 3 months after the bilateral occipitoparietal scalp-lift. The frontoparietal advancement lift is used for hairline development for those who wish to forgo hair transplantation frontally. A delay is performed 2 weeks before the actual lift, and two scalp-lifts are usually necessary for the hairline to be fully developed.

TEMPOROPARIETO-OCCIPITAL FLAPS

The temporoparieto-occipital flap (TPO or Juri flap)[16] is a pedicled transposition flap based on the superficial temporal artery (Tables 27–16 through 27–19). Before planning this 4.0-cm wide flap, the superficial temporal artery must be identified by Doppler ultrasonography, making certain that the artery traverses the center of the flap. The base of the flap should begin approximately 3 cm above the root of the helix and should incline about 40 degrees in a posterosuperior direction. The flap is designed to mildly arch superiorly into the parietal scalp and then curve posteriorly and inferiorly toward the hairline of the nape, making certain not to cross the midline. The flap length is determined by measuring the base of the flap to the distal end of the hairline and adding approximately 4.0 cm to adjust for dog-ear formation (Fig. 27–14A).

TABLE 27–15. Scalp-lifting: Postoperative Care

Pain Management
Oxycodone (Percocet) (1–2 every 3 hours) as needed
Extra-strength acetaminophen every 4–6 hours to augment the Percocet
Dressings
One 6-inch Ace wrap
Eight gynecologic pads
4 × 4-inch gauze pad stacks to be placed over the drains
Four Kling rolls (4 inch)
One stretch Kling roll placed loosely around the bandage and under the chin
Two nonadherent (Telfa) pads
Cervical collar
Next day dressing:
    One 6-inch Ace wrap
    Three gynecologic pads
    4 × 4-inch gauze pads to place over drain sites
    K-Y Jelly over incisions
Complications
Necrosis
    Keep clean with hydrogen peroxide solution until crust falls off.
    Revise during donor harvest procedure for minigrafting.
Remainder same as punch hair-grafting and scalp reduction

TABLE 27–16. Temporoparieto-occipital Flaps: Indications, Contraindications, Limitations

Indications
For patients who have no desire for hair-grafting
For patients not projected to develop posterior baldness
Contraindications
Projected extensive baldness
Caution with previously hair-grafted patients
Limitations
Backward direction of the hair
Scar at anterior hairline
Abrupt hairline
Elevated periauricular and nape hairline
Permanent hypesthesia
Two delays and a dog-ear revision must be performed

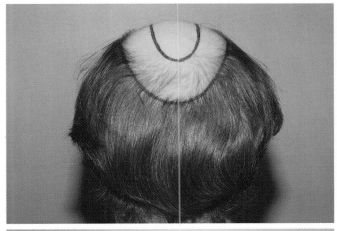
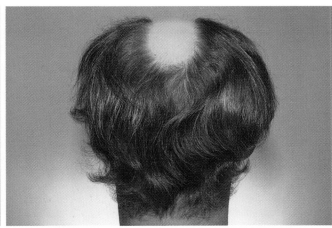
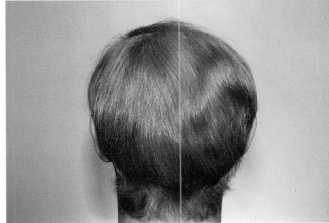

CASE 5

FIGURE 27–13. Scalp-lifting, *A,* A patient with extensive baldness immediately before a bilateral occipitoparietal scalp-lift. The area to be removed is marked with blue lines on the scalp. *B,* Appearance after the bilateral occipitoparietal lift and before the bitemporal lift. Note the 5.0-cm elevation into the crown. *C,* Appearance after the bilateral occipitoparietal and bitemporal lifts. Note the lack of slot formation because of the posterior elevation and the veer into the donor dominant scalp.

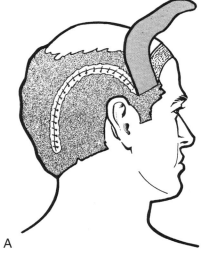
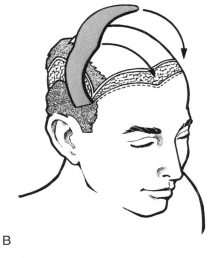

FIGURE 27–14. Temporoparieto-occipital flap. *A,* The donor site is closed after extensive undermining to the postauricular sulcus and past the hairline of the nape. *B,* The flap is transposed anteriorly. The anterior 1.0 mm of the flap is de-epithelialized, and the posterior alopecia excised. The dog-ear is revised in 6 weeks.

TABLE 27–17. Temporoparieto-occipital Flaps: Patient Preoperative Discussion

1. Same as for scalp-lifting (see Table 27–13).
2. A dog-ear that develops will be revised 6 weeks after the flap.

TABLE 27–18. Temporoparieto-occipital Flaps: Operative Issues

Preoperative Evaluation
Wet the hair to make certain that posterior baldness is not going to develop.
Same as scalp-lifting (see Table 27–14)
Preoperative Equipment Needs
Same as scalp-lifting (see Table 27–14)
Intraoperative Needs
Same as scalp-lifting (see Table 27–14)

There are four stages to performing this procedure. The first stage involves the incision of the proximal three fourths of the flap (without elevation). One week later, the distal 5.0 cm of the flap is incised, elevated, and sutured back down into place. The occipital neurovascular bundle that lies under this distal end is cauterized or ligated at this time. One week after the second delay, the flap is elevated in a subgaleal plane and is transposed to lie across the frontal area. Undermining adjacent to the donor site is performed superiorly as far as needed, laterally to the postauricular sulcus, and inferiorly past the hairline of the nape toward the clavicle. After it is determined that a loose closure is achievable, the wound is closed in a double layer and the flap is transposed anteriorly (Fig. 27–14). It is important to bevel the forehead skin edge and de-epithelial-

ize the anterior 1.0 mm of the flap edge so that hair grows through the anterior scar. Any overlapping alopecia posterior to the flap is then excised, making certain to avoid tension on the flap. Dog-ear formation that develops at the transposition site is revised 6 weeks after rotating the flap (Case 6, Fig. 27–15). If a second flap is desired, it is placed 4.0 cm behind the first flap in 3 months. The bald space between the two flaps can then be reduced with scalp reductions.

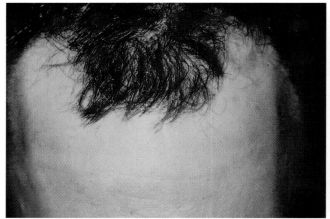

A

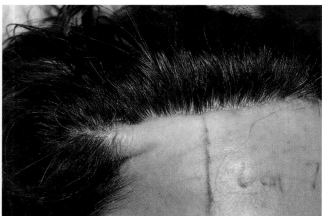

B

C

CASE 6

FIGURE 27–15. Temporoparieto-occipital flap. *A*, Patient with frontal baldness. *B*, Appearance after a temporoparieto-occipital flap with the dog-ear present at the temporal recession of the hairline. *C*, Appearance after dog-ear revision. (*A* to *C*, Courtesy of Raymond Konior, M.D.)

TABLE 27-19. Temporoparieto-occipital Flaps: Postoperative Care

Pain Management

Same as scalp-lifting (see Table 27-15)

Dressings

Same as scalp-lifting (see Table 27-15)

Complications

Same as scalp-lifting (see Table 27-15)

Injury to the spinal accessory nerve could induce weakness to the trapezius muscle.

References

1. Orentreich N. Autographs in alopecias and other selected dermatological conditions. Ann NY Acad Sci 1959;83:463.
2. Stough DB III, Berger RA, Orentreich N. Surgical improvement of cicatricial alopecia of diverse etiology. Arch Dermatol 97:331,1968.
3. Stough DB IV. Why does transplanted hair have a different quality? The electron microscope gives the answer. Presented before the First World Congress of the International Society of Hair and Scalp Surgery. Dallas, Texas, April 30–May 2, 1993.
4. Nordstrom REA. Hyperpigmentation of transplanted terminal hairs after punch hair grafting. J Dermatol Surg Oncol 1982;8:787–789.
5. Bradshaw W. Quarter grafts. Presented before the International Congress on Hair Replacement Surgery. New York: American Academy of Cosmetic Surgery, 1984.
6. Brandy DA. A new instrument for the expedient production of minigrafts. J Dermatol Surg Oncol 1992;18:487–492.
7. Brandy DA. A three-step systematic incisional-slit minigrafting approach. J Dermatol Surg Oncol 1993;19:421–426.
8. Brandy DA. A stencil for the improved accuracy, speed and aesthetics in slit-minigrafting. J Dermatol Surg Oncol, in press.
9. Nordstrom REA. Scalp kinetics in multiple excisions for correction of male pattern baldness. J Dermatol Surg Oncol 1984;10:991–995.
10. Nordstrom REA. Stretch-back in scalp reductions for male pattern baldness. Plast Reconstr Surg 1984;73:422–426.
11. Brandy DA. Circumferential scalp reduction: the application of the principles of extensive scalp-lifting for the improvement of scalp reduction surgery. J Dermatol Surg Oncol, 1994;20:277–284.
12. Frechet P. A new method for correction of the vertical scar observed following scalp reduction for extensive alopecia. J Dermatol Surg Oncol 1990;16:640–644.
13. Brandy DA. The use of retention sutures and tensed Silastic-Dacron strips for the prevention of stretch-back after alopecia reducing procedures. J Dermatol Surg Oncol, 1994;20:277–284.
14. Frechet P. Scalp extension. J Dermatol Surg Oncol 1993;19:616–622.
15. Brandy DA. Scalp-lifting: An 8 year experience with 1,231 cases. J Dermatol Surg Oncol, 1993;19:1005–1014.
16. Juri J. Use of parieto-occipital flaps in the surgical treatment of baldness. Plast Reconstr Surg 1975;55:456.

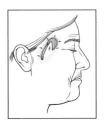

chapter 28

Liposuction

WILLIAM P. COLEMAN, III

Liposuction is one of the most commonly requested cosmetic surgical procedures.[1-3] This technique involves removal of fat cells from areas of excess fat storage (Fig. 28–1; see Cases 1 through 3, Figs. 28–3 through 28–5).[4] These localized adiposities are presumably sites of genetically determined excessive fat storage (Table 28–1).[5-14]

The tumescent anesthetic technique is used to obtain anesthesia and vasoconstriction. A solution of 0.1% lidocaine, 1:1,000,000 epinephrine, and 10 mEq/L of sodium bicarbonate is injected into the subcutaneous tissue until it becomes quite firm (Tables 28–2 and 28–3). Usually several hundred to thousands of milliliters of the fluid is

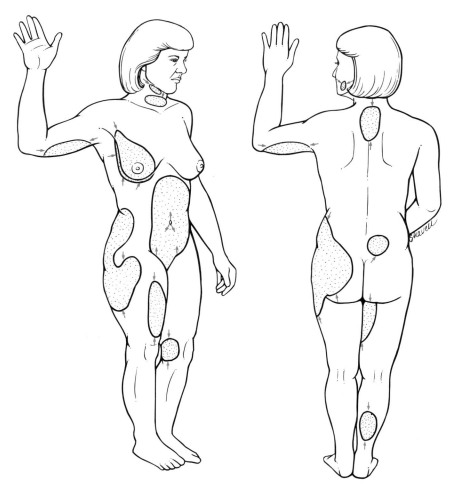

FIGURE 28–1. Areas of the body commonly exhibiting excess fat storage. Arrows indicate the predominant direction of motion of the cannula and the sites of incision to allow entry of the cannula. It is better to maintain a head-to-foot tunneling orientation when possible. This diminishes the chance of surface creases and ripples as tunnels contract postoperatively.

TABLE 28–1. Liposuction: Indications, Contraindications, Limitations

Indications

Excessive fat (see Case 2, Fig. 28–4)
Lipomas[6,7]
Hyperhidrosis[8,9]
Apocrine hidradenitis
Pseudogynecomastia[10]
Subcutaneous debulking to assist in flap movement[11,12]

Contraindications

Impaired wound healing
Poor clotting ability[13]

Limitations

Fat can only be removed in localized areas
May result in dimples or surface irregularities and/or loose overlying skin[14]

TABLE 28–2. Formula for Tumescent Solution

Ingredient	Amount
Lidocaine 0.05%	500 mg (50 mL of 1% solution)
Epinephrine 1:1,000,000	1 mg (1 mL of 1:1000 solution of epinephrine)
Sodium bicarbonate	12.5 mEq (12.5 mL of 8.4% solution)
Normal saline	1000 mL of 0.9% NaCl solution

needed to obtain proper tumescence. The safe maximum dose of lidocaine using the tumescent technique is 35 mg/kg. If the area is not sufficiently firm, vasoconstriction and anesthesia will be incomplete. Tumescent anesthesia decreases the surgical risk of correcting for loss of fluid. The tumescent anesthetic solution is best injected from the intended sites of cannula entry. Ten-mL syringes attached to an 18-gauge spinal needle are an efficient way to inject small amounts of the fluid. As each syringe is emptied, the assistant hands the surgeon a new full syringe to attach to the needle, which remains inserted in the tissue. Larger volumes require pumping the fluid through a 12- to 14-gauge injection cannula. A mechanical blood pump or electrical pump is commonly used.

After approximately 5 minutes intense vasoconstriction of the skin overlying the tumesced areas assures the surgeon that the tissues are properly anesthetized. The tumescent anesthesia bloats the fatty layer and makes it easy to guide the cannula through the proper plane without injuring underlying structures.

Liposuction is a closed surgical technique in which a cannula is inserted through a small incision and used to create tunnels through the adipose tissue (Fig. 28–2A; Tables 28–4 and 28–5).[15–22] After surgical scrubbing of the surgical site, a No. 11 scalpel blade is used to make a stab wound in one of the preselected sites. A blunt cannula is carefully inserted just under a 1-cm buffer layer of fat. A suction machine or syringe is used to create negative pressure to carry away the avulsed fat cells. The tunnels are collapsed by the use of postoperative compression garments (Fig. 28–2B; Table 28–6). Healing leads to a gradual diminution in the size of the adiposities (Cases 1 to 3, Figs. 28–3 through 28–5).

For apocrine hidradenitis and hyperhidrosis (Case 4, Fig. 28–6), the axilla may be shaved in preparation for the procedure. To identify the location of the glands, corn starch and iodine are applied. The apocrine glands responsible for the disease are dyed black, thus defining the area to be removed. The dark stain washes off during surgery; therefore, it is necessary to outline the area for treatment with gentian violet.

In treating these diseases of the axilla, a 4-mm blunt or flat cannula removes superficial fat in a "windshield wiper" motion throughout the entire axilla (see Fig. 28–6B). In contrast to treating adiposities, close attention is directed to remove as much fat adherent to the dermis as

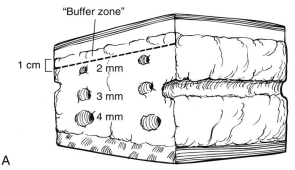

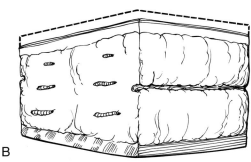

FIGURE 28–2. *A,* Under a buffer zone of 1.0 cm of the superficial fat, multiple parallel tunnels trace the course of the cannula through the deep fat. Larger-diameter cannulas are employed in the deep fat with progressively smaller-diameter cannulas in the superficial fat. *B,* Compression garments, tape, and bandages collapse the tunnels and reduce the thickness of the fat layer after completion of liposuction surgery.

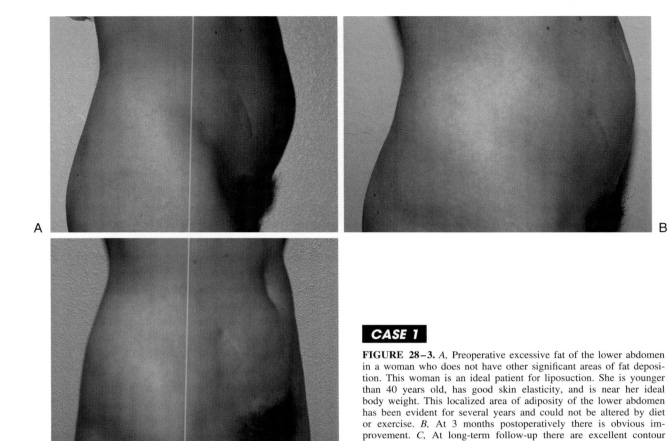

CASE 1

FIGURE 28–3. *A,* Preoperative excessive fat of the lower abdomen in a woman who does not have other significant areas of fat deposition. This woman is an ideal patient for liposuction. She is younger than 40 years old, has good skin elasticity, and is near her ideal body weight. This localized area of adiposity of the lower abdomen has been evident for several years and could not be altered by diet or exercise. *B,* At 3 months postoperatively there is obvious improvement. *C,* At long-term follow-up there are excellent contour changes. The dimple of the lower right quadrant is the top of the appendectomy incision that is present preoperatively.

possible. This maximizes the reduction of apocrine and eccrine glands. In treating apocrine hidradenitis, after the cannula has been used to separate the dermis from the superficial subcutaneous tissue, the aperture of the instrument is turned up toward the skin and the cannula is used to scrape the overlying dermis in an attempt to injure any superficially residing apocrine glands. Once the entire axilla has been treated from one entry site, the cannula is withdrawn and the same procedure is performed from the opposite side of the axilla. Only one axilla is treated at a time. This crisscross technique assures the surgeon that the entire axilla is adequately treated. This use of the cannula is in marked contrast to the usual liposuction technique that creates tunnels in the deeper fat for removal of excessive fat deposited in localized areas. After completing the procedure, the incision is sutured.

TABLE 28–3. Tumescent Anesthesia: Volumes of Tumescent Solution

Area	Amount (mL)
Abdomen	1000–2000
Lateral or posterior flanks	800–1200
Lateral thighs	1000–2000
Anterior thighs	1000–2000
Medial thighs	500–1000
Knees	500–1000
Male breasts	800–1200
Submental chin	100–250
Cheeks and jowls	200–400

TABLE 28–4. Liposuction: Patient Preoperative Discussion

1. Rest is required the first postoperative day.
2. Most patients are sore for 2 or 3 days postoperatively.
3. A special compression garment must be worn for at least 2 weeks after surgery.
4. Sutures are required, usually in multiple sites. Antibiotic ointments must be applied to these and the sutures removed after 1 week.
5. Swelling will often persist for several months.
6. You may not be able to see the final result of the procedure for 3 or more months.

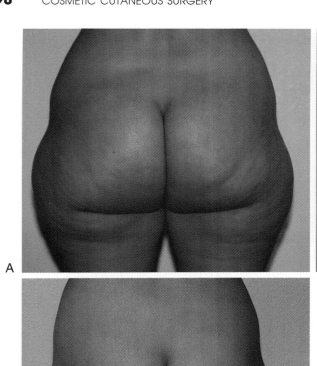
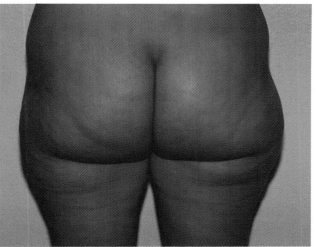
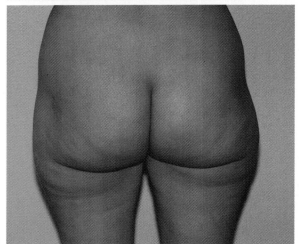
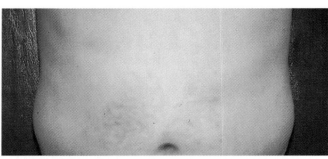

CASE 2

FIGURE 28–4. *A,* Preoperative marked fat deposition of the upper thighs and buttocks demonstrates the "violin deformity" in this woman. *B,* One month after liposuction surgery there is some improvement. *C,* Eight months postoperatively, dramatic improvement in the contour of this difficult area is seen.

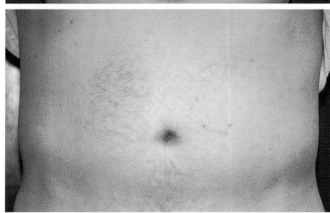

CASE 3

FIGURE 28–5. *A,* Preoperative marked fat deposition in this man demonstrates "love handle" deformity. *B,* Nine months after liposuction of the flanks and lower abdomen there is an excellent contour improvement.

TABLE 28-5. Liposuction: Operative Issues

Preoperative Evaluation

History of bleeding diathesis. Workup includes a complete blood cell count, platelet count, prothrombin time, partial thromboplastin time, and chemistry profile.

Preoperative Equipment Needs

Suction machine or appropriate syringe system
Various suction cannulas, No. 11 blade
Sterile drapes, gown, and gloves
Tumescent anesthetic solution including 0.05% to 0.1% lidocaine, 1:1,000,000 fresh epinephrine, 10 mEq sodium bicarbonate[18-20]
Topical antibacterial scrubs

Intraoperative Needs

Blood pumps, injection gun, or peristaltic pumps to deliver anesthetic fluid[21]
Reservoir bottle for fat
Pulse oximeter, cardiac monitor, and standby intravenous line may be needed when respiratory depressants are used in addition to local anesthesia.[22]

TABLE 28-6. Liposuction: Postoperative Care

Pain Management

Acetaminophen is often sufficient; class III or IV pain relievers may be required for some patients.
Ice packs should be used through the first postoperative day.

Dressings

Cover suture sites with antibiotic ointment and multiple layers of gauze to absorb leaking anesthetic tumescent fluid.
Prescribe custom girdle or tight-fitting garment.

Complications

Early Sequelae

Adequate attention to fluid and electrolytes must be maintained to prevent hypovolemic shock.[13]
Visceral penetration is possible, especially near scars from previous surgery.[23]
Pulmonary and fat emboli are possible in liposuctions combined with other procedures, especially abdominoplasty.[24,25]
Death has occurred secondary to complications from general or intravenous anesthesia.[26]
Patients should be examined 2 or 3 days postoperatively to check for infection, hematoma, or seroma.
Hematomas or seromas should be drained by needle aspiration; compression is continued for 5-7 more days.

Later Sequelae

Skin waviness and surface contour irregularities especially of the extremities and abdomen may be the result of overaggressive liposuction surgery with larger cannulas or performing liposuction too superficially. This is less of a problem now that smaller cannulas are used. Cannulas smaller than 3 mm are used in the upper layers of subcutaneous tissue with avoidance of the dermal fat junction.
Excessive liposuction in an area unbalances the body contour. Correction is by sculpting the remaining areas with liposuction.
Paresthesias—usually temporary
Persistent edema for 6 months in the area of surgery
Ptosis of gluteal fold due to suctioning the inferior buttress of the fold (Case 5, Fig. 28-7)
Creation of ``banana fold'' under the buttocks.
Suctioning of areas above and below the gluteal fold without vertical suctioning of the fold leaves an area of protuberant fat.

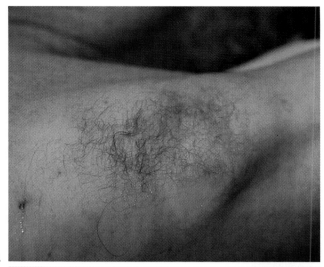

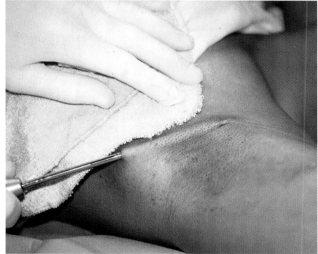

CASE 4

FIGURE 28-6. *A,* Tumescent anesthesia is of great benefit in the axilla because the volume injected below the skin raises the adnexal structures away from the deeper contents of the axillary vault (e.g., the brachial plexus). Extreme fullness of the axillary vault and intense vasoconstriction are present before starting liposuction surgery. *B,* The cannula is very superficially placed and moves in a ``windshield wiper'' motion. After the cannula separates the dermis from the superficial subcutaneous tissue, the aperture of the instrument is used to scrape the underside of the dermis, removing any remaining apocrine glands.

Because the dermis is treated aggressively during the treatment of apocrine hidradenitis, necrosis of the skin of the vault of the axilla may occur. Often a grayish color or bruising appears on the second or third postoperative day. It is possible that focal dermal ulcerations could occur in these sites, although this has not been reported. Even if scarring were to ensue from such an ulcer, this would be far preferable to the eventual scarring of the disease.

An interesting new use of liposuction is the treatment of sites of extravasation of chemotherapeutic agents. Immediately after the extravasation is recognized the region is flushed with saline and the fluid removed with liposuction.[27]

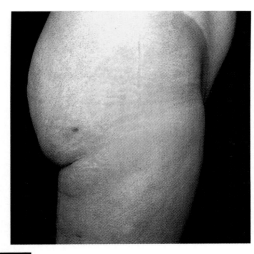

CASE 5

FIGURE 28-7. Ptosis of the buttocks after liposuction resulting from too aggressive surgery in the infragluteal fold.

References

1. Coleman WP III. The history of dermatologic liposuction. Dermatol Clin 1990;8:381–383.
2. Newman J. Liposuction surgery: Past, present, future. Am J Cosmet Surg 1984;1:1.
3. Asken S. Liposuction Surgery and Autologous Fat Transplantation. East Norwalk, CT: Appleton & Lange, 1988.
4. Coleman WP III. Liposuction surgery. In: Demis J, ed. Clinical Dermatology, 15th revision, unit 37-3. Philadelphia: JB Lippincott, 1988:1–9.
5. Brownell K, Steen S. Modern methods for weight control: The physiology and psychology of dieting. Phys Sports Med 1987;15(12):122–137.
6. Pinski K, Roenigk H. Liposuction for lipomas. Dermatol Clin 1990;8:483–492.
7. Narins R. Liposuction surgery of a buffalo hump, secondary to Cushing's disease. J Am Acad Dermatol 1989;21:307.
8. Coleman WP III. Liposuction for hyperhidrosis. In: Robins P, ed. Surgical Gems in Dermatology, vol 2. New York, Journal Publishing, 1992;100–103.
9. Lillis P, Coleman WP III. Liposuction for treatment of axillary hyperhidrosis. Dermatol Clin 1990;8:479–482.
10. Coleman WP III. Non-cosmetic applications of liposuction. J Dermatol Surg Oncol 1988;14:1085–1090.
11. Field L, Spinowitz A. Flap elevation and mobilization by blunt liposuction cannula dissection in reconstructive surgery. Dermatol Clin 1990;8:493–499.
12. Field L, Skouge J, Anhalt T, et al. Blunt liposuction cannula dissection with and without suction assisted lipectomy in reconstructive surgery. J Dermatol Surg Oncol 1988;14:1116–1122.
13. Chrisman B, Coleman WP III. Determining safe limits for untransfused outpatient liposuction: Personal experience and review of the literature. J Dermatol Surg Oncol 1988;14:1095–1102.
14. Teimourin B, Rogers WB. A national survey of complications associated with suction lipectomy: A comparative study. Plast Reconstr Surg 1989;84:628–631.
15. Fischer A, Fischer G. First surgical treatment for molding body's cellulite with three 5-mm incisions. Bull Int Acad Cosmet Surg 1976;3:35.
16. Illouz Y. Body contouring by lipolysis: A 5-year experience with over 3000 cases. Plast Reconstr Surg 1983;72:511–524.
17. Ottani F, Fournier P. A history and comparison of suction techniques until their debut in North America. In: Hetter G, ed. Lipoplasty: The Theory and Practice of Blunt Suction Lipectomy. Boston: Little, Brown, 1984:19–23.
18. Klein J. The tumescent technique: Anesthesia and modified liposuction technique. Dermatol Clin 1990;8:425–437.
19. Lillis PJ. The tumescent technique for liposuction surgery. Dermatol Clin 1990;8:439–450.
20. Klein JA. Tumescent technique for regional anesthesia permits lidocaine doses of 35 mg/kg for liposuction: Peak plasma lidocaine levels are diminished and delayed 12 hours. J Dermatol Surg Oncol 1990;16:248–263.
21. Coleman WP III, Badame A, Phillips H. A new technique for injection of tumescent anesthetic mixtures. J Dermatol Surg Oncol 1991;17:535–537.
22. American Academy of Dermatology. Guidelines of care for liposuction. J Am Acad Dermatol 1991;24:489–494.
23. Teimourian B. Complications associated with suction lipectomy. Clin Plast Surg 1989;16:385–394.
24. Christman K. Death following suction lipectomy and abdominoplasty (letter). Plast Reconstr Surg 1986;78:428.
25. Coleman WP III. Liposuction. In: Coleman WP III, Hanke CW, Alt T, Asken S, eds. Cosmetic Surgery of the Skin. Philadelphia: BC Decker, 1991:213–238.
26. Bernstein G, Hanke CW. Safety of liposuction: A review of 9478 cases performed by dermatologists. J Dermatol Surg Oncol 1988;14:1112–1114.
27. Gault DT. Extravasation injuries. Br J Plast Surg 1993;46:91.

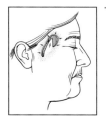

chapter 29

Blepharoplasty

PAUL S. COLLINS

Upper eyelid blepharoplasty is performed to eliminate fat protrusions and to reestablish the upper eyelid crease that has been obliterated by tissue ptosis. Lower eyelid blepharoplasty is typically performed to eliminate fat protrusions that give a "tired appearance."

ANATOMY OF THE EYELID

The upper eyelid is divided into an orbital (preseptal) and a tarsal portion. The orbital portion lies between the orbital rim and the superior border of the tarsus (Fig. 29–1A). The tarsal portion of the eyelid overlies the tarsal plate. The upper eyelid crease (superior palpebral fold), 8 to 11 mm above the eyelid margin, is formed by the attachment of the levator aponeurosis (Fig. 29–1B). Above the eyelid crease in the septal portion of the eyelid there are seven major layers: skin, orbicularis muscle, orbital septum, orbital fat, levator aponeurosis, Müller's muscle, and conjunctiva. The lower lid tarsus is smaller (4 to 5 mm at the central lid) than the upper lid tarsus (8 to 10 mm at the central lid).

INDICATIONS

Upper lid blepharoplasty is indicated in those patients who have redundancy of the upper eyelid tissues (dermochalasis) with or without fat protrusions that obliterates the natural sulcus found between the eyelid and orbital rim (Figs. 29–2 through 29–4; Case 1, Fig. 29–5). Some patients will have an upper or a lateral visual field defect due to the ptotic skin. Fat pad protrusion is the usual indication for a lower lid blepharoplasty (Figs. 29–6 through 29–11; Case 2, Fig. 29–12). One can also achieve some skin tightening and correct an incipient lid laxity with a muscle suspension flap.

CONTRAINDICATIONS

Blepharoplasty is a cosmetic procedure, but it can be a corrective procedure when lid ptosis interferes with upper and lateral visual fields. A medical problem takes precedence. Once stable, the blepharoplasty can be considered. When in doubt as to the significance of a medical problem, a consultation requesting suitability to perform surgery should be obtained.

There are several local orbital problems that should also preclude surgery. Acute glaucoma is a contraindication. Ectropion is a relative contraindication depending on its severity and the ability of the surgeon to perform a lid-shortening procedure. Naturally any local infection, uncontrolled skin disease, or recent local surgery (cataract surgery) should delay surgery. Some physicians will not perform the procedure in patients who are legally blind in one eye. If a complication occurs in the "good" eye, there is the risk of total blindness.

LIMITATIONS

Elimination of rhytides in the orbital region, either laterally (crow's feet) or from the inferior eyelid region, is a frequent request. Although there will usually be some improvement of the inferior eyelid rhytides, the lateral rhytides will remain unchanged. The patient should be informed not to expect the rhytides to disappear. The procedure will also not correct hyperpigmentation (dark circles under the eyes) nor eliminate chronic edema or festoons, which are also common treatment requests by patients. Lower lid laxity and ectropion are not corrected by the standard blepharoplasty.

Text continued on page 305

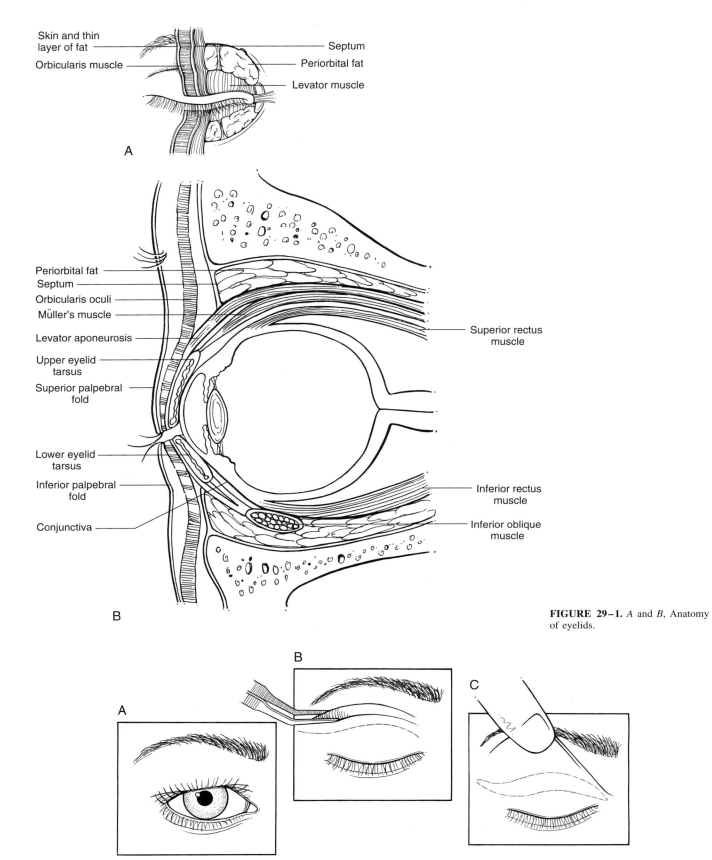

FIGURE 29–1. *A* and *B*, Anatomy of eyelids.

FIGURE 29–2. Upper eyelid blepharoplasty. *A,* Redundant skin hoods the eye. *B,* The eyelid crease, where the fine lid skin meets the heavier orbit skin, may be used to mark the incision line. Forceps grasp the redundant skin in increasing quantities until the eyelid is forced open. *C,* The tissue is marked by the area pinched up by the forceps. The superior and inferior borders of the incision conform to the area of redundant skin. The widest portion of the S-shaped ellipse is just lateral to the pupil. The medial end of the incision is rounded.

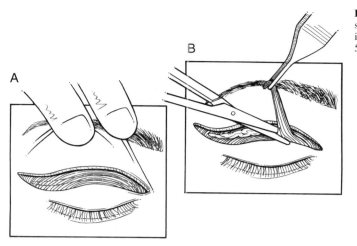

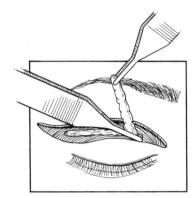

FIGURE 29–3. Upper eyelid blepharoplasty. *A,* After removal of the skin, the underlying muscle is exposed. The area of muscle to be removed is estimated. *B,* The muscle is tented up with a fine-toothed forceps, and a 5- to 8-mm wide strip of muscle is excised with scissors.

FIGURE 29–4. The fat is raised with a forceps, and the base of the elevated fat is grasped with bipolar forceps and cauterized. The excess fat is then excised with scissors superior to the line of cauterization.

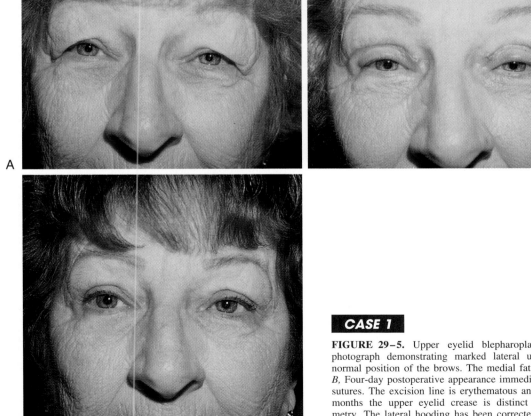

CASE 1

FIGURE 29–5. Upper eyelid blepharoplasty. *A,* Preoperative photograph demonstrating marked lateral upper lid ptosis with normal position of the brows. The medial fat pads are protuberant. *B,* Four-day postoperative appearance immediately after removal of sutures. The excision line is erythematous and edematous. *C,* At 3 months the upper eyelid crease is distinct with minimal asymmetry. The lateral hooding has been corrected by extension of the upper eyelid incision onto the temporal orbital region.

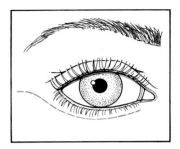

FIGURE 29–6. Lower eyelid blepharoplasty. Placement of the incision is lateral to the puncta and extends beyond the orbital rim with an upward arch before it reaches the lateral palpebral angle.

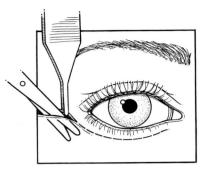

FIGURE 29–7. The skin–muscle flap is gently raised with blunt scissors.

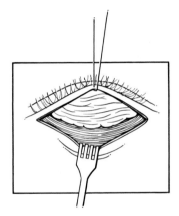

FIGURE 29–8. A suture is placed through the eyelid margin and the lid is pulled over the globe, exposing the underlying muscle. Blunt dissection continues caudally to the infraorbital rim. The wound edge is held back with a multipronged hook.

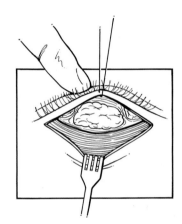

FIGURE 29–9. Gentle pressure on the globe pushes the fat anteriorly so that it bulges below the orbital septum. The three compartments of fat (medial, middle, and lateral) are accessed gently and the fat is teased out.

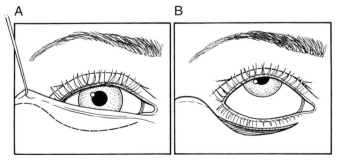

FIGURE 29–10. Lower eyelid blepharoplasty. *A,* The flap is draped in a superior and lateral direction over the incision line. *B,* To accurately measure the amount of the flap to be resected, the patient looks up to the top of the head. The area to be excised is indicated by the broken red line.

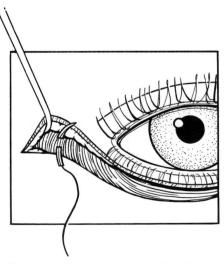

FIGURE 29–11. A 6-0 permanent suture attaches the muscle to the periosteum of the lateral orbital bone, thus supporting the flap.

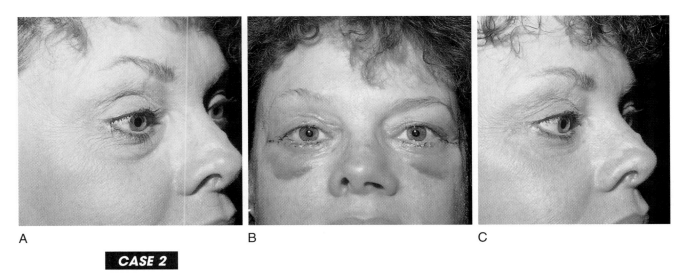

A   B   C

CASE 2

FIGURE 29–12. Lower eyelid blepharoplasty. *A,* The lower eyelids have protuberant fat pads, the primary indication for lower lid blepharoplasty. *B,* Four-day postoperative appearance before removal of the sutures. Bruising is typically more extensive with lower lid blepharoplasty. *C,* Four-month postoperative appearance shows flattening of the lower lid tissues and maturation of the incision lines.

EXPECTED CHANGES AND DURATION OF CHANGES

The eyes are a main focal point of the face, and any change by blepharoplasty can produce dramatic results. The surgery beautifies the eyes by removing redundant tissue, altering the slit-like appearance, and thereby enlarging the appearance of the eyes. The "tired" look is corrected with removal of the fat pads. This is especially noticeable with the lower eyelids where the fat pads produce a tired, sleepless, and aged appearance. The upper lid lateral bulky tissue, producing hooding and a "sad eye," can also be dramatically improved.

The duration of change of the upper eyelid is dependent on stability of the brow and the frontalis muscle. With aging, ptosis will become more prominent, the forehead tissue sinking further over the orbital rim into the orbital socket, compromising the previous upper lid surgery. The medial fat pad, frequently overlooked, may not be removed with the first procedure and becomes overtly protuberant with time.

Since the major changes of aging found in the lower eyelids are due to the fat protrusions, lower lid blepharoplasty changes have a longer duration (Case 2, Fig. 29–12A). Thus the requirement for additional lower eyelid surgery is usually due to a failure of adequate removal of the medial or lateral fat pads.

PREOPERATIVE EVALUATION

Medical History

The medical history, including allergies and medications, is reviewed to ensure there are no risks to the proposed surgery (Table 29–1).

Patients with an allergic history may be plagued by recurrent or permanent periorbital edema and blepharochalasis. Thyroid disease is associated with ophthalmopathy. Hyperthyroidism can produce exophthalmos. Hypothyroidism (myxedema) produces edema with thickening of the eyelid skin that leads to drooping and bagginess. The patient may even be euthyroid and still have ophthalmic involvement, including scleral show (vertical retraction of the lower eyelids), chemosis, persistent eyelid edema, lagophthalmos, and proptosis. Multiple sclerosis can be aggravated by stress such as surgery and lead to loss of visual acuity. Incipient glaucoma, provoked and masked by symptoms incorrectly associated with the surgery, may eventuate in visual loss before the disease is discovered. Keratoconjunctivitis sicca, associated with Sjögren's disease, produces the dry eye syndrome. An aggressive surgical blepharoplasty can aggravate the already dry eye, aggravating symptoms. Preoperative ophthalmologic examination will verify these potential problems as well as any lenticular opacities or retinal pathology. It is important to inquire as to the use of contact lenses, which after surgery may not be used for several weeks.

Uncontrolled hypertension, coagulation disorders, and atherosclerotic disease can increase the risk of bleeding with the threat of retrobulbar hematoma. Diabetes mellitus will increase the incidence for postoperative infection, while smoking exacerbates local edema, is associated with poor wound healing, and increases blood pressure and the pulse rate, thus augmenting bleeding.

Medications

Any medication that increases the tendency for bleeding should be eliminated before surgery. Aspirin and aspirin-containing medications are the most common surgical causes of excess surgical bleeding and subsequent hematoma formation.

TABLE 29–1. Blepharoplasty: Preoperative Evaluation, Laboratory Results, Preoperative and Intraoperative Equipment Needs

Preoperative Evaluation

Medical History

Systemic disease
  Recent myocardial infarction or unstable angina pectoris
  Congestive heart failure
  Uncontrolled hypertension
  Diabetes mellitus
  Thyroid disease
  Multiple sclerosis
Ocular disease
  Glaucoma
  Blindness or severely compromised visual acuity
  Dry eye syndrome
  Allergies
  Inflammatory eye disease
  Previous orbital surgery
Bleeding diathesis and medications that enhance bleeding

Orbital Examination

General examination
  Position of brow
  Asymmetries
  Prominence of brow and orbital bones
  Position of eyeball and sockets
  Lateral rhytides (crow's feet)
  Ocular diseases, inflammations, tumors, and abnormalities
Upper eyelid
  Redundancy of skin
  Fat pads, medial and middle
  Prominence of lacrimal gland
  Presence of lateral fat pad
  Lateral hooding
  Levator ptosis
  Skin tumors
Lower eyelid
  Laxity of lower eyelid
  Fat pads, medial, middle, and lateral
  Prominence of orbicularis oculi muscle
  Presence of festoons, pigmentation, and edema

Laboratory Results

Complete blood cell count
Platelet count
Prothrombin time
Partial thromboplastin time
Chemistries
Thyroid function tests

Preoperative Equipment Needs

Electrosurgical machine with bipolar coagulator capabilities
Adson bipolar forceps
Delicate needle holder for 6-0 and 7-0 suture
Fine mosquito forceps
Skin retractors: three or four prong, blunt
Scissors: baby Metzenbaum, curved plastic scissors, iris or Kaye scissors
Silk suture, 6-0 and 7-0, and Prolene suture, 6-0, with plastic needles

Intraoperative Needs

Sterile drapes
Adequate operating room lighting
Skin marking pen
Suction (optional)
Cotton-tipped applicators
Ophthalmic antibiotic ointment

Hypertensive patients may be taking a nonselective β-adrenergic blocker, such as propranolol, which protects the heart against the deleterious effects of catecholamines.[2,3] Cardiac blood vessels have only β-receptors, while peripheral vessels have both β- and α-receptors. Patients taking propranolol may respond to epinephrine by paradoxically developing a marked hypertensive episode followed quickly by a reflex bradycardia. This combination can potentially cause a cardiac arrest. Selective β-blockers do not cause this interaction and are safe to use. Most studies indicate that no arrhythmias occur with epinephrine doses of 5 μg/mL. A concentration of 1 : 200,000 epinephrine equals 5 μg/mL. Usually the volume of anesthetic with epinephrine used in blepharoplasty is small and not of consequence even in the presence of nonselective β-adrenergic blocker. Caution must be followed if several simultaneous procedures are being performed and the volume of epinephrine is significant. Sudden cessation of propranolol can produce a rebound adrenergic excess and increased angina.[1]

Prior Surgery in the Region

A previous blepharoplasty or periorbital surgery may have left significant scar tissues that will lead to a tendency to excess bleeding. The previous surgery may also have weakened the lower lid structures, resulting in a propensity to ectropion. Exophthalmos can be either familial or secondary to hyperthyroidism. This can limit the improvement sought. Asymmetry is common but usually not overtly obvious and may be hidden by fat protrusions or ptotic skin. It may then be unmasked by the surgery, and, unless the patient had been prewarned, its appearance may be attributed to poor surgical technique. The presence of deep-seated or "sunken" eyeballs may be exaggerated and become unsightly after blepharoplasty. Surgery in these individuals is usually not recommended. In eyelid surgery, errors of omission carry far fewer consequences than errors of commission. It is wiser to remove too little than too much skin, particularly from the lower lid, and less radical removal of fat is more desirable than removal of an excessive amount, which will produce a sunken, cadaverous appearance.

Physical Examination

The patient should first undergo a limited general physical examination, including determination of blood pressure and pulse rate and cardiac and lung auscultation. Patients with complicated medical histories may require evaluation by a consultant physician to determine their ability to undergo surgery.

Eyelids and Periorbital Region

Evaluation of the surgical site should first include a general examination of both orbital regions, followed by specific evaluation of upper and then lower eyelids. The general examination will determine the symmetry of the bony orbit, eyelids, and eyes. Considerable asymmetry can be camouflaged by presence of redundant skin and/or periorbital fat and may not become evident until after surgery. The patient will then incorrectly assume the surgery was the cause. The orbital rim may be prominent, especially laterally, encroaching on the globe and lids, thus inhibiting the ability to create a distinct upper eyelid crease. One eye may be larger than the other, or the sockets themselves may vary in size or position. The eyeball sockets may be sunken or cadaverous, rendering surgical correction difficult and possibly exaggerating this anatomic variation.

The brows may be asymmetrical, or even ptotic, owing to previous temporal nerve damage. Particular attention should be given to the horizontal rhytides of the forehead. Arching of these creases above the brow indicates frontalis muscle contraction in an attempt to elevate ptotic eyebrows. The action of the frontalis muscles can be assessed by having the patient direct the eyes into downward gaze and by massaging the forehead in a downward direction to relax the muscles.[4] The significance of the brow ptosis into the orbital region can now be correctly analyzed.

The presence of eyelid edema, lateral eyelid rhytides (crow's feet), or festoons should be recorded since they will not be corrected by the surgery. The conjunctiva and sclera should be clear and without evidence of inflammation or abnormalities, and the patient's visual acuity should be checked. A preoperative ophthalmic consultation will evaluate these areas in greater detail and report the presence of any retinal disease and glaucoma. Finally, the skin should be examined for any blemishes or tumors, such as xanthelasma, milia, or syringoma.

The Upper Eyelid Examination

The fullness of the upper eyelids is directly influenced by the brow. The ideal position of the eyebrow is at the level of the superior orbital rim in men and slightly above the superior orbital rim in women. The degree of any brow ptosis must be evaluated and determined if its influence on the upper eyelids is of significance. A major portion of upper eyelid ptosis may be entirely due to the effect of a ptotic brow rolling over the bony orbital rim and impinging into the orbital socket. Unless the brow is lifted, ptosis will recur after blepharoplasty because removal of the eyelid tissue will allow the ptotic brow tissue to fall even farther into the orbital socket. Compounding this mistake is the unpleasant fact that once the blepharoplasty has been completed, there may be paucity of orbital tissue remaining. An attempt now at lifting the brow will produce lagophthalmos of the upper eyelid because of a deficiency of eyelid tissue.

The upper lid should be examined for symmetry and to ensure there is no levator muscle ptosis with its resultant lid ptosis. The normal covering of the upper cornea is about 1 mm with the eyes in the primary position. Deviation greater than 1 mm may suggest levator muscle malfunction. Additionally, one can measure the vertical eyelid fissure opening, which is the distance from the lower eyelid margin to the upper eyelid margin at its greatest dimension. The greatest height of the eyelid fissure is generally on the nasal edge of the pupil. Normal vertical eyelid fissure is 7 to 10 mm for men and 8 to 12 mm for women. Again, deviation from normal requires further evaluation of levator muscle function. A standard blepharoplasty will not correct ptosis due to levator malfunction.

The presence of bulging fat pads (medial and middle) is to be noted. The lateral upper eyelid region may bulge from a protruding orbital lobe of the lacrimal gland or occasionally from the presence of a lateral fat pad.[5] Lateral fat pads are correctable while lacrimal gland ptosis may not be. Lateral hooding should be recorded and noted to the patient. Correction will require extension of the upper eyelid excision onto the temporal skin. Sometimes the lateral upper eyelid tissue is heavy and thickened, lending to the exaggerated hooded appearance. Awareness will enable the surgeon to carefully trim the subcutaneous tissue in this region resulting in a more satisfying cosmetic appearance. The temporal excision will heal slower and with more significant and prolonged erythema than the orbital excision. Upper eyelid skin tumors, such as xanthelasma or seborrheic keratosis, may require treatment before the blepharoplasty procedure.

The Lower Eyelid Examination

Evaluation of the lower eyelid is more critical than that of the upper lid. The presence of scleral show, lid laxity, ectropion or entropion, pigmentation, fat protrusions, orbicularis oculi muscle hypertrophy, eyelid edema, and festoons or malar pouches should be recorded in detail.[6] Lower eyelid malposition is a serious complication of blepharoplasty, and thus the integrity of the lower eyelid must be carefully evaluated. Eyelid laxity is probably the result of stretching of the lateral and/or medial canthal tendon as opposed to actual tarsal lengthening. Differential forces between the anterior (skin and orbicularis muscle) and the posterior lamella (tarsus and eyelid retractors) help determine if ectropion or entropion will result. Horizontal lid laxity is determined by pulling the lower eyelid in a horizontal direction. Normal excursion is less than 8 mm, and abnormal excursion is a function of a redundant and stretched lower eyelid.[7] After the gentle flicking down of the lower eyelid, there should be a brisk ''snap back'' to its position against the globe without blinking. If blinking is necessary, then laxity is present. These are valuable, simple tests that assess the function of the lower eyelid and will help the physician avoid unforeseen complications postoperatively. Scleral show may be present. It is commonly caused by a previous lower eyelid blepharoplasty.

Orbicularis oculi muscle hypertrophy of the lower eyelid is more prominent in younger patients. The ''muscle roll'' of the orbicularis oculi muscle is accentuated by animation of the face. However, it is a normal variant and the patient must understand that blepharoplasty will not eliminate the roll. Careful trimming of the muscle, without concomitant excision of the overlying skin, can improve but not necessarily eliminate the extent of prominence.

Redundant skin of the lower eyelid usually does not require significant excision. Indeed, excessive trimming will induce scleral show or eyelid malposition. The skin laxity will improve when the fat pads are removed and the skin falls into the resultant hollow. By having the patient look superiorly toward the top of the head, a true evaluation of skin redundancy can be accurately made perioperatively. It is surprising how the excess skin suddenly disappears when the eyes gaze superiorly. It is wiser to err with excess skin (often improved with a chemical peel) than to deal with an ectropion.

There are three fat pads in the lower eyelid (see Fig. 29–9). The middle pad is the most prominent. The lateral fat pad is oriented more superiorly than the medial and middle lower lid fat pads. This superior location may cause this pad to be overlooked during surgery, leaving a bulge at the lateral lower eyelid postoperatively. The lower eyelid medial fat pad is simpler to discover and thus is seldom erroneously bypassed, unlike the upper medial fat pad.

Lower eyelid hyperpigmentation will respond to a chemical peel, either trichloroacetic acid or a phenol formula. Orbital rim pouches, palpebral bags, malar pouch, or festoons may be the result of chronic pockets of edema with eventual fibrosis and recurrent edema. They are not corrected by blepharoplasty.

Preoperative Discussion of Benefits and Risks of the Procedure

Patient discussion is a critical stage of the preoperative evaluation. If rapport cannot be developed during this time, the procedure should be delayed or possibly not considered. During the consultation, it is important to realize the patient concerns and desires, and the physician must not assume anything during this discussion. The patient's personality and motives must be carefully evaluated. Unrealistic expectations should be noted and discussed before surgery. The use of a mirror will facilitate the anatomic findings of concern to the patient and enable the physician to specifically point out what is less likely to be corrected by the surgery. It is paramount the patient understands not only what the planned surgery will accomplish but also its limitations and failures. It is emphasized that blepharoplasty may not result in symmetry, be free of scarring, or eliminate puffy eyelids due to edema. Since postoperative edema can be significant and persistent, this sequelae is emphasized. These shortcomings must be relayed to all individuals, and especially to those who express grandiose speculation of the accomplishments of blepharoplasty surgery. Severe complications and imperfect results are to be detailed to a patient with unrealistic expectations, while, with others, these are noted but their uncommonness is expressed.

The typical expected time of recovery is outlined (Table 29–2). The possible additional recovery time necessary when significant sequelae or even complications occur is discussed. The patient is reminded that it is impossible to predict the future and therefore no promises of exact recovery time can ever be given. A thorough explanation of the sequelae (occurrences inherent to the procedure such as bruising, pain, edema, surgical scars) and complications (occurrences not normally expected such as hematoma, wound dehiscence, or allergic reactions) will enable the patient to make an informed decision. Discussion also includes the most serious complications: blindness of one or both eyes and severe allergic reactions. This is not to discourage but to emphasize to the patient that this surgery should not be taken lightly or without adequate preparation (Table 29–3).

It is the patient who must determine whether to undergo the procedure with its risk of sequelae, complications, and delay in recovery. A photograph album of the surgeon's previous results, both excellent and average, will demonstrate the expected surgical outcome. Presenting photographs of other physicians' results can be misleading to patients and makes it seem that you have greater surgical skills than your level of proficiency.

The medications to be used during the procedure are explained to the patient, who may suddenly remember an incompatibility. After review of the medical history and physical evaluation, the surgeon then can make his or her recommendations, explain any shortcomings, and request pertinent additional information or consultations before performing surgery.

Finally, at the conclusion of the consultation and the physical examination, the patient is given instructional sheets on the preoperative and postoperative surgical course and care, a list of medications to avoid, the total fees involved, a surgical consent form, and a risk form explaining possible sequelae and complications of blepharoplasty.

PERFORMING BLEPHAROPLASTY

Knowledge of orbital anatomy (see Fig. 29–1) and a complete understanding of the potential for complications and their causes will enable dissection with absolute hemostasis. The surgical cavity must not contain any foreign material such as stray cotton from a cotton-tipped applicator or fragments of gauze that can stimulate edema, granulation, or scar tissue. Fluid or blood that accumulates under the lower lid flap can subsequently produce contracture of the flap and an ectropion. Hemosiderin deposition can also result in unsightly hyperpigmentation. Even the preoperative surgical scrub must be meticulous, with avoidance of eye contact with chlorhexidine (Hibiclens), a known corneal irritant and clouding agent.

Bleeding with the threat of retrobulbar hematoma has its highest incidence within the first few hours after the surgery. Immediate decompression of the orbital septum by removal of sutures and a reopening of the wound followed by pinpoint coagulation of any bleeding vessels is paramount. The surgeon must be within instant communication and in close proximity to the surgical operatory to prevent this potential disaster. Postoperatively the incidence of this severe complication exponentially decreases after several hours.

TABLE 29-2. Blepharoplasty: Patient Information Sheet: Preoperative and Postoperative Care

Eyelid Surgery Instructions
Before Your Operation:

Preliminary:
1. No aspirin or medicines containing aspirin for 2 weeks before surgery. These medicines can interfere with normal blood clotting, can cause excess bleeding that may result in complications including blindness and scarring. If needed, use acetaminophen instead. No vitamin E for 2 weeks before surgery.
2. It is necessary to have an ophthalmologic (eye) examination including a glaucoma test before surgery.
3. Laboratory work is required for the surgery.
4. Smokers should stop smoking for 2 days before surgery and for 2 days after surgery. Smoking interferes with healing and causes postoperative bleeding. PLEASE DO NOT SMOKE.
5. Arrange for someone to drive you to your home, hotel, or motel after surgery.

Day of Surgery:
1. Do not wear any make-up, mascara, or eye shadow. Do not apply cream to your face.
2. Do not wear your contact lenses to the office or for the first week after surgery.
3. Sips of water and a light breakfast of toast can be taken the morning of the surgery unless instructed otherwise. Avoid drinking coffee and tea. They contain caffeine, which can raise your blood pressure and cause excess bleeding.
4. Do not take medication of any kind (unless instructed by your physician). Your preoperative medications will be given to you on arrival.
5. Wear comfortable, loose-fitting clothes that do not have to be pulled over your head. Pantyhose should not be worn because you must lower your head to tug them on.
6. You may wish to bring sunglasses to wear after your operation.
7. You must have a responsible person drive you after surgery. On arrival at the office, leave your driver's name and phone number, as well as the address and phone number of where you will be staying the night after surgery. We often call to check your progress and answer any questions you may have that first night.
8. You must have someone spend the first 24 hours with you. Medications given during the surgery may make you drowsy, confused, and dizzy, leading to falls and injuries. Your vision will be blurred, which will make walking without help difficult. Additional instructions and prescriptions can be given to the person staying with you. Such prescriptions should be filled promptly.
9. If you have any questions before your operation, please call our office.

After Your Operation:
1. Bed rest for the first 48 hours. Do not strain, bend over, or do any physical work. This will cause increased bruising and swelling that will compromise your healing and surgical results.
2. Take medications according to instructions. You will be given an ophthalmic antibiotic ointment after your surgery. Please apply the antibiotic ointment as often as needed to keep the eyelid incisions moist. This prevents crusting, which interferes with healing and causes scarring. Also apply the ointment directly to the eye at night for lubrication, which prevents drying and corneal abrasions.
3. Apply cool compresses to your eyelids consisting of gauze pads or a clean washcloth soaked in dilute salt water (1 level teaspoon of salt to 1 quart of water). It does not have to be iced. This is soothing and helps control swelling. Do not use hot or warm compresses!
4. No smoking for 48 hours after your operation because it will interfere with healing and cause excess bleeding.
5. No alcohol for 5 days after surgery. Alcohol will also cause excess bleeding and interfere with healing.
6. You can expect:
   a. Moderate discomfort along the incisions and at the corner of your eyes. Use acetaminophen or the pain medicine prescribed. Most of the discomfort will occur the first day of surgery. Take the acetaminophen or pain medication as soon as you experience discomfort. By waiting for the discomfort to become intolerable, you will actually decrease the effectiveness of the medication.
   b. Moderate swelling that will last several days.
   c. Black and blue discoloration that can last several weeks.
   d. Bloodshot eyes. Usually only one eye is involved and while it may look terrible it is not harmful.
   e. Moderate bleeding from wound edges during the first 24 hours. It is better to have the blood seep from the incisions than collect under the skin and prolong the black and blue discoloration.
7. Please call if you have
   a. Pain not responding to medication.
   b. Marked swelling or obviously more swelling on one side than the other.
   c. Significant changes in vision (anything more than mild blurring).
   d. If any other question or problem arises.
8. You may read or watch television if you wish, although you can expect to have blurred vision for the first several days. Intermittent mild visual blurring can occur for several weeks after surgery. Repetitive eye blinking will help clear these blurring episodes.
9. You may wear eye make-up on the sixth day after surgery.
10. Avoid prolonged exposure to sun until all bruising has resolved. This may cause unsightly pigmentation that can last for months.
11. Avoid eating salty foods, which will cause fluid retention and excess swelling.

Office Visits:
First: 4 days after surgery at which time your sutures will be removed.
Second: 1 week to 10 days after your surgery. Additional visits will be determined by your physician.

TABLE 29-3. Blepharoplasty: Risks

You and your doctor are considering a plastic surgery procedure to remove skin and fat from your eyelids. This operation is called a ''blepharoplasty'' and is also known as an ''eye lift.'' This type of operation is done by making surgical cuts at the eyelids and adjacent facial skin. This is an elective and not emergency surgery. It is not necessary to improve or protect your physical health. It is possible that your appearance will be unlike your expectations and therefore less pleasing after the operation than it is now. Because of these facts, your doctor cannot guarantee a favorable result from the operation you are considering. Furthermore, even if the surgery is successful, the results will not be permanent due to natural aging. Although complications and adverse results are uncommon from this type of operation, they do sometimes occur. Doctor _____ will do his best to avoid any possible complications but he cannot guarantee they will not occur.

Some of the possible complications of eyelid surgery are as noted:
Bleeding, abnormal collections of blood underneath the skin of the eyelids and face, discoloration of the eyelids and face, nerve damage causing temporary and permanent loss of feeling and weakness of the eyelids, infection, prolonged pain, swelling of portion or all of the eyelids, drooping of the eyelids, and insufficient or excessive amount of wrinkle removal, and even blindness are some of the possible complications of this surgery. Personality changes and mental difficulties following the surgery sometimes occur even when the operation has been a cosmetic success. Allergic or other adverse reactions to one or more of the substances and medications used in the operation can also occur.
Complications of this operation can cause the need for further surgery. Some of the complications can cause prolonged illness, visual problems, dry and irritated eyes, draining wounds, unsightly and painful scars, weakened and drooping eyelids, and permanent deformity of the eyelids and inconvenience. Allergic reactions have been known to cause death. There are also other rare complications from this operation in addition to the ones noted above. However, it is not possible to advise you of every conceivable complication. The purpose of this form is not to frighten you or upset you. The complications stated above are very unlikely to occur. The purpose of this form is merely to ensure that your decision to have this operation is not made in ignorance of the risks of a blepharoplasty, also known as an eye lift surgery. No promise can be made that complications will not occur.

INTRAOPERATIVE NEEDS AND SPECIAL INSTRUMENTS AND EQUIPMENT

An electrosurgical machine with bipolar coagulating capability and Adson bipolar forceps are mandatory to obtain complete hemostasis. A fine needle holder for handling 6-0 and 7-0 suture is advisable. Several types of scissors can be used during the operation. Straight, 5-inch, baby Metzenbaum with round blades (for blunt dissection and tissue trimming); plastic curved scissors, 5 to 6 inches, with blunted point (to trim lower lid tissue with the curve paralleling the natural curve of the eyelid); and iris or Kaye 4-inch scissors (to dissect and separate muscle tissue for the suspending suture and fine undermining of the lateral region of the eyelid incision) will facilitate the surgical procedure. Retractors, with three or four blunt prongs, will minimize tissue trauma while facilitating tissue exposure. Finally, curved mosquito hemostat forceps can be used for clamping fat before excision and cauterization (I do not clamp fat but use the bipolar Adson forceps to cauterize the fat and then excise the excess fat above the burnt tissue). A hemostat also secures the suture retraction of the lower eyelid to the head dressing. Silk suture, 6-0 or 7-0, and Prolene, 6-0, for the lower lid suspension, are required.

UPPER EYELID BLEPHAROPLASTY PROCEDURE

The quantity of upper eyelid redundant tissue to be removed can be estimated by careful observation (Fig. 29–2A; Case 1, Fig. 29–5). Fine, redundant, crinkled skin can be observed above the eyelid crease within the superior palpebral fold. Where the fine skin meets the heavier skin of the orbit marks the superior incision line. Alternately, or as a method of verification, utilizing forceps, the upper tissue is grasped in increasing quantities until the eyelid is forced open (Fig. 29–2B). The tissue is then marked, establishing the superior border of the incision (Fig. 29–2C).

The upper lid tarsal plate is 8 to 11 mm wide, with the upper eyelid crease marking the attachment of the levator aponeurosis to the plate. The location and marking of the crease is important in indicating the inferior edge of the upper eyelid incision. An important factor in upper eyelid blepharoplasty is the eyelid crease since a well-formed eyelid crease will mask many other imperfections. The widest portion of ellipse should be located just lateral to the pupil (Fig. 29–2C).

One of the most offensive signs of aging to most patients is lateral hooding of the upper eyelids. Most hooding problems can be corrected by extending the lateral incision beyond the orbital rim. It is important that the lower incision not be placed low into a natural crease. It must be higher so that the final incision is more horizontal than S-shaped. A low incision will pull the lateral eyebrow and supraorbital skin downward. The more superior the final lateral incision closure, the more support can be expected from above. This lateral incision is into facial skin, and healing required for this extension contrasts sharply to the minimal time required for healing of the eyelid skin. The lateral extension may remain erythematous for a month or more. The lateral eyelid ideally is free of hooding and wrinkling and demarcated by a lateral eyelid sulcus. There is a clear definition of a sulcus between the lateral eyelid as it joins the upper lateral quadrant of the bony orbital rim. Removal of the muscle from the center of lateral aspect of the incisional blepharoplasty defect will create a eyelid-rim sulcus on final healing.

The medial incision markings should be rounded. This allows the skin to fall naturally into the defect created when fat and muscle have been removed. The surgeon may remove just the skin or both the skin and the overlying muscularis at the same time (Fig. 29–3). Usually I remove the skin first and then use scissors to cut the underlying muscularis tented up with the utilization of a fine-toothed forceps. This prevents accidental injury to the underlying levator muscle. A 5- to 8-mm wide strip of orbicularis muscle is excised just superior to the upper border of the tarsal plate (Fig. 29–3B). Removal of a strip of the orbicularis muscle will allow skin to adhere to the underlying levator aponeurosis. This will improve the definition of the supratarsal sulcus and the lid crease and form a natural-appearing eyelid. The male eyelid does not require the quantity of skin and muscle tissue removal expected in the female eyelid. Overzealous removal can feminize the eye. The same may apply for elderly patients who just require an improvement of their upper lid ptosis which is obstructing part of the visual field.

Once the muscle is removed the orbital fat will extrude through the opening in the attenuated orbital septum. Pressure placed on the eyelid as it is pulled downward will bulge the septum forward, delineating the underlying fat. There are two fat compartments in the upper lid, the medial and the middle. Occasionally one can encounter fat laterally in the area of the superior lacrimal gland. Lacrimal gland tissue is paler in color and does not desiccate and shrink. When and if there is fullness of the lateral eyelid temporal region, excision of the subcutaneous muscle and fascia will decrease the bulk, lending to the cosmetic result.

The overlying septum may require splitting open (with blunt scissors) to expose the fat lobules. The excess fat is gently teased out with the use of forceps and a cotton-tipped applicator, which gently separates the fat from the surrounding tissue. Light pressure on the globe will accentuate the fat pads that require treatment. I prefer to raise the fat up and, utilizing the bipolar forceps, crush and then cauterize the fat (Fig. 29–4). The excess is excised with scissors just superior to the line of cauterized, crushed fat. Some surgeons will clamp the fat, excise the excess, and then cauterize the stump before releasing the clamp. The idea is to remove the excess but not to excessively remove the fat. Medial fat should be removed if noted on examination. It is not unusual for the middle fat to produce some medial bulging. The medial fat often has a cap of membranous tissue that must be excised for the fat to come forward. The medial fat typically is more whitish than the middle fat.

After complete hemostatis is obtained, with most bleeding due to the orbicularis muscle, the skin can be closed. Neither the septum nor the orbicularis muscle is anastomosed. Starting medially I use either 6-0 or 7-0 silk interlocking the suture. Occasionally over the middle of the incision an interrupted suture may be required to ensure complete anastomosis of the wound. It is not unusual to observe 1 or 2 mm of lagophthalmos on completion. This is due to edema and partial muscle paresis and quickly resolves. The conjunctiva sac is cleansed of all blood and debris with sterile eye-irrigating solution. Antibiotic ointment is placed within the sac, and a damp gauze sponge is placed over the eye (without pressure or taping) to absorb any oozing blood and to keep the wound moist. The lagophthalmos will disappear within several hours.

LOWER EYELID BLEPHAROPLASTY PROCEDURE

A line is drawn just lateral to the puncta medially to the lateral orbital rim and beyond. The line is placed within the first natural skin crease below the eyelid margin and is thus located 2 to 3 mm below the eyelid margin (infraciliary). The lateral lower eyelid incision arches upward before it reaches the lateral palpebral angle (Fig. 29–6; Case 2, Fig. 29–12). The incision thus is placed higher on the orbital rim. Although initially more obvious, this incision places the incision into the eyelid area where dark eye shadow makeup use is acceptable, allowing for early camouflage beginning on the fifth or sixth postoperative day. Second, the final scar does not amplify an existing lateral orbital crease. However, the incision, to minimize pouching at the angle of the eye, should not have a sharp vertical angulation.

The scalpel incision is superficial below the eyelid but deep lateral at the orbital rim. Curved scissors complete the incision, separating the skin from the lid margin. The tissue is raised laterally with forceps, and the suborbicularis muscle plane is located by a blunt scissors incision. The scissors are then placed into the plane and used to separate the skin–muscle flap from the lower eyelid by gently opening the blades (Fig. 29–7). A suture is placed through the lid margin, and the lid is pulled up over the globe, exposing the underlying tissue while protecting the globe from injury (Fig. 29–8). The skin–muscle flap can now be elevated, and blunt dissection is continued caudal to the infraorbital rim. The wound edge is then held down by an assistant's dull multipronged hook (Fig. 29–8).

Gentle pressure on the globe will push the fat anteriorly so that it bulges below the orbital septum (Fig. 29–9). The orbital septum is opened, and the fat is gently teased out. I use blunt or fine-toothed forceps to hold the fat while gently separating surrounding tissue from it with the use of a cotton-tipped applicator. This minimizes trauma and bleeding. The lower eyelid has three compartments: medial, middle, and lateral. The lateral compartment is located superior and lateral to the middle fat. A more vascular tissue often overlies the lateral compartment. Complete hemostasis is mandatory to prevent persistent oozing or even brisk bleeding later. If the incision is not extended medially, the medial fat compartment is not accessible. Once the fat has been separated, it is injected with a minute quantity of anesthetic and then cauterized with the bipolar forceps while being held outward with the forceps. The cauterized stump is partially cut with scissors and the remaining portion of the stump is again cauterized with the bipolar coagulating forceps. Finally the fat is excised completely and discarded.

The amount of intraorbital fat is not related to body habitus, and right and left orbits in the same cadaver can demonstrate unequal amounts of fat. Thus I do not routinely compare the quantity of fat removed from each side. Instead, after carefully redraping the loosened lower eyelid flap, any bulges that signify excess fat are noted and, if present, additional fat removed. Another method of determining the presence of fat excess is by gentle pressure on the globe, which will magnify the orbital fat present.

It is possible to overdo excision of fat in the upper eyelid, while it is not very possible to do the same in the lower eyelid. The reason is that the eyeball settles downward when the patient stands up and makes the upper eyelid sulcus deeper.

On completion of fat removal, the operative site is carefully examined for any bleeding. The flap is then released and allowed to settle back onto the lower eyelid site. The flap is smoothed over the surgical site, and the presence of any unusually protrusions is noted. This usually implies the presence of fat pockets not adequately removed.

The flap is draped in a superior and lateral direction (Fig. 29–10A). The flap draped laterally to the eye is trimmed while minimal flap resection is done inferior to the eye. To accurately measure the quantity of flap to be resected, the patient is told to look superiorly to the top of the head (Fig. 29–10B). With the eyes extended in this direction, much of the apparent excess skin will fall into the gap now produced. Although the patient with marked fat protrusions may appear to have excess skin, this is often not the case since the skin will fall back into the cavity now created by the removal of the fat.

At a superior position in relation to the line of excision, sharp scissors are used to expose the periosteum of the lateral orbital bone. A 6-0 permanent suture is buried, attaching the muscle to the periosteum of the lateral orbital bone (Fig. 29–11). This supports the lateral flap and minimizes the formation of a ''rounded eye.'' The placement of the suture is critical. If it is not attached to the periosteum, tension on the suture will result in movement. It is this anchoring that maintains the position of the flap and prevents downward migration.

Several interrupted sutures are placed to secure the position of the lateral eyelid skin before the entire flap is sutured. Lastly, a running 6-0 silk suture, loosely placed, is used to close the lower eyelid. Wet sponges are applied, without pressure or tape, to supply moisture to the wound and absorb the expected oozing of blood from the superficial tissues.

POSTOPERATIVE SEQUELAE

Even the normal expected occurrences after the surgery may require care to prevent progression to complications. Bleeding from the suture line is typical the first few hours. It is better for the blood to ooze from the surgical wounds than to remain within the wound producing ecchymoses and bruising. Bruising is expected and typically reaches its

zenith the second or third day. It resolves sufficiently within 2 weeks to be unobtrusive. Many patients will have only a yellowish hue present in their cheeks after 1 week. Wet dressings of cotton gauze placed over the eyes will absorb the bloody discharge and soothe the wounds. The dressing is applied without pressure or taping. Discomfort and soreness is also normal and may last for several days. Acetaminophen is adequate for most patients, but a non-aspirin codeine compound may be added for the first day only for added comfort. Pain is unusual and should be investigated. Eye pain must be immediately investigated because it is a sign of an emerging hematoma.

Generalized edema is expected (see Fig. 29–5B). It is worse on awakening because the orbital socket is a dependent area. Edema can be severe and may close the eyes. Edema may also be localized, asymmetrical, and exasperatingly slow to resolve. Edema of the lower lid can cling along the incision line and remain for weeks. Furthermore, asymmetrical edema of the lower lid is not uncommon. The edema can involve a section of or the entire lower lid and cause a significant dissimilarity from the other lower lid for months. Blepharoplasty can also induce malar edema that can persist for weeks or months. All this will alarm the patient, who may perceive its presence as the part of the final surgical result. Reassurance is necessary and a delay in treatment the wisest choice since it will usually spontaneously resolve. Premature treatment of an edematous area can result in rapid correction, now rendering other areas more noticeably edematous, with additional complaints.

The use of a dilute corticosteroid (triamcinolone [Kenalog-10] diluted to a 10% solution) injection into the site of edema will hasten resolution if deemed necessary. Uncommonly the swellings can last for months and be very distressing to both the patient and physician. Extreme care in limiting the strength of the solution and the interval between injections is paramount to avoid unnecessary and permanent subcutaneous atrophy. The extent and severity of edema is often secondary to excessive electrocoagulation of blood vessels or fat and extensive skin–muscle flap dissection. It is more common when surgery is done on all four lids.

Blurring of vision and dryness of the eyes are common. This is due to the surgical ''widening of the eyes'' with exposure to the elements. The eye must now adjust to an insufficient blink reflex and the resultant dry tear film. The precorneal tear film is normally quite unstable. It relies on effective eyelid closure and adequate blink rates to remain protective. If blinking is prevented, observable areas of desiccation appear on the corneal surface. This may predispose to more corneal desiccation and, eventually, epithelial damage. Patients are instructed to blink several times rapidly when they experience either visual blurring or grittiness (dryness) of the eyes. Lagophthalmos can also compound this problem and is due to muscle trauma and local anesthetics. Ophthalmic antibiotic ointment must be applied into the conjunctival sac for lubrication before sleeping the first week to prevent dryness during sleep when both the blink reflexes are diminished and the lid closure is defective. These will resolve within several days to weeks when a new frequency of blink reflex is established. Blurred vision makes reading difficult the first few days and is a function of a dry tear film as well as the film of ophthalmic antibiotic ointment applied to the wounds and conjunctiva sac during sleep.

Epiphora (excessive tearing) may be seen in the immediate postoperative period.[8] Most tears are lost by evaporation, with the rest drained through the lacrimal system. After surgery the lower puncta and canaliculi may be compromised by edema and inflammation. The excessive tearing is transient.

Several frightening occurrences may be seen within the first several postoperative days. The conjunctiva of one, or rarely, both eyes may become suffused with bright red blood. This will resolve without complication within 1 to 2 weeks, but the patient will require reassurance. Since it is frightening, the patient is forewarned of this possible sequelae. Chemosis (excessive edema of the ocular conjunctiva with actual bulging of the tissue over the lower lid) may persist for several weeks. Resolution may be hastened by the use of antibiotic ophthalmic ointment in conjunction with Cortisporin ophthalmic ointment (a combination product of hydrocortisone, neomycin, and polymyxin B) applied three times daily.

COMPLICATIONS AND TREATMENT

Minor Complications

Sutures usually are removed on the fourth or fifth day. Occasionally, when there is excessive tension, partial dehiscence of wound may occur. Dehiscence may also be caused by the presence of a small wound hematoma. Treatment is simple, either application of Steri-Strips or allowing the wound to granulate is all that is necessary. Milia formation is common if sutures are not removed within 5 days. Milia can also occur even in those patients who have their sutures removed within 4 days. These can be incised with a No. 11 blade.

Skin excisions from the upper eyelids can be quite generous without producing lagophthalmos. Overly enthusiastic removal in an attempt to achieve perfection can result in lagophthalmos. Temporary lagophthalmos is not unusual in the first 12 hours. Permanent lagophthalmos is uncommon and can lead to corneal drying and ulceration. Treatment would require replacement of the skin by grafting.

Carelessly left debris, coagulated blood, and strands of material from sponges and cotton-tipped applicators may irritate the conjunctiva and cause hypertrophic changes laterally within the sac. Cleansing and the use of a topical antibiotic and corticosteroid will correct this irritation.

Surgical omissions are not uncommon in this exacting surgical procedure. A difference of 1 or 2 mm in the upper lid is noticeable to the discerning patient. Correction is simple with additional resection once all upper lid edema has resolved. This may take several months, and it is wise to defer removal until normal tissue turgor is present. Incomplete fat pad removal is usually seen with the medial pads of both upper and lower lids and with the lateral pad of the lower eyelid. A wide stab wound over the offending fat pad will leave a small but inconspicuous scar. The surgical site should be carefully marked before anesthetic infiltration, which will obscure the offending bulging fat.

Major Complications

Retrobulbar Hematoma and Blindness

The most serious complication of blepharoplasty is blindness. Fortunately it is rare.[9] The ultimate event leading to permanently impaired vision is ischemia. The incidence is higher for lower lid surgery but has occurred with only upper lid surgery. Retrobulbar hematoma is the feature common to most cases (Fig. 29–13). The appearance of proptosis, eye pain, and/or visual disturbances is evidence of increased pressure and requires immediate reopening of the wound with evacuation of hematoma, if present, and precise electrocoagulation of any bleeding vessels. The patient's head should be elevated, and some surgeons advocate the utilization of steroids to minimize edema. Ophthalmic consultation is imperative if symptoms are not immediately ameliorated or if there is progression of visual symptoms. I routinely obtain a preoperative consultation before surgery, for not only a full ocular evaluation but also to be familiar with the patient's ophthalmologist should assistance be required. Needle injection trauma, rough handling of the intraorbital fat, blood vessel spasm from trauma or vasopressor agents (epinephrine injected into a blood vessel), and exacerbating factors such as uncontrolled hypertension and coagulation disorders caused by medications have been cited as the causes of retrobulbar

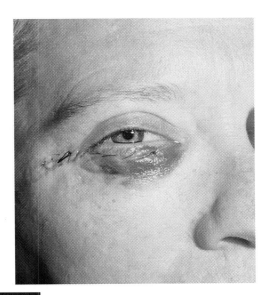

CASE 3

FIGURE 29–13. Postoperative periorbital hematoma with swelling of the lower right eyelid accompanied by pain and blurring of vision. Immediate opening of the wound and careful hemocoagulation of all bleeding vessels reversed all symptoms. Recovery then proceeded uneventfully.

hematoma. Pressure from the ensuing hematoma causes progressive ischemia of the optic nerve and vessels. The most important factor in preventing retrobulbar hemorrhage and blindness, beside the elimination of medical causes, is the careful handling of intraorbital fat. Fortunately, most cases of retrobulbar hematoma rarely lead to blindness.[10]

Lid Retraction and Ectropion

Ectropion, after blepharoplasty, can be temporary or permanent and range in severity from mild lower lid retraction to frank ectropion with marked, symptomatic, lower lid retraction.[11] Etiologies of potentially irreparable postblepharoplasty ectropion include failure to correct a preexisting eyelid laxity, excessive skin removal, and anatomic factors (proptosis or exophthalmus). Ectropion in all these cases is due to a failure to recognize these preoperative problems. Now the surgeon is faced with the unenviable task of correcting a difficult complication.

There are remediable causes of ectropion that can resolve without surgical intervention. These include wound edema, dystonic orbicularis oculi muscle function (from the anesthetic and muscle trauma), scar contracture, adhesions of the orbital septum, and hematoma. Good postoperative care (wound care, massage, taping the eyelid up) and the additional use of steroids will often correct or markedly improve the lid laxity. Persistent ectropion will require a lid-shortening procedure. Ectropion due to medial tendon laxity is a more difficult problem, usually requiring the assistance of an ophthalmic plastic surgeon. Thus it is important to diagnose this complication before blepharoplasty.

Ptosis

Ptosis due to edema and the anesthetic effects on the ocular muscle is common the first few hours and even days after surgery. Unrecognized preoperative ptosis due to levator aponeurosis dehiscence is a serious problem. It may be attributed to the surgery. It may also become overtly present secondary to edema, hematoma, or excess cautery.

PHOTOGRAPHS: BEFORE AND AFTER SURGERY AND LONG TERM

Documentation of the presurgical condition and the final surgical results is achieved approximately 1 to 2 months later. The standard photographic views utilized are primary gaze, upgaze, and downgaze and left and right modified side views. Any unusual sequelae or complications should also be photographed, including the subsequent phases of recovery. This will record your care in resolving the condition and can document any problems the patient may have induced.

POSSIBLE ADDITIONAL OPERATIONS

Occasionally after the edema has settled, it may become obvious that the surgeon has not resected adequately skin from the upper lateral eyelid region, thereby leaving lateral hooding. This is resolved easily by resection of a thin strip of lateral eyelid skin with suture removal 4 to 5 days later. One should wait for at least 2 months, or longer if necessary, after the initial surgery to allow all postoperative edema to resolve. The medial fat pad of the upper eyelid and the lateral fat pad of the lower eyelid (occasionally the medial lower fat pad) are occasionally overlooked and not resected, thus leaving a bulge postoperatively. This is usually hidden by postoperative edema and may not appear until months after the surgery. A wide stab wound directly over the fat protrusion (carefully marked before local infiltration) will allow removal.

References

1. Elliot DL, et al. Medical considerations in ambulatory surgery. Clin Plast Surg 1983;10:295.
2. Foster CA, Aston SJ. Propranolol–epinephrine interaction: A potential disaster. Plast Reconstr Surg 1983;72:74.
3. Gradinger GP. Preoperative Considerations in Blepharoplasty. In: Kaye BL, Gradinger GP, eds. Symposium on Problems and Complications in Aesthetic Plastic Surgery of the Face, vol 23. St. Louis: CV Mosby, 1984:195–207.
4. Wolfley DE, Guibor P. Preoperative evaluation of the blepharoplasty patient. Facial Plast Surg 1984;1:284–291.
5. Owsley JQ. Resection of the prominent lateral fat pad during upper lid blepharoplasty. Plast Reconstr Surg 1980;65:4.
6. Rees TD, Tabbal N. Lower blepharoplasty with emphasis on the orbicularis muscle. Clin Plast Surg 1981;8:643–662.
7. Shagets FW, Shore JW. The management of eyelid laxity during lower eyelid blepharoplasty. Arch Otolaryngol Head Neck Surg 1986;112:729–732.
8. Adams B, Feurstein S. Complications of Blepharoplasty. Ear Nose Throat J 1986;65:11.
9. Mahaffey PJ, Wallace AF. Blindness following cosmetic blepharoplasty: A review. Br J Plast Surg 1986;39:213.
10. DeMere M, Wood T, Austin W. Eye complications with blepharoplasty or other eyelid surgery. Plast Reconstr Surg 1974;53:634.
11. McGraw BL, Adamson PA. Postblepharoplasty ectropion. Arch Otolaryngol Head Neck Surg, 1991;117:852.

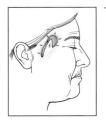

chapter 30

Browlift Surgery

PAUL S. COLLINS

Browlift surgery can be accomplished by several procedures, each having its own benefits and risks. Each procedure raises the forehead tissue off the superior orbital rim and elevates the position of the eyebrow while increasing the vertical height of the orbit. Surgical correction may be approached by procedures at the brow, mid forehead, or forehead hairline junction or within the scalp. Browlift surgery seeks to achieve the return of the brow to its ideal location (Fig. 30–1).

INDICATIONS

Browlift surgery is indicated in those patients who experience a redundancy of the tissues of the upper orbit due primarily from ptosis of the forehead. The ptotic forehead tissue produces a low-lying brow, with the forehead brow tissue protruding over the orbital rim (Fig. 30–2). The brow and forehead tissue sits on the upper orbital tissue, which amasses over the upper eyelid, reducing the upper and lateral visual fields. Cosmetically this produces a fatigued, aged appearance to the face. Functionally, the forehead ptosis impinges on the upper eyelids and produces a significant visual field defect that is pronounced on upward gaze. Browlift surgery can correct the visual field impairment (Fig. 30–2; Case 4, Fig. 30–13).

CONTRAINDICATIONS

When the true cause of upper orbital fullness was a ptotic brow, an upper eyelid blepharoplasty may have been performed unnecessarily. The quantity of upper eyelid tissue sacrificed during the blepharoplasty may preclude any brow elevation without causing lagophthalmos.

Medical complications and diseases should take precedence over a cosmetic procedure. If there is doubt as to the significance of a medical problem, a medical consultation can determine the surgical risk.

Cosmetic tattooing of the eyebrows may have been done either to camouflage natural loss of eyebrow hair or to place a brow in a higher, more aesthetically pleasing position in response to eyebrow ptosis and hair plucking. If the ptotic forehead tissue is raised, the permanently tattooed eyebrow will be repositioned in an unnaturally high location. The patient will then have a ''surprised'' countenance.

LIMITATIONS

Improvement of forehead rhytides due to ptosis is expected. If the individual has forehead folds secondary to familial inherited frontalis muscle hypertrophy, the prominent rhytides will remain. Correction requires intervention with the frontalis muscle. Furthermore, glabellar rhytides will also remain prominent unless a myectomy of the corrugator muscles is performed.

Each forehead procedure has its own specific limitations. No single procedure is suitable for all patients. At times it may be necessary to recommend a procedure that is less likely to correct the problem because it has fewer undesirable secondary effects. The direct brow or a midforehead procedure requires surgical intervention through glabrous forehead tissue. A prominent, erythematous surgical excision line will require weeks or even months before it matures. The final surgical scar can remain prominent, negating the final result. A lateral upper or hairline forehead lift procedure cannot provide adequate medial brow elevation in those patients who suffer from medial brow ptosis. Extending the procedure across the forehead will correct this, but at the expense of increasing the extent of permanent anesthesia of the scalp by cutting the sensory nerves. If the surgery is performed in a supramuscular plane, loss of cutaneous sensation can be avoided but there

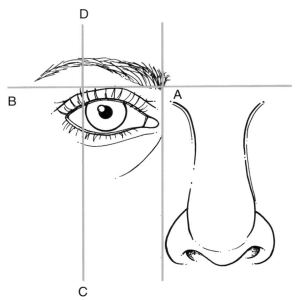

FIGURE 30–1. The ideal brow is arched above the orbital rim in women and at the rim in men. The apex of the arch is directly above the lateral limbus (*line CD*) and is about 10 mm from the midpoint of the limbus to the inferior aspect of the brow in white women. The medial aspect of the brow is directly over the alar base (*point A*). The lateral aspect of the brow (*point B*) lies on a line drawn from the nasal ala through the lateral canthus and is level with the medial aspect of the brow (*line AB*).

is greater risk of injury to the cutaneous forehead tissue and subsequent scarring. Coronal forehead surgery can produce an undesirably wide line of alopecia. It may raise the forehead to an unnatural position unless the patient preoperatively has a low forehead. Lastly, recession of frontal and temporal hair is common in aging in both men and women. With aging, a previously aesthetic coronal forehead lift may now result in an exaggerated elevated hairline due to the receding hair. The hairline is now located above the frontal eminence, thus elongating the forehead and unbalancing the facial measurements.

EXPECTED CHANGES AND DURATION OF CHANGES

The orbital region is the main focal point of the face. Any change that enlarges the orbital vertical distance and enlarges the appearance of the eyes produces dramatic results. The duration of change is dependent on the extent of correction and on the stability of the newly positioned brow. Failure to overcorrect and firmly secure the elevated tissue will result in the sliding forward of the forehead tissues, negating some of the initial improvement. The extent of overcorrection necessary is somewhat dependent on the procedure chosen, the general laxity of the individual's skin, and the mobility of the scalp tissue, which can allow it to slide forward in response to the surgical tightening of the forehead tissue. With aging over several decades, it is possible for forehead ptosis to become more prominent, with forehead tissue again sinking farther over the orbital rim into the orbital socket.

PREOPERATIVE EVALUATION

Medical History

Systemic disease can affect the surgical outcome by either interfering with the ability to correct the anatomic findings or resulting in complications that compromise the surgical results. The American Society of Anesthesiology (ASA) classification of physical status is a recognized measure of the potential for perioperative complications and the use of conscious sedation (Table 30–1). There are two general areas of assessment critical in the preoperative evaluation: (1) identification of risks related to underlying medical disorders and (2) evaluation for potential bleeding and coagulation problems (Table 30–2). Therefore, laboratory tests should include a complete blood cell test, chemistry profile with liver function tests (if the medical history warrants evaluation), prothrombin time, partial thromboplastin time, and, where appropriate, request for an electrocardiogram and medical clearance for surgery. The patient should be either in good general health or have stable

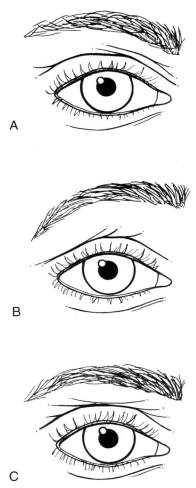

FIGURE 30–2. *A,* Brow ptosis may be medial, producing an angry look. *B,* Lateral brow ptosis produces a sad look. *C,* Universal brow ptosis gives a tired appearance. Surgical correction must be individualized to the brow deformity that is present.

TABLE 30–1. American Society of Anesthesiology Classification of Physical Status

Class 1: A normal, healthy patient; may have localized pathologic processes; does not have systemic disease
Class 2: Mild systemic disease (no limit to normal activity) (i.e., mild asthma)
Class 3: Not incapacitating severe systemic disease (i.e., uncontrolled hypertension, diabetes mellitus, or the presence of acquired immunodeficiency syndrome)
Class 4: Incapacitating severe systemic disease that is a constant threat to life (i.e., significant congestive heart failure)
Class 5: Moribund (i.e., not expected to survive 24 hours)

systemic disease. Patients with severe systemic disease (hepatitis) or unstable disease (congestive heart failure, a recent myocardial infarction, or psychiatric problems) should not undergo the procedure until the illness is stabilized. Infectious diseases such as hepatitis B surface antigen and acquired immunodeficiency syndrome or a positive human immunodeficiency virus test may warrant reevaluation of the patient risks and reclassification to an ASA class 3, thereby precluding elective cosmetic surgery. Outpatient cosmetic surgery is usually limited to patients with an ASA classification of 1 or 2 (Table 30–1).

The most significant cardiac risk factors during surgery and general anesthesia are uncompensated congestive heart failure and myocardial infarction within the past 6 months. Smoking, hypertension, stable exertional angina, mitral valve disease, cardiomegaly, and conducting system disease do not correlate with increased cardiac risk, although they can have an adverse effect on the surgical results. Blood pressure should be evaluated during the initial consultation. Hypertension is stabilized before scheduling surgery because it can increase bleeding especially perioperatively and increase the risk of postoperative hematoma.

Cosmetic surgery patients should minimize smoking for several days before surgery and, if possible, eliminate any smoking for several days after. Smoking can increase skin flap morbidity, exacerbate local edema, increase blood pressure and the pulse rate, thus augmenting bleeding, and is associated with poor wound healing. As with blepharoplasty patients, thyroid ophthalmopathy may produce periorbital abnormalities that may not be corrected by surgery.

Medications

Medication that increases the tendency for bleeding should be stopped before the surgical procedure. Aspirin and aspirin-containing medications are the most common causes of excess surgical bleeding and subsequent hematoma formation. Alcohol, which has a synergistic effect with aspirin, and vitamin E should be stopped.

Hypertensive patients, who are taking a nonselective β-adrenergic blocker such as propranolol, may respond to epinephrine with an episode of markedly elevated hypertension followed quickly by a reflex bradycardia. This combination can potentially cause a cardiac arrest. β-adrenergic blockers protect the heart against the deleterious

effects of catecholamines.[2] Cardiac blood vessels have only β-receptors, while peripheral vessels have both β- and α-receptors. Nonselective β-blockers affect all β-receptors, thus allowing epinephrine to react unopposed with the α-receptors. Dilute (1:800,000) concentrations of epinephrine provide adequate cutaneous hemostasis. Most studies indicate that no arrhythmias occur with epinephrine doses of 5 μg/mL. A concentration of 1:200,000 epinephrine equals 5 μg/mL. Usually the volume of anesthetic with epinephrine used in blepharoplasty is small and not of consequence even in the presence of nonselective β-adrenergic blocker. Caution must be followed when several simultaneous procedures are being performed and the volume of epinephrine is significant. Propranolol must be tapered in decreasing doses. Sudden cessation of propranolol can produce a rebound adrenergic excess and increased angina.[1]

Prior Surgery in the Region

A previous upper lid blepharoplasty with removal of excessive eyelid tissue allows the ptotic brow tissue to fall even farther into the orbital socket and results in a paucity

TABLE 30–2. Browlift Surgery: Operative Issues

Preoperative Evaluation
Medical History
Systemic disease:
  Recent myocardial infarction or unstable angina pectoris
  Congestive heart failure
  Uncontrolled hypertension
  Diabetes mellitus
Bleeding diathesis and medications that enhance bleeding
Examination of the Upper Face
Position of brows
Asymmetries of the brows and orbital bones
Prominence of brow and orbital bones
Presence of rhytides of the forehead, glabella, and lateral eyelids (crow's feet)
Presence of brow tattooing
Presence and extent of scalp laxity
Previous eyelid surgery
Redundancy of eyelid skin and presence of upper eyelid fat pads
Levator ptosis and asymmetrical eyelids
Intraoperative Equipment Needs
Electrosurgical machine with bipolar coagulator capabilities
Adson bipolar forceps
Needle holders for 4-0, 5-0, and 6-0 suture
Hemostats
Skin retractors, three or four prong, blunt
Scissors: long Metzenbaum curved scissors
Nylon suture, 5-0 and 6-0, and Prolene suture 4-0 with plastic surgery needles
Sterile field drapes, OR lights, skin marking pens, suction
Oximeter, blood pressure cuff, pulse or cardiac monitor
Laboratory Examination
Complete blood cell count
Platelets
Prothrombin time
Partial thromboplastin time
Chemistries

of orbital upper eyelid tissue. A subsequent attempt at lifting the brow will produce lagophthalmos of the upper eyelid. In this situation brow surgery is contraindicated.

Physical Examination

Ideally the normal female eyebrow lies in a high-arched position, well above the orbital rim. The apex of the brow's arch is at a line perpendicular to the temporal limbus (scleral-pupillary border) of the eye (Fig. 30–1). Here the brow lies approximately 1 cm above the orbital rim. The medial brow begins at a vertical line drawn from the ala of the nose, while the lateral border terminates at a line drawn from the nasal ala through the lateral canthus. There is a well-defined upper lid cleft, and no hooding is present in the lateral canthal area. The male brow, in contrast, has a middle-age configuration. It is heavier in hair content, begins more medially, occupies a more caudal position along the supraorbital rim, and has less lateral arch than the female brow. There is less upper lid cleft definition with mild hooding of the lateral canthal area. Persons with ptotic brows commonly attempt to elevate the brow by effecting excessive forehead animation. The greater the ptosis and resultant visual field obstruction, the greater the subconscious compensation of habitually raising the forehead and subsequent horizontal forehead wrinkling.[3-5]

Eyebrow ptosis can be familial or acquired. Acquired ptosis is usually associated with aging and occurs when the forehead loses its elasticity and sags with descent of the forehead tissues. As the severity of ptosis increases, the brow descends over the orbital rim. As the ptosis increases, the brow becomes incorporated into the upper part of the orbital cavity, finally impinging on the upper eyelids. This can produce a partial obstruction of the superior visual fields. Unilateral ptosis may be the result of nerve paralysis. Familial brow ptosis is noticeable at an early age and produces the same tired appearance. The descent of the eyebrow tissues below the supraorbital margins gives the eyes a tired, crowded appearance, decreasing their relative size. The ptosis can be lateral (hooding of the lateral canthal area producing a "sad look"), midlateral (only the medial brow remains at its normal height), medial (imparting an "angry look"), or universal (a "tired" appearance) (Fig. 30–2).[6]

Brow elevation procedures should be performed before upper eyelid blepharoplasty, thereby facilitating judgment as to the precise amount of upper lid skin to be excised. Brow elevation will always reduce the quantity of redundant upper lid tissue and may make upper lid blepharoplasty unnecessary. A common mistake is a misidentification of brow ptosis, incorrectly interpreting the redundancy due to the upper lid. Upper eyelid blepharoplasty does not completely remedy the problem and allows additional thick eyebrow skin to settle down onto the eyelids. The blepharoplasty also leads to inferior displacement of the eyebrow by closure of the excisional defects and secondarily by scar contraction. The eyebrow is drawn nearer the lid margin, obliterating the infrabrow cleft, and a smaller, squinting eye results. The patient will compensate subconsciously by tilting his head backward and habitually raising the forehead, which will produce horizontal wrinkles. The preoperative level of the brow is the most useful parameter in deciding whether a blepharoplasty, a browlift, or a combination of procedures will be required.[6]

The patient who has had a previous blepharoplasty will require a more conservative approach when performing the eyebrow lift for ptotic eyebrows. Too much skin removal will make it impossible for the lids to close, causing a permanent lagophthalmos of the eyelids.[7] Patients with prominent upper orbital rims and deep upper palpebral sulci will usually achieve significant improvement from a browlift while those with small orbits may not.

The surgeon must differentiate between several variations of upper face ptosis. It is important to recognize the difference between ptosis of the brow, temple, forehead, and glabella when planning the corrective surgery.[5] Forehead ptosis produces a low hairline with tissue redundancy of the medial brow and glabellar regions. In contrast, there is no redundancy of the supraciliary tissues with a familial low forehead and hairline. Ptosis of the temple will lower the temporal hairline and produce sagging of the lateral brow. Universal ptosis, as it implies, involves both the forehead and temple. Lastly, ptosis can be isolated to the glabella and medial brow. The presence of asymmetrical brows should be investigated for possible temporal nerve damage.

Finally, evaluation of the upper face for the suitability of a brow elevation should also include a critical examination of the orbital region. As has been noted, previous surgery of the orbital region, especially an upper lid blepharoplasty, can preclude or contraindicate the proposed brow surgery. The symmetry of the bony orbit, eyelids, and eyes needs to be ascertained. Considerable asymmetry of the orbital region can be camouflaged by presence of redundant skin and/or periorbital fat and may not become evident until after surgery. The patient will then incorrectly assume the surgery was the cause. The orbital rim may be prominent, especially laterally; one eye may be larger than the other, or the sockets may vary in size or position. A blepharoplasty may render less than ideal surgical results if the eyeball sockets are sunken or cadaverous and can possibly exaggerate this anatomic variation. Conversely, a browlift may give improvement to some patients. The skin should be examined for any blemishes or tumors, such as xanthelasma, milia, or syringoma that may require removal before the browlift.

Proposed Brow Elevation Measurement

Critical evaluation, including assessment of the eyebrow position, height, and shape, is carried out with the patient sitting and in repose. It is extremely important that preoperative analysis be done with complete relaxation of the forehead muscles to allow an accurate assessment of the brow in repose. The height of the desired brow elevation must be determined before commencement of the surgical procedure.

Particular attention should be given to the horizontal rhytides of the forehead. Arching of these creases above the brow indicates frontalis muscle contraction and elevation of the ptotic eyebrows. This positions the eyebrows superior to their true height. The influence of the frontalis muscles on the brow can be assessed by having the patient direct the eyes in a downward gaze. The forehead is then massaged in a downward direction to relax the muscles.[8] By manually elevating the brow, with the patient gazing straight ahead, a tentative judgment can be made of the favorable effect of brow elevation on the aesthetic unit of the eye and the orbit (Fig. 30–3). The significance of the frontalis muscle on brow ptosis can now be correctly analyzed, and any excess eyelid fullness that is due to the eyebrow and/or forehead ptosis will become apparent.

The degree of tissue prolapse is measured with the patient sitting with gaze forward and the forehead in repose. The brow is lifted to an elevation slightly above its desired position and the height of the lift is measured. The maximal brow height measurement should be made at a line perpendicular to the lateral limbus of the cornea. This height of the proposed lift should also be measured from the superior or forehead border of the brow. As the compressed brow is lifted, it widens dramatically. Measurement from the inferior border will not result in a correct measurement of the ptosis while that of the superior border will (Fig. 30–3).

Ideally, the brow should be surgically placed at an exaggerated level. Postoperatively there will be a relaxation of the overlying tissues and a decrease in operative edema with the resultant descent in the height of the corrected brow. An overcorrection of 0.5 to 1.0 cm is necessary owing to this postoperative descent of forehead tissues. The brow will typically take several weeks to arrive at its final destination. The female brow should aesthetically be placed at a higher level than the male brow. Therefore, it is wiser, when measuring the desired height, to overestimate the elevation of the female brow and, conversely, to underestimate the male brow.

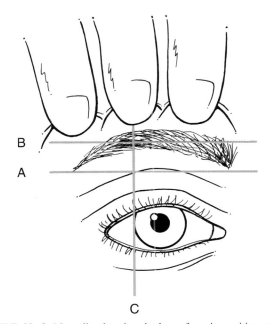

FIGURE 30–3. Manually elevating the brow from its position at repose (*line A*) to a proposed position of the brow (*line B*) assists in making a tentative judgment of the effect of brow elevation. Line C is tangential to the lateral limbus of the eye and assists in placing the arch of the brow at its maximum point of elevation.

Preoperative Discussion of Benefits and Risks of the Procedure

Patient discussion is always a critical stage of the preoperative evaluation (see Table 29–2). Most patients do not perceive that forehead ptosis is the cause of the fullness of the upper eyelids. Unlike the widely known procedures for blepharoplasty or lower face rhytidectomy, the forehead lift is a new concept to most patients. An important aspect of the consultation is the education of the patient as to the expectations of forehead lift surgery.

The use of a mirror will facilitate the anatomic findings of concern to the patient and enable the physician to specifically point out what is less likely to be corrected by the surgery. It is paramount that the patient understands not only what the planned surgery will accomplish but also its limitations and failures. The procedure should be delayed or possibly not considered if rapport cannot be developed during the interview.

All patients need to understand that forehead surgery may not produce perfect surgical results, be free of scarring, or eliminate all rhytides. The typical expected time of recovery of 10 to 14 days is noted. Additional recovery time may be necessary if significant sequelae or complications occur. The expected occurrences inherent to the procedure, such as bruising, pain, edema, and surgical scars, and occurrences not normally expected, such as hematoma, wound dehiscence, or allergic reactions are explained to the patient so he or she can make an informed decision. Discussion should include the possible serious complications: temporal nerve damage, severe bruising, prominent scarring, hair loss, and severe allergic reactions. A photograph album of previous surgical results, both excellent and average, will demonstrate the expected outcome of the procedure. Instructional sheets outlining both the preoperative and postoperative surgical course and care (see Table 29–2), a list of medications to avoid, the total fees involved, a surgical consent form, and a risk form explaining possible sequelae and complications of browlift surgery are given to the patient.

PERFORMING BROWLIFT SURGERY

Intraoperative Needs and Special Instruments and Equipment

An electrosurgical machine with bipolar coagulating capability and the use of Adson bipolar forceps are mandatory to obtain complete hemostasis. Several types of scissors can be used during the operation. Long (8 inch) straight Metzenbaum scissors with round blades are necessary for blunt dissection to the orbital rim. Retractors, with three or four blunt prongs, will minimize tissue trauma while facilitating tissue exposure. Hemostats may be necessary for clamping any bleeding vessels. Needle holders for handling 6-0, 5-0, and 4-0 suture are advisable. Nylon suture (4-0, 5-0 and 6-0) for cutaneous closure as well as Prolene (4-0 or 5-0) for buried suspension sutures are required.

An oximeter will assure that the patient is oxygenating adequately, while a pulse monitor will note any rhythm abnormalities. While not necessary for most patients, this equipment may be required for the elderly or for patients with underlying medical problems. Its use is recommended when intravenous sedation is utilized.

Anesthesia

Certainly all but a coronal lift can be accomplished with the use of local anesthesia. With longer procedures, a mixture of equal parts of lidocaine and bupivacaine will provide extended local anesthesia. Intramuscular meperidine and promethazine with oral diazepam or intramuscular midazolam can be used for additional comfort or as a supplement in those patients requiring additional sedation. Intravenous sedation with midazolam or diazepam is used for anxious patients. It is highly unusual to need intravenous narcotics.

Forehead Anatomy

Surgery for correction of brow ptosis may be approached from one of three anatomically distinct directions: the frontotemporal, the temporal, or the suprabrow areas. Each surgical approach has its own specific anatomic features and hazards (Figs. 30–4 and 30–5).

Frontotemporal Anatomy

The tissue layers of the frontotemporal area are similar whether over the anterior scalp or at the forehead hairline. The tissues encountered at the forehead are the skin, subcutaneous fat, superficial frontalis fascia, frontalis muscle, deep frontalis fascia, periosteum, and bone. Significantly, the overlying superficial fascia is not only adherent to the underlying frontalis muscle but also forms a firm fibrofatty

layer of tissue adherent to the skin. This layer inserts into the skin of the eyebrows and the root of the nose and is part of the superficial musculoaponeurotic system (SMAS). At the anterior scalp, the frontalis muscle and its fascia are replaced by the galea aponeurotica. The galea interdigitates with the frontalis fascia, connecting it to the fascia of the occipital muscle. This inelastic aponeurotic tissue is attached to the bony orbital rim by fibrous adhesions that prevent upward movement of the soft tissues of the supraorbital regions over the orbital rim.[10]

The surgical plane of dissection in the frontotemporal approach will be in the supraperiosteal-subgaleal space. Dissection in this relatively avascular plane avoids the motor and sensory nerves of this region, which are located in the supragaleal tissues until the orbital region. The supraorbital and supratrochlear neurovascular bundles leave their respective foramen and immediately pierce the frontalis fascia and muscle (Fig. 30–4).

At the inferior temporal region above the zygomatic process, the SMAS interdigitates with the fascial envelope of the frontalis muscle. The temporal branch of the facial nerve enters the inferolateral border of the frontalis muscle in the SMAS, which originates over the zygomatic arch (Fig. 30–5). Therefore, when the approach is from a superior direction, a subaponeurotic plane of dissection will diminish risk to the temporal branch of the facial nerve until the border of the zygomatic arch is reached.[11–13]

The corrugator supercilii muscles arise from the medial end of the superciliary ridge of the frontal bone (Fig. 30–4). Their action pulls the eyebrows medially, producing vertical wrinkles at the glabella and a resultant frowning expression. The procerus muscle, originating from the lower part of the nasal bone and upper lateral nasal cartilage, creates transverse wrinkles at the nasofrontal angle, drawing the eyebrows inferiorly. Both of these muscles must be isolated from the supraorbital and supratrochlear neurovascular bundles before resection.

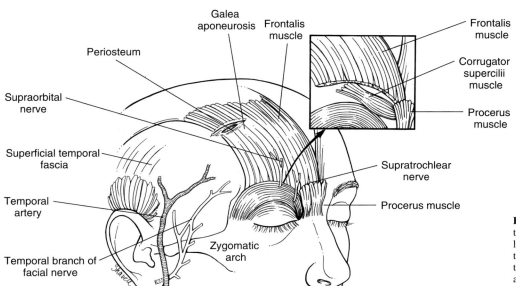

FIGURE 30–4. Relevant anatomy of the forehead and orbit with the brow-lift incision placed at the hairline in the frontotemporal area. Dissection in the subgaleal (supraperiosteal) plane avoids injury to the temporal branch of the facial nerve.

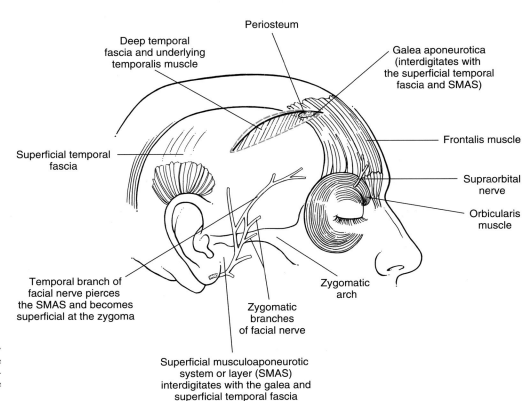

Periosteum

Deep temporal
fascia and underlying
temporalis muscle

Galea aponeurotica
(interdigitates with
the superficial temporal
fascia and SMAS)

Superficial temporal
fascia

Frontalis muscle

Supraorbital
nerve

Orbicularis
muscle

Temporal branch of
facial nerve pierces
the SMAS and becomes
superficial at the zygoma

Zygomatic
arch

Zygomatic
branches
of facial nerve

Superficial musculoaponeurotic
system or layer (SMAS)
interdigitates with the galea and
superficial temporal fascia

FIGURE 30–5. Relevant anatomy of the forehead and orbit with the browlift incision placed at the hairline in the temporal area or in the scalp.

Suprabrow Anatomy

The following layers of tissue are seen immediately superior to the brow: skin, subcutaneous fat, superficial fascia, muscle (interdigitating fibers from both the orbicularis and frontalis muscle), fascia with associated neurovascular bundles (supraorbital and supratrochlear), galea–frontalis aponeurosis, and septa of the galea–frontalis aponeurosis that attach to the underlying periosteum and within which lies the fat pad of the eyebrow, periosteum, and bone. Two neurovascular bundles traverse in the fascia located below the muscle layer (medially the supraorbital and laterally the temporofrontalis). Incisions made through the muscle and underlying fascia at the brow will place the supraorbital neurovascular bundle at risk. The temporofrontalis nerve curves medially around the lateral brow as it innervates the frontalis muscle. A deep incision superior to the lateral brow may injure the temporofrontalis nerve. Brow hairs grow obliquely downward. An incision made at the brow line must be angled acutely oblique upward to prevent sectioning of the brow hair bulbs.[14]

Temporal Anatomy

Forehead lifting procedures initiated at the temporal area are either within the scalp or at the border of hair-bearing skin. Here an incision will transect the skin, subcutaneous fat, temporoparietal fascia, temporalis muscle (which is enveloped by the temporalis fascia), and finally expose the periosteum and temporal bone (Fig. 30–5). The temporoparietal fascia represents an extension of the SMAS and is in continuity with the galea above. This fascial layer caudally lies superficial to the zygomatic arch and contains both the temporofrontalis nerve and temporal vessels. An avascular subaponeurotic plane separates the temporoparietal fascia from the temporal fascia and muscle. This is a safe plane of dissection that extends from the temple and scalp region to an area immediately superior to the zygoma.[11]

The temporal branch of the facial nerve, which courses within the SMAS-temporoparietal fascia, travels within a distinct zone. This zone extends in a line, measuring 2 cm wide, from a point 0.5 cm below the tragus of the ear to a point 2.0 cm above the lateral eyebrow.[12] Within this danger zone, which includes the area located superolateral to the brow, an incision into the fascial layer can sever the temporal branch of the facial nerve.[13]

Forehead Lift Procedures

Browlifting can be accomplished by several different procedures. Each procedure has its benefits, limitations, and disadvantages.[15] Although there is no ideal procedure, there are ideal surgical candidates for each specific procedure. The surgeon has the following procedures to choose from: direct brow lift, midforehead lift, upper forehead lift, temple lift (temporal scalp approach), and coronal forehead lift.

Direct Browlift

Local anesthesia for the direct brow is adequate or can be supplemented with intramuscular meperidine and promethazine or with oral diazepam. The direct browlift is the simplest of all the surgical procedures for correcting brow ptosis. The surgeon can individualize the lifting of each brow by creating an individual excisional design pattern and by varying the height of elevation (Fig. 30–6). Asymmetrical brows can be corrected since each brow can be

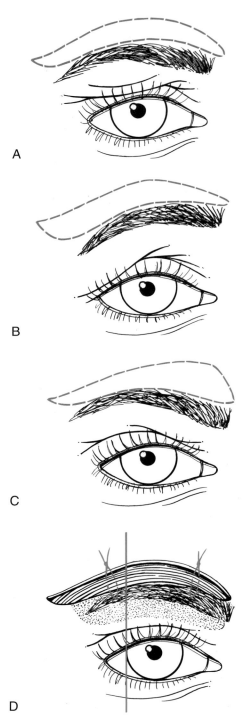

FIGURE 30–6. Direct browlift excisional designs differ for different types of brow ptosis. *A,* Universal ptosis. *B,* Lateral ptosis. *C,* Medial ptosis. *D,* The orbicularis muscle is pulled up and sutured to the frontalis muscle with 4-0 nonabsorbable suture.

lifted independently of the other. This browlift is ideally suited for lateral and middle ptosis of the brow with minimal effect on medial ptosis and glabellar rhytides.

A distinct disadvantage of the direct browlift is the surgical scars. A woman's forehead skin is thinner, softer, and less sebaceous and heals with finer, less noticeable scars (Case 1, Fig. 30–10). The application of cosmetic products can also camouflage the scar. In contrast, men have thicker, sebaceous skin that heals with erythematous, prominent scarring. Application of cosmetic coverups is not a usual alternative for men. In time, these scars will improve and can become inconspicuous. The hairs in a distinct, bushy eyebrow aid in concealing the scar located along the brow border (Case 4, Fig. 30–13). Placing the incision in a deep transverse rhytid superior to the brow can also provide an excellent location for concealing the browlift scar in some men without a heavy glabrous component of the skin.[4] The direct browlift is also a reasonable option in the glabrous-skinned man. The procedure may cause slight thinning of the eyebrow hair and occasionally fifth cranial nerve neuralgia from injury to the supratrochlear, supraorbital, or zygomaticotemporal nerves.[14] It may aggravate an obviously low temporal hairline by shortening the distance between the hairline and the brow.

Operative Procedure. The outline of the elliptical excision is now designed with careful measurement of the height of the ellipse. The excision design is individualized to the type of brow ptosis (Fig. 30–6*A* through *C*). Placement of the brow should be at an exaggerated elevation to compensate for the normal inferior drift of the forehead tissue and brow. Immediately postoperative, the brow will appear to be too high. Overcorrection is necessary with all browlifting procedures and can be especially noticeable with a direct browlift. The brow is lifted by the surgeon, with the forehead in repose, to the desired height. The measurement is made at the inferior border of the lifted brow. The maximal elevation of the proposed excision (height of brow elevation) is marked along a line located between the lateral limbus and lateral canthus of the eye. This peak height of the ellipse is vertically above the lateral canthus. An elliptical excision is designed extending from the medial border of the brow past the lateral margin of the ptotic eyebrow. Failure to extend the excision past the border of the lateral brow will result in an inadequate lateral lift and a brow that curves downward.

The lower border of the excision is within the most superior brow hairs. This will ensure that as the surgical scar matures it will remain at the brow border and be less conspicuous. An excision above the border of the brow can drift superiorly as the scar matures and becomes visually obvious.[16] The brow hair bulbs lie obliquely and exit in a caudal direction. The inferior incision must be sharply beveled away from the brow hair to avoid injury to the hair follicles, which lie at a level higher than where the hair exits through the skin (Fig. 30–7). The corresponding upper portion of the incision is also beveled to match the lower portion, allowing better apposition during closure.

The skin is resected to a level just above the frontalis and orbicularis occuli muscles. An incision through the underlying muscle could endanger the supraorbital and supratrochlear neurovascular bundles. At the lateral third of the brow, the temporofrontalis nerve is at risk.[14] The brow

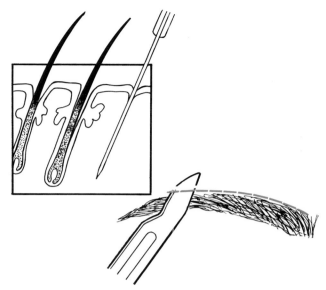

FIGURE 30–7. The incision of the direct browlift is beveled to avoid injury to the hair follicles.

is adherent to the orbital rim by fibrous attachments and cannot be lifted unless it is freed from the underlying tissues. Directly beneath the brow, submuscular dissection with blunt scissors will free the brow and avoid injury to the hair follicles. The orbicularis muscle layer can now be lifted separately from the skin and tacked superiorly into the frontalis muscle-fascia or periosteum.[17] This plication of the orbicularis muscle is based on the similar principle of SMAS plication in lower face rhytidectomy. The skin is separated from the muscle 0.5 cm below and above the excisional border.

With the use of sharp scissors, the frontalis muscle fibers are separated, exposing the underlying fascia at four to five points 1.0 to 1.5 cm apart under the superior margin of the excision.[18] A nonabsorbable 4-0 suture is passed vertically into the orbicularis muscle underlying the brow. The orbicularis is then pulled up and sutured onto the frontalis muscle at the site of maximal brow elevation (Fig. 30–6D). The remaining plicating sutures are then placed, raising the brow as a single skin–muscle unit while anastomosing the skin edges. The overlying skin, which has previously been separated from the muscle, is now closed as a separate layer. Meticulous placement of vertical mattress sutures evert the skin edges. Wound eversion will minimize scar stretch and skin depression. Sutures are removed in 4 to 5 days, and adhesive strips are applied for support.

Buried absorbable sutures are not used because they will not result in a permanent fixation. The absorbable suture is absorbed before scar tissue that is strong enough to support the brow at its new position is produced. Nonabsorbable buried suture and the scar tissue it induces will give support to the elevated tissues. I prefer propylene glycol suture (Prolene) because stitch abscess and spitting have been rare.

Initially the brow will be at an exaggerated level but will sink in 3 to 4 weeks to its final destination. Cosmetics can be used to camouflage the scar at day 10. The scars may take 6 months or longer to mature. Light dermabrasion can be performed as early as 6 to 8 weeks after suture removal to hasten scar maturity. However, with time, most scars will mature, fade, and mimic a rhytid. Overzealous abrasion of the scar can result in persistent erythema and demarcation lines.

Upper Forehead Browlift

The upper forehead approach to brow ptosis offers several surgical advantages.[19] The incision is located at the hairline (Fig. 30–8), and the surgical scar is hidden in or along the hairline (Case 2, Fig. 30–11). In glabrous men, the incision is above the forehead boss where the forehead slants back and thus in a less noticeable site (Case 3, Fig. 30–12). It avoids a scar at the eyebrow, which may be objectionable to men who do not use cosmetic coverups. Dissection is subfascial to the frontalis muscle in a relatively avascular space. The temporal branch of the facial nerve is superior to the muscle fascia in the area of dissection.[13] The brow, which is firmly attached to the supraorbital rim, can be released, thus enabling adequate elevation. Ptosis that is lateral or universal can be corrected with the incision limited to the lateral forehead. Conversely, a complete forehead incision is required to improve medial and glabellar ptosis.

This surgical approach does have its limitations. The use of bilateral lateral forehead incisions will only correct lateral and midlateral ptosis. Limiting the incisions to the lateral hairlines produces a scar that is well camouflaged. Neither procerus nor corrugator muscle ablation for glabellar rhytids can be performed from this approach. Extending the incision across the entire hairline enables the surgeon to lift the entire brow region, including the glabella. The disadvantage is a more visible scar. Permanent cutaneous anesthesia is common when a supraperiosteal dissection is done, while with a subcutaneous dissection it is unlikely. Myectomies of the corrugator and frontalis muscles can result in deformities of the skin contour.

Operative Procedure. The length of the proposed forehead hairline excision is determined by the extent and type of brow ptosis. The excisional site is tapered laterally, extending into the lateral scalp hair where it can extend down at a midauricular vertical line if a supraperiosteal plane of dissection is used.[10] The supraorbital notch is palpated and its location marked on the overlying skin for the ensuing surgery.

The procedure can be performed under local anesthesia with additional intramuscular and, in a few individuals, intravenous sedation. The eyebrow tissues and the temporal region lateral to the brow are infiltrated first with 1% lidocaine hydrochloride with 1:100,000 epinephrine. The incisional site and forehead tissues are then anesthetized.

The surgeon has the choice of two planes of surgical dissection: the classic supraperiosteal dissection or a subcutaneous dissection plane.[20] A supraperiosteal plane of dissection is used when the incision is carried down to the supraperiosteal plane lying under the galea. This is the same surgical plane as used in a coronal forehead lift.[12,21] The incisional site is usually vascular. Bleeding is usually controlled with meticulous electrocoagulation, but occa-

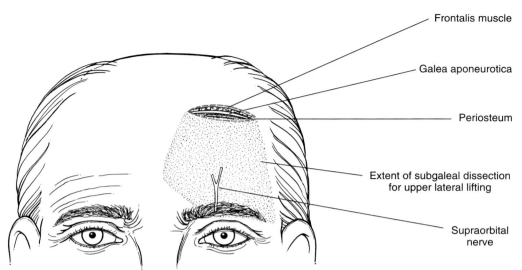

Frontalis muscle

Galea aponeurotica

Periosteum

Extent of subgaleal dissection
for upper lateral lifting

Supraorbital
nerve

FIGURE 30-8. Extent of subgaleal dissection for the upper forehead browlift.

sionally brisk hemorrhaging requires hemostatic clamping before electrocoagulation. Dissection then proceeds in the relatively bloodless supraperiosteal plane. A long-handled Metzenbaum scissors is used to separate the overlying frontalis fascia and muscle from the periosteum inferiorly to the lateral brow area.

The brow, adherent to the orbital rim by fibrous attachments, is separated from the superior bony orbit. This will allow the brow and forehead tissues to be lifted to their new position. Failure to separate the brow from the orbital rim will prevent upward mobility of the brow when the incisional site tissues are anastomosed. The brow is initially separated at the lateral orbital rim where there are no neurovascular bundles in the dissection plane. Dissection continues medially along the orbital rim while carefully avoiding transection of the supraorbital nerve and vessels (Fig. 30-8). Careless dissection to loosen the medial brow from the orbital rim can place this nerve at risk. With lateral forehead excisional sites, the tissues located in the middle of the forehead can be dissected free, aiding lifting of the glabellar region while avoiding injury to the neurovascular bundles. When the forehead excision is extended across the forehead, the surgeon can now expose the glabellar region with the neurovascular bundles and muscles. Myectomies of the corrugator muscle by resection of a strip of the muscle will ameliorate the frown lines.

The flap is now pulled superiorly, lifting the brow over the orbital rim to a slightly overcorrected position. The surgeon can determine if adequate dissection has been completed by attempting, from the incisional site on the upper lateral forehead, to pull the forehead tissue and brow up. Inability to raise the brow means that it is still adherent to the orbital rim and further dissection is required. With the use of 4-0 nonabsorbable suture, the frontalis fascia and/or galea is closed, raising the brow to its new position. During closure, the overlying skin edges are anastomosed, facilitating cutaneous closure. The skin edges are everted with a 5-0 vertical mattress suture with the knot tied superiorly to the incision. A running cutaneous 6-0 suture completes closure.

Sutures are removed in approximately 5 days and Steri-Strips are applied. The eyebrows will settle to their final position in several weeks. Postoperative edema of the glabella and brow regions is not uncommon, and it may not appear until several days after the surgery. Corticosteroids administered during, or immediately after, the surgery will decrease the anticipated tissue edema. There will be improvement of the rhytids located above the brow since the need for compensatory muscle movement to lift the brow is no longer necessary.

The subcutaneous forehead lift separates the skin from the underlying frontalis muscle and dissection continues beneath the brows.[20] Separation of the tissue planes is vascular and dissection is more tedious than in a supraperiosteal plane. The corrugator and procerus muscles can be viewed from above and myectomies performed as needed. Or the frontalis muscle can be incised and the muscles approached as described in the midforehead lift. The advantage of this approach is the effectiveness of correcting forehead rhytides and the relative lack of permanent cutaneous anesthesia, although initial anesthesia is to be expected. Tissue necrosis due to vascular compromise, although very unlikely, is a potential risk.

The Midforehead Browlift

The midforehead lift is well suited for individuals who have overactive frontalis, procerus, or corrugator muscles; high or sparse frontal hairline; midforehead frown lines; glabellar ptosis; and brow ptosis.[22] Relative contraindications for this procedure include an unfurrowed forehead, a low forehead, and sebaceous skin. The incision site may be extremely hyperemic for an inordinate period of time, and there may be delayed healing at the site of the incision. Awaiting scar maturation can be extremely anxiety provoking to both patient and surgeon.[23] Even though the incision site can be hyperemic, hypertrophic scarring is extremely uncommon. The planned forehead excision can use one of several different designs (Fig. 30-9A through

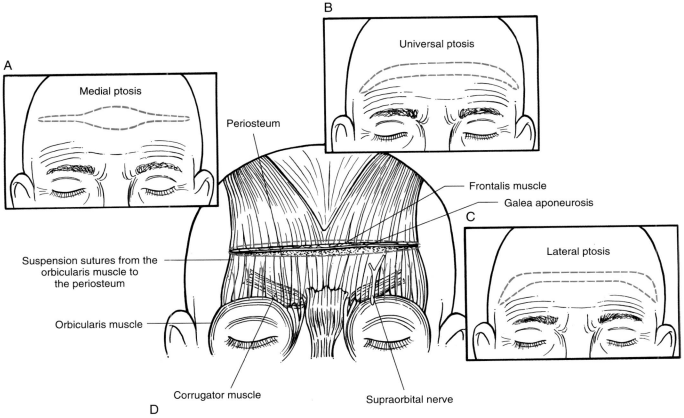

FIGURE 30–9. Excisional designs for the midforehead browlift. *A,* Medial ptosis. *B,* Universal ptosis. *C,* Lateral ptosis. *D,* Position of suspension sutures from the orbicularis muscle to the periosteum.

C). It may vary in width if some areas of the forehead are to be elevated more than others. For instance, if relatively greater elevation of the glabellar area is desired, the excision will be wider here than over the lateral brow. Conversely, lateral brow ptosis will require greater elevation and therefore greater width of the designed forehead excision laterally.[22]

Operative Procedure. The excision is planned so that the resultant scar will lie in one of the forehead rhytids. The upper limb of the planned excision should be in a horizontal furrow even if the furrow is not symmetrical across the forehead. Thus the surgical scar will ultimately mimic a forehead rhytid. The vertical width will be a function of the proposed brow elevation required at that

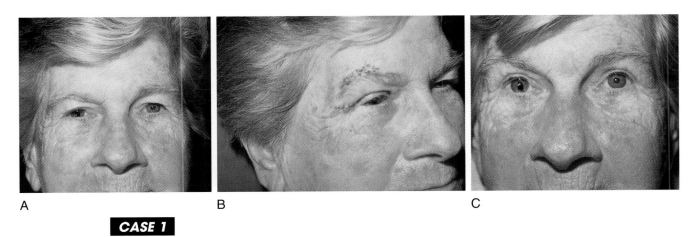

CASE 1

FIGURE 30–10. Direct brow lift. *A,* Preoperative brow ptosis and dermatochalasis. *B,* The incision is at the immediate superior hair line and is sharply beveled to avoid injury to the hair bulbs. *C,* At 3 months after surgery there is an elevated symmetric brow. The scar line is hidden by the superior brow hairs.

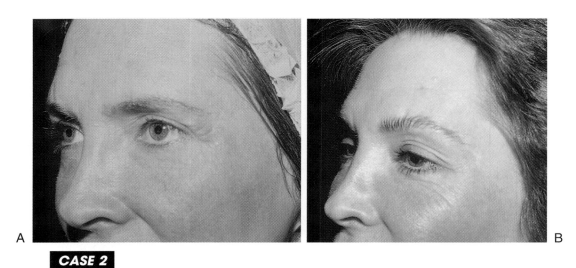

A   B

CASE 2

FIGURE 30–11. Upper forehead lift. *A,* Preoperative lateral view of the brow ptosis. *B,* After surgery there is elevation of the brow above the orbital bony ridge. This opens the eye allowing greater visual expression.

point. The height of brow correction desired is measured, and overcorrection (as with all types of brow surgical procedures) of 0.5 to 1.0 cm is desirable owing to postoperative descent.

The outlined skin is excised, leaving the underlying adherent frontalis muscle intact. The forehead skin is literally stripped off the underlying frontalis muscle by lifting up from one end of the incised skin. This is a safe excision and does not transect the cutaneous nerves. If the excision included the frontalis muscle, the sensory branches supplying the forehead skin would be transected. Anesthesia would be complete and extremely unsettling to the patient. Cutaneous sensation may return in time but will probably be incomplete.

At this point, one of several surgical techniques may be followed. In the simplest technique, minimal if any undermining is performed at the inferior border. By using a series of buried intradermal sutures, the excisional site is anastomosed, bringing the skin edges together. This raises the brow up. Cutaneous closure is completed with vertical mattress sutures, which evert the skin edges. A continuous running cutaneous closure further immobilizes the skin edges.

In another variation, the forehead is meticulously undermined at a subdermal plane to the supraorbital rims. Dissection is superior to the frontalis muscle, which is tightly adherent to the overlying skin. Dissection is usually bloody if the underlying frontalis muscle is violated. By remaining above the muscle there is no danger of damage to the supraorbital and supratrochlear nerves as they lie at a deeper level. Dissection is continued under the brow, exposing the orbicularis muscle. The upper margin of the orbicularis muscle is now imbricated using 4-0 nonabsorbable suture. It is tacked superiorly with three or four sutures to the underlying frontalis fascia or periosteum, raising the brow. Dissection can also continue to the glabella and onto the nasal root, allowing this lax skin to be lifted.

In patients who exhibit deep glabellar furrows, the procerus and corrugator muscles are trimmed from above by utilizing an electrosurgical cutting current.[20,23] Subcutaneous buried sutures are used to anastomose the skin edges. Meticulous skin closure is mandatory.

Another technique differs slightly from the previously discussed technique. After undermining the skin at a suprafrontalis plane of dissection to the orbital rims, a transverse incision is carried through the frontalis muscle at a level 3 to 4 cm superior to the nasal root. This incision does not extend laterally beyond the previously carefully marked supraorbital notches. Through this incision, the flap is undermined in a plane just above the periosteum to the nasal root and medial supraorbital rims. The medial ends of the corrugator muscles are identified and isolated while avoiding injury to the supraorbital and supratrochlear neurovascular bundles (see Fig. 30–9D). A small section (0.5 cm) of the corrugator muscle is resected bilaterally utilizing an electrosurgical cutting current. Similarly, the procerus muscle is also divided by a cutting current. The incision into the frontalis muscle is now repaired. Failure to anastomose the frontalis muscle will result in an unsightly bulge and depression on the forehead. The depression is due to the gap in the frontalis muscle, and the bulge is from the contracted edge of the muscle.[22]

In each of the above techniques, anastomosis of the skin edges must be meticulous to minimize cutaneous scarring since the surgical site is conspicuously placed. The wound is covered with antibiotic ointment and a forehead surgical dressing. The dressing should be supportive but not too constrictive as to impede circulation. The sutures are removed in 3 to 4 days, and the wound is splinted with supportive flesh-tone adhesive tape for an additional 2 or 3 weeks. Women may apply a light makeup over the tape. The forehead takes 2 to 3 weeks to settle from its overcorrected position, and complete maturation of the scar may take 6 months.

POSTOPERATIVE SEQUELAE AND COMPLICATIONS

The following normal occurrences are expected after the surgery. Mild bruising is common. Most patients will develop only a yellowish hue, typically present in the orbital region. However, its appearance may not be seen until several days after the surgery. Its late occurrence is attributable to the time it takes the blood to seep and settle in this caudal location.

Discomfort and soreness are also normal and may last for several days. Acetaminophen or a mild narcotic is adequate for direct browlift procedures. When subgaleal dissection is performed, a narcotic (e.g., codeine or propoxyphene) is necessary for added comfort. Pain is unusual and should be investigated since it is a sign of an emerging hematoma.

Edema is common and worse on awakening. It may be located on the forehead, at the glabellar region, or within the upper orbital socket. Edema can be greatest at the glabella and/or upper eyelids, where it can impair vision. The onset of the edema can be delayed until the third or fourth day after surgery. Its delay can be disconcerting and alarming to the uninformed patient.

Inadequate hemostasis before wound closure can allow extensive bruising with the blood seeping, by gravity, through the plane dissected into the upper and lower orbital tissue. Here the bruising may take several weeks to dissipate. Hematomas are relatively uncommon because the site is amendable to pressure dressings.

The scalp in some persons is very mobile and can be forcefully moved significantly in an anterior direction. These patients may exhibit stretch-back of the tissues, thereby negating what initially appeared to be excellent results. Surgical overcorrection can decrease the negative effects of the scalp tissue sliding forward; however, the initial surgical correction must be exaggerated elevation of the brows.

Sutures are usually removed on the fourth or fifth day. Occasionally, if there is excessive tension and there is inadequate subcutaneous wound support, partial dehiscence may occur. Dehiscence can also be due to a hematoma present at the site of the incision. Extensive dehiscence should be closed with suture after the hematoma has been evacuated. Application of Steri-Strips or allowing the wound to granulate may be all that is necessary when the dehiscence is in a cosmetically unimportant site. Uncommonly the buried Prolene suspension suture will ''spit'' or form a stitch abscess. Treatment is removal of the suture.

Inadequate lifting of the brows may be due to a poorly planned procedure or underestimation of tissue stretch-back after surgery. Inadequate lifting of the brow can sometimes be compensated by an upper eyelid blepharoplasty. This is appropriate in those cases in which the brow has been obviously elevated but not to the ideal height. Lifting an unrecognized asymmetry of the forehead and brows will be exaggerated at the upper eyelids. The asymmetrical tissue is manifested as a difference in the tissue bulk between upper eyelids. Unless there is blatant asymmetry of the brows, correction is simply obtained with an upper eyelid blepharoplasty.

Lagophthalmos can occur if browlifting is incorrectly performed after, instead of before, upper eyelid blepharoplasty. Removal of the excess upper eyelid tissue will actually produce greater brow ptosis, with the inability now to raise the brow to its correct position due to a lack of

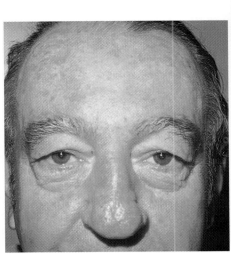 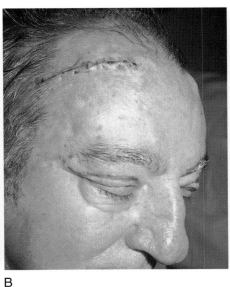 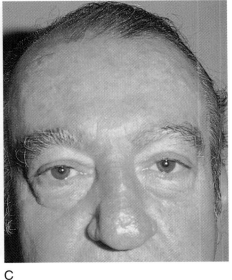

A   B   C

CASE 3

FIGURE 30–12. Upper lateral forehead lift. *A,* Ptosis of the brows with dermatochalasis of the upper eyelids. *B,* Incision on the upper lateral forehead with upper lid blepharoplasty. *C,* Mature upper lateral forehead scar is above the bossing of the forehead. The brows are in the appropriate position, and the upper lid dermatochalasis has been corrected.

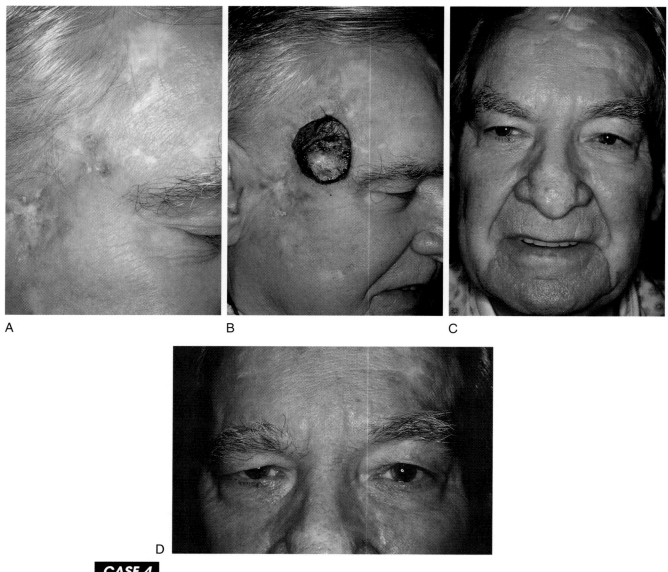

A B C

D

CASE 4

FIGURE 30–13. Correction of unilateral ptotic brow resulting from resection of cancer with loss of temporal branch of facial nerve. *A,* An elderly man has a recurrent basal cell carcinoma of the right temple superior to the poikilodermatous changes of an area treated 10 years earlier with radiation therapy. *B,* Resection with Mohs' micrographic surgery is carried through the muscle with ligation of the temporal artery and loss of the temporal branch of the facial nerve. The wound heals by second intention. *C,* Two months after resection the wound has healed. The right brow ptosis is beginning to interfere with upward gaze. *D,* Seven months after surgery the right brow ptosis has progressed to impair both upward and lateral gaze.

tissue. A previous blepharoplasty done in the presence of brow ptosis may also preclude adequate browlifting owing to a paucity of upper eyelid tissue.

Direct Browlift Complications

The direct browlift is relatively free of bleeding complications because of the site and superficial depth of the excision. At risk are the neurovascular bundles that can be transected if the frontalis muscle is violated. This can result in loss of cutaneous sensation or, more seriously, in sectioning of the temporal branch of the facial nerve at the lateral brow.

The visual position of the direct browlift scar makes it susceptible to poor surgical technique. Incorrectly placing the incision above the brow can produce a scar that, during healing, will drift superiorly into a visually conspicuous

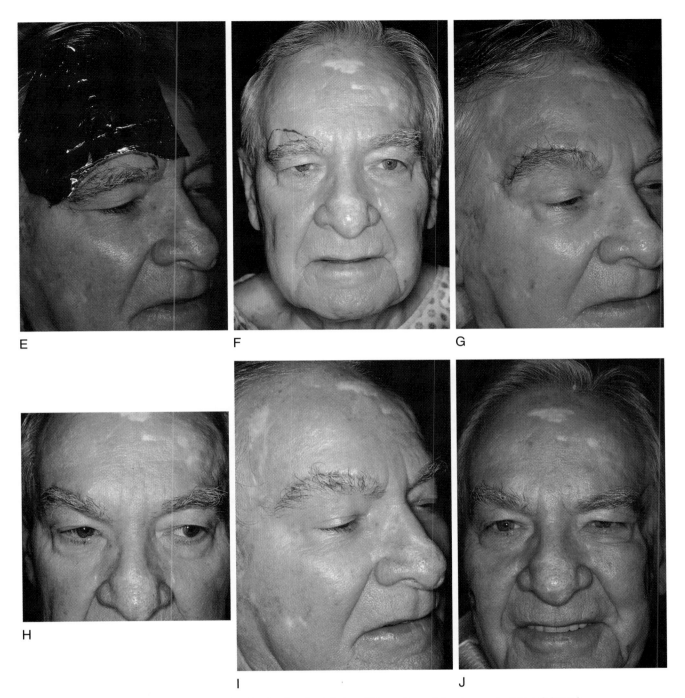

FIGURE 30–13 *Continued E,* In planning the right browlift, a pattern of the placement of the left brow is made and flipped over. The distance from the temporal and frontal hairline is accurately measured with this pattern. The upper gentian violet line represents the ideal placement of the brow. A method to measure the amount of ptosis is especially important for positioning unilateral brow ptosis. *F,* While there is universal right brow ptosis, the lateral ptotic portion interferes with lateral gaze; thus, the dimensions of the planned excision are altered over the lateral brow to give more lift to that portion. *G,* The incision of the direct browlift is placed within the upper aspect of the brow. The periosteal tacking sutures give extreme elevation of the upper lid. This patient will not have a subsequent blepharoplasty. *H,* At the time of suture removal in 5 days the arch of the right brow is a bit pronounced in comparison with the left. *I,* At 2 weeks, the pronounced arch has flattened somewhat and the incision line outlined with gentian violet is hidden by bushy brows. *J,* Two years later the right browlift remains in position, preserving upward and lateral gaze. Eighteen months after the right browlift the patient developed a squamous cell carcinoma of the left temple. Now, 6 months after resection of the left temple lesion, he has left brow ptosis, which interferes with upward gaze. The concavity of the left temple is the site of the resection and repair with a split-thickness skin graft. In the near future a left browlift will be considered. (*A* to *J* courtesy of June K. Robinson, M.D.)

site. Excessive wound tension will also result in a wide and conspicuous scar. Meticulous closure and eversion of the wound edges will minimize this complication. A poorly designed repair can result in improperly shaped eyebrows.

Postsurgical neuralgia is a relatively common sequela. Spontaneous shooting pains can start above the eyebrow or be felt in the anterior scalp and can last for several months before resolving. Intralesional corticosteroids (triamcinolone diluted to 5 mg/mL), injected weekly, if necessary, at the trigger point will hasten resolution when the neuralgia warrants treatment.

Upper Forehead Browlift Complications

This incision is partially hidden by the scalp hair but is exposed when the hair is swept back. Meticulous closure of the fascial layer will oppose the skin edges. Eversion of the wound edges can then be accomplished without tension. This will minimize the occurrence of a wide, atrophic scar on the forehead skin and loss of hair in the scalp portion of the wound.

The brow tissues must be freed from the orbital rim by releasing the fibrous adhesions. Failure to release these septa will make it difficult to raise the brow and close the surgical forehead wound without tension. The frontalis muscle must also be separated from the periosteum above the medial portion of the brow to allow lifting of the medial brow area as the wound is closed. If dissection is not completed medially, there may be excessive lift laterally. This will produce eyebrows that slant medially, imparting a ''Mr. Spock'' appearance.

When the brow is freed from the orbital rim, careful dissection is necessary to avoid sectioning of the supraorbital neurovascular bundle (Fig. 30–4). The tissue is carefully freed by blunt dissection. It is surprising that careful dissection can continue almost to the medial border of the brow without serious neurovascular damage. Firm pressure for several minutes will usually stop any bleeding that serves as a warning that dissection should cease in this area.

As the wound at the hairline heals, hairs may become embedded within the scar line. A foreign body reaction with inflammation may occur.

Midforehead Browlift Complications

The surgical scar across the forehead will be conspicuous and hyperemic for months before it matures and fades. Failure to place the upper incision site within a forehead rhytid will enhance the conspicuousness of the scar. Improper technique in the subcutaneous and cutaneous closure will cause similar complications.

Hematoma formation is prevented by meticulous electrocoagulation and application of a supportive dressing. However, a strangulating surgical dressing may result in flap necrosis and skin ulceration.

Dissection must be above the frontalis muscle to avoid nerve sectioning and the resultant anesthesia. When the subgaleal space is entered, the incision must be placed between the supraorbital and supratrochlear neurovascular bundles. The same care must also be taken during the isolation and cutting of the corrugator and procerus muscles to avoid damage to the supraorbital and supratrochlear neurovascular bundles (Fig. 30–4).

Possible Additional Operations

After the edema has settled, it may become obvious that the browlift was not adequate. Patients are usually not concerned about a low-lying brow but rather about fullness of the upper orbital rim as manifested by eyelid ptosis. This is easily resolved by resection of the upper eyelid skin. Obvious asymmetry of the brow is unusual unless the surgeon has grossly miscalculated the proposed height of the lift on one side. Surgery should be delayed (for 6 to 8 weeks) until all edema has settled and the brow has reached its final resting position. Resolution of the edema may result in improvement of the asymmetry, obviating additional surgery.

REFERENCES

1. Elliot DL, et al. Medical considerations in ambulatory surgery. Clin Plast Surg 1983;10:295.
2. Foster CA, Aston SJ. Propranolol–epinephrine interaction: A potential disaster. Plast Reconstr Surg 1983;72:74.
3. Ellenbogen R. Transcoronal eyebrow lift with concomitant upper blepharoplasty. Plast Reconstr Surg 1983;71:490–499.
4. Rafaty MF, Brennan HG. Current concepts of browpexy. Arch Otolaryngol 1983;109:152–154.
5. Brennan HG. Correction of the ptotic brow. Otolaryngol Clin North Am 1980;13:265–273.
6. Webster RC, Fanous N, Smith RC. Blepharoplasty: When to combine it with brow, temple, or coronal lift. J Otolaryngol 1979;8:339–343.
7. Dicker PL, Syracuse VR. Adjunctive procedures to maximize the result of cosmetic eyelid surgery. Otolaryngol Head Neck Surg 1981;89:504–510.
8. Wolfley DE, Guibor P. Preoperative evaluation of the blepharoplasty patient. Facial Plast Surg 1984;1:284–291.
9. Beeson WH, McCollough EG. Complications of the forehead lift. Ear Nose Throat J 1985;64:527.
10. Viñas JC, Caviglia C, Cortiñas JL. Forehead rhytidoplasty and brow lifting. Plast Reconstr Surg 1976;57:445–454.
11. Stuzin JM, Wagstrom L, Kawamoto HK, Wolfe SA. Anatomy of the frontal branch of the facial nerve: The significance of the temporal fat pad. Plast Reconstr Surg 1989;83:265–271.
12. Pitanguy I. Indications for and treatment of frontal and glabellar wrinkles in an analysis of 3,404 consecutive cases of rhytidectomy. Plast Reconstr Surg 1981;67:157–166.
13. Liebman E, Webster RC, Berger A, DellaVechia M. The frontalis nerve in the temporal brow lift. Arch Otolaryngol 1982;108:232–235.
14. Johnson CM, Anderson JA, Katz RB. The browlift 1978. Arch Otolaryngol 1979;105:124–126.
15. Collins PS. Surgical procedures for correction of the ptotic brow. In: Coleman WP, et al. eds. Cosmetic Surgery of the Skin. Philadelphia, BC Decker, 1991:317–333.
16. Dicker PL, Syracuse VR. Adjunctive procedures to maximize the result of cosmetic eyelid surgery. Otolaryngol Head Neck Surg 1981;89:504–510.
17. Lewis JR. A method of direct eyebrow lift. Ann Plast Surg 1983;10:115–119.
18. Chrisman BB. Blepharoplasty and brow lift. In: Wheeland RG, ed.

Cutaneous Surgery. Philadelphia, WB Saunders Co. 1994:568–586.

19. Collins PS. The upper lateral forehead brow lift. Presented before the 15th Annual Clinical and Scientific Meeting of the American Society of Dermatologic Surgery, Monterey, California, April 1988.

20. Wolfe SA, Baird WL. The subcutaneous forehead lift. Plast Reconstr Surg 1989;83:251–256.

21. Toledo GA, Tate JL. Coronal approach for rejuvenation of the eyes and forehead. Arch Otolaryngol Head Neck Surg 1986;112:738.

22. Johnson CM, Waldman SR. Midforehead lift. Arch Otolaryngol 1983;109:155–159.

23. Brennan HG, Rafaty FM. Midforehead incisions in treatment of the aging face. Arch Otolaryngol 1982;108:732–734.

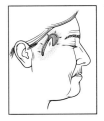

chapter 31

Dermabrasion

JOHN M. YARBOROUGH and
WILLIAM P. COLEMAN, III

Dermabrasion is a technique for removing the epidermis and a portion of the dermis using an abrasive wheel driven by a high-speed rotary engine.[1] Although originally developed for the treatment of acne scars, dermabrasion is also used successfully to remove benign and premalignant skin lesions, tattoos, wrinkles, and rhinophyma (Tables 31–1 and 31–2).[2,3] If the pathologic process does not extend below the deep reticular dermis, complete removal of the disease is possible.[6,10,11] Facial skin can heal without visible scarring if the dermabrasion is limited to the dermis above the deep reticular layer.

The skin is anesthetized using local anesthesia or a cryogenic spray (Figs. 31–1 and 31–2). A diamond fraise or a wire brush is employed as the abrasive instrument (Table 31–3; Fig. 31–3). Either instrument can be attached to a hand engine developing 15,000 to 20,000 rpm. The wire brush abrades more deeply more easily, whereas the diamond fraise is easier to control.[8] The surgeon must take great care to abrade the proper depth for the specific pathologic condition. Most dermabrasion is carried to the mid dermis. Scarring is more common when dermabrasion is performed on nonfacial areas.[6]

Postoperatively, biosynthetic dressings are useful especially for the first 24 hours (Table 31–4).[9] After this application of bland ointments, frequent washing is recommended. Reepithelialization takes 7 to 10 days to complete. Erythema may last for an additional 2 to 12 weeks. Patients remain hypersensitive to sun exposure for several months after dermabrasion and need to use sun protection for 6 months after dermabrasion. Depending on the depth of the dermabrasion, there may be permanent change in skin texture. There is evidence that improvement in the appearance of abraded skin correlates with histologic evidence of new collagen formation in the dermis.[10,11]

TABLE 31–1. Dermabrasion: Indications, Contraindications, Limitations

Indications[2,3]

Benign

Scars (acne (Cases 1 and 2, Figs. 31–4 and 31–5), traumatic (Case 3, Fig. 31–6), or other diseases)
Seborrheic keratosis
Epidermal nevi (Case 4, Fig. 31–7)
Trichoepitheliomas
Adenoma sebaceum
Rhinophyma
Wrinkles
Tattoos
Hailey-Hailey disease[6]

Premalignant

Actinic keratosis (Cases 5 and 6, Figs. 31–8 and 31–9)

Malignant

Superficial basal cell carcinoma
Squamous cell carcinoma in situ

Contraindications

Impaired wound healing
Recent treatment with isotretinoin (Accutane)[4,5]
Keloid diathesis
Prior radiation therapy or deep thermal or chemical burns
Active herpes warts or bacterial infection within the area to be dermabraded
Psychosis

Limitations

Removal of scars or lesions may be incomplete, requiring additional dermabrasion.
Cosmetic results are unsatisfactory in locations other than on the face.

Text continued on page 343

TABLE 31-2. Dermabrasion: Patient Preoperative Discussion

1. You will receive a sedative before surgery. Please come with a responsible driver.
2. Initial healing may take up to 2 weeks. You should remain home until crusting and scabbing have stopped.
3. Final healing may take several months, and you may have to disguise areas of redness.
4. Some patients develop hyperpigmentation in the early postoperative period and require therapy with bleaching agents.[3]
5. Long-lasting hyperpigmentation or hypopigmentation may result in treated areas. Cosmetics may be used to camouflage this.
6. Frequent office visits will be required during the early postoperative phase.
7. Final results may not be apparent for several months.
8. Additional treatment with other modalities or subsequent dermabrasion may be required to achieve the best possible result.

TABLE 31-3. Dermabrasion: Operative Issues

Preoperative Evaluation

History:
    Bleeding diathesis
    Hepatitis
    Human immunodeficiency virus infection
    Herpes simplex virus infection
    Prior radiation
    Immunosuppression
    Keloiding tendency
    Prior isotretinoin (Accutane) therapy
    Examine prior scars for clues to healing

Preoperative Equipment Needs

Hand engine capable of 15,000 rpm or more
Appropriate-sized diamond fraise or wire brush
Extensive barrier protection for the surgeon and staff
Local anesthesia or cryosprays, preoperative chilling with ice packs

Intraoperative Needs

Suture tray if simultaneous scar excision is planned
Terrycloth towels
Additional faceshields when initial one becomes obscured

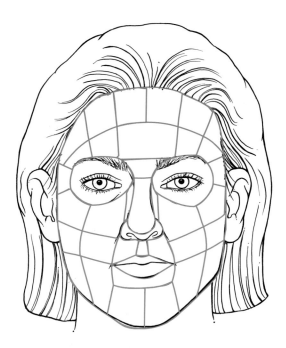

FIGURE 31-1. An imaginary grid pattern is planned to obtain local anesthesia by freezing the skin with a cryogenic spray. The grid size is generally 4 to 5 cm². The more dependent areas of the face are treated first. This allows uniform freezing of areas without warming by blood flow from contiguous dermabraded skin. The size of the imaginary grid (*red lines*) is limited by the technique of the surgeon. If freezing the larger size areas is performed and thawing occurs before completion of dermabrasion of that unit, then the units may be subdivided. Freezing lasts about 10 seconds. As the surgeon becomes more experienced, larger areas are frozen at a time. Although partial facial dermabrasions may be performed, at least a whole cosmetic unit is abraded. Usually symmetrical cosmetic units are dermabraded (e.g., both cheeks). Dermabrasion of entire cosmetic units avoids demarcation by changes in pigmentation. Dermabrasion of cheeks is extended to just beneath the jaw line, out to the preauricular area, and up to the suborbital area to ensure a uniform texture and appearance.

FIGURE 31-2. After preoperative analgesia is achieved with oral, intramuscular, or intravenous agents and with or without facial nerve blocks, each unit of the imaginary grid is frozen. A unit (*red outline*) is isolated by towels, and traction is applied at its borders. Either the surgeon or the assistant may spray the cryogenic agent. After the skin becomes white, the surgeon may gently press on the frozen area to determine the firmness of the skin. No indentation should occur within the frozen area. Gauze sponges are not used to isolate skin units because they can become entangled on the instrument during the procedure.

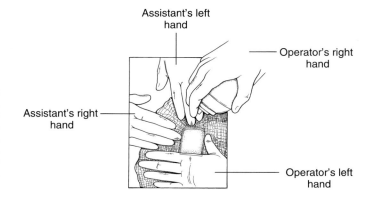

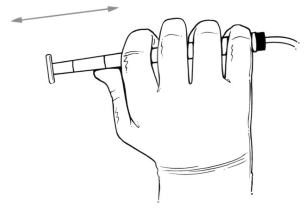

FIGURE 31–3. A firm grip using the thumb to stabilize the shaft of the instrument is essential. This particular grip on the handle allows rapid lifting of the handpiece in a move familiar to all as "the dermabrader's reflex." If the feel of the instrument in the hand becomes wrong, the handpiece is rapidly withdrawn from contact with the patient. The placement of the fingers on the handle depends on the instrument and the individual surgeon. For an instrument without a protective fender over the top of the fraise or brush, the surgeon's hand is placed farther back on the handle. The handle of the device is held parallel to the skin surface. No gauze pads are used, and all hair is taped out of the field. Both gauze pads and hair can catch in the rapidly spinning wire brush or diamond fraise.

The wire brush tends to grab and pull the skin more than the fraise. To minimize this pulling, the instrument is carried over the surface of the skin in a direction perpendicular to the rotation of the brush (*red arrows*). Strokes are directed parallel (left to right) or obliquely to the surgeon's body (from his body and away). The wire brush requires almost no pressure. Circular movements may gouge the skin. Special attention must be paid to fixing the lip by traction when dermabrading this area. It is sometimes useful to place a finger inside the patient's mouth to maintain control of the lip while dermabrading this area. Firm traction and a delicate touch are also required when dermabrading the lower eyelid.

TABLE 31–4. Dermabrasion: Postoperative Care

Pain Management
Acetaminophen is sufficient.
Narcotics may be required for some patients.

Dressings
Vigilon, Omniderm, or other biological dressing is applied first.
Nonstick pads overlie this.
Precut masks or gauze secure the pads.

Complications
Focal persistent erythema (Case 8, Fig. 31–11) may indicate incipient hypertrophic scars. Early treatment with topical steroids or steroid-impregnated tape is usually successful (Case 9, Fig. 31–12), (Case 14, Fig. 31–17).
True hypertrophic scars must be managed with intralesional steroids and/or silicone sheeting (Case 10, Fig. 31–13).
Hemorrhagic reaction follows Valsalva maneuver in postoperative period.
Postinflammatory hyperpigmentation appears in some patients at the third to fourth week postoperatively. Early treatment with 4% hydroquinone creams usually controls this tendency but often must be continued for 3 to 4 months postoperatively (Case 11, Fig. 31–14).
Hypopigmentation: use cosmetics; blend edges with chemical peel (Case 12, Fig. 31–15)
Bacterial or viral infections may occur in the initial postoperative phase and can be treated appropriately using systemic and topical agents.

Expected Sequela of Limited Duration
Milia at 3 to 4 weeks; treat with tretinoin (Retin-A) cream or needle extraction.
Rebound oiliness of skin
Mild acneiform eruption (folliculitis) (Case 13, Fig. 31–16)

CASE 1

FIGURE 31–4. *A*, This man has multiple, broad-based acne scars of the cheeks. *B*, One year after dermabrasion the scars are markedly improved.

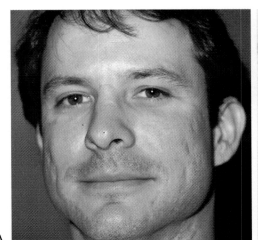

A

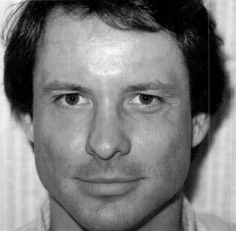

B

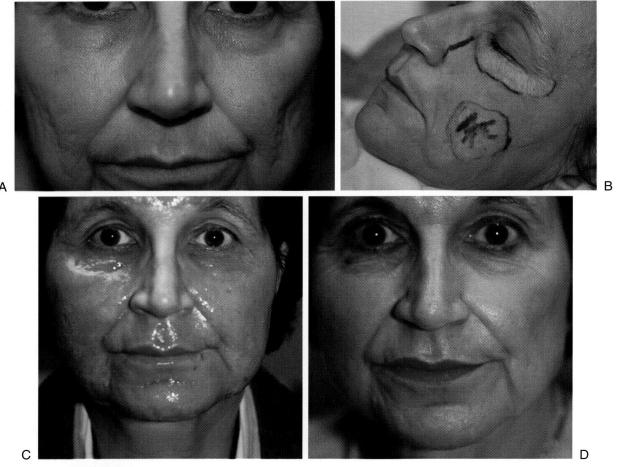

A

B

C

D

CASE 2

FIGURE 31–5. *A,* Ice-pick type acne scars of the cheeks have become more prominent with aging in this woman. In addition, the patient is concerned about the dark circles under her eyes. She has some photodamage with sallowness of the skin of the face. *B,* Before dermabrasion, a chemical peel of the lower eyelids is done to blend the line of demarcation with the dermabraded skin. It is also possible that the peel will improve her dark circles. When combining peeling with dermabrasion, it is important to do the peel before doing the dermabrasion. The area delineated by the peel can be avoided in doing the dermabrasion. If the two procedures are performed in the reverse order, the chemical agent frequently "wicks" or "bleeds" into the freshly dermabraded skin. This can unfortunately cause greater depth of injury to the skin with resultant pigmentary changes. The area of greatest concentration of acne scars is marked for special attention to go deeper during the dermabrasion. The whole anatomic unit of the cheek will be abraded, not just the isolated area marked. In this candidate with photoaged sallow skin, dermabrasion limited to just the cheeks would result in lines of demarcation with the lips, chin, and forehead; therefore, these areas are included in the dermabrasion. *C,* Five days after the procedure, she has slight edema but all areas have nearly epithelialized. *D,* One year postoperatively the acne scars have almost completely disappeared.

FIGURE 31–6. *A,* Extensive facial scars of the left nasal dorsum, left cheek, left upper lip, left lower lip, and chin after a bicycle accident 6 weeks previously. Dermabrasion performed in a favorable time period 4 to 8 weeks after traumatic scarring assists in remodeling of dermal collagen with remarkable improvement in the anticipated scarring. *B,* Four months after dermabrasion of the entire face. The entire face was dermabraded to try to prevent differences in pigmentation.

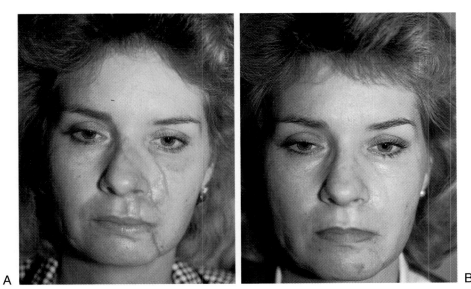

A

B

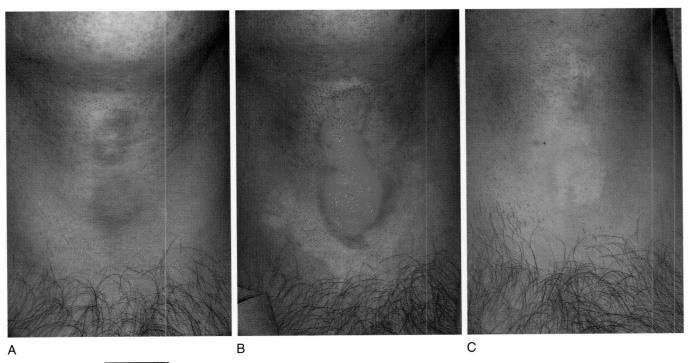

A

B

C

FIGURE 31–7. *A,* An epidermal nevus of the anterior neck of a young man was sampled with a spot dermabrasion in the center of the superior area before treating the whole area with dermabrasion. *B,* The dermabrasion with a diamond fraise was performed under local anesthesia with 1% lidocaine with epinephrine. The blanching of the skin from the epinephrine accentuates the 1- to 2-mm rim of epidermal nevus that remains. This nevus was left in the hope of decreasing the visibility of the line of demarcation on the neck. *C,* Two years later the remaining nevus has not progressed. (*A* to *C* courtesy of June K. Robinson, M.D.)

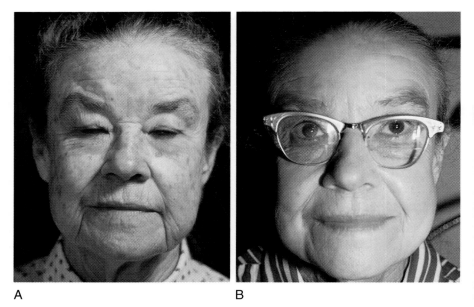

A

B

FIGURE 31–8. Dermabrasion for actinic damage. *A,* This older woman has extensive photodamage with multiple, poorly demarcated actinic keratoses. *B,* Two years after dermabrasion of all facial areas except the eyelids, she has no return of actinic keratoses. She does have slight hypopigmentation of areas that were dermabraded. Careful placement of the line of demarcation of the dermabrasion just slightly below the mandibular line makes the contrast with the photodamaged skin of the neck less noticeable. There may be slower healing in older patients with thinned, actinically damaged skin. Preconditioning with topical retinoic acid for 2 weeks before dermabrasion may enhance healing.

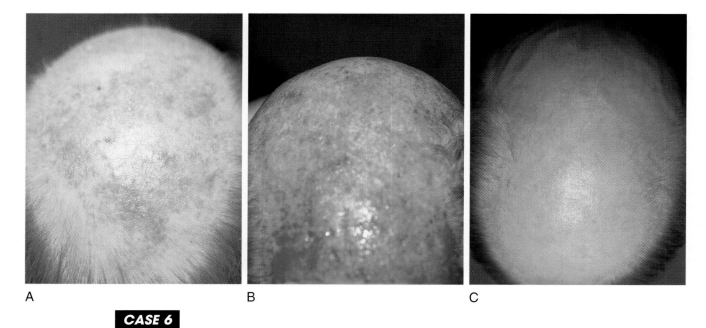

A

B

C

CASE 6

FIGURE 31–9. *A,* Severe actinic damage with multiple actinic keratoses of the bald scalp extends down to the fringe of hair. *B,* Immediately after dermabrasion of forehead and scalp, the bleeding indicates a relatively superficial abrasion was achieved. *C,* Three months after dermabrasion there are no remaining keratoses and the skin color is uniform over the scalp. There is mild erythema of the forehead.

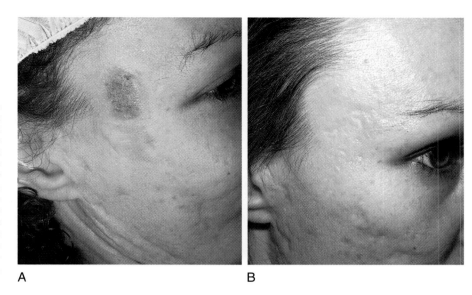

A **B**

CASE 7

FIGURE 31–10. Spot dermabrasion. *A,* Some dermatologic surgeons use a test spot to predict the patient's ability to tolerate the procedure and the risk of untoward sequelae in that person. The test spot serves as a way to educate the patient about the procedure and allows the patient to decide whether to have a larger area of one or more cosmetic units treated. The test spot is located in the temporal concavity near to the hairline and a diamond fraise is used. *B,* Three months later there is no visible color change at the test site; however, acne scars of the cheeks are hyperpigmented. The patient decided to proceed with full-face dermabrasion for acne scarring. (*A* and *B* courtesy of June K. Robinson, M.D.)

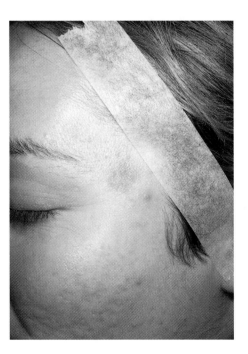

CASE 8

FIGURE 31–11. This patient experienced persistent erythema at the site of the test spot dermabrasion that was done 3 months before with a diamond fraise. The patient and physician decided not to perform the full-face dermabrasion. (Courtesy of June K. Robinson, M.D.)

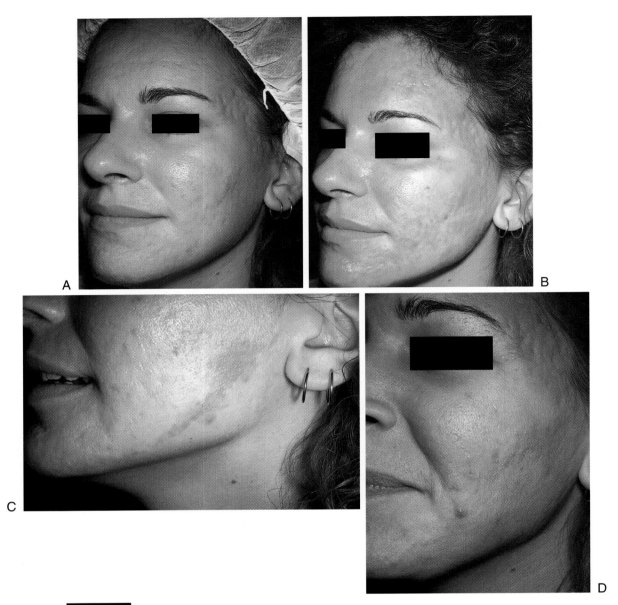

FIGURE 31–12. Linear focal erythema. *A,* The left cheek of this young woman before dermabrasion for acne scarring. *B,* One month after dermabrasion there is mild erythema and some edema. *C,* Six weeks after dermabrasion, she developed over the left cheek a single linear area of erythema that was palpable. This was believed to represent incipient hypertrophic scar formation. The area was treated with corticosteroid-impregnated tape daily for 3 weeks. The area was occluded with tape 24 hours a day. This case occurred before the existence of silicone gel sheeting, which is now another treatment option. *D,* Six months after the dermabrasion the area resolved without hypertrophic scar formation. (*A* to *D* courtesy of June K. Robinson, M.D.)

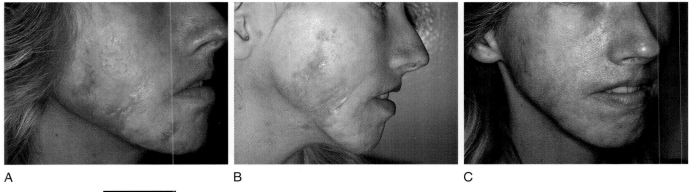

A   B   C

CASE 10

FIGURE 31–13. Hypertrophic scars. *A,* Focal erythema and telangiectasia over the right mandible appears 6 weeks after a dermabrasion performed by another surgeon. Patient partially conceals it with cosmetics at the time of the consultation visit. *B,* Three months of use of topical corticosteroid cream failed to abort the process of developing hypertrophic scars. Intralesional corticosteroid injections with triamcinalone starting at 10 mg/mL and tapering to 5 mg/mL at 4-week intervals were started. *C,* After 8 months of intralesional injections, the hypertrophic scars improved somewhat. (*A* to *C* courtesy of June K. Robinson, M.D.)

CASE 11

FIGURE 31–14. *A,* Hyperpigmentation of the right cheek and eye junction area 5 years after dermabrasion performed by another surgeon. The hyperpigmentation was not responsive to a 6-week course of sun protection and 4% topical hydroquinone cream that was prescribed at the time of the consultation visit. *B,* The hyperpigmented areas were peeled with 25% trichloroacetic acid solution. The frosting of the peel and reactive erythema is apparent. When peeling for hypopigmentation or hyperpigmentation after dermabrasion, it is best to wait at least 1 year after dermabrasion to allow full recovery of the dermis. *C,* In the immediate period after peeling hyperpigmentation may appear. As soon as the skin epithelializes after peeling, topical 4% hydroquinone is started. Two months after the first peel, this patient had some blending of the color variations. *D,* The patient had two more peels with the same agent followed by 4% hydroquinone. Five years after the first peel, she wears only light cosmetics and has very little visible pigmentary change. (*A* to *D* courtesy of June K. Robinson, M.D.)

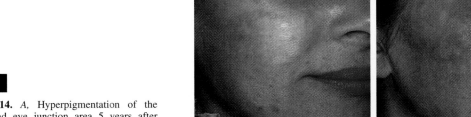

A   B

C   D

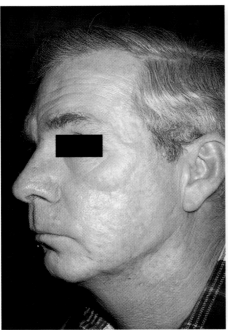

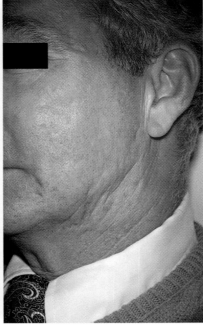

A

B

FIGURE 31–15. *A,* Hypopigmentation of the face and neck resulted from a dermabrasion performed by another surgeon 20 years before the patient was seen in consultation about ways to improve the noticeable area of color demarcation on his neck. *B,* After use of opaque cosmetics, the hypopigmentation of the neck is less apparent. (*A* and *B* courtesy of June K. Robinson, M.D.)

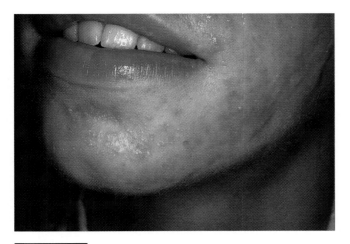

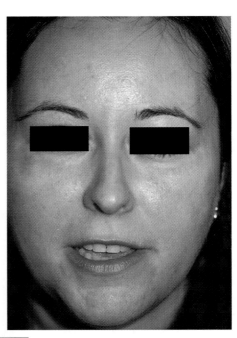

FIGURE 31–16. Milia within the area of dermabrasion is an expected sequela of limited duration. It can be treated with topical tretinoin cream or needle extraction.

FIGURE 31–17. Persistent erythema of the malar area 90 days after dermabrasion. If not treated with topical steroid creams and/or tape, hypertrophic scarring may ensue. Early management of such cases will usually result in complete clearing of the erythema.

When dermabrasion is performed skillfully by an experienced surgeon on a good candidate, improvement in acne scarring is obtained (Case 1, Fig. 31–4). Scar revision by scar excision, or punch elevation and grafting may assist with deep acne scars that cannot be improved by dermabrasion alone.

Among the other therapeutic uses of dermabrasion are treatment of numerous actinic keratosis and diffuse photodamage (Cases 5 and 6, Figs. 31–8 and 31–9). Such patients are at risk of developing squamous cell carcinoma in preexisting actinic keratosis. Dermabrasion treats many actinic keratoses and the entire photodamaged epidermis in a single procedure. Since regeneration of the epidermis occurs from the less actinically damaged adnexal structures, there is less risk of developing subsequent actinic keratosis.[10,12] Clinical improvement is associated with histologic replacement of elastotic material in the upper dermis with newly formed collagen.[10,13] However, actinic keratosis can occur in previously abraded skin.[14]

A new therapeutic use of dermabrasion is the remodeling of traumatic facial scars by dermabrasion within 4 to 8 weeks after the injury (Case 3, Fig. 31–6). Dermabrasion has been performed soon after traumatic injury to remove particulate matter such as gunpowder tattoo. Today, dermabrasion after traumatic injury may also improve contour deformities. New indications are evolving for the use of this older technique.

References

1. Roenigk HH. Dermabrasion: Rejuvenation and scar revision. In: Roenigk RK, Roenigk HH, eds. Surgical Dermatology. London: Martin Dunitz, 1993:509–516.
2. Alt TH, Coleman WP III, Hanke CW, Yarborough JM. Dermabrasion. In: Coleman WP III, Hanke CW, Asken S, Alt TH, eds. Cosmetic Surgery of the Skin. Philadelphia: BC Decker, 1991:147–196.
3. Yarborough JM. Dermabrasive surgery: State of the art. Clin Dermatol 1987;5:75–80.
4. Roenigk HH Jr, Pinski JB, Robinson JK, Hanke CW. Acne, retinoids, and dermabrasion. J Dermatol Surg Oncol 1985;11:396–398.
5. Rubenstein R, Roenigk HH, Stegman SJ, Hanke CW. Atypical keloids after dermabrasion of patients taking isotretinoin. J Am Acad Dermatol 1986;15:280–285.
6. Hamm H, Metze D, Bröcker EB. Hailey-Hailey disease: Eradication by dermabrasion. Arch Dermatol 1994;130:1143–1149.
7. Hanke CW, O'Brian JJ. A histologic evaluation of the effects of skin refrigerants in an animal model. J Dermatol Surg Oncol 1987;31:664–669.
8. Yarborough JM. Dermabrasion by wire brush. J Dermatol Surg Oncol 1987;31:610–615.
9. Pinski JB. Dressing for dermabrasion: Occlusive dressings and wound healing. Cutis 1986;37:471–476.
10. Nelson BR, Majmudar G, Griffiths CEM, et al. Clinical improvement following dermabrasion of photoaged skin correlates with synthesis of collagen. Arch Dermatol 1994;130:1136–1142.
11. Frank W. Therapeutic dermabrasion, back to the future. Arch Dermatol 1994;130:1187–1189.
12. Burks JQ, Marascalo J, Clark WH. Half-face planning of precancerous skin after 5 years. Arch Dermatol 1963;88:572–585.
13. Benedetto AY, Griffen TD, Benedetto EA, Humeniuk H. Dermabrasion: Therapy and prophylaxis of the photoaged face. J Am Acad Dermatol 1992;27:439–447.
14. Ayres S III, Wilson JW, Luikart R II. Dermal changes following dermabrasion. Arch Dermatol 1959;79:553–568.

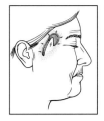

Superficial Chemical Peels with α-Hydroxy Acids

LAWRENCE S. MOY

Chemical peeling (chemexfoliation) entails the use of a chemical agent (Table 32–1) to cause controlled destruction of the outer layers of skin for the treatment of certain skin diseases or conditions (Table 32–2) and for aesthetic improvement. The destruction of portions of the epidermis and/or dermis with these chemical agents results in regeneration of new epidermal and dermal tissues.

With superficial peeling, epidermal wounding is obtained. The therapeutic agents used include resorcinol as a 10% to 50% paste, Jessner's solution or Combes' mixture, 50% salicylic ointment under occlusion for nonfacial areas, 10% to 25% trichloroacetic acid and α-hydroxy acids (e.g., glycolic acid, lactic acid).[1] Tretinoin or 10% to 15% α-hydroxy acid gels may be used at home by the patient before chemical peeling to prepare the skin. Various agents and concentrations may be combined to enhance the depth of the peel. For instance, while 10% to 25% trichloroacetic acid is usually a superficial peel, 35% trichloroacetic acid may be a deeper peel when used as multiple applications or in combination with Jessner's solution. Jessner's solution or Combes' peel is 14% each of salicylic acid, lactic acid, and resorcinol in 95% alcohol.

Glycolic acid is one of a class of compounds called α-hydroxy acids or "fruit acids." Initial work found that glycolic acid can modify the stratum corneum and stratum spinosum.[2] α-Hydroxy acids decrease epidermal cohesiveness by disrupting the keratinocyte bonds.[3,4] Glycolic acid will smooth and remove many keratotic lesions, including actinic keratoses, seborrheic keratoses, and flat warts.[5,6] It has been suggested that glycolic acid may play a role in the stimulation of collagen synthesis by an effect on fibroblasts and alteration of the ground substance in the dermis.[7] α-Hydroxy acids are used in unbuffered and buffered forms. The formulation and extent of the buffering influences the reproducible nature of the results.

TABLE 32–1. Agents Used in Chemical Peeling

Formulations	When Used	How Applied
10% glycolic acid	2 weeks before peel	Daily by patient
Alcohol or acetone 50% glycolic acid	Skin preparation Peel	2 × 2-inch gauze pad
70% glycolic acid	Peel	Large cotton-tipped applicator
Cool tap water	Stopping the peel	Gauze and running water
Antibiotic ointment Mild cortisone ointment	Post-peel care	To crusted areas To erythematous areas

PATIENT INFORMATION

The patient should understand several features of the glycolic acid peel. First, glycolic acid peels are a chemical peel with similar risks and side effects as other peels. These risks are minimized because glycolic acid is a superficial peel and does not penetrate as deeply as other peeling agents. However, it is important to communicate

TABLE 32–2. Timing of Glycolic Acid Peel

Condition	Skin Preparation	Strength of Glycolic Acid	Time (minutes)
Acne	Alcohol	50%	1–2
Melasma	Alcohol	50%	2–4
Actinic keratoses	Acetone	70%	4–8
Fine rhytids	Acetone	70%	4–8
Solar lentigines	Acetone	70%	4–8

that glycolic acid is a variation of a chemical peel. Glycolic acid has a key role in improving the skin for certain conditions and certain patients.

Second, glycolic acid may have some unique capabilities to stimulate the cells in the skin to produce some skin components (i.e., collagen or glycosaminoglycans). Because glycolic acid is a natural product, it has structural similarities to other natural chemicals, such as ascorbic acid.[6]

Glycolic acid may smooth out the surface of the skin and lighten pigmentation of sunspots and other causes of pigmentation.[8] Fine wrinkles can also be improved with the glycolic acid peel. Deeper lines and more severe sun damage should be treated with a deeper peeling agent, such as trichloroacetic acid peel or phenol peel or other methods. The glycolic acid peel does not replace the other peels in improving the face.

Side effects occur with glycolic acid. Hyperpigmentation or dark spots can result if the skin becomes too sensitive during the peel. Combination bleaching agents will lighten these spots. Persistent redness may last for weeks but will resolve over time. Several patients have experienced a flare of acne, but these improve in a few weeks. If cold sores are common, the glycolic acid peels can induce the herpes lesions.

After the peel, the face is lubricated with an emollient to aid healing. There will be flaking of the skin for 3 to 5 days after the peel. Sunscreens should be used for 4 to 6 weeks after peeling.

PROCEDURE

The manner of application and selection of defatting agents affects the evenness of the application and the penetration of the peeling agents. Very thick keratoses may be cauterized or treated with cryosurgery before applying peeling agents.

The skin should be cleansed to remove cosmetic products, skin oils, and keratin debris (Fig. 32–1A). For treatment of acne and epidermal problems, the skin is scrubbed gently with an alcohol-soaked gauze pad. For photodamage problems, a more vigorous scrubbing with acetone-soaked gauze pads is more appropriate.

A large cotton-tipped applicator or cotton ball should be heavily soaked in the glycolic acid (Fig. 32–1B) and wrung out to prevent dripping during application. The 50 to 70% glycolic acid is applied to individual anatomic units separately to ensure complete coverage of the skin. For instance, one whole cheek can be treated, then the forehead, and then the other cheek (Fig. 32–1C). Perioral and perinasal areas can be treated last. It should take 20 to 30 seconds to apply the solution to each cosmetic unit of the face. Specific lesions or problem areas can be rubbed vigorously with more glycolic acid to accentuate the effect in those areas (Fig. 32–1D). The glycolic acid peel is carefully timed (see Fig. 32–1E) from the initial contact to the skin to the time that the material is washed off (see Table 32–2). With prolonged contact, deeper penetration may occur. Usually the glycolic acid is left intact for up to 8 minutes.

Glycolic acid peels can be repeated every 2 to 6 weeks

TABLE 32–3. Clinical and Histologic Characteristics That Affect the Glycolic Acid Peel

Clinical	Histologic
1. For acne and melasma: stop the peel when erythema first appears.	1. Both the 50% and 70% glycolic acid peels easily penetrate through the epidermis if left on for enough time.
2. For photodamage: stop the peel when pinpoint epidermolysis appears	2. The 70% glycolic acid will penetrate to over twice the depth of 50% glycolic acid peels.
3. Glycolic acid may exhibit further penetration even after the peel is stopped.	

depending on the depth of peeling and the condition being treated. Additional peeling with glycolic acid can be very helpful in obtaining gradual improvement. Glycolic acid chemical peels react differently than other chemical peels (Table 32–3). When treating acne and pigmentation, the peel should be stopped when erythema appears. The 70% glycolic acid can penetrate much deeper than 50% glycolic acid and should be used for more pronounced photodamage problems.

The peel is stopped primarily by a dilutional effect of washing with liberal amounts of water. A water-soaked gauze pad should be used to remove the majority of the glycolic acid and then the patient rinses the skin with running tap water (Table 32–4).

After care consists of lubrication with emollients. Desquamation begins within 3 days and resembles a mild sunburn. Healing is completed in 5 days.

Glycolic acid chemical peels are versatile modalities to treat the skin in a safe manner and improve certain conditions that are not easily treated with other chemical peels. Although caution is always warranted, glycolic acid can be used on all Fitzpatrick skin types with minimal risk of side effects. As shown in Table 32–5, glycolic acid chemical peels can be highly effective for a variety of facial skin conditions.[9] Acne, disorders of pigmentation, photodamage, and actinic keratoses are treated with minimal discomfort to the patient.

For acne, glycolic acid has been successful in cases that

TABLE 32–4. Chemical Peeling: Operative Issues

1. Checking of concentration of the formula and its date before application
2. Neutralizing agents readily available (e.g., water for α-hydroxy acids)
3. Eyewash irrigation set-up in the room to use if chemical is accidentally placed in eye
4. Technique that prevents spillage onto patient or staff and monitors procedure with a stopwatch or timer
5. Periorbital area is treated separately using a semi-moist cotton-tipped applicator to ensure that the agent does not get into the eyes. The eyes are kept closed during the procedure. Tears are wiped dry to avoid capillary attraction into the eye. The application ceases 4 to 5 mm from the eyelash line.

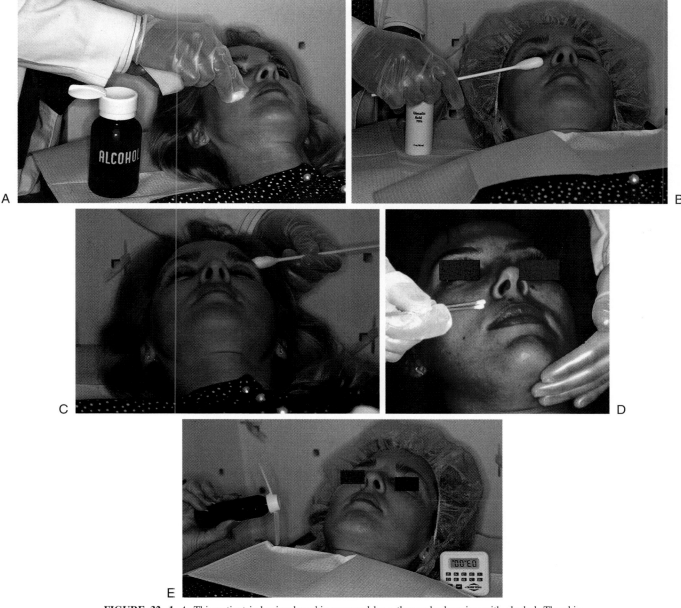

FIGURE 32–1. *A,* This patient is having her skin prepared by a thorough cleansing with alcohol. The skin is firmly rubbed and cleansed to remove surface oils, debris, and excess cells. Skin preparation makes the peel penetrate properly and evenly. *B,* The glycolic acid peel is applied with a large cotton-tipped applicator that is heavily soaked with the peeling solution. A liberal amount of the glycolic acid is layered onto the skin during peel application. The glycolic acid is applied in firm, broad strokes for consistent and expedient peeling. *C,* The peel is applied to the other side of the face. The glycolic acid can be most easily applied in a clockwise manner around the face to ensure that the peel is applied completely around the face. The total time to apply the glycolic acid in an even coat usually takes 15 to 20 seconds per cosmetic unit. *D,* During the peel application, a small cotton-tipped applicator can be used to intensify the peel. More glycolic acid can be applied and repeatedly rubbed into the area to focus the glycolic acid into local keratoses or furrows. *E,* The timer is started at the beginning of applying glycolic acid to the skin. The peel is carefully timed because of the critical time dependency for the glycolic acid peel penetration into the skin. A small battery fan can be held by the patient to self-direct the fan to areas that sting. The fan provides a cooling effect to comfort the patient.

are recalcitrant to common, combination therapies, including oral therapy (Case 1, Fig. 32–2). The glycolic acid chemical peel probably acts by penetrating the pores and causing keratinocyte disadhesion in the comedomal lesions.[10,11] Clinically, patients may have a mild flare of papules and pustules during initial use of glycolic acid. With repeated peels, the initial treatment flare will quickly resolve. Patients are warned about the flare. Combination therapy with topical antibiotics and mild benzoyl peroxide agents appears to be helpful with the glycolic acid.

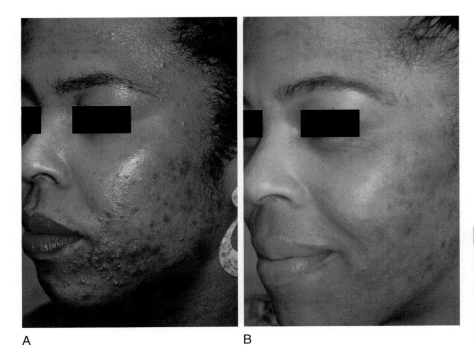

CASE 1

FIGURE 32–2. *A,* This young, black woman had cystic and pustular acne that was leading to prominent acne hyperpigmentation. She had one glycolic acid 50% peel for 2 minutes and a 10% glycolic acid gel. No other medication or treatment was given. *B,* After 5 months, the acne has markedly improved. The pigmentation has significantly lightened and continues to improve.

When treating pigmentation, glycolic acid can be more effective for certain cases that are not improved with other treatments (Cases 2 and 3, Figs. 32–3 and 32–4).[12] As with the peels for acne, glycolic acid peels for pigmentation should be light and should be repeated for optimal results. Caution should be used to minimize the nonspecific damage of a glycolic acid chemical peel to reduce the risk of postinflammatory hyperpigmentation from the treatment.[13]

Photodamage composed of actinic keratoses, rhytids, lentigines, and rough texture can be treated with a deeper peeling effect than when treating acne or pigmentation disorders. Thus, 70% glycolic acid or pyruvic acid is rec-

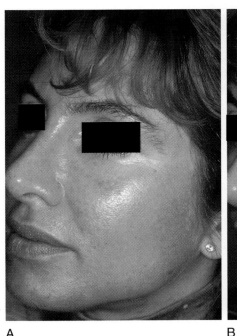

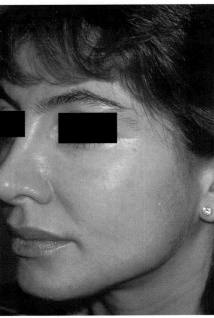

CASE 2

FIGURE 32–3. *A,* This young woman has melasma that is symmetrically across her cheeks, especially her upper cheek. Pigmentation also exists on her upper lip, forehead, and nose. She had two 50% glycolic acid chemical peels. Each peel was left on for 1½ minutes and was performed at 1-month intervals. *B,* At 3 weeks after the second glycolic acid chemical peel, the pigmentation has cleared dramatically. The pigmentation remained gone over 1 year.

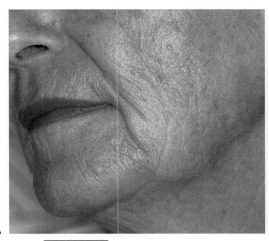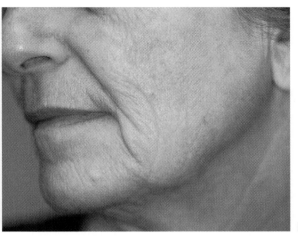

A B

CASE 3

FIGURE 32–4. *A,* This patient is an older woman with sun damage composed of wrinkles, rough texture, and lentigines. She had two 70% glycolic acid chemical peels 1 month apart. The patient also was using 10% glycolic acid for 3 months. *B,* After the glycolic acid treatment, improvements in wrinkles and lentigines are seen. The skin appears smoother and more even. (*A* and *B* from Moy LS, Murad H, Moy RL. Superficial chemical peels. In: Wheeland RG, ed. Cutaneous Surgery. Philadelphia; WB Saunders Co., 1994:464.)

ommended for treatment of significant photodamage.[2] The glycolic acid can also be left on the skin for an extended amount of time, as indicated in Table 32–2. More severe photodamage will tolerate repeated chemical peeling by the glycolic acid.

The most common side effect that occurs with glycolic acid procedures is postinflammatory hyperpigmentation (Table 32–6). To avoid problems, the glycolic acid peel should be monitored by the physician throughout the peel. In addition, the patient should understand that the glycolic acid procedure is a type of chemical peel and has some risks similar to other chemical peels.

Glycolic acid may have a stimulatory effect on connective tissue components, as demonstrated by laboratory and histologic studies on glycolic acid and related compounds.[7] These effects suggest a direct mechanism of action that may specifically enhance the activity of the dermal fibroblasts to produce certain proteins. Additionally, it has been found that glycolic acid histologically will thin the stratum corneum and also thicken the granular layer, which suggests that glycolic acid enhances or upregulates other layers of the epidermis.[8]

The spectrum of use of α-hydroxy acids is evolving. Higher concentrations, prolonged contact, and combination with other agents are expected to change the usual superficial depth of α-hydroxy acids as peeling agents. The risks and benefits of these adaptations remain to be defined. The α-hydroxy acids may ultimately be most useful for pretreatment of the skin before application of lower-strength trichloroacetic acid.

TABLE 32–5. Chemical Peeling: Indications and Contraindications

Indications	Relative Contraindications
Acne	Extreme skin sensitivity
Comedomal	
Inflammatory	Photosensitivity drugs
Cystic	
Pigmentation	Recurrent herpetic outbreaks
Melasma	
Acne hyperpigmentation	Dermatitis
Photodamage, mild	
Fine wrinkles	Recent heavy sun exposure
Actinic keratoses	
Solar lentigines	

TABLE 32–6. Chemical Peeling: Side Effects

Side Effect	Treatment
Hyperpigmentation	Mild cortisones for the first few days, then a combination lotion of glycolic acid and hydroquinone later with protection from exposure to ultraviolet light.
Persistent erythema	Mild cortisone for 2 weeks and strict sun protection
Herpetic flares	Pre-peel acyclovir tablets.
Depressed scars	Mild cortisone; possible repeeling to even the edges later.

References

1. Brody HJ. Chemical Peeling. Chicago: Mosby–Year Book, 1992.
2. Griffin TD, Van Scott EJ. Use of pyruvic acid in the treatment of actinic keratoses: A clinical and histopathologic study. Cutis 1991; 47:325–329.
3. Van Scott EJ, Yu RJ. Hyperkeratinization, corneocyte cohesion and alpha hydroxy acids. J Am Acad Dermatol 1984;11:867–879.
4. Van Scott EJ, Yu RJ. Substances that modify the stratum corneum by modulating its formulation. In: Frost P, Horwitz SN, eds. Principles of Cosmetics for the Dermatologist. St. Louis: CV Mosby, 1982: 70–74.
5. Moy LS, Murad H, Moy RL. Glycolic acid therapy: Evaluation of efficacy and techniques in treatment of photodamage lesions. Am J Cosmet Surg 1993;10:9–13.
6. Van Scott EJ, Yu RJ. Alpha hydroxy acids: Procedures for use in clinical practice. Cutis 1989;43:222–228.
7. Moy LS, Howe K, Moy RL. Stimulation of collagen synthesis by glycolic acid. J Am Acad Dermatol, submitted for publication.
8. Newman N, Newman A, Moy LS, et al. Clinical improvement of photoaged skin with 50% glycolic acid: A double-blind vehicle-controlled study. J Dermatol Surg Oncol, submitted for publication.
9. Moy LS, Murad H, Moy RL. Glycolic acid peels for the treatment of wrinkles and photoaging. J Dermatol Surg Oncol 1993;19:243–246.
10. Van Scott EJ, Yu RJ. Control of keratinization with alpha hydroxy acid and related compounds. Arch Dermatol 1974;110:58–690.
11. Murad H, Shamban A, Moy LS. Acne improves with glycolic acid regimen. Cosmet Dermatol 1993;32–35.
12. Murad H, Shamban A, Moy LS. Polka-dot syndrome: A more descriptive name for a common problem. Cosmet Dermatol 1993;6: 57–58.
13. Haas JE. The effect of ascorbic acid and potassium ferri-cyanide as melanogenesis inhibitors on the development of pigmentation in Mexican axolotols. Am Osteopath, 1974;73:674.

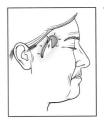

chapter 33

Chemical Peels

SETH L. MATARASSO, HAROLD J. BRODY,
and RICHARD G. GLOGAU

Chemical peels are defined as the application of a caustic agent to the skin resulting in partial-thickness injury and varying amounts of necrosis. Wound healing consists of epidermal regeneration and migration from adnexal appendageal structures and new dermal connective tissue formation. The result is an overall rejuvenation and improvement in surface topography. The major indications for chemical peels are intrinsic and premature photoaging secondary to excess exposure to ultraviolet light, as manifested by dyschromia and rhytides (Cases 1 through 3, Fig. 33–1 through Fig. 33–3).

Peels are broadly categorized based on the histologic depth of injury produced by the peeling agents (Table 33–1; Fig. 33–4). However, there are a host of factors, ranging from individual operator philosophy to patient skin type, that can alter the penetration of the peeling agent such that the depth becomes superficial, medium, or deep (Table 33–2). As such, although fairly well entrenched in the literature, this classification scheme should be seen as somewhat arbitrary and used primarily as a guideline and a means of communicating information about various peeling agents. Superficial chemical peels are discussed in Chapter 32.

PATIENT SELECTION

When evaluating the patient, it is important initially to qualify what the patient's therapeutic goals are. Patient selection is the key to success. Patients are given a mirror and asked to identify precisely their concerns. Although other areas, such as the upper chest, dorsa of the hands, and dorsal forearms, may also be areas of concern, the facial photodamage is usually why the patient seeks care.

As aging begins, at first wrinkles appear only when the face is in motion, usually as expression lines parallel to the melolabial folds, the corners of the mouth (marionette lines), and the lateral canthal areas (crow's feet). As photoaging proceeds, these areas of wrinkles persist when the face is at rest. Gradually the wrinkles may increase in number and cover larger facial areas. In general, the lighter peels are appropriate for early changes and the medium and deeper peels for later changes of photoaging.

Patient goals and what can actually be accomplished with a chemical peel are often incongruous, and it is critical that all involved agree on expectations (Table 33–5). The ideal candidate is a well-informed, fair-skinned (Fitzpatrick type I–III, blond hair, blue eyes) white woman with intact adnexal structures with fine rhytides and superficial pigmentary changes. Conversely, a less than optimal candidate is a darker-complexioned patient (Fitzpatrick type V–VI) with deep furrows with few vellus hairs and decreased sebaceous gland activity and inappropriate expectations. Men's skin can be peeled, but men are at a slight disadvantage because their skin is thicker and therefore more resistant to peel penetration and they cannot use makeup during recuperation or postoperatively to conceal color discrepancies. As a general rule, patients with Fitzpatrick skin types I through III will tolerate peeling without significant risk of color change. Although chemical peeling can be done in those with Fitzpatrick skin types IV through VI, the risk of pigmentary change is much greater than in those with types I to II; and the patient should be so informed. If the patient is an acceptable candidate phenotypically (Table 33–6), by Fitzpatrick skin type (Table 33–7), and by type of photoaging (Glogau classification [Table 33–8]) and behaviorally, other medical and psychological criteria must also be considered (Table 33–9).

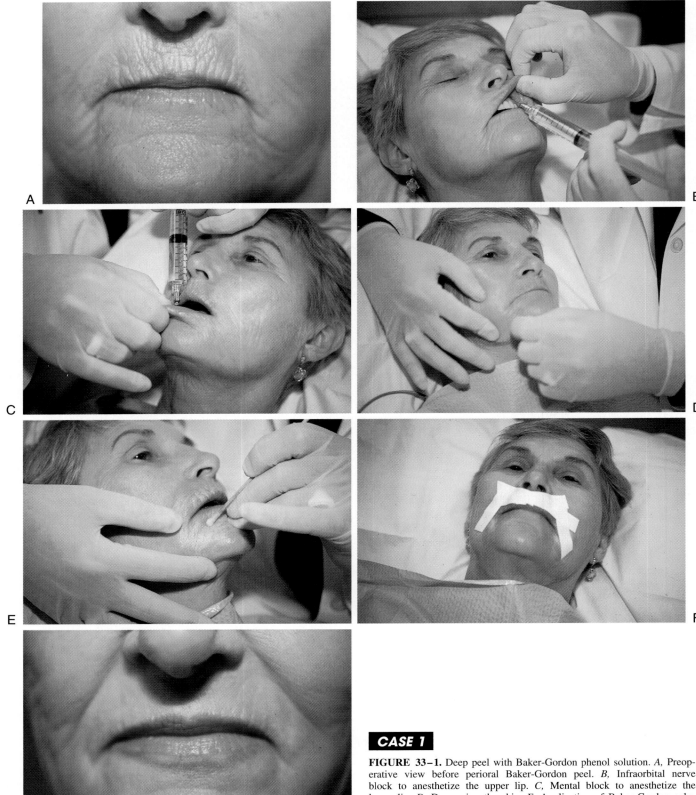

FIGURE 33–1. Deep peel with Baker-Gordon phenol solution. *A,* Preoperative view before perioral Baker-Gordon peel. *B,* Infraorbital nerve block to anesthetize the upper lip. *C,* Mental block to anesthetize the lower lip. *D,* Degreasing the skin. *E,* Application of Baker-Gordon solution with a single cotton-tipped applicator with immediate appearance of frost. *F,* Layered application of occluded tape dressing. *G,* Appearance 1 month after peel.

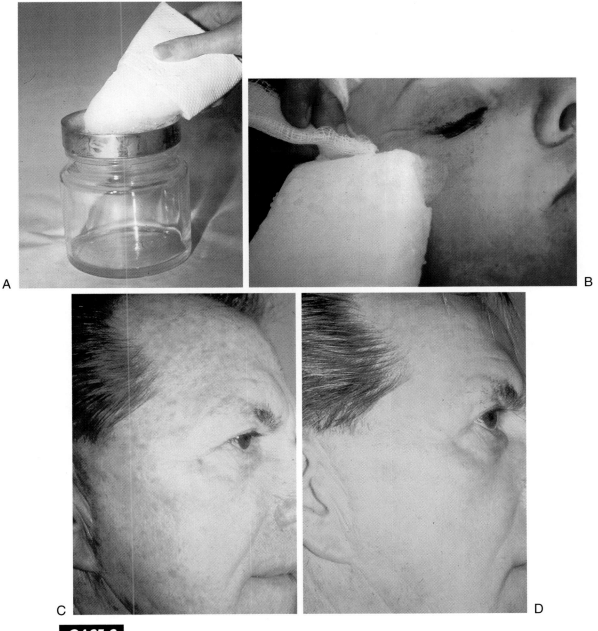

CASE 2

FIGURE 33–2. Medium depth peel with carbon dioxide followed by 35% trichloroacetic acid. *A*, Solid carbon dioxide combined with 3 : 1 acetone and alcohol. *B*, Carbon dioxide slush applied to the skin before application of trichloroacetic acid. *C*, Preoperative appearance before application of carbon dioxide followed by two applications of 35% trichloroacetic acid with a gauze sponge. *D*, Postoperative appearance with improvement of solar elastosis and actinic keratoses.

Once the patient understands the procedure inclusive of the risks, alternatives, and techniques (including recuperative period), an optional peel test spot can be placed and the patient is begun on a preoperative skin preparation routine (Table 33–10). The test spot placed inconspicuously near the hairline, albeit optional, does provide some relevant information. It gives the patient some idea about healing, and it allows the physician to evaluate the duration of erythema and potential for postoperative pigmentation. Observation of the test spot should last 4 to 6 weeks, during which time the patient can initiate the preoperative skin preparatory regimen. Chemical peels are ideally performed when patients have adequate time to heal and during winter or fall months when sun exposure can be kept to a minimum in a climate with seasonal changes in incident ultraviolet light.

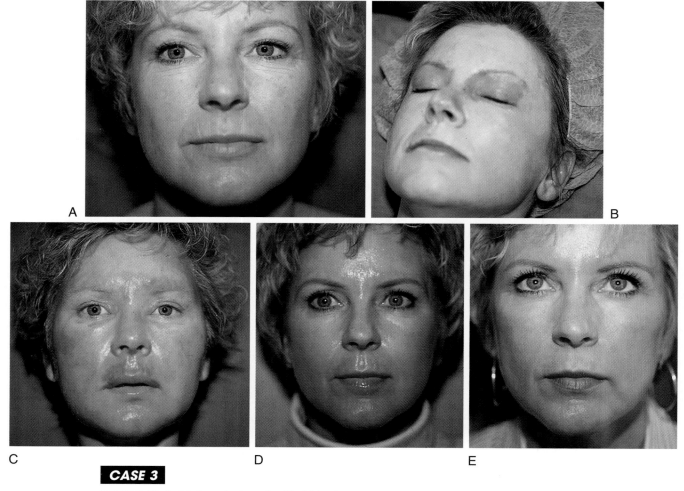

CASE 3

FIGURE 33–3. Medium depth peel with 35% trichloroacetic acid. *A,* Preoperative view before 35% trichloroacetic acid peel. *B,* Homogeneous white frost produced with 35% trichloroacetic acid applied with a gauze sponge. *C,* Postoperative appearance after 72 hours. *D,* Postoperative appearance after 10 days. *E,* Postoperative appearance after 6 weeks.

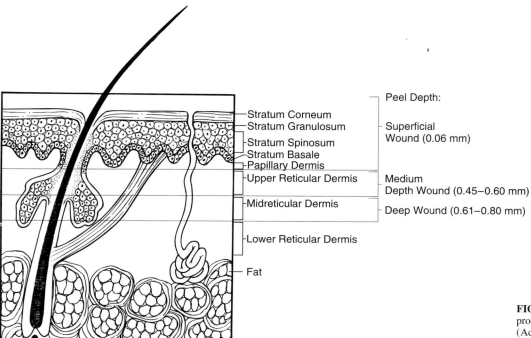

Peel Depth:

Stratum Corneum
Stratum Granulosum

Superficial
Wound (0.06 mm)

Stratum Spinosum
Stratum Basale
Papillary Dermis

Upper Reticular Dermis

Medium
Depth Wound (0.45–0.60 mm)

Midreticular Dermis

Deep Wound (0.61–0.80 mm)

Lower Reticular Dermis

Fat

FIGURE 33–4. Depth of injury produced by chemical peels. (Adapted from Brody HJ. Chemical Peeling. St. Louis: Mosby–Year Book, 1992.)

TABLE 33-1. Indications and Depths of Chemical Peels

Type of Peel	Chemical Formula	Indications
Deep	Baker-Gordon formula (occluded or unoccluded): 3 mL 88% phenol 3 drops croton oil 8 drops Septisol 2 mL distilled water	Rhytidosis (moderate) Actinic damage Superficial neoplasms Pigmentary anomalies (melasma, ephelides, lentigines) Epidermal lesions (seborrheic keratoses) Adjunct to aesthetic procedures (rhytidectomy, blepharoplasty, dermabrasion)
Medium	88% phenol 50% trichloroacetic acid 35% trichloroacetic acid ± initial keratolytic: Jessner's (Combes') solution Carbon dioxide (solid) Glycolic acid Pyruvic acid	Rhytidosis (mild) Photodamage (poikiloderma) Pigmentary changes Epidermal and premalignant lesions
Superficial	α-Hydroxy acids Azelaic acid Carbon dioxide 5-Fluorouracil Jessner's (Combes') solution* Resorcinol Retinoic acid Salicylic acid Trichloroacetic acid (10%–25%) Unna's paste	Rhytidosis (fine) Acute actinic damage Pigmentary changes (postinflammatory) Acne vulgaris or rosacea

* Jessner's solution: resorcinol, 14.0 g; salicylic acid, 14.0 g; lactic acid, 14.0 g; and ethanol (95%), quantity sufficient to add up to 100 mL.

PROCEDURE OF CHEMICAL PEELING

Medium- and deep-depth peels are usually performed as a single therapeutic procedure. If medium-depth peels are to be repeated, an interval of at least 6 months is recommended to allow regeneration and maturation of upper dermal collagen.

The standard medium-depth peeling agent is 35% trichloroacetic acid with or without an initial keratolytic or plain 88% phenol (Table 33–2). A single application of 35% trichloroacetic acid with a gauze square or lightly wrung cotton-tipped applicator produces an even frost within 10 to 15 seconds of application. The frost fades to erythema within 30 minutes. The peeling agent is applied to aesthetic units in a sequential manner (Tables 33–4 and 33–11; Fig. 33–5).

The discomfort produced by 35% trichloroacetic acid is intense for a few minutes but is relieved by cold compresses and a fan. Peeling with 88% phenol produces less intense pain than trichloroacetic acid and it fades more slowly than with trichloroacetic acid.

Medium-depth peels are done without tape occlusion. Surgeons seeking deeper penetration may immediately apply a second coat to produce a denser frost. This is especially true in areas of deeper rhytides (e.g., lateral canthal crow's feet).

With medium-depth peels, edema and crusting appear within 48 to 72 hours and improve in 7 days (Table 33–12). Postoperative care is detailed in Table 33–14. Erythema fades over 2 to 3 weeks. During this time protection from ultraviolet light is necessary to avoid irregular pigmentation.

Patient monitoring because of potential systemic cardiotoxicity and adequate patient hydration are necessary when using 88% phenol and Baker-Gordon formula. Intraoperative technique in using phenol involves the careful use of one or two cotton-tipped applicators rather than a broad brush or gauze square. This limits the cumulative phenol exposure as it is applied in segments over 15-minute intervals, thus lessening chances of systemic toxicity (see

TABLE 33-2. Chemical Peel: Operative Issues

The patient should eat a light meal 3 hours before surgery and be accompanied by a responsible individual to provide transportation.

1. The patient arrives without makeup and wearing a loose shirt that does not need to be pulled over the head
2. Review of goals, medical history, and patient questions
3. Obtain written consent and photos
4. Sedation and analgesia:
   a. Trichloroacetic acid—diazepam (Valium)
   b. Phenol—diazepam (Valium), meperidine (Demerol), nerve blocks
      Cardiac monitoring and IV access (full-face phenol peels)
5. Patient supine with head slightly elevated (45 degrees), mark mandible line
6. Skin degreased; in case of accidental spills, irrigation agents; water for trichloroacetic acid and α-hydroxy acids; vegetable oil for phenol; eye wash station should be immediately available
7. Acid applied sequentially to aesthetic units:
   a. Trichloroacetic acid—cotton-tipped applicator(s), 2×2-inch gauze pads
      Phenol solutions—15-minute break between cosmetic units, one cotton-tipped applicator
   b. Feather—hair-bearing regions (scalp, sideburns, and eyebrows), earlobe, and over mandibular ramus
8. Cool compresses and aeration; adequate ventilation for phenol peels
9. Immediately before discharge: emollient and review of postoperative instructions

TABLE 33-3. Factors Determining Depth of Peel

Agent
Solution (superficial, medium, deep)
Concentration
Number of applications (multiple frosts)
Frequency
Duration

Integrity of Epidermal Barrier

Pretreatment
Retinoic acid
α-Hydroxy acids

Degreasing
Acetone
Alcohol
Ether

Epidermal Abrasion
Mechanical
α-Hydroxy acids
Carbon dioxide
Jessner's solution

Skin Type
Atrophy:

Skin Type *(cont.)*
  Actinic
  Radiation
  Senile
  Steroid
Density and number of pilosebaceous units
Epidermal lesions
Fitzpatrick skin type
Gender
Location: facial vs. nonfacial
Thickness of dermis
Cicatrix

Physician
Pressure
Mode of application:
  Number of cotton applicators
  Gauze
  Swab
  Paint brush
Occlusion:
  Tape (porous vs. nonporous)
  Ointment

Tables 33–4 and 33–11). Phenol is expected to produce some permanent hypopigmentation.

Deeper peels with the Baker-Gordon formula require special attention to technique (see Table 33–4). The solution (see Table 33–1) is not miscible and must be constantly stirred to keep components from separating. General anesthesia or light sedation with intravenous analgesics or sedatives combined with regional nerve blocks of the face are necessary to control the intense pain associated with the procedure. Cardiac monitoring and intravenous hydration are necessary safety measures. One or two cotton-tipped applicators are placed in freshly stirred solution, lightly wrung out against the side of the container, and then evenly applied to the skin. After the entire face is painted, occlusive plastic tape may be applied for 24 hours. This occlusion provides deeper penetration. At 24 hours, the tape usually spontaneously separates during the initial washing with water. Some prefer not to tape the Baker-Gordon peel and believe that depth of penetration may be enhanced by prepeel preparation of the skin with tretinoin or by defatting the skin with acetone. Deep peels are rarely repeated.

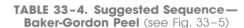

TABLE 33-4. Suggested Sequence— Baker-Gordon Peel (see Fig. 33–5)

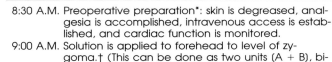

8:30 A.M. Preoperative preparation*: skin is degreased, analgesia is accomplished, intravenous access is established, and cardiac function is monitored.
9:00 A.M. Solution is applied to forehead to level of zygoma.† (This can be done as two units (A + B), bisecting the forehead at the midline.)
9:15 A.M. First cheek (C) is peeled from the lateral aspect of the nose to the tragus of the ear and from the infraorbital rim to the mandibular margin.‡ Peel solution is applied over the mandibular border but not onto the neck.
9:30 A.M. Contralateral cheek (D) is similarly treated.
9:45 A.M. Nose and glabella are treated (E).
10:00 A.M. Perioral (chin + cutaneous upper and lower lips) area and vermilion are treated (F).
10:15 A.M. Lower eyelids (eyes directed superiorly) are peeled, preserving 1.0–3.0 mm at margin (G).§
10:30 A.M. Upper eyelids (eyes closed) are peeled, feathering into eyebrow and maintaining 1.0–3.0 mm margin at the ciliary border (H).
11:00 A.M. Patient is observed and monitored for additional 30 minutes postoperatively. Wound can then be dressed and patient discharged.

---

* Schedule in the morning: increased patient pain threshold and tolerance; increased observation period immediately postoperatively.
† Solution is an emulsion and needs agitation before application.
‡ A fresh applicator should be used each time solution is applied.
§ Wet applicator should be rolled on dry gauze before treating the eyelids.

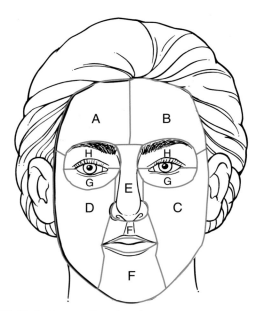

FIGURE 33–5. Face peeling chart becomes a permanent part of the patient's record and indicates order of areas and time treated. Feathering should extend into hair of scalp, sideburns, and eyebrows. Regions peeled are indicated by solid red lines. Sequence of application of the chemical peeling agent begins with location A and moves through to location H.

TABLE 33-5. Patient Handout: Chemical Peel Fact Sheet

Objective

Physicians have been performing chemical peels for many years to rejuvenate and improve skin damaged from excess sun exposure. Peels are routinely performed on sun-damaged skin of the face, neck, chest, and hands. Light or superficial peels correct mild defects, medium-depth peels correct moderate defects, and deep peels correct severe defects. The goal of chemical peels is to improve skin color, soften wrinkles, and impart a fresher appearance to the skin. They are not a substitute but are an adjunct to other rejuvenative surgery. Similarly, they are not the treatment of choice for deep acne scarring or pore size.

Procedure

Patients will start on a home skin preparation regimen that will begin 2 to 3 weeks before the peel and resume upon complete healing. Daily use of nonirritating soaps, sunscreens, exfoliants, and bleaching creams will aid in healing and sustain peel results. On the day of surgery, patients should arrive accompanied by someone to provide transportation, without makeup, and in loose, easy-to-remove clothing. All routine medications should be taken, and a light meal can be eaten up to 3 hours preoperatively. After photographs are taken and pain medication is administered, the skin will be cleansed. An acid will then be applied, and the accompaning discomfort is tolerable with fans and cool compresses. Over the next 7 to 10 days, the skin will become swollen and turn from red to brown and then peel off in pieces. Although tempting, you are not to assist in the removal of "dead skin." Rather, help the skin heal with frequent washing. The skin is freshly injured and very susceptible to the sun and, therefore, should be protected at all times. You will be seen in follow-up during the next week, but do not hestitate to contact the office should concerns arise. Wearing of makeup and return to work and social functions can generally be resumed in 7 to 10 days. A green-based makeup is helpful to hide any residual redness.

Complications

Chemical peels are not risk free, and the potential for complications generally increases with the depth of the peel. Complications include pigmentary changes, scarring, and patient dissatisfaction from prolonged healing and unmet expectations. Scarring and pigment can be unpredictable but have been associated with infection from poor wound care and premature exposure to the sun. After aesthetic surgery it is not uncommon to have high expectations. It is important to remember that healing can take a long time. Disappointment can be avoided if you precisely express your goals and concerns and ask questions—any and all questions are welcome!

RISKS OF MEDIUM AND DEEP CHEMICAL PEELS

The risk of complications (Table 33–13; Cases 4 through 8; Figs. 33–6 through 33–10) increases proportionately with the depth of the wound and ranges from systemic toxicity to emotional lability. Adequate preoperative counseling and patient selection can assist in avoiding complications. By far the most common local complication is aberrant pigmentation. Generally, lighter peels are associated with hyperpigmentation and deeper peels with hypopigmentation. Hyperpigmentation can be temporary (postinflammatory) or permanent and can occur in irregular patterns (see Fig. 33–10). Time, sun protection, and judicious use of preoperative and postoperative (Retin-A) and hydroquinone reduce hyperpigmentation. Some amount

of pigment loss is routinely associated with phenol peels and should be anticipated. Mottled uneven pigment can result from inadequate degreasing, skip areas, or lack of blending into adjacent anatomic areas. Spot "touch-up" peeling can correct this once wound healing and inflammation have resolved. Postoperative erythema is a normal sequela. However, prolonged erythema (greater than 6 weeks) may be a sign of contact dermatitis, delayed wound healing, or pending scar formation and should be addressed. It is therefore important to be able to distinguish standard wound healing from frank or pending complications (see Tables 33–12 and 33–13).

Scarring is one of the most dreaded complications of chemical peels, and unfortunately its precise etiology remains elusive (see Figs. 33–8 and 33–9). Manifested as localized subcutaneous indurated nodules with erythema,

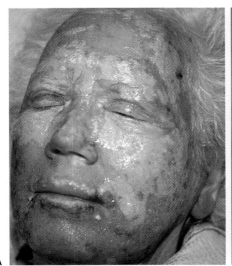
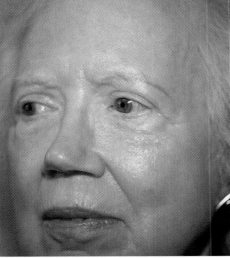

CASE 4

FIGURE 33–6. Complication. *A, Pseudomonas aeruginosa* infection manifested by a green color and fruity odor. *B,* Complete resolution with aggressive acetic acid soaks and systemic ciprofloxacin.

A

B

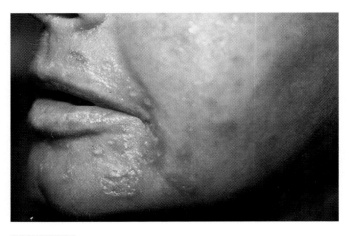

CASE 5

FIGURE 33–7. Complication. Heralded by unusual and unexpected post-peel pain, a herpetic flare is evident. After treatment with oral acyclovir healing generally occurs without scar formation.

TABLE 33-6. Factors in Patient Evaluation

Age and actinic damage
Blue eyes and blond hair
Color (skin) and use of cosmetics
Density of pilosebaceous glands
Epidermal topography
Fitzpatrick skin type
Glogau photoaging classification (I–IV)

TABLE 33-7. Fitzpatrick Skin Type

Skin Type	Description
I	Always burns easily, never tans
II	Always burns easily, tans minimally
III	Burns moderately, tans gradually and uniformly (light brown)
IV	Burns minimally, always tans well (moderate brown)
V	Rarely burns, tans profusely (dark brown)
VI	Never burns, deeply pigmented (black)

Note: The ability of the skin to burn is measured in the first 60 minutes of sun exposure after winter or no sun exposure.

TABLE 33-8. Glogau Photoaging Classification

Group	Keratoses	Wrinkling	Scarring	Makeup
I (Mild, age 28–35 years)	None	Little	None	Little to none
II (Moderate, age 35–50 years)	Early Slight yellow skin discoloration	Early Parallel smile lines	Mild	Little
III (Advanced, age 50–60 years)	Keratoses Yellow discoloration Telangiectasia	Present at rest	Moderate	Always
IV (Severe, age 60–75 years)	Keratoses Skin cancers	Much cutis laxa: actinic, gravitational, and dynamic	Severe	Cakes on

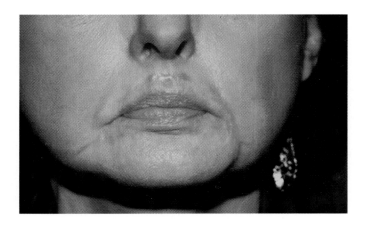

CASE 6

FIGURE 33–8. Complication. Hypertrophic perioral scarring following application of a high-concentration of trichloroacetic acid.

scars usually appear within the first 3 postoperative months. Treatment includes early recognition and must be prompt. Compression and massage encourage spontaneous resolution and may improve small scars. Larger scars, however, require the addition of fluorinated corticosteroids. Depending on both size and location, intralesional triamcinolone in concentrations of 5 mg/mL to 40 mg/mL is used. Full-thickness skin necrosis and contractural scarring can also occur. Usually full-thickness skin necrosis is due to vascular compromise from recent undermining of facial skin performed during blepharoplasty or rhytidectomy. It is wise to allow a 30- to 90-day interval between facial surgery and chemical peels.

Patients often become frightened and intimidated by their postoperative appearance and respond with inadequate wound care. This can lead to bacterial colonization and infection, which can eventuate in scarring (see Fig. 33–6). It is therefore crucial for patients to have adequate follow-

TABLE 33-9. Relative Medical and Psychological Contraindications for Peels

Medical

Phenol Peels

Cardiac disease
Renal disease
Hepatic disease
Recent extensive facial surgery with undermining

All Peels

Herpes simplex infection or warts in area to be peeled
Hormonal therapy
    Estrogen
    Progesterone
Continuous or prolonged ultraviolet light exposure
Decreased sebaceous gland density:
    Recent use of isotretinoin
    Previous ionizing radiation therapy
Skin type IV to VI
Predisposition to keloid formation
Anatomic locations with few adnexa
Ectropion before periorbital peeling

Psychological: Potential Problem Patients*

The patient with unrealistic expectations
The obsessive-compulsive patient
The sudden whim patient
The indecisive patient
The rude patient
The overflattering patient
The overly familiar patient
The unkempt patient
The patient with minimal or imagined deformity
The careless or poor historian
The VIP patient
The uncooperative patient
The overly talkative patient
The surgeon shopper
The depressed patient
The ''plastic surgicoholic''
The price haggler
The patient involved in litigation
The patient you or your staff dislike

---

* From Tardy ME. Klimsensmith in face-lift surgery: Principles and variations. In: Roenigk RK, Roenigk HH, eds. Dermatologic Surgery. New York: Marcel Dekker, 1988.

TABLE 33-10. Chemical Peels: Preoperative Care

Preparatory Regimen

_A.M._

Bland cleanser: unscented Dove, Purpose, or soap substitute (Cetaphil)
10%–14% glycolic acid lotion (can be compounded with hydroquinone)
Sunscreen SPF ≥ 15
Acyclovir, 200 mg orally four times per day
    (2–3 days pre- and postoperative)*

_P.M._

Bland cleanser
0.025%–0.1% tretinoin (Retin-A) (based on patient tolerance)
4% hydroquinone cream

Preoperative Skin Preparation

1. Checks the level of patient motivation and eliminates noncompliant patients
2. Stimulates epidermal turnover and aids uniform peel application and speeds reepithelialization
3. Eliminates potential confusion between normal postoperative erythema and an irritant dermatitis
4. May reduce the total number of complications
5. Sustains the results of the peel

---

* With positive history of herpes simplex.

up and understand the role of aggressive postoperative hygiene (Table 33–14). Reactivation of herpes simplex virus can occur with any peel (see Fig. 33–7). Acyclovir (Zovirax), 200 to 400 mg three times per day, controls the infection and allows delayed healing without scar formation. Because many patients are unaware of their history of herpes (cold sores, fever blisters), it may be useful to use acyclovir prophylactically in all chemical peel patients.

CASE 7

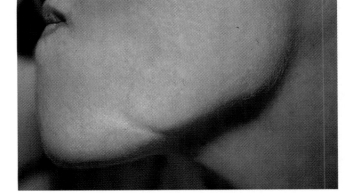

FIGURE 33-9. Complication. Atrophic scarring following 35% trichloroacetic acid application.

TABLE 33–11. Operative Report and Sequence—Baker-Gordon Peel

Name_____ Age_____ Date_____

□ Consent_____ □ Photographs

Medical Clearance □ CBC □ SMAC □ EKG Comments_____

Skin degreasing: □ Alcohol □ Acetone

Anesthesia:

Time	Type	Amount	Vital Signs

Dressing: □ Ointment (brand)_____

□ Occlusion (type)_____

□ Full face

□ Regional (area)

Postoperative Medication: Analgesia_____

Antibiotics_____

Comments: Feathering (location and solution)_____

Condition upon discharge_____

Follow-up appointment_____

_____   _____
Physician   Assistant

TABLE 33–12. Chemical Peel: Normal Sequelae

1. On peel application, appearance of white frost (the deeper the peel, the faster and more intense the frost)
2. First 24 hours: dusky erythema and edema
3. 48 hours: skin is brown
4. Third day: skin is mask-like—beginning to desquamate
5. Days 4 to 7: trichloroacetic acid—skin exfoliation phenol—maceration
6. Days 7 to 12: resolving erythema

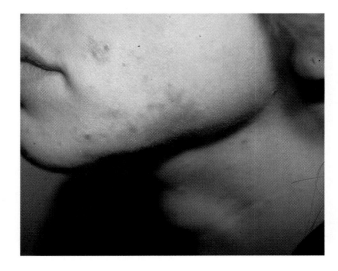

CASE 8

FIGURE 33–10. Complication. Postinflammatory hyperpigmentation 1 month after trichloroacetic acid peel.

TABLE 33-13. Chemical Peel: Complications

Systemic (Phenol)	Cutaneous		Infectious		Miscellaneous
	Pigmentary	*Scarring**	*Bacterial*	*Viral*	**Miscellaneous**
Cardiac	Depigmentation	Keloid	*Staphylococcus*	Herpes simplex	Milia
Renal	Hypopigmentation	Hypertrophic	*Streptococcus*	Verruca	Pruritus
Hematologic	Uneven pigmenta-	Atrophic	*Pseudomonas*	Epstein-Barr keratitis	Increase in pore size
	tion (streaking,	Full thickness skin	Toxic shock syn-		Increase in amount of
	mottled, blotchy)	necrosis	drome		telangiectasia
	Lines of demarca-	Structural:			Laryngeal edema
	tion	Ectropion			Temperature sensitivity
	Accentuation of	Eclabium			Neuropsychiatric:
	nevi				Depression
	Erythema				Destabilization of
	Persistent flushing				compensated
					psyche

* Risk factors for scarring:
Hereditary predisposition
Quality and quantity of adnexa (radiation therapy, time interval between systemic isotretinoin use, previous dermabrasion, or deep peel)
Wounding agent (excess volume, concentration, occlusion)
Location and actinic dermal quality of the skin
Quality of postoperative peel care (infection, excoriation)
Interference with lymphatic or vascular supply (edema, recent subcutaneous undermining)
?Post-peel facial movement or local skin tension

CONCLUSION

Results from chemical peels run the gamut from gratifying to disastrous. The risk of complications can be reduced, however, if a few basic tenets are observed: strict adherence to patient selection, careful evaluation of skin type, selection of appropriate agent for each indication, and careful assessment of patient expectations. The technique, applying a uniform coat of acid, is deceptively simple, and many of the nuances to the art of chemical peeling are not adequately appreciated. It is therefore prudent to begin conservatively with mild agents, drier applicators, and mild manual pressure. More aggressive peels can be undertaken with increased experience.

TABLE 33-14. Chemical Peel: Postoperative Wound Care

1. Analgesia: aspirin, acetaminophen (with or without co-deine), and/or sedatives*
2. Decrease edema:
   a. Head elevation
   b. Decrease facial movement
3. Frequent cleaning (three to five times per day): tap water, ⅙ strength boric acid, ¼% acetic acid, povidone-iodine (Betadine)
4. Emollients: Crisco, Preparation H, antibiotic (Bactroban), or 1% hydrocortisone ointments
5. Sun avoidance: Topical sunscreen and physical protection
6. No premature eschar removal
7. Resume topical preparatory regimen on complete reepithelialization
8. "Talkasthesia"

* If undue pain or pruritus persists, may signal fever blister—needs immediate attention.

References

1. Asken S. Unoccluded Baker/Gordon phenol peels: Review and update. J Dermatol Surg Oncol 1989;15:998-1008.
2. Baker TJ. Chemical face peeling in rhytidectomy. Plast Reconstr Surg 1962;29:199-207.
3. Brody HJ. Variations and comparisons in medium-depth chemical peeling. J Dermatol Surg Oncol 1989;15:953-963.
4. Brody HJ. Chemical Peeling. St. Louis: Mosby-Year Book, 1992.
5. Coleman WP, Futrell JM. The glycolic acid trichloroacetic acid peel. J Dermatol Surg Oncol 1994;20:76-80.
6. Hevia O, Nemeth AJ, Taylor JR. Tretinoin accelerates healing after trichloroacetic acid chemical peel. Arch Dermatol 1991;127:678-682.
7. Matarasso SL, Salman SM, Glogau RG, Rogers GS. The role of chemical peeling in the treatment of photodamaged skin. J Dermatol Surg Oncol 1990;16:945-954.
8. Matarasso SL, Glogau RG. Chemical face peels. Clin Dermatol 1991;9:131-150.
9. Monheit G. Jessner's plus TCA peel: A medium-depth chemical peel. J Dermatol Surg Oncol 1989;15:945-950.
10. Rubin MG. Trichloroacetic acid and other nonphenol peels. Clin Plast Surg 1992;19:525-536.
11. Stegman SJ. A comparative histologic study of the effects of three peeling agents and dermabrasion on normal and sundamaged skin. Aesthetic Plast Surg 1982;6:121-135.
12. Tardy ME. Klimsensmith in face-lift surgery: Principles and variations. In: Roenigk RK, Roenigk HH, eds. Dermatologic Surgery. New York: Marcel Dekker, 1988.

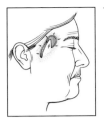

chapter 34

Soft Tissue Augmentation Techniques

RICHARD G. GLOGAU and SETH L. MATARASSO

Three methods of correction of soft tissue loss from aging or disease are widely available: injectable collagen implants, gelatin matrix implants, and autologous fat implantation. Innovative techniques and implants are continuously being developed.

Expanded polytetrafluorethylene (Gore-Tex) is an experimental implant that is introduced as strips by a trocar into the nasolabial fold, lips, and glabellar folds.[1] It is approved for use in deficiencies of the bone or cartilage such as augmentation of the nasal dorsum or chin region. The implant is placed in the subcutaneous layer and not in the dermis. Dermal placement may result in surface irregularities. Hylan gel, a viscoelastic derivative of hyaluronan polymer, is used experimentally for dermal augmentation. It is approved for use as a viscoelastic tool in ophthalmology for cataract surgery and retinal detachment surgery.[2]

Safety and efficacy with emerging procedures and materials remain to be defined. In this chapter, details of correction of soft tissue deficiencies are provided for those techniques whose safety and efficacy are well described.

INJECTABLE COLLAGEN IMPLANTS (ZYDERM, ZYPLAST)

Zyderm I and Zyderm II Collagen Implants (Collagen Corporation, Palo Alto, CA) are injectable suspensions of type I and type III bovine collagen.[3] Zyderm I has a concentration of 35 mg/mL and Zyderm II is 65 mg/mL of solubilized bovine collagen. Zyplast Collagen Implant is solubilized collagen that has been treated with glutaraldehyde during processing to increase the cross-linking between collagen strands, thereby delaying the rate of biologic degradation of the implant by the host.

These materials are in common use in dermatology and cosmetic surgery to treat premature aging of the skin and some types of dermal scarring secondary to cystic acne (Table 34–1; Cases 1 through 3, Figs. 34–1 through 34–3).[4–6] The material is injected with a small-gauge needle and provides temporary, repeatable dermal augmentation.

TABLE 34–1. Injectable Collagen Implants (Zyderm, Zyplast): Indications, Contraindications, and Limitations

Indications
Soft, shallow, distensible acne scars (Fig. 34–1)
Deep nasolabial or melolabial fold lines (Fig. 34–2)
Perioral parallel ``smile'' lines, perioral ``marionette'' lines (Fig. 34–3)
Solitary rhytids or creases
Augmentation of the lips*

Contraindications
``Ice pick'' acne scars
Most varicella scars
Nondistensible or rigid scars of any kind
Rhytids that do not improve with lateral stretch or distention of the skin
Active herpes simplex infections
Prior history of allergy to Zyderm/Zyplast
Unrealistic expectations

Limitations
Variable response of vertical glabellar creases
Variable response horizontal creases on forehead
Length of time for correction varies from weeks to months.
Implant may produce beading if placed too superficially in dermis
Expensive

*Not approved by the Food and Drug Administration.

363

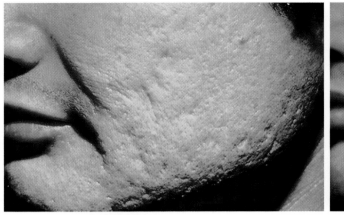
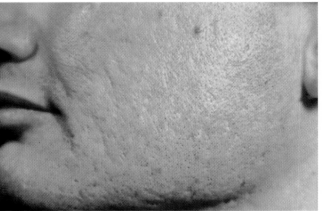

CASE 1

FIGURE 34–1. Dramatic amelioration of moderately severe acne scarring with Zyderm II. *A*, Appearance before treatment. *B*, Six-month follow-up photograph.

Zyderm I and Zyderm II are placed with a serial puncture technique, introducing the 30-gauge needle at a 10- to 20-degree angle to the plane of the skin, making multiple punctures along the desired line or scar. With each puncture a small amount of collagen is injected, producing an almost immediate visible blanch and elevation in the skin. The material is placed high in the dermis, well into the papillary dermis (Fig. 34–4). Because a significant portion of Zyderm I and Zyderm II is water, overcorrection is commonly utilized to maximize residual aesthetic correction (Table 34–2).

Zyderm FL, or "fine line" collagen, is injected in very small lines, such as the lateral crow's feet or the fine rhytids of the upper lip. It is placed high in the dermis, using a 32-gauge needle provided with the product.

Zyplast is injected with the needle at more of a 45- to 90-degree angle into the scar or line and is placed deeper in the dermis (Fig. 34–5). Multiple punctures are used to place multiple discrete amounts along the line of injection. Zyplast, if placed properly, does not cause immediate blanching but usually a more subtle and somewhat delayed blanching. Overcorrection is avoided with Zyplast since the

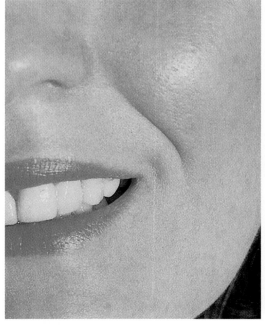
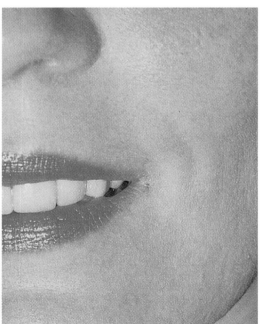

CASE 2

FIGURE 34–2. *A* and *B*, Softening the nasolabial fold with Zyplast.

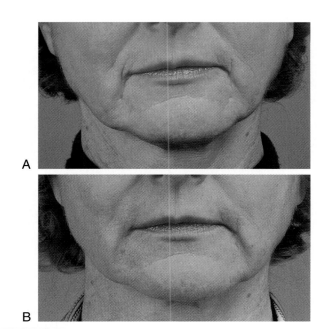

CASE 3

FIGURE 34–3. "Marionette lines" at the lower corners of the mouth before *(A)* and after *(B)* treatment on only one side (the right).

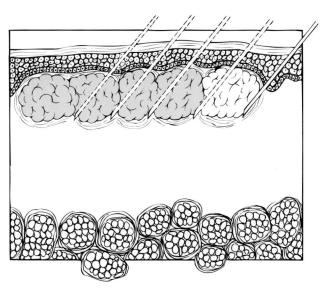

FIGURE 34–4. Serial puncture technique is used to place small amounts of Zyderm I or II into the papillary dermis. Red areas of implant associated with dotted outlines of the needle indicate serial puncture technique.

material will typically show less loss of correction than Zyderm. Zyplast may be molded with finger pressure immediately after serial injections to fit the shape of the defect.

The different types of collagen implant may be used together to achieve a "layered" effect that is particularly useful when the cosmetic defect is the result of deep grooving from underlying muscle action and fine lines secondary to photoaging. Zyplast is placed first, in the deeper dermis, and Zyderm is layered above it, in the superficial dermis (Fig. 34–6).

Although patient satisfaction is a complex mix of patient expectations, physician attitude and technique, and the product profile, about 10% of patients treated express some reservations about the degree of cosmetic success of treatment (Table 34–3). Some of this limitation is due to the inability of the dermal implant to completely repair the creases and lines due to photoaging, which require resurfacing techniques such as chemical peeling and/or dermabrasion. Some may be related to the high cost of the material that affects the perceived value. But as an average, at least half of the patients treated usually go on to have at least one further treatment, and one fourth will repeat the treatments at regular intervals. Obviously this is subject to marketing and economic forces beyond the scope of this discussion.

True classic delayed hypersensitivity to the implants develops in about 1% of those patients whose skin tests are negative and who receive treatment. The reaction is manifested by redness, firmness, and swelling at the treatment sites, and usually the skin test site, which develop from 2 days to several weeks after the treatment. Such reactions resolve spontaneously and are best treated with time, reassurance, and makeup. Nonsteroidal anti-inflammatory drugs

and, rarely, intralesional injections of triamcinolone acetonide (Kenalog, 2 mg/mL) may provide the temporary amelioration needed to attend significant social occasions while waiting for the reaction to subside. If the reaction is left untreated, there is almost invariably complete resolution with no permanent untoward effect but the erythema may wax and wane for months (Table 34–4).

Sudden development of pain accompanied by skin blanching during injection heralds the potential onset of vascular occlusion or compression, which may lead to localized cyanosis, ecchymosis, eschar, and dermal slough with scarring. Immediate cessation of injection followed by massage, nitroglycerin paste, ice compresses, and supportive wound care with bio-occlusive dressings (Vigilon, Duoderm) and silicone gel sheeting (Epiderm, Biodermis, Las Vegas, NV) may minimize the damage. This phenom-

TABLE 34–2. Injectable Collagen Implants (Zyderm, Zyplast): Operative Issues

Preoperative Evaluation

History
 No prior reactivity
 Allergies (esp. beef)
 Negative skin test(s)
 Informed consent

Preoperative Equipment Needs

Camera for optional preoperative photos
EMLA cream to diminish the discomfort of injection

Intraoperative Needs

Alcohol swabs
Adequate lighting
Chair or table with the patient sitting up
1–2× optical loupes
Dry cotton
Ice compresses

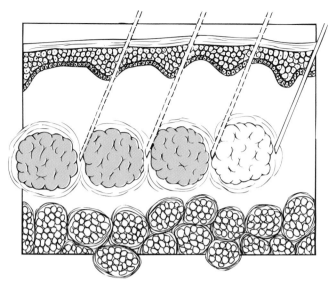

FIGURE 34–5. Serial puncture technique is used to place small amounts of Zyplast *(red)* into the deep reticular dermis. Massage is used to help even the distribution of the material.

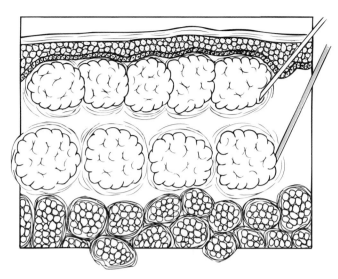

FIGURE 34–6. Both Zyderm and Zyplast may be used together in the same cosmetic defect, layering one above the other as shown. The Zyplast *(red)* is always placed deeply first, then followed with the more superficial Zyderm.

TABLE 34-3. Injectable Collagen Implants (Zyderm, Zyplast): Patient Preoperative Discussion

1. Correction is temporary, usually measured in weeks to months, depending on the amount of movement in and around the treated area. Typically, re-treatment is necessary to maintain correction within 1 to 3 months. Occasionally, correction in some areas will last longer, but on average, one needs re-treatment three to four times per year to maintain correction.
2. Because of a recognized incidence of allergy, prior skin testing with at least one test dose is mandatory, together with a 4-week observation period before beginning therapy. A second skin test with a 1-week observation period is commonly offered to prospective patients but is not required by Food and Drug Administration–sanctioned treatment protocol.[7] Be sure to report to the physician any sign of redness, swelling, discoloration, itching, or increase in firmness at the test site.
3. The physician may massage the treated area after injection. There is some degree of minor trauma to the skin coincident with injection as might be expected with multiple hypodermic needle punctures even though a 30- or 32-gauge needle is used. Minor bruising and some minimal swelling can be expected. Ice compresses may be used to minimize chances of bruising and edema. Always plan on receiving injections about 2 days ahead of any important social appearances if possible. Usually makeup can be reapplied within an hour of injection.
4. Native delayed hypersensitivity to the implants in the nonexposed population appears to range between 1% and 3%.[8,9] In 1% to 2% of patients with negative skin tests who are treated, delayed hypersensitivity reactions to the material will develop at some point during repeated exposure to the material.[10] Therefore, no guarantee can be made that a patient will not develop an allergy to the material, in spite of negative skin tests and successful previous treatments.
5. If at all possible, avoid aspirin products, nonsteroidal anti-inflammatory drugs, and anything else that promotes anticoagulation for a week to 10 days before treatment.
6. Although there has been much speculation on the possible link between the use of collagen implants and autoimmune disease, there is no credible medical evidence establishing a causal relationship between the two.[8,11]

enon has been reported with both Zyderm and Zyplast and appears to be more common in the glabellar area, but it has been seen elsewhere on the face, especially at the angle of the mouth or in the lip. It is technically easier to produce with Zyplast since this material is less viscous and injects with much less pressure, making inadvertent overinjection or rapid injection more likely.

Rare cystic reactions have been reported with the implants (see Table 34–4).[12] The incidence appears to be in the magnitude of 1 in 10,000 treatments. These reactions are characterized by the sudden onset of pain, usually days to weeks after injection, followed shortly by tense edema and erythema, with characteristic fluctuant deep nodules. The pain is the cardinal sign, often requiring narcotic analgesia. The lesions should be treated as foreign body abscesses with attempted drainage using a 16- to 18-gauge needle or a No. 11 blade. Intralesional steroids are helpful. Permanent scarring may result.

GELATIN MATRIX IMPLANT (FIBREL)

Fibrel is a purified and denatured gelatin powder mixed with ϵ-aminocaproic acid that is combined with the patient's plasma to produce an injectable gelatin matrix.[13,14]

TABLE 34-4. Injectable Collagen Implants: Postoperative Care

Pain Management
Acetaminophen
Dressings
None
Complications
Patient dissatisfaction, 10%
Classic delayed hypersensitivity, 1%
Cystic reactions, 0.05%
Vascular occlusion and slough, 0.05%

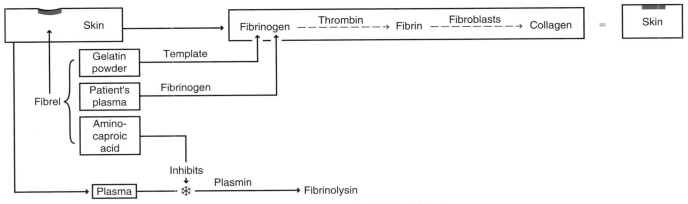

FIGURE 34–7. The pathway and proposed site of activity of the Fibrel implant.

When the matrix is placed in the dermis, it appears to stimulate new fibroblast collagen formation, which eventually replaces the implant at the injection site. Theoretically the Fibrel has a clot-stabilizing effect by interfering with the activity of plasmin and tissue plasminogen activator, enhancing collagen synthesis (Fig. 34–7).

Fibrel has the theoretical advantage of avoiding allergic complications since it is essentially an autograft, using the patient's own plasma as the only protein constituent. The Food and Drug Administration has given the current man-ufacturer (Mentor, Santa Barbara, CA) approval for marketing the implant as a "two year correction" (1987).

Since the technique requires phlebotomy and centrifugation to obtain plasma, and the company markets the material in vials that yield essentially 1 mL of injectable material, the process is cumbersome. Obtaining more than 1 mL of injectable material requires use of more than one kit, mixing each milliliter from an individual kit (Tables 34–5 through 34–7).

The manufacturer recommends a technique, utilizing a 25-gauge needle, in which a pocket is created in the dermis to receive the implant. The needle tip is used to break up fibrous bands in the dermis and to create a potential space for the implant. This technique can produce significant ecchymosis (Table 34–8).

TABLE 34–5. Gelatin Matrix Implants (Fibrel): Indications, Contraindications, and Limitations

Indications
Soft, shallow, distensible scars

Contraindications
"Ice pick" acne scars
Most varicella scars
Nondistensible or rigid scars of any kind
Active herpes simplex infections
Unrealistic expectations

Limitations
Significant postinjection edema and erythema that can last for weeks
Requires phlebotomy
Expensive
Cumbersome to produce more than 1 mL at a time for injection

TABLE 34–6. Gelatin Matrix Implants (Fibrel): Patient Preoperative Discussion

1. Skin testing with the gelatin powder is performed before undertaking treatment. The skin test is observed for 4 weeks. Reactivity to any of the components is unlikely.
2. Significant swelling, edema, and temporary bruising can occur after Fibrel implantation. You should not plan on achieving a "normal" appearance for about 2 weeks.
3. Makeup may be applied within 1 hour of treatment, and ice compresses may be used to minimize swelling and discomfort. Acetaminophen and nonsteroidal anti-inflammatory drugs may be used but aspirin should be avoided.

TABLE 34–7. Gelatin Matrix Implants (Fibrel): Operative Issues

Preoperative Evaluation
History
  No previous reactions to Fibrel
  No bleeding diathesis

Preoperative Equipment Needs
Skin test kit containing one vial of gelatin powder and
  ε-aminocaproic acid and one vial of normal saline for
  mixing

Intraoperative Needs
Fibrel gelatin matrix implants kit
Alcohol swabs
Dry cotton
Ice compresses

TABLE 34–8. Gelatin Matrix Implants (Fibrel): Postoperative Care

Pain Management
Acetaminophen
Ice compresses

Dressings
None

Complications
Patient dissatisfaction, 10%
Persistent edema and erythema for 2 weeks or more, 35%
Significant ecchymosis and eschar, 1%

TABLE 34-9. Autologous Fat Implantation (Microlipoinjection): Indications, Contraindications, and Limitations

Indications

Broad areas of skin depression

Areas of distinct lipoatrophy secondary to trauma, disease, or steroid atrophy

Cosmetic units subject to loss of subcutaneous volume associated with aging (e.g., nasolabial folds, perioral skin, lips, malar cheeks, temples, and dorsal hands) (Figs. 34–8 and 34–9)

Contraindications

Small or superficial scars

History of panniculitis

Active herpes simplex infections

Unrealistic expectations

Limitations

Significant postinjection edema and erythema that can last for several days

Requires anesthesia and trauma to donor site

Expensive

Cumbersome and time consuming

Inability to predict percentage of graft survival and longevity of correction

TABLE 34-10. Autologous Fat Implantation: Patient Preoperative Discussion

1. The donor sites commonly used are the upper hip and buttock, abdomen, and median knees. The donor site will be anesthetized with an injection of local anesthetic solution that is diluted. A small puncture incision is made in the skin, and the fat is harvested with a syringe and needle, moving the needle rapidly up and down into the fat. The small incision is closed with either a single suture or small tape strips.

2. The treatment sites will be anesthetized with a small injection of anesthetic. You will feel some discomfort, lasting only a few seconds, as the fat is injected underneath the skin. After injection there will be some swelling and minimal if any bruising. Several days will be required for your appearance to be normal.

3. The principal problem with fat grafting is the inability to predict what percentage of the graft will be maintained. Many investigators now believe that serial injections over time provide the most satisfactory and long-lasting results.[19-21]

4. Antibiotics are given to minimize chances of infection. Avoid aspirin to minimize chances of bruising and bleeding.

AUTOLOGOUS FAT IMPLANTATION (MICROLIPOINJECTION)

Autologous fat injection as an outgrowth of work in liposuction[15] has revived interest in the use of fat for soft tissue augmentation.[16,17] Theoretical advantages include the avoidance of allergy since it is an autograft, relative abundance of graft supply, relative ease in addressing volume correction when Zyderm or Fibrel would be prohibitively expensive, and possibility of permanent correction.[18-21]

Theoretical disadvantages include the inability to place material into the dermis to address fine lines and wrinkles or small scars; the cumbersome aspects of harvesting the fat, including potential exposure of health care personnel to blood and tissue products; and the inability to predict the percentage of graft survival (Tables 34–9 and 34–10; Cases 4 and 5, Figs. 34–8 and 34–9).

The technique we currently use is modified from that of Fournier[22] and Asken[23] and involves injection of dilute 0.05% lidocaine with epinephrine 1 : 1,000,000 into the proposed donor site. A 13-gauge needle with a 45-degree

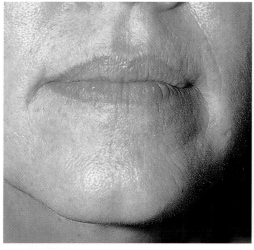
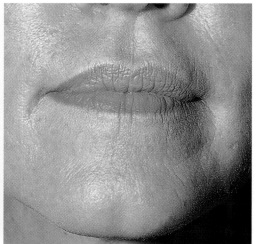

CASE 4

FIGURE 34–8. Before *(A)* and after *(B)* treatment with microlipoinjection of the upper lip. (From Glogau RG. Microlipoinjection. Arch Dermatol 1988;124:1341–1343. Copyright 1988, American Medical Association.)

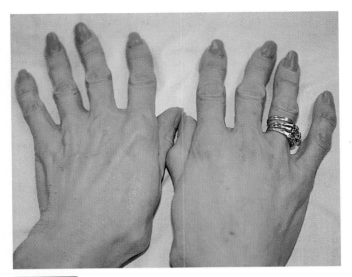

CASE 5

FIGURE 34–9. Severely arthritic hands with marked subcutaneous atrophy secondary to aging. Just the right hand was treated with 7 mL of injected fat.

TABLE 34–11. Autologous Fat Implantation: Operative Issues

Preoperative Evaluation

Broad areas of contour deformity as opposed to discrete dermal depressions are most logical candidates for fat grafting.

Preoperative Equipment Needs

Photographs
Local anesthesia
    0.05% lidocaine with epinephrine 1 : 1,000,000 infiltrated into donor area with 18-gauge spinal needle
    Recipient area at injection site: 1% lidocaine with epinephrine 1 : 100,000

Intraoperative Needs

13-gauge, 2-inch needle with bevel cut at 45 degrees
20-mL syringes for harvesting; 10-mL syringes for reinjecting
Ringer's lactate to "wash" fat
Local anesthesia
Luer-Lok transfer adapter

---

bevel-cut tip is used with a 20-mL syringe "primed" with 2 mL of Ringer's lactate to eliminate air deadspace. The tip of the needle is introduced into the subcutaneous compartment through a skin incision made with a No. 11 blade. The plunger of the syringe is extended with the thumb or mechanical clips made for that purpose while the syringe and needle are rapidly and repeatedly moved back and forth, perpendicular to the plane of the skin into the fat (Fig. 34–10). The fat will come into the syringe with relatively little blood. In a sterile fashion, Ringer's lactate is drawn into the syringe and the mixture allowed to settle. The infranatant is discarded and the "washing" repeated until the fat is no longer blood tinged. The donor site is closed with a single suture or Steri-Strip (Table 34–11).

With the use of sterile technique the fat is transferred to smaller syringes (usually 3 to 10 mL) for injection. A 16- or 18-gauge needle is used for the injections. A small wheal of 1% lidocaine is raised at the proposed needle-entry site. The needle is introduced, and advanced subcutaneously to the limit of the proposed treatment area; the plunger is drawn back to check for inadvertent intravascular injection; and the fat is injected as the needle is withdrawn. After removal of the needle, the area can be massaged to move the fat to the desired position and consistency. Pressure is used over the puncture site, and ice can be applied to minimize swelling. Postoperative antibiotics are given for 3 days, (usually cephalexin [Keflex], 1 g per day in divided doses). Non–aspirin-containing analgesics may be given as needed (Table 34–12).

The technique of microlipoinjection is relatively free of significant complications although glabellar injections have been reported to cause blindness.[24,25] Calcification has been noted in the female breast as a complication of augmentation.[26] Survival of the graft remains the major point of contention.[27,28] Clinical investigations are underway to determine the practicality and implications of harvesting fat and using freezing techniques to provide future treatment resources without reharvesting.

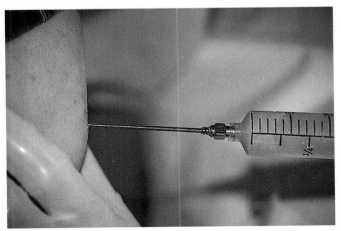

FIGURE 34–10. Harvesting the fat using a syringe. Two important points are to "prime" the syringe with a little Ringer's lactate and to keep the motion of the needle perpendicular to the plane surface of the skin, while grasping and lifting the fat with the free hand.

TABLE 34–12. Autologous Fat Implantation: Postoperative Care

Pain Management

Acetaminophen
Ice compresses

Dressings

Steri-strips

Complications

Bruising at recipient site
Patient dissatisfaction, 10%
Persistent edema and erythema for 2 weeks or more, 35%
Disappearance of graft, 50%

References

1. Schoenrock LD, Reppucci AD. Gore-Tex in facial plastic surgery. Int J Aesthet Reconstr Surg 1993;1:63–68.
2. Nussbaum JJ, Roarte J. Hylan gel and retinal detachment surgery (abstract). Invest Ophthalmol Vis Sci 1991;32(Suppl):880.
3. McPherson JM, Wallace DG, Piez KA. Development and biochemical characterization of injectable collagen. J Dermatol Surg Oncol 1988;14(Suppl 1):13–20.
4. DeLustro F, Condell RA, Nguyen MA, McPherson JM. A comparative study of the biologic and immunologic response to medical devices derived from dermal collagen. J Biomed Mater Res 1986;20:109–120.
5. Stegman SJ, Tromovitch TA. Implantation of collagen for depressed scars. J Dermatol Surg Oncol 1980;6:450–453.
6. Yarborough JM. The treatment of soft tissue defects with injectable collagen. Am J Med Sci 1985;290:28–31.
7. Klein AW. In favor of double testing (editorial). J Dermatol Surg Oncol 1989;15:263.
8. Cooperman L, Michaeli D. The immunogenicity of injectable collagen: I. A 1-year prospective study. J Am Acad Dermatol 1984;10:638–646.
9. Cooperman L, Michaeli D. The immunogenicity of injectable collagen: II. A retrospective review of seventy-two tested and treated patients. J Am Acad Dermatol 1984;10:647–651.
10. Clark DP, Hanke CW, Swanson NA. Dermal implants: Safety of products injected for soft tissue augmentation. J Am Acad Dermatol 1989.
11. Klein AW. Bonfire of the wrinkles (editorial). J Dermatol Surg Oncol 1991;17:543–544.
12. Hanke CW, Higley HR, Jolivette DM, Swanson NA, Stegman SJ. Abscess formation and local necrosis after treatment with Zyderm or Zyplast collagen implant. J Am Acad Dermatol 1991;25:319–326.
13. Gottlieb SK. Soft tissue augmentation: The search for implantation materials and techniques. Clin Dermatol 1987;5:128–134.
14. Milikan L. Long-term safety and efficacy with Fibrel in the treatment of cutaneous scars: Results of a multicenter study. J Dermatol Surg Oncol 1989;15:837–842.
15. Illouz YG. The fat cell ''graft'': A new technique to fill depressions (letter). Plast Reconstr Surg 1986;78:122–123.
16. Peer LA. Transplantation of Tissues, Transplantation of Fat. Baltimore: Williams & Wilkins, 1959.
17. Newman J, Ftaiha Z. The biographical history of fat transplant surgery. Am J Cosmet Surg 1987;4:85–87.
18. Glogau RG. Microlipoinjection: Autologous fat grafting. Arch Dermatol 1988;124:1340–1343.
19. Hambley RM, Carruthers JA. Microlipoinjection for the elevation of depressed full-thickness skin grafts on the nose. J Dermatol Surg Oncol 1992;18:963–968.
20. Pinski KS, Roenigk HH Jr. Autologous fat transplantation: Long-term follow-up (comments). J Dermatol Surg Oncol 1992;18:179–184.
21. Asaadi M, Haramis H. Successful autologous fat injection at 5 year follow-up (letter). Plast Reconstr Surg 1993;91:755–756.
22. Fournier PF. Microlipoextraction et microlipoinjection. Rev Chir Esthet Lang Fr 1985;10:40.
23. Asken S. Facial liposuction and microlipoinjection. J Dermatol Surg Oncol 1988;14:297–305.
24. Dreizen NG, Framm L. Sudden unilateral visual loss after autologous fat injection into the glabellar area. Am J Ophthalmol 1989;107:85–87.
25. Teimourian, Bahman. Blindness following fat injections (letter). Plast Reconstr Surg 1988;82:361–362.
26. Bircoll M. Reply (letter). Plast Reconstr Surg 1987;80:647.
27. Horl HW, Feller AM, Biemer E. Technique for liposuction fat reimplantation and long-term volume evaluation by magnetic resonance imaging. Ann Plast Surg 1991;26:248–258.
28. Liang MD, Narayanan K, Davis PL, Futrell JW. Evaluation of facial fat distribution using magnetic resonance imaging. Aesthet Plast Surg 1991;15:313–319.

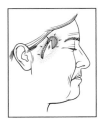

chapter 35

Surgical Wound Dressing

WILLIAM J. GRABSKI and MARTIN B. GIANDONI

The wound dressing is an integral part of the overall surgical treatment of a patient. Surgical dressings perform several important functions (Table 35–1).

The design of an appropriate surgical dressing often involves the use of multiple layers (Table 35–2). Although not every dressing will require all of these components, certain principles of applications of dressings are pertinent to all dressings.

Dressings should apply gentle pressure and immobilize the area but must not be so tight or occlusive that circula-tion is impeded or other problems develop (Table 35–3). Bandages should be unrolled flat against the skin and kept taut without allowing wrinkles that will place undue pres-sure in certain areas. The patient is instructed to look for and report pallor, duskiness, numbness, coldness, or swell-ing. If a patient travels a great distance to the physician's office, it may be advisable to have the patient wait until local anesthetic dissipates and to check the area distal to the dressing for numbness before the patient leaves the office.

TABLE 35–1. Surgical Dressings

Function	Benefit
Cover wound	Decrease contamination, decrease trauma
Absorb wound drainage	Decrease infection
Apply pressure	Increase hemostasis, decrease hematoma
Immobilize area	Increase hemostasis, decrease dehiscence
Provide moist environment	Increase rate of healing, increase cosmesis

TABLE 35–2. Components of Wound Dressing

Layer	Material
Ointment	Bacitracin
	Erythromycin
	Garamycin
	Petrolatum
Contact layer	Nonadherent pads (Telfa, Release, N-terface)
	Hydrocolloid dressing (Duoderm, Ultec)
	Films (Op-Site, Tegaderm)
	Hydrogels (Vigilon, Nu-Gel)
Absorbent layer	Gauze pads
Contouring layer	Dental rolls, cotton balls, gauze pads
Securing layer	Tape
	Elastic gauze rolls (Kerlix, Kling)
	Tubular gauze (X-span)
	Elastic bandages (Ace)
	Nonwoven, adhesive bandage (Cover Roll Stretch, Hypafix)

TABLE 35–3. Wound Dressing Complications

Dressing Problem	Complication
Excessive pressure of dressing	Bulla, ulcer, flap/graft failure
Insufficient pressure or ineffective contouring layer	Increased risk of bleeding/hematoma
Excessive occlusion	Gram-negative infection, *Candida* infection
Inappropriate contact layer	Pain and bleeding with dressing changes
Adhesive tape reactions	Irritant/allergic contact dermatitis

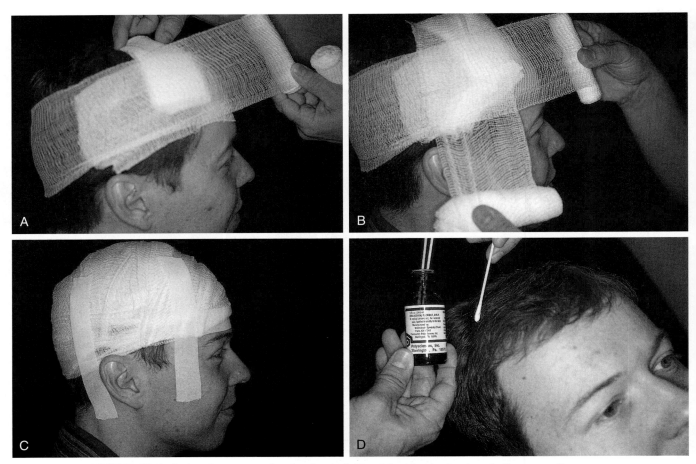

FIGURE 35–1. *A,* A turban compression dressing is fashioned by interweaving two elastic gauze rolls. *B,* One roll circles the scalp and repeatedly interlocks with the other traversing back and forth across the crown. *C,* The dressing is anchored in place with tape. *D,* After 24 hours, if there is no significant bleeding, then the wound can be painted with flexible collodion.

The generic standard postoperative surgical dressing includes a layer of antibiotic ointment, a nonadherent pad, several layers of gauze pads, and adhesive tape. To increase the holding property of tape, especially when working on a mobile or sebaceous region, the area can be degreased with acetone or alcohol and prepped with liquid adhesive (Mastisol). Hairy areas over which tape is to be applied should be shaved, but avoid shaving or clipping eyebrows. After 24 hours, if no significant bleeding has occurred, then a lighter dressing composed of an antibiotic ointment layer, a nonadherent pad, and adhesive tape is used and changed daily until the time of suture removal. Special dressings can be fashioned for certain anatomic sites, including the scalp, nose, ear, and digits (Figs. 35–1 through 35–7).

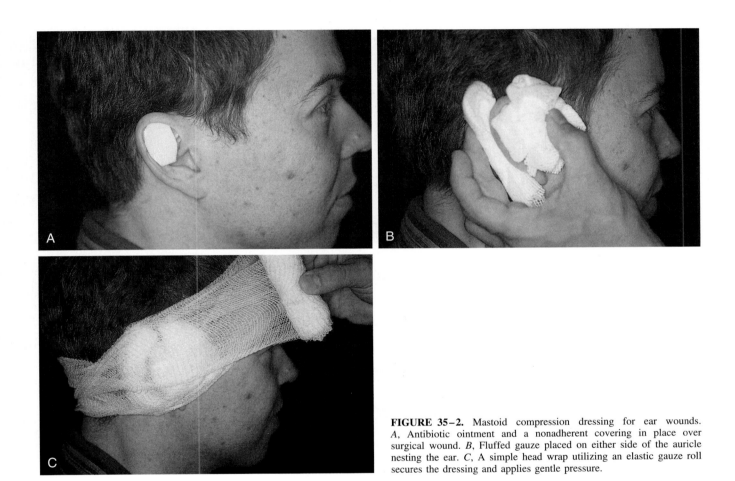

FIGURE 35–2. Mastoid compression dressing for ear wounds. *A,* Antibiotic ointment and a nonadherent covering in place over surgical wound. *B,* Fluffed gauze placed on either side of the auricle nesting the ear. *C,* A simple head wrap utilizing an elastic gauze roll secures the dressing and applies gentle pressure.

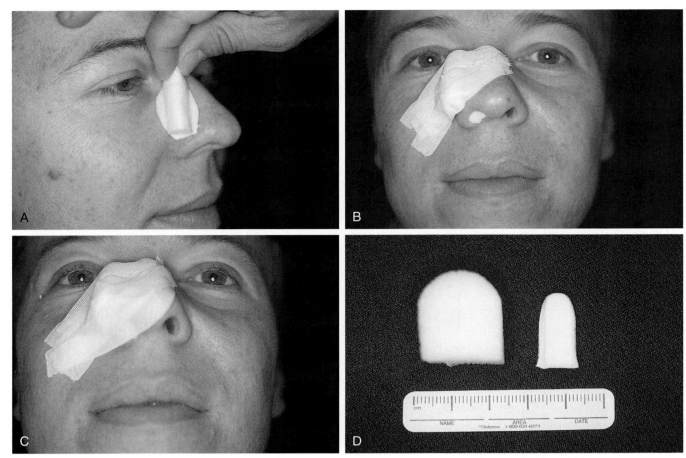

FIGURE 35–3. Dressings on the nose must accommodate complex contours and soft regions. *A*, Additional contour material (dental rolls) is often necessary to apply effective pressure over concavities. *B*, A nasal tampon can be placed in the nostril for stabilization and counterpressure of surgical wounds near the ala. *C*, Additional tape holding nasal tampon in place. *D*, Expanded and unexpanded nasal tampon (Merocel Brand surgical sponge). Nasal tampons are available with a central breathing tube (not illustrated). The unexpanded tampon is placed intranasally and is moistened with saline to expand the sponge.

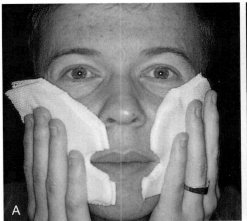

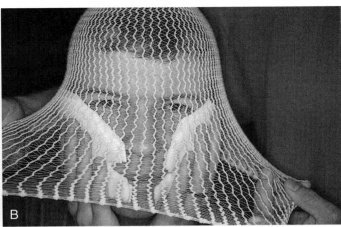

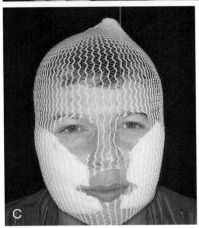

FIGURE 35-4. Facial dressing. *A*, Ointment, contact, and absorptive layers held in place by the patient. *B*, X-span tubular dressing (size 6) pulled over face and dressings. Before placement a knot is tied at one end and the dressing is turned inside out. *C*, Slits are made in tubular dressing to accommodate eyes and mouth.

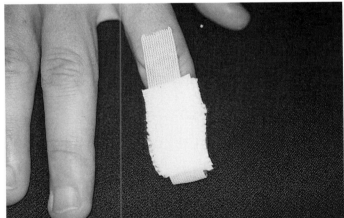

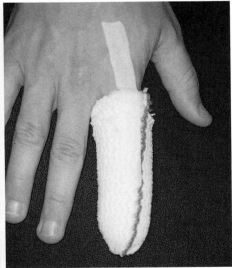

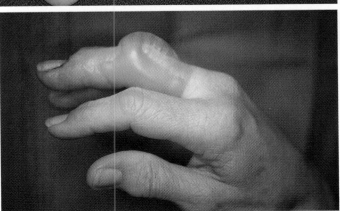

FIGURE 35-5. Dressing for digits. *A*, A layer of antibiotic ointment, a nonadherent pad, and surgical gauze are taped over the surgical site. Note that the tape is not placed circumferentially around the digit. *B*, Two layers of X-span tubular gauze are placed over the primary dressing. This will cushion and immobilize the digit. Always examine the final dressing to make sure it is not too tight. *C*, Ischemic injury with bulla formation 24 hours after removal of a constricting dressing of the digit composed of several layers of tubular gauze.

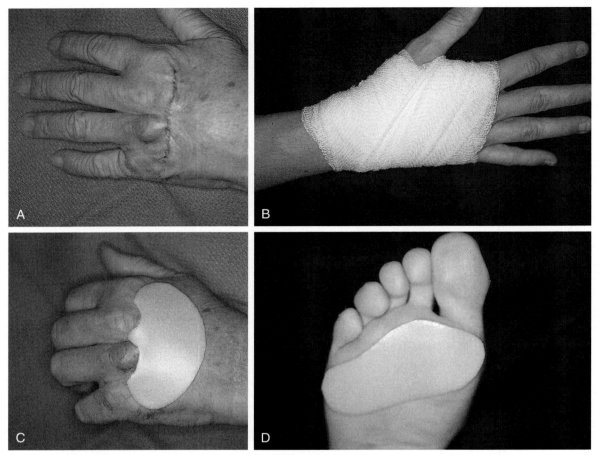

FIGURE 35–6. Hand dressing. *A,* Primary closure of a defect across the dorsum of the hand. *B,* After a standard inner dressing, a roll of tubular gauze is wrapped in a figure-of-eight fashion to cushion and immobilize the hand. *C,* At 24 hours, if no significant bleeding has occurred, the area can be covered with a custom-fit hydrocolloid dressing patch. This protects the wound and allows the patient normal function. *D,* A similar hydrocolloid dressing patch can be fashioned for the plantar surface of the foot. These dressings can remain in place until the time of suture removal. They require minimal care and can be held in place by painting the periphery of the surgical site with liquid adhesive (Mastisol).

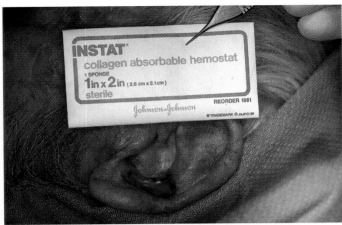

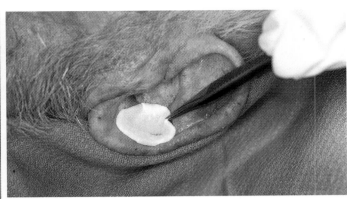

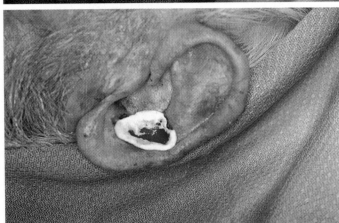

FIGURE 35–7. Wounds healing by second intention.

A, Defects healing secondarily in vascular areas such as the ear have a tendency to bleed excessively despite a standard pressure dressing. This problem can be minimized by using a collagen absorbable hemostatic sponge.

B, The collagen hemostatic sponge is cut to fit the defect and placed in the wound.

C, The sponge quickly becomes saturated with blood, and since it is composed of collagen, it does not need to be removed from the wound. A standard dressing can then be applied over this hemostatic layer.

Selected Readings

1. Bennett RG. Dressings and miscellaneous surgical materials. In: Bennett RG. Fundamentals of Cutaneous Surgery. St. Louis: CV Mosby, 1988:310–351.
2. Carver N, Leigh IM. Synthetic dressings. Int J Dermatol 1992;31:10–18.
3. Winton GB. Wound dressings for Mohs micrographic surgery. In: Mikhail GR, ed. Mohs Micrographic Surgery. Philadelphia: WB Saunders Co., 1991:207–221.
4. Winton GB, Salasche SJ. Wound dressings for dermatologic surgery. J Am Acad Dermatol 1985;13:1026–1044.
5. Zitelli JA. Wound healing and dressings. In: Roenigk RK, Roenigk HH, Jr, eds. Dermatologic Surgery, Principles and Practice. New York: Marcel Dekker, 1989:97–135.

Index

Note: Page numbers in *italics* indicate illustrations; those followed by t refer to tables.

ISBN 0-7216-5404-5